Lippincott®
Illustrated Reviews:
Pharmacology
Seventh Edition

D1346838

Lippincott®
Illustrated Reviews:
Pharmacology
Seventh Edition

Karen Whalen, PharmD, BCPS, FAPhA

Clinical Professor
Department of Pharmacotherapy and Translational Research
College of Pharmacy
University of Florida
Gainesville, Florida

Collaborating Editors

Carinda Feild, PharmD, FCCM

Clinical Associate Professor
Department of Pharmacotherapy and Translational Research
College of Pharmacy
University of Florida
St. Petersburg, Florida

Rajan Radhakrishnan, BPharm, MSc, PhD

Professor of Pharmacology
College of Medicine
Mohammed Bin Rashid University of Medicine and Health Sciences
Dubai, United Arab Emirates

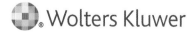

Philadelphia • Baltimore • New York • London
Buenos Aires • Hong Kong • Sydney • Tokyo

Not authorised for sale in United States, Canada, Australia, New Zealand, Puerto Rico, and U.S. Virgin Islands.

Acquisitions Editor: Matt Hauber
Development Editor: Andrea Vosburgh
Editorial Coordinator: Kerry McShane
Editorial Assistant: Brooks Phelps
Production Project Manager: Barton Dudlick
Design Coordinator: Stephen Druding
Art Director: Jennifer Clements
Manufacturing Coordinator: Margie Orzech
Marketing Manager: Michael McMahon
Prepress Vendor: SPi Global

KEELE UNIVERSITY
LIBRARY

2 4 JUN 2019

POL-15262

Seventh Edition

Copyright © 2019 Wolters Kluwer

Copyright © 2015 Wolters Kluwer, © 2012 Wolters Kluwer Health / Lippincott Williams & Wilkins, Copyright © 2009 Lippincott Williams & Wilkins, a Wolters Kluwer business, Copyright © 2006, 2000 Lippincott Williams & Wilkins, Copyright © 1997 Lippincott-Raven Publishers, Copyright © 1992 J. B. Lippincott Company. All rights reserved. This book is protected by copyright. No part of this book may be reproduced or transmitted in any form or by any means, including as photocopies or scanned-in or other electronic copies, or utilized by any information storage and retrieval system without written permission from the copyright owner, except for brief quotations embodied in critical articles and reviews. Materials appearing in this book prepared by individuals as part of their official duties as U.S. government employees are not covered by the above-mentioned copyright. To request permission, please contact Wolters Kluwer Health at Two Commerce Square, 2001 Market Street, Philadelphia, PA 19103, via email at permissions@lww.com, or via our website at lww.com (products and services).

9 8 7 6 5 4 3 2 1

Printed in China

Library of Congress Cataloging-in-Publication Data
Names: Whalen, Karen, editor. | Feild, Carinda, editor. | Radhakrishnan, Rajan, editor.
Title: Pharmacology / [edited by] Karen Whalen ; collaborating editors, Carinda Feild, Rajan Radhakrishnan.
Other titles: Pharmacology (Whalen) | Lippincott's illustrated reviews.
Description: Seventh edition. | Philadelphia : Wolters Kluwer, [2019] | Series: Lippincott illustrated reviews | Includes bibliographical references and index.
Identifiers: LCCN 2018030673 | ISBN 9781496384133 (pbk.)
Subjects: | MESH: Pharmacology | Examination Questions | Outlines
Classification: LCC RM301.14 | NLM QV 18.2 | DDC 615/.1076—dc23 LC record available at https://lccn.loc.gov/2018030673

This work is provided "as is," and the publisher disclaims any and all warranties, express or implied, including any warranties as to accuracy, comprehensiveness, or currency of the content of this work.

This work is no substitute for individual patient assessment based upon healthcare professionals' examination of each patient and consideration of, among other things, age, weight, gender, current or prior medical conditions, medication history, laboratory data and other factors unique to the patient. The publisher does not provide medical advice or guidance and this work is merely a reference tool. Healthcare professionals, and not the publisher, are solely responsible for the use of this work including all medical judgments and for any resulting diagnosis and treatments.

Given continuous, rapid advances in medical science and health information, independent professional verification of medical diagnoses, indications, appropriate pharmaceutical selections and dosages, and treatment options should be made and healthcare professionals should consult a variety of sources. When prescribing medication, healthcare professionals are advised to consult the product information sheet (the manufacturer's package insert) accompanying each drug to verify, among other things, conditions of use, warnings and side effects and identify any changes in dosage schedule or contradictions, particularly if the medication to be administered is new, infrequently used or has a narrow therapeutic range. To the maximum extent permitted under applicable law, no responsibility is assumed by the publisher for any injury and/or damage to persons or property, as a matter of products liability, negligence law or otherwise, or from any reference to or use by any person of this work.

LWW.com

RRS1807

In Memoriam

Richard A. Harvey, PhD

1936–2017

Co-creator and series editor of the *Lippincott Illustrated Reviews* series, in collaboration with Pamela C. Champe, PhD (1945–2008).

Illustrator and co-author of the first books in the series: *Biochemistry, Pharmacology, and Microbiology and Immunology.*

Katherine Vogel Anderson, PharmD, BCACP
Associate Professor
Colleges of Pharmacy and Medicine
University of Florida
Gainesville, Florida

Shawn Anderson, PharmD, BCACP
Clinical Pharmacy Specialist—Cardiology
NF/SG Veterans Medical Center
Adjunct Clinical Assistant Professor
College of Pharmacy
University of Florida
Gainesville, Florida

Angela K. Birnbaum, PhD
Professor
Department of Experimental and Clinical Pharmacology
College of Pharmacy
University of Minnesota
Minneapolis, Minnesota

Nancy Borja-Hart, PharmD
Associate Professor
The University of Tennessee Health Science Center
College of Pharmacy
Nashville, Tennessee

Lindsey Childs-Kean, PharmD, MPH, BCPS
Clinical Assistant Professor
College of Pharmacy
University of Florida
Gainesville, Florida

Jonathan C. Cho, PharmD, MBA
Clinical Assistant Professor
The University of Texas at Tyler
Tyler, Texas

Michelle Chung, PharmD
Clinical Pharmacy Specialist—Cardiology
NF/SG Veterans Medical Center
Gainesville, Florida

Jeannine M. Conway, PharmD
Associate Professor
College of Pharmacy
University of Minnesota
Minneapolis, Minnesota

Kevin Cowart, PharmD, MPH, BCACP
Assistant Professor
College of Pharmacy
University of South Florida
Tampa, Florida

Zachary L. Cox, PharmD
Associate Professor
College of Pharmacy
Lipscomb University
Heart Failure Clinical Pharmacist
Vanderbilt University Medical Center
Nashville, Tennessee

Stacey Curtis, PharmD
Clinical Assistant Professor
College of Pharmacy
University of Florida
Gainesville, Florida

Eric Dietrich, PharmD, BCPS
Clinical Assistant Professor
College of Pharmacy
University of Florida
Gainesville, Florida

Lori Dupree, PharmD, BCPS
Clinical Assistant Professor
College of Pharmacy
University of Florida
Jacksonville, Florida

Eric F. Egelund, PharmD, PhD
Clinical Assistant Professor
College of Pharmacy
University of Florida
Jacksonville, Florida

Carinda Feild, PharmD, FCCM
Clinical Associate Professor
Department of Pharmacotherapy and Translational Research
College of Pharmacy
University of Florida
St. Petersburg, Florida

Chris Giordano, MD
Associate Professor
Department of Anesthesiology
College of Medicine
University of Florida
Gainesville, Florida

Benjamin Gross, PharmD, MBA
Associate Professor
College of Pharmacy
Lipscomb University
Nashville, Tennessee
Clinical Pharmacist
Maury Regional Medical Group
Columbia, Tennessee

Jennifer Jebrock, PharmD, BCPS
Liver and GI Transplant Clinical Pharmacist
Jackson Memorial Hospital
Miami, Florida

Sandhya Jinesh, BPharm, MS, PharmD, RPh
Chief Pharmacist
West Haven Pharmacy
West Haven, Connecticut

Jacqueline Jourjy, PharmD, BCPS
Clinical Assistant Professor
College of Pharmacy
University of Florida
Orlando, Florida

Adonice Khoury, PharmD, BCPS
Clinical Assistant Professor
College of Pharmacy
University of Florida
UF Health Shands Hospital
Clinical Pharmacy Specialist
Gainesville, Florida

Jamie Kisgen, PharmD
Pharmacotherapy Specialist—Infectious Diseases
Sarasota Memorial Health Care System
Sarasota, Florida

Kenneth P. Klinker, PharmD
Clinical Associate Professor
College of Pharmacy
University of Florida
Gainesville, Florida

Kourtney LaPlant, PharmD, BCOP
Clinical Pharmacy Program Manager—Oncology
Department of Veterans Affairs
Gainesville, Florida

Robin Moorman Li, PharmD, BCACP, CPE
Clinical Associate Professor
College of Pharmacy
University of Florida
Jacksonville, Florida

Brandon Lopez, MD
Clinical Assistant Professor
Department of Anesthesiology
College of Medicine
University of Florida
Gainesville, Florida

Paige May, PharmD, BCOP
Oncology Pharmacy Specialist
Malcom Randall VA Medical Center
Clinical Assistant Professor
University of Florida
Gainesville, Florida

Kyle Melin, PharmD, BCPS
Assistant Professor
School of Pharmacy
University of Puerto Rico
San Juan, Puerto Rico

Shannon Miller, PharmD, BCACP
Clinical Associate Professor
College of Pharmacy
University of Florida
Orlando, Florida

W. Cary Mobley, BS Pharmacy, PhD
Clinical Associate Professor
College of Pharmacy
University of Florida
Gainesville, Florida

Cynthia Moreau, PharmD, BCACP
Assistant Professor
College of Pharmacy
Nova Southeastern University
Fort Lauderdale, Florida

Carol Motycka, PharmD, BCACP
Clinical Associate Professor
College of Pharmacy
University of Florida
Jacksonville, Florida

Joseph Pardo, PharmD, BCPS-AQ ID, AAHIVP
Infectious Diseases Clinical Specialist
North Florida/South Georgia Veterans Health System
Gainesville, Florida

Kristyn Pardo, PharmD, BCPS
Ambulatory Care Clinical Specialist
Department of Pharmacy
North Florida/South Georgia VA Medical Center
Gainesville, Florida

Charles A. Peloquin, PharmD
Professor
College of Pharmacy
University of Florida
Gainesville, Florida

Joanna Peris, PhD
Associate Professor
College of Pharmacy
University of Florida
Gainesville, Florida

Rajan Radhakrishnan, BPharm, MSc, PhD
Professor of Pharmacology
College of Medicine
Mohammed Bin Rashid University of Medicine and
Health Sciences
Dubai, United Arab Emirates

Jane Revollo, PharmD, BCPS
Kidney/Pancreas Transplant Clinical Pharmacist
Jackson Memorial Hospital
Miami, Florida

Jose A. Rey, MS, PharmD, BCPP
Professor
Nova Southeastern University
Davie, Florida
Clinical Psychopharmacologist
South Florida State Hospital
Pembroke Pines, Florida

Karen Sando, PharmD, BCACP, BC-ADM
Associate Professor
College of Pharmacy
Nova Southeastern University
Fort Lauderdale, Florida

Elizabeth Sherman, PharmD
Associate Professor
Nova Southeastern University
Fort Lauderdale, Florida
HIV/AIDS Clinical Pharmacy Specialist
Division of Infectious Disease
Memorial Healthcare System
Hollywood, Florida

Kaylie Smith, PharmD
Instructor
College of Pharmacy
University of Florida
Gainesville, Florida

Dawn Sollee, PharmD
Assistant Director
Florida/USVI Poison Information Center—Jacksonville
Associate Professor
Department of Emergency Medicine
College of Medicine
University of Florida
Jacksonville, Florida

Joseph Spillane, PharmD, DABAT
Courtesy Associate Professor
Department of Emergency Medicine
College of Medicine
University of Florida
Jacksonville, Florida

Amy Talana, BS, PharmD
Instructor
College of Pharmacy
University of Florida
Gainesville, Florida

Veena Venugopalan, PharmD
Clinical Assistant Professor
College of Pharmacy
University of Florida
Gainesville, Florida

Karen Whalen, PharmD, BCPS, FAPhA
Clinical Professor
Department of Pharmacotherapy and Translational
Research
College of Pharmacy
University of Florida
Gainesville, Florida

Emily Jaynes Winograd, PharmD
Clinical Toxicology/Emergency Medicine Fellow
Florida/USVI Poison Information Center—Jacksonville
Jacksonville, Florida

Marylee V. Worley, PharmD, BCPS
Assistant Professor
College of Pharmacy
Nova Southeastern University
Fort Lauderdale, Florida

Venkata Yellepeddi, BPharm, PhD
Associate Professor
Department of Pediatrics
School of Medicine
University of Utah
Salt Lake City, Utah

Reviewers

Faculty Reviewers

Ronald Bolen, RN, BSN, CFRN, CEN, CCRN, EMT-P
Flight Nurse
Vanderbilt University LifeFlight
Nashville, Tennessee

Mary G. Flanagan, MS, PA-C
Associate Director
PA Program
Touro College
New York, New York

Eyad Qunaibi, PhD

Student Reviewers

Sarah Corral
Yewande Dayo
Wanda Lai
Lorenzo R. Sewanan
Melissa M. Vega

Illustration and Graphic Design

Michael Cooper
Cooper Graphic
www.cooper247.com

Claire Hess
hess2 Design
Louisville, Kentucky

Contents

Go to http://thePoint.lww.com/activate and use the scratch-off code on the inside cover this book to access the following electronic chapters:

Pharmacokinetics

1

Venkata Yellepeddi

I. OVERVIEW

Pharmacokinetics refers to what the body does to a drug, whereas pharmacodynamics (see Chapter 2) describes what the drug does to the body. Four pharmacokinetic properties determine the onset, intensity, and duration of drug action (Figure 1.1):

- **Absorption:** First, absorption from the site of administration permits entry of the drug (either directly or indirectly) into plasma.

- **Distribution:** Second, the drug may reversibly leave the bloodstream and distribute into the interstitial and intracellular fluids.

- **Metabolism:** Third, the drug may be biotransformed through metabolism by the liver or other tissues.

- **Elimination:** Finally, the drug and its metabolites are eliminated from the body in urine, bile, or feces.

Using knowledge of pharmacokinetic parameters, clinicians can design optimal drug regimens, including the route of administration, dose, frequency, and duration of treatment.

II. ROUTES OF DRUG ADMINISTRATION

The route of administration is determined by properties of the drug (for example, water or lipid solubility, ionization) and by the therapeutic objectives (for example, the need for a rapid onset, the need for long-term treatment, or restriction of delivery to a local site). Major routes of drug administration include enteral, parenteral, and topical, among others (Figure 1.2).

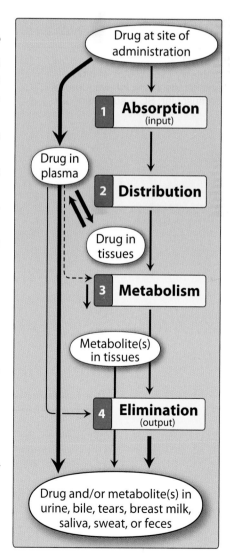

Figure 1.1
Schematic representation of drug absorption, distribution, metabolism, and elimination.

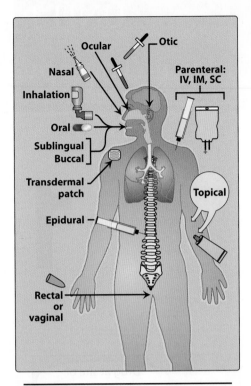

Figure 1.2
Commonly used routes of drug administration. IV = intravenous; IM = intramuscular; SC = subcutaneous.

A. Enteral

Enteral administration (administering a drug by mouth) is the most common, convenient, and economical method of drug administration. The drug may be swallowed, allowing oral delivery, or it may be placed under the tongue (sublingual) or between the gums and cheek (buccal), facilitating direct absorption into the bloodstream.

1. **Oral:** Oral administration provides many advantages. Oral drugs are easily self-administered, and toxicities and/or overdose of oral drugs may be overcome with antidotes, such as activated charcoal. However, the pathways involved in oral drug absorption are the most complicated, and the low gastric pH inactivates some drugs. A wide range of oral preparations is available including enteric-coated and extended-release preparations.

   a. **Enteric-coated preparations:** An enteric coating is a chemical envelope that protects the drug from stomach acid, delivering it instead to the less acidic intestine, where the coating dissolves and releases the drug. Enteric coating is useful for certain drugs (for example, *omeprazole*) that are acid labile, and for drugs that are irritating to the stomach, such as *aspirin*.

   b. **Extended-release preparations:** Extended-release (abbreviated ER, XR, XL, SR, etc.) medications have special coatings or ingredients that control drug release, thereby allowing for slower absorption and prolonged duration of action. ER formulations can be dosed less frequently and may improve patient compliance. In addition, ER formulations may maintain concentrations within the therapeutic range over a longer duration, as opposed to immediate-release dosage forms, which may result in larger peaks and troughs in plasma concentration. ER formulations are advantageous for drugs with short half-lives. For example, the half-life of oral *morphine* is 2 to 4 hours, and it must be administered six times daily to provide continuous pain relief. However, only two doses are needed when extended-release tablets are used.

2. **Sublingual/buccal:** The sublingual route involves placement of drug under the tongue. The buccal route involves placement of drug between the cheek and gum. Both the sublingual and buccal routes of absorption have several advantages, including ease of administration, rapid absorption, bypass of the harsh gastrointestinal (GI) environment, and avoidance of first-pass metabolism (see discussion of first-pass metabolism below).

B. Parenteral

The parenteral route introduces drugs directly into the systemic circulation. Parenteral administration is used for drugs that are poorly absorbed from the GI tract (for example, *heparin*) or unstable in the GI tract (for example, *insulin*). Parenteral administration is also used for patients unable to take oral medications (unconscious patients) and in circumstances that require a rapid onset of action. Parenteral administration provides the most control over the dose of drug delivered to the body. However, this route of administration is irreversible and may cause pain, fear, local tissue damage, and infections. The four major parenteral routes are intravascular (intravenous or intra-arterial), intramuscular, subcutaneous, and intradermal (Figure 1.3).

1. **Intravenous (IV):** IV injection is the most common parenteral route. It is useful for drugs that are not absorbed orally, such as the neuromuscular blocker *rocuronium*. IV delivery permits a rapid effect and a maximum degree of control over the amount of drug delivered. When injected as a bolus, the full amount of drug is delivered to the systemic circulation almost immediately. If administered as an IV infusion, the drug is infused over a longer period, resulting in lower peak plasma concentrations and an increased duration of circulating drug.

2. **Intramuscular (IM):** Drugs administered IM can be in aqueous solutions, which are absorbed rapidly, or in specialized depot preparations, which are absorbed slowly. Depot preparations often consist of a suspension of drug in a nonaqueous vehicle, such as polyethylene glycol. As the vehicle diffuses out of the muscle, drug precipitates at the site of injection. The drug then dissolves slowly, providing a sustained dose over an extended interval.

3. **Subcutaneous (SC):** Like IM injection, SC injection provides absorption via simple diffusion and is slower than the IV route. SC injection minimizes the risks of hemolysis or thrombosis associated with IV injection and may provide constant, slow, and sustained effects. This route should not be used with drugs that cause tissue irritation, because severe pain and necrosis may occur.

4. **Intradermal (ID):** The intradermal (ID) route involves injection into the dermis, the more vascular layer of skin under the epidermis. Agents for diagnostic determination and desensitization are usually administered by this route.

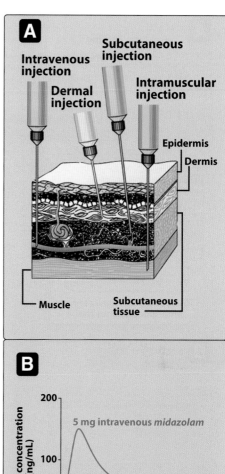

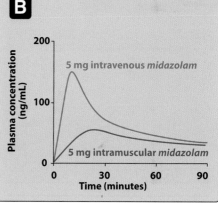

Figure 1.3
A. Schematic representation of subcutaneous and intramuscular injection. **B.** Plasma concentrations of *midazolam* after intravenous and intramuscular injection.

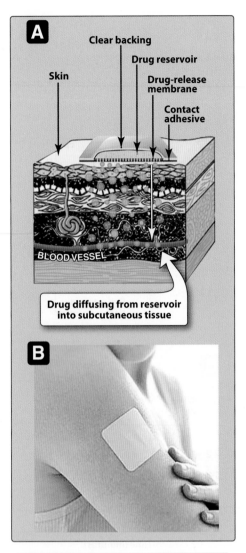

Figure 1.4
A. Schematic representation of a transdermal patch. **B.** Transdermal nicotine patch applied to the arm.

C. Other

1. **Oral inhalation and nasal preparations:** Both the oral inhalation and nasal routes of administration provide rapid delivery of drug across the large surface area of mucous membranes of the respiratory tract and pulmonary epithelium. Drug effects are almost as rapid as are those with IV bolus. Drugs that are gases (for example, some anesthetics) and those that can be dispersed in an aerosol are administered via inhalation. This route is effective and convenient for patients with respiratory disorders such as asthma or chronic obstructive pulmonary disease, because drug is delivered directly to the site of action, thereby minimizing systemic side effects. The nasal route involves topical administration of drugs directly into the nose, and it is often used for patients with allergic rhinitis.

2. **Intrathecal/intraventricular:** The blood–brain barrier typically delays or prevents the absorption of drugs into the central nervous system (CNS). When local, rapid effects are needed, it is necessary to introduce drugs directly into the cerebrospinal fluid.

3. **Topical:** Topical application is used when a local effect of the drug is desired.

4. **Transdermal:** This route of administration achieves systemic effects by application of drugs to the skin, usually via a transdermal patch (Figure 1.4). The rate of absorption can vary markedly, depending on the physical characteristics of the skin at the site of application, as well as the lipid solubility of the drug.

5. **Rectal:** Because 50% of the drainage of the rectal region bypasses the portal circulation, the biotransformation of drugs by the liver is minimized with rectal administration. The rectal route has the additional advantage of preventing destruction of the drug in the GI environment. This route is also useful if the drug induces vomiting when given orally, if the patient is already vomiting, or if the patient is unconscious. Rectal absorption is often erratic and incomplete, and many drugs irritate the rectal mucosa. Figure 1.5 summarizes characteristics of the common routes of administration, along with example drugs.

III. ABSORPTION OF DRUGS

Absorption is the transfer of a drug from the site of administration to the bloodstream. The rate and extent of absorption depend on the environment where the drug is absorbed, chemical characteristics of the drug, and the route of administration (which influences bioavailability). Routes of administration other than intravenous may result in partial absorption and lower bioavailability.

ROUTE OF ADMINISTRATION	ABSORPTION PATTERN	ADVANTAGES	DISADVANTAGES	EXAMPLES
Oral	• Variable; affected by many factors	• Safest and most common, convenient, and economical route of administration	• Limited absorption of some drugs • Food may affect absorption • Patient compliance is necessary • Drugs may be metabolized before systemic absorption	• *Acetaminophen* tablets • *Amoxicillin* suspension
Sublingual	• Depends on the drug: Few drugs (for example, *nitroglycerin*) have rapid, direct systemic absorption Most drugs erratically or incompletely absorbed	• Bypasses first-pass effect • Bypasses destruction by stomach acid • Drug stability maintained because the pH of saliva relatively neutral • May cause immediate pharmacological effects	• Limited to certain types of drugs • Limited to drugs that can be taken in small doses • May lose part of the drug dose if swallowed	• *Nitroglycerin* • *Buprenorphine*
Intravenous	• Absorption not required	• Can have immediate effects • Ideal if dosed in large volumes • Suitable for irritating substances and complex mixtures • Valuable in emergency situations • Dosage titration permissible • Ideal for high molecular weight proteins and peptide drugs	• Unsuitable for oily substances • Bolus injection may result in adverse effects • Most substances must be slowly injected • Strict aseptic techniques needed	• *Vancomycin* • *Heparin*
Intramuscular	• Depends on drug diluents: Aqueus solution: prompt Depot preparations: slow and sustained	• Suitable if drug volume is moderate • Suitable for oily vehicles and certain irritating substances • Preferable to intravenous if patient must self-administer	• Affects certain lab tests (creatine kinase) • Can be painful • Can cause intramuscular hemorrhage (precluded during anticoagulation therapy)	• *Haloperidol* • *Depot medroxy-progesterone*
Subcutaneous	• Depends on drug diluents: Aqueous solution: prompt Depot preparations: slow and sustained	• Suitable for slow-release drugs • Ideal for some poorly soluble suspensions	• Pain or necrosis if drug is irritating • Unsuitable for drugs administered in large volumes	• *Epinephrine* • *Insulin* • *Heparin*
Inhalation	• Systemic absorption may occur; this is not always desirable	• Absorption is rapid; can have immediate effects • Ideal for gases • Effective for patients with respiratory problems • Dose can be titrated • Localized effect to target lungs; lower doses used compared to that with oral or parenteral administration • Fewer systemic side effects	• Most addictive route (drug can enter the brain quickly) • Patient may have difficulty regulating dose • Some patients may have difficulty using inhalers	• *Albuterol* • *Fluticasone*
Topical	• Variable; affected by skin condition, area of skin, and other factors	• Suitable when local effect of drug is desired • May be used for skin, eye, intra-vaginal, and intranasal products • Minimizes systemic absorption • Easy for patient	• Some systemic absorption can occur • Unsuitable for drugs with high molecular weight or poor lipid solubility	• *Clotrimazole* cream • *Hydrocortisone* cream • *Timolol* eye drops
Transdermal (patch)	• Slow and sustained	• Bypasses the first-pass effect • Convenient and painless • Ideal for drugs that are lipophilic and have poor oral bioavailability • Ideal for drugs that are quickly eliminated from the body	• Some patients are allergic to patches, which can cause irritation • Drug must be highly lipophilic • May cause delayed delivery of drug to pharmacological site of action • Limited to drugs that can be taken in small daily doses	• *Nitroglycerin* • *Nicotine* • *Scopolamine*
Rectal	• Erratic and variable	• Partially bypasses first-pass effect • Bypasses destruction by stomach acid • Ideal if drug causes vomiting • Ideal in patients who are vomiting, or comatose	• Drugs may irritate the rectal mucosa • Not a well-accepted route	• *Bisacodyl* • *Promethazine*

Figure 1.5
The absorption pattern, advantages, and disadvantages of the most common routes of administration.

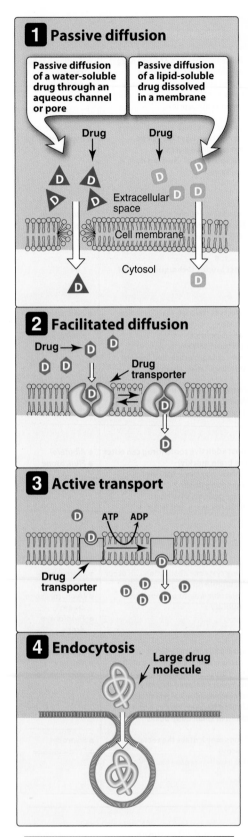

1 Passive diffusion

| Passive diffusion of a water-soluble drug through an aqueous channel or pore | Passive diffusion of a lipid-soluble drug dissolved in a membrane |

Drug

Drug

Extracellular space

Cell membrane

Cytosol

2 Facilitated diffusion

Drug

Drug transporter

3 Active transport

ATP   ADP

Drug transporter

4 Endocytosis

Large drug molecule

Figure 1.6
Schematic representation of drugs crossing a cell membrane. ATP = adenosine triphosphate; ADP = adenosine diphosphate.

A. Mechanisms of absorption of drugs from the GI tract

Depending on their chemical properties, drugs may be absorbed from the GI tract by passive diffusion, facilitated diffusion, active transport, or endocytosis (Figure 1.6).

1. **Passive diffusion:** The driving force for passive diffusion of a drug is the concentration gradient across a membrane separating two body compartments. In other words, the drug moves from an area of high concentration to one of lower concentration. Passive diffusion does not involve a carrier, is not saturable, and shows low structural specificity. The vast majority of drugs are absorbed by this mechanism. Water-soluble drugs penetrate the cell membrane through aqueous channels or pores, whereas lipid-soluble drugs readily move across most biologic membranes due to solubility in the membrane lipid bilayers.

2. **Facilitated diffusion:** Other agents can enter the cell through specialized transmembrane carrier proteins that facilitate the passage of large molecules. These carrier proteins undergo conformational changes, allowing the passage of drugs or endogenous molecules into the interior of cells. This process is known as facilitated diffusion. It does not require energy, can be saturated, and may be inhibited by compounds that compete for the carrier.

3. **Active transport:** This mode of drug entry also involves specific carrier proteins that span the membrane. However, active transport is energy dependent, driven by the hydrolysis of adenosine triphosphate (ATP). It is capable of moving drugs against a concentration gradient, from a region of low drug concentration to one of higher concentration. The process is saturable. Active transport systems are selective and may be competitively inhibited by other cotransported substances.

4. **Endocytosis and exocytosis:** This type of absorption is used to transport drugs of exceptionally large size across the cell membrane. Endocytosis involves engulfment of a drug by the cell membrane and transport into the cell by pinching off the drug-filled vesicle. Exocytosis is the reverse of endocytosis. Many cells use exocytosis to secrete substances out of the cell through a similar process of vesicle formation. Vitamin B_{12} is transported across the gut wall by endocytosis, whereas certain neurotransmitters (for example, norepinephrine) are stored in intracellular vesicles in the nerve terminal and released by exocytosis.

B. Factors influencing absorption

1. **Effect of pH on drug absorption:** Most drugs are either weak acids or weak bases. Acidic drugs (HA) release a proton (H^+), causing a charged anion (A^-) to form:

$$HA \rightleftarrows H^+ + A^-$$

Weak bases (BH^+) can also release an H^+. However, the protonated form of basic drugs is usually charged, and loss of a proton produces the uncharged base (B):

$$BH^+ \rightleftarrows B + H^+$$

A drug passes through membranes more readily if it is uncharged (Figure 1.7). Thus, for a weak acid, the uncharged, protonated HA can permeate through membranes, and A⁻ cannot. For a weak base, the uncharged form B penetrates through the cell membrane, but the protonated form BH⁺ does not. Therefore, the effective concentration of the permeable form of each drug at its absorption site is determined by the relative concentrations of the charged and uncharged forms. The ratio between the two forms is, in turn, determined by the pH at the site of absorption and by the strength of the weak acid or base, which is represented by the ionization constant, pK_a (Figure 1.8). [Note: The pK_a is a measure of the strength of the interaction of a compound with a proton. The lower the pK_a of a drug, the more acidic it is. Conversely, the higher the pK_a, the more basic is the drug.] Distribution equilibrium is achieved when the permeable form of a drug achieves an equal concentration in all body water spaces.

2. **Blood flow to the absorption site:** The intestines receive much more blood flow than does the stomach, so absorption from the intestine is favored over the stomach. [Note: Shock severely reduces blood flow to cutaneous tissues, thereby minimizing absorption from SC administration.]

3. **Total surface area available for absorption:** With a surface rich in brush borders containing microvilli, the intestine has a surface area about 1000-fold that of the stomach, making absorption of the drug across the intestine more efficient.

4. **Contact time at the absorption surface:** If a drug moves through the GI tract very quickly, as can happen with severe diarrhea, it is not well absorbed. Conversely, anything that delays the transport of the drug from the stomach to the intestine delays the rate of absorption. [Note: The presence of food in the stomach both dilutes the drug and slows gastric emptying. Therefore, a drug taken with a meal is generally absorbed more slowly.]

5. **Expression of P-glycoprotein:** P-glycoprotein is a transmembrane transporter protein responsible for transporting various

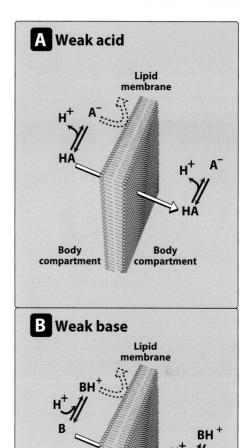

Figure 1.7
A. Diffusion of the nonionized form of a weak acid through a lipid membrane.
B. Diffusion of the nonionized form of a weak base through a lipid membrane.

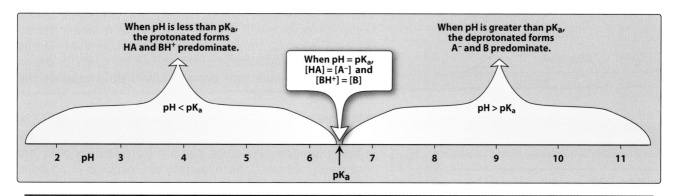

Figure 1.8
The distribution of a drug between its ionized and nonionized forms depends on the ambient pH and pK_a of the drug. For illustrative purposes, the drug has been assigned a pK_a of 6.5.

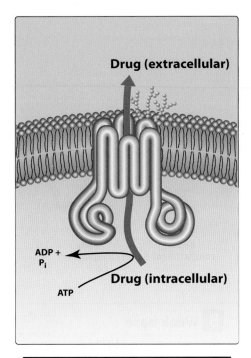

Figure 1.9
The six membrane-spanning loops
of the P-glycoprotein form a central
channel for the ATP-dependent pumping
of drugs from the cell.

molecules, including drugs, across cell membranes (Figure 1.9). It is expressed in tissues throughout the body, including the liver, kidneys, placenta, intestines, and brain capillaries, and is involved in transportation of drugs from tissues to blood. That is, it "pumps" drugs out of cells. Thus, in areas of high expression, P-glycoprotein reduces drug absorption. In addition to transporting many drugs out of cells, it is also associated with multidrug resistance.

C. Bioavailability

Bioavailability is the rate and extent to which an administered drug reaches the systemic circulation. For example, if 100 mg of a drug is administered orally and 70 mg is absorbed unchanged, the bioavailability is 0.7 or 70%. Determining bioavailability is important for calculating drug dosages for nonintravenous routes of administration.

1. **Determination of bioavailability:** Bioavailability is determined by comparing plasma levels of a drug after a particular route of administration (for example, oral administration) with levels achieved by IV administration. After IV administration, 100% of the drug rapidly enters the circulation. When the drug is given orally, only part of the administered dose appears in the plasma. By plotting plasma concentrations of the drug versus time, the area under the curve (AUC) can be measured. A schematic depiction of determination of bioavailability is provided in Figure 1.10.

2. **Factors that influence bioavailability:** In contrast to IV administration, which confers 100% bioavailability, orally administered drugs often undergo first-pass metabolism. This biotransformation, in addition to chemical and physical characteristics of the drug, determines the rate and extent to which the agent reaches the systemic circulation.

   a. **First-pass hepatic metabolism:** When a drug is absorbed from the GI tract, it enters the portal circulation before entering the systemic circulation (Figure 1.11). If the drug is rapidly metabolized in the liver or gut wall during this initial passage, the amount of unchanged drug entering the systemic circulation is decreased. This is referred to as first-pass metabolism. [Note: First-pass metabolism by the intestine or liver limits the efficacy of many oral medications. For example, more than 90% of *nitroglycerin* is cleared during first-pass metabolism. Hence, it is primarily administered via the sublingual, transdermal, or intravenous route.] Drugs with high first-pass metabolism should be given in doses sufficient to ensure that enough active drug reaches the desired site of action.

   b. **Solubility of the drug:** Very hydrophilic drugs are poorly absorbed because of the inability to cross lipid-rich cell membranes. Paradoxically, drugs that are extremely lipophilic are also poorly absorbed, because they are insoluble in aqueous body fluids and, therefore, cannot gain access to the surface of cells. For a drug to be readily absorbed, it must be largely lipophilic, yet have some solubility in aqueous solutions. This is one reason why many drugs are either weak acids or weak bases.

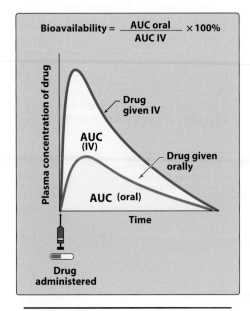

$$\text{Bioavailability} = \frac{\text{AUC oral}}{\text{AUC IV}} \times 100\%$$

Figure 1.10
Determination of the bioavailability
of a drug. AUC = area under curve;
IV = intravenous.

   c. Chemical instability: Some drugs, such as *penicillin G*, are unstable in the pH of gastric contents. Others, such as *insulin*, are destroyed in the GI tract by degradative enzymes.

   d. Nature of the drug formulation: Drug absorption may be altered by factors unrelated to the chemistry of the drug. For example, particle size, salt form, crystal polymorphism, enteric coatings, and the presence of excipients (such as binders and dispersing agents) can influence the ease of dissolution and, therefore, alter the rate of absorption.

D. Bioequivalence and other types of equivalence

Two drug formulations are bioequivalent if they show comparable bioavailability and similar times to achieve peak blood concentrations. Two drug formulations are therapeutically equivalent if they are pharmaceutically equivalent (that is, they have the same dosage form, contain the same active ingredient at the same strength, and use the same route of administration) with similar clinical and safety profiles. Thus, therapeutic equivalence requires that drug products are bioequivalent and pharmaceutically equivalent.

IV. DRUG DISTRIBUTION

Drug distribution is the process by which a drug reversibly leaves the bloodstream and enters the extracellular fluid and tissues. For drugs administered IV, absorption is not a factor, and the initial phase immediately following administration represents the distribution phase, during which the drug rapidly leaves the circulation and enters the tissues (Figure 1.12). The distribution of a drug from the plasma to the interstitium depends on cardiac output and local blood flow, capillary permeability, tissue volume, degree of binding of the drug to plasma and tissue proteins, and relative lipophilicity of the drug.

A. Blood flow

The rate of blood flow to the tissue capillaries varies widely. For instance, blood flow to "vessel-rich organs" (brain, liver, and kidney) is greater than that to the skeletal muscles. Adipose tissue, skin, and viscera have still lower rates of blood flow. Variation in blood flow partly explains the short duration of hypnosis produced by an IV bolus of *propofol* (see Chapter 13). High blood flow, together with high lipophilicity of *propofol*, permits rapid distribution into the CNS and produces anesthesia. A subsequent slower distribution to skeletal muscle and adipose tissue lowers the plasma concentration so that the drug diffuses out of the CNS, down the concentration gradient, and consciousness is regained.

B. Capillary permeability

Capillary permeability is determined by capillary structure and by the chemical nature of the drug. Capillary structure varies in terms of the fraction of the basement membrane exposed by slit junctions between endothelial cells. In the liver and spleen, a significant portion of the basement membrane is exposed due to large, discontinuous capillaries

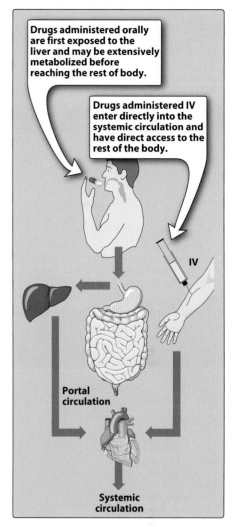

Figure 1.11
First-pass metabolism can occur with orally administered drugs. IV = intravenous.

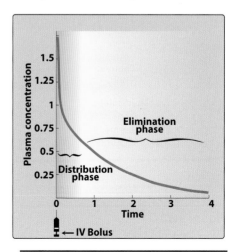

Figure 1.12
Drug concentrations in serum after a single injection of drug. Assume that the drug distributes and is subsequently eliminated.

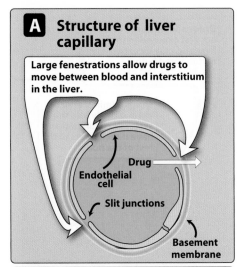

A Structure of liver capillary

Large fenestrations allow drugs to move between blood and interstitium in the liver.

Drug

Endothelial cell

Slit junctions

Basement membrane

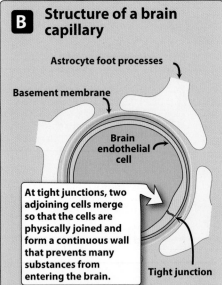

B Structure of a brain capillary

Astrocyte foot processes

Basement membrane

Brain endothelial cell

At tight junctions, two adjoining cells merge so that the cells are physically joined and form a continuous wall that prevents many substances from entering the brain.

Tight junction

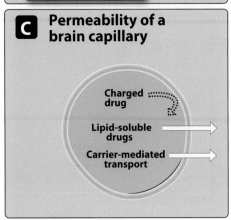

C Permeability of a brain capillary

Charged drug

Lipid-soluble drugs

Carrier-mediated transport

Figure 1.13
Cross section of liver and brain capillaries.

through which large plasma proteins can pass (Figure 1.13A). In the brain, the capillary structure is continuous, and there are no slit junctions (Figure 1.13B). To enter the brain, drugs must pass through the endothelial cells of the CNS capillaries or undergo active transport. For example, a specific transporter carries *levodopa* into the brain. Lipid-soluble drugs readily penetrate the CNS because they dissolve in the endothelial cell membrane. By contrast, ionized or polar drugs generally fail to enter the CNS because they cannot pass through the endothelial cells that have no slit junctions (Figure 1.13C). These closely juxtaposed cells form tight junctions that constitute the blood–brain barrier.

C. Binding of drugs to plasma proteins and tissues

1. **Binding to plasma proteins:** Reversible binding to plasma proteins sequesters drugs in a nondiffusible form and slows transfer out of the vascular compartment. Albumin is the major drug-binding protein, and it may act as a drug reservoir. As the concentration of free drug decreases due to elimination, the bound drug dissociates from albumin. This maintains the free-drug concentration as a constant fraction of the total drug in the plasma.

2. **Binding to tissue proteins:** Many drugs accumulate in tissues, leading to higher concentrations in tissues than in interstitial fluid and blood. Drugs may accumulate because of binding to lipids, proteins, or nucleic acids. Drugs may also undergo active transport into tissues. Tissue reservoirs may serve as a major source of the drug and prolong its actions or cause local drug toxicity. (For example, acrolein, the metabolite of *cyclophosphamide*, can cause hemorrhagic cystitis because it accumulates in the bladder.)

D. Lipophilicity

The chemical nature of a drug strongly influences its ability to cross cell membranes. Lipophilic drugs readily move across most biologic membranes. These drugs dissolve in the lipid membranes and penetrate the entire cell surface. The major factor influencing the distribution of lipophilic drugs is blood flow to the area. By contrast, hydrophilic drugs do not readily penetrate cell membranes and must pass through slit junctions.

E. Volume of distribution

The apparent volume of distribution, V_d, is defined as the fluid volume that is required to contain the entire drug in the body at the same concentration measured in the plasma. It is calculated by dividing the dose that ultimately gets into the systemic circulation by the plasma concentration at time zero (C_0).

$$V_d = \frac{\text{Amount of drug in the body}}{C_0}$$

Although V_d has no physiologic or physical basis, it can be useful to compare the distribution of a drug with the volumes of the water compartments in the body.

1. **Distribution into the water compartments in the body:** Once a drug enters the body, it has the potential to distribute into any one

of the three functionally distinct compartments of body water or to become sequestered in a cellular site.

a. **Plasma compartment:** If a drug has a high molecular weight or is extensively protein bound, it is too large to pass through the slit junctions of the capillaries and, thus, is effectively trapped within the plasma (vascular) compartment. As a result, it has a low V_d that approximates the plasma volume, or about 4 L in a 70-kg individual. *Heparin* (see Chapter 21) shows this type of distribution.

b. **Extracellular fluid:** If a drug has a low molecular weight but is hydrophilic, it can pass through the endothelial slit junctions of the capillaries into the interstitial fluid. However, hydrophilic drugs cannot move across the lipid membranes of cells to enter the intracellular fluid. Therefore, these drugs distribute into a volume that is the sum of the plasma volume and the interstitial fluid, which together constitute the extracellular fluid (about 20% of body weight or 14 L in a 70-kg individual). Aminoglycoside antibiotics (see Chapter 30) show this type of distribution.

c. **Total body water:** If a drug has a low molecular weight and has enough lipophilicity, it can move into the interstitium through the slit junctions and pass through the cell membranes into the intracellular fluid. These drugs distribute into a volume of about 60% of body weight or about 42 L in a 70-kg individual. *Ethanol* exhibits this apparent V_d. [Note: In general, a larger V_d indicates greater distribution into tissues; a smaller V_d suggests confinement to plasma or extracellular fluid.]

2. **Determination of V_d:** The fact that drug clearance is usually a first-order process allows calculation of V_d. First order means that a constant fraction of the drug is eliminated per unit of time. This process can be most easily analyzed by plotting the log of the plasma drug concentration (C_p) versus time (Figure 1.14). The concentration of drug in the plasma can be extrapolated back to time zero (the time of IV bolus) on the Y axis to determine C_0, which is the concentration of drug that would have been achieved if the distribution phase had occurred instantly. This allows calculation of V_d as

$$V_d = \frac{Dose}{C_0}$$

For example, if 10 mg of drug is injected into a patient and the plasma concentration is extrapolated back to time zero, and C_0 = 1 mg/L (from the graph in Figure 1.14B), then V_d = 10 mg/1 mg/L = 10 L.

3. **Effect of V_d on drug half-life:** V_d has an important influence on the half-life of a drug, because drug elimination depends on the amount of drug delivered to the liver or kidney (or other organs where metabolism occurs) per unit of time. Delivery of drug to the organs of elimination depends not only on blood flow but also on the fraction of drug in the plasma. If a drug has a large V_d, most of the drug is in the extraplasmic space and is unavailable to the excretory organs. Therefore, any factor that increases V_d can increase the half-life and extend the duration of action of the drug. [Note: An exceptionally large V_d indicates considerable sequestration of the drug in some tissues or compartments.]

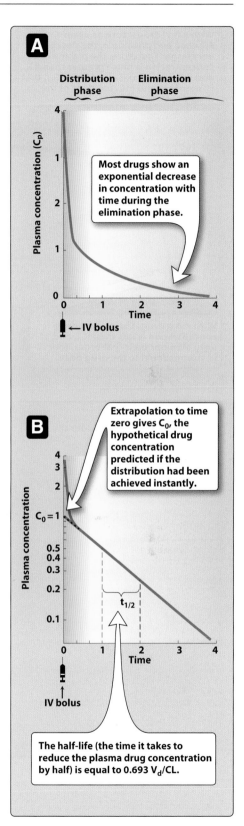

Figure 1.14
Drug concentrations in plasma after a single injection of drug at time = 0. **A.** Concentration data are plotted on a linear scale. **B.** Concentration data are plotted on a log scale.

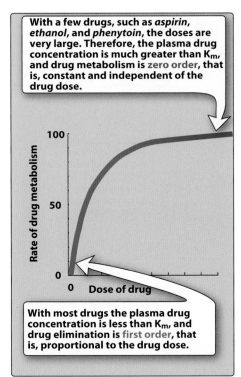

With a few drugs, such as *aspirin*, *ethanol*, and *phenytoin*, the doses are very large. Therefore, the plasma drug concentration is much greater than K_m, and drug metabolism is zero order, that is, constant and independent of the drug dose.

With most drugs the plasma drug concentration is less than K_m, and drug elimination is first order, that is, proportional to the drug dose.

Figure 1.15
Effect of drug dose on the rate of metabolism.

V. DRUG CLEARANCE THROUGH METABOLISM

Once a drug enters the body, the process of elimination begins. The three major routes of elimination are hepatic metabolism, biliary elimination, and urinary excretion. [Note: Elimination is irreversible removal of drug from the body. It involves biotransformation (drug metabolism) and excretion. Excretion is removal of intact drug from the body.] Together, these elimination processes decrease the plasma concentration exponentially. That is, a constant fraction of the drug is eliminated in a given unit of time (Figure 1.14A). Metabolism results in products with increased polarity, which allows the drug to be eliminated. Clearance (CL) estimates the volume of blood from which the drug is cleared per unit of time. Total CL is a composite estimate reflecting all mechanisms of drug elimination and is calculated as follows:

$$CL = 0.693 \times V_d / t_{1/2}$$

where $t_{1/2}$ is the elimination half-life, V_d is the apparent volume of distribution, and 0.693 is the natural log constant. Drug half-life is often used as a measure of drug CL, because, for many drugs, V_d is a constant.

A. Kinetics of metabolism

1. **First-order kinetics:** The metabolic transformation of drugs is catalyzed by enzymes, and most of the reactions obey Michaelis-Menten kinetics, where K_m is Michaelis constant (the substrate concentration at half maximal velocity).

$$v = \text{Rate of drug metabolism} = \frac{V_{max}[C]}{K_m + [C]}$$

In most clinical situations, the concentration of the drug, [C], is much less than the Michaelis constant, K_m, and the Michaelis-Menten equation reduces to

$$v = \text{Rate of drug metabolism} = \frac{V_{max}[C]}{K_m}$$

That is, the rate of drug metabolism and elimination is directly proportional to the concentration of free drug, and first-order kinetics is observed (Figure 1.15). This means that a constant fraction of drug is metabolized per unit of time (that is, with each half-life, the concentration decreases by 50%). First-order kinetics is also referred to as linear kinetics.

2. **Zero-order kinetics:** With a few drugs, such as *aspirin*, *ethanol*, and *phenytoin*, the doses are very large. Therefore, [C] is much greater than K_m, and the velocity equation becomes

$$v = \text{Rate of drug metabolism} = \frac{V_{max}[C]}{[C]} = V_{max}$$

The enzyme is saturated by a high free drug concentration, and the rate of metabolism remains constant over time. This is called zero-order kinetics (also called nonlinear kinetics). A constant amount of drug is metabolized per unit of time. The rate of elimination is constant and does not depend on the drug concentration.

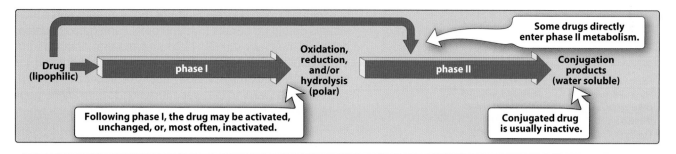

Figure 1.16
The biotransformation of drugs.

B. Reactions of drug metabolism

The kidney cannot efficiently excrete lipophilic drugs that readily cross cell membranes and are reabsorbed in the distal convoluted tubules. Therefore, lipid-soluble agents are first metabolized into more polar (hydrophilic) substances in the liver via two general sets of reactions, called phase I and phase II (Figure 1.16).

1. **Phase I:** Phase I reactions convert lipophilic drugs into more polar molecules by introducing or unmasking a polar functional group, such as $-OH$ or $-NH_2$. Phase I reactions usually involve reduction, oxidation, or hydrolysis. Phase I metabolism may increase, decrease, or have no effect on pharmacologic activity.

   a. **Phase I reactions utilizing the P450 system:** The phase I reactions most frequently involved in drug metabolism are catalyzed by the cytochrome P450 (CYP) system. The P450 system is important for the metabolism of many endogenous compounds (such as steroids, lipids) and for the biotransformation of exogenous substances (drugs, carcinogens, and environmental pollutants). CYP is a superfamily of heme-containing isozymes located in most cells, but primarily in the liver and GI tract.

   [1] **Nomenclature:** The family name is indicated by the Arabic number that follows CYP, and the capital letter designates the subfamily, for example, CYP3A (Figure 1.17). A second number indicates the specific isozyme, as in CYP3A4.

   [2] **Specificity:** Because there are many different genes that encode multiple enzymes, there are many different P450 isoforms. These enzymes have the capacity to modify a large number of structurally diverse substrates. In addition, an individual drug may be a substrate for more than one isozyme. Four isozymes (CYP3A4/5, CYP2D6, CYP2C8/9, and CYP1A2) are responsible for the vast majority of P450-catalyzed reactions (Figure 1.17). Considerable amounts of CYP3A4 are found in intestinal mucosa, accounting for first-pass metabolism of drugs such as *chlorpromazine* and *clonazepam*.

   [3] **Genetic variability:** P450 enzymes exhibit considerable genetic variability among individuals and racial groups. Variations in P450 activity may alter drug efficacy and the risk of adverse events. CYP2D6, in particular, exhibits genetic polymorphism. CYP2D6 mutations result in very low

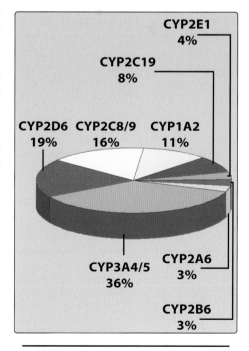

Figure 1.17
Relative contribution of cytochrome P450 (CYP) isoforms to drug biotransformation.

Isozyme: CYP2C9	
COMMON SUBSTRATES	INDUCERS
Celecoxib Glimepiride Ibuprofen Phenytoin Warfarin	Carbamazepine Phenobarbital Rifampin

Isozyme: CYP2D6	
COMMON SUBSTRATES	INDUCERS
Fluoxetine Haloperidol Paroxetine Propranolol	None*

Isozyme: CYP3A4/5	
COMMON SUBSTRATES	INDUCERS
Carbamazepine Cyclosporine Erythromycin Nifedipine Simvastatin Verapamil	Carbamazepine Dexamethasone Phenobarbital Phenytoin Rifampin

Figure 1.18
Some representative cytochrome P450 isozymes. CYP = cytochrome P. *Unlike most other CYP450 enzymes, CYP2D6 is not very susceptible to enzyme induction.

capacities to metabolize substrates. For example, some individuals obtain no benefit from the opioid analgesic *codeine*, because they lack the CYP2D6 enzyme that activates the drug. Similar polymorphisms have been characterized for the CYP2C subfamily of isozymes. For instance, *clopidogrel* carries a warning that patients who are CYP2C19 "poor metabolizers" have a diminished antiplatelet effect when taking this drug and an alternative medication should be considered. *Clopidogrel* is a prodrug, and CYP2C19 activity is required to convert it to the active metabolite.

[4] **CYP inducers:** The CYP450-dependent enzymes are an important target for pharmacokinetic drug interactions. Certain drugs (for example, *phenobarbital*, *rifampin*, and *carbamazepine*) are capable of inducing CYP isozymes. This results in increased biotransformation of drugs and can lead to significant decreases in plasma concentrations of drugs metabolized by these CYP isozymes, often with concurrent loss of pharmacologic effect. For example, *rifampin*, an antituberculosis drug (see Chapter 32), significantly decreases the plasma concentrations of human immunodeficiency virus (HIV) protease inhibitors, thereby diminishing the ability to suppress HIV replication. Figure 1.18 lists some of the more important inducers for representative CYP isozymes.

[5] **CYP inhibitors:** Inhibition of drug metabolism can lead to significant increases in plasma drug concentration and resultant adverse effects or drug toxicity. The most common form of inhibition is through competition for the same isozyme. Some drugs, however, are capable of inhibiting reactions for which they are not substrates (for example, *ketoconazole*), leading to drug interactions. Numerous drugs inhibit one or more of the CYP-dependent biotransformation pathways of *warfarin*. For example, *omeprazole* is a potent inhibitor of three CYP isozymes involved in *warfarin* metabolism. When taken with *omeprazole*, plasma concentrations of *warfarin* increase, which leads to greater anticoagulant effect and increased risk of bleeding. [Note: The more important CYP inhibitors are *erythromycin*, *ketoconazole*, and *ritonavir*, because they each inhibit several CYP isozymes.]

b. **Phase I reactions not involving the P450 system:** These include amine oxidation (for example, oxidation of catecholamines or histamine), alcohol dehydrogenation (for example, *ethanol* oxidation), esterases (for example, metabolism of *aspirin* in the liver), and hydrolysis (for example, of *procaine*).

2. **Phase II:** This phase consists of conjugation reactions. If the metabolite from phase I is sufficiently polar, it can be excreted by the kidneys. However, many phase I metabolites are still too lipophilic to be excreted. A subsequent conjugation reaction with an endogenous substrate, such as glucuronic acid, sulfuric acid, acetic acid, or an amino acid, results in polar, usually more water-soluble compounds that are often therapeutically inactive. A notable exception is *morphine-6-glucuronide*, which is more potent than *morphine*. Glucuronidation is the most common and

the most important conjugation reaction. [Note: Drugs already possessing an –OH, –NH$_2$, or –COOH group may enter phase II directly and become conjugated without prior phase I metabolism (Figure 1.16).] The highly polar drug conjugates are then excreted by the kidney or in bile.

VI. DRUG CLEARANCE BY THE KIDNEY

Drugs must be sufficiently polar to be eliminated from the body. Removal of drugs from the body occurs via a number of routes; the most important is elimination through the kidney into the urine. Patients with renal dysfunction may be unable to excrete drugs and are at risk for drug accumulation and adverse effects.

A. Renal elimination of a drug

A drug passes through several processes in the kidney before elimination: glomerular filtration, active tubular secretion, and passive tubular reabsorption.

1. **Glomerular filtration:** Drugs enter the kidney through renal arteries, which divide to form a glomerular capillary plexus. Free drug (not bound to albumin) flows through the capillary slits into the Bowman space as part of the glomerular filtrate (Figure 1.19). The glomerular filtration rate (GFR) is normally about 120 mL/min/1.73m^2 but may diminish significantly in renal disease. Lipid solubility and pH do not influence the passage of drugs into the glomerular filtrate. However, variations in GFR and protein binding of drugs do affect this process.

2. **Proximal tubular secretion:** Drugs that were not transferred into the glomerular filtrate leave the glomeruli through efferent arterioles, which divide to form a capillary plexus surrounding the nephric lumen in the proximal tubule. Secretion primarily occurs in the proximal tubules by two energy-requiring active transport systems: one for anions (for example, deprotonated forms of weak acids) and one for cations (for example, protonated forms of weak bases). Each of these transport systems shows low specificity and can transport many compounds. Thus, competition between drugs for these carriers can occur within each transport system. [Note: Premature infants and neonates have an incompletely developed tubular secretory mechanism and, thus, may retain certain drugs in the blood.]

3. **Distal tubular reabsorption:** As a drug moves toward the distal convoluted tubule, its concentration increases and exceeds that of the perivascular space. The drug, if uncharged, may diffuse out of the nephric lumen, back into the systemic circulation (Figure 1.20). Manipulating the urine pH to increase the fraction of ionized drug in the lumen may be done to minimize the amount of back diffusion and increase the clearance of an undesirable drug. Generally, weak acids can be eliminated by alkalinization of the urine, whereas elimination of weak bases may be increased by acidification of the urine. This process is called "ion trapping." For example, a patient presenting with *phenobarbital* (weak acid) overdose can be given *bicarbonate*, which alkalinizes the urine and keeps the drug ionized, thereby decreasing its reabsorption.

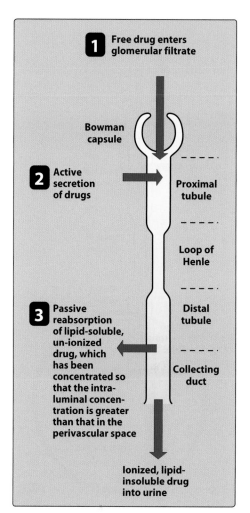

Figure 1.19
Drug elimination by the kidney.

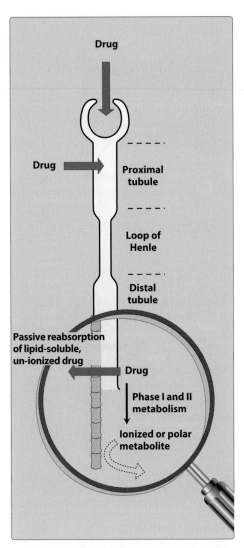

Figure 1.20
Effect of drug metabolism on reabsorption in the distal tubule.

VII. EXCRETION BY OTHER ROUTES

Drug excretion may also occur via the intestines, bile, lungs, and breast milk, among others. Drugs that are not absorbed after oral administration or drugs that are secreted directly into the intestines or into bile are excreted in the feces. The lungs are primarily involved in the elimination of anesthetic gases (for example, *desflurane*). Elimination of drugs in breast milk may expose the breast-feeding infant to medications and/or metabolites being taken by the mother and is a potential source of undesirable side effects to the infant. Excretion of most drugs into sweat, saliva, tears, hair, and skin occurs only to a small extent. Total body clearance and drug half-life are important measures of drug clearance that are used to optimize drug therapy and minimize toxicity.

A. Total body clearance

The total body (systemic) clearance, CL_{total}, is the sum of all clearances from the drug-metabolizing and drug-eliminating organs. The kidney is often the major organ of excretion. The liver also contributes to drug clearance through metabolism and/or excretion into the bile. Total clearance is calculated using the following equation:

$$CL_{total} = CL_{hepatic} + CL_{renal} + CL_{pulmonary} + CL_{other}$$

where $CL_{hepatic} + CL_{renal}$ are typically the most important.

B. Clinical situations resulting in changes in drug half-life

When a patient has an abnormality that alters the half-life of a drug, adjustment in dosage is required. Patients who may have an increase in drug half-life include those with 1) diminished renal or hepatic blood flow, for example, in cardiogenic shock, heart failure, or hemorrhage; 2) decreased ability to extract drug from plasma, for example, in renal disease; and 3) decreased metabolism, for example, when a concomitant drug inhibits metabolism or in hepatic insufficiency, as with cirrhosis. These patients may require a decrease in dosage or less frequent dosing intervals. In contrast, the half-life of a drug may be decreased by increased hepatic blood flow, decreased protein binding, or increased metabolism. This may necessitate higher doses or more frequent dosing intervals.

VIII. DESIGN AND OPTIMIZATION OF DOSAGE REGIMEN

To initiate drug therapy, the clinician must select the appropriate route of administration, dosage, and dosing interval. Selection of a regimen depends on various patient and drug factors, including how rapidly therapeutic levels of a drug must be achieved. Therapy may consist of a single dose of a drug, for example, a sleep-inducing agent, such as *zolpidem*. More commonly, drugs are continually administered, either as an IV infusion or in IV or oral fixed-dose/fixed-time interval regimens (for example, "one tablet every 4 hours"). Continuous or repeated administration results in accumulation of the drug until a steady state occurs. Steady-state concentration is reached when the rate of drug elimination is equal to the rate of drug administration, such that plasma and tissue levels remain relatively constant.

A. Continuous infusion regimens

With continuous IV infusion, the rate of drug entry into the body is constant. Most drugs exhibit first-order elimination, that is, a constant fraction of the drug is cleared per unit of time. Therefore, the rate of drug elimination increases proportionately as the plasma concentration increases.

1. **Plasma concentration of a drug following continuous IV infusion:** Following initiation of a continuous IV infusion, the plasma concentration of a drug rises until a steady state (rate of drug elimination equals rate of drug administration) is reached, at which point the plasma concentration of the drug remains constant.

   a. **Influence of infusion rate on steady-state concentration:** The steady-state plasma concentration (C_{ss}) is directly proportional to the infusion rate. For example, if the infusion rate is doubled, the C_{ss} is doubled (Figure 1.21). Furthermore, the C_{ss} is inversely proportional to the clearance of the drug. Thus, any factor that decreases clearance, such as liver or kidney disease, increases the C_{ss} of an infused drug (assuming V_d remains constant). Factors that increase clearance, such as increased metabolism, decrease the C_{ss}.

   b. **Time to reach steady-state drug concentration:** The concentration of a drug rises from zero at the start of the infusion to its ultimate steady-state level, C_{ss} (Figure 1.21). The rate constant for attainment of steady state is the rate constant for total body elimination of the drug. Thus, 50% of C_{ss} of a drug is observed after the time elapsed, since the infusion, t, is equal to $t_{1/2}$, where $t_{1/2}$ (or half-life) is the time required for the drug concentration to change by 50%. After another half-life, the drug concentration approaches 75% of C_{ss} (Figure 1.22). The drug concentration is 87.5% of C_{ss} at 3 half-lives and 90% at 3.3 half-lives. Thus, a drug reaches steady state in about 4 to 5 half-lives.

   The sole determinant of the rate that a drug achieves steady state is the half-life ($t_{1/2}$) of the drug, and this rate is influenced

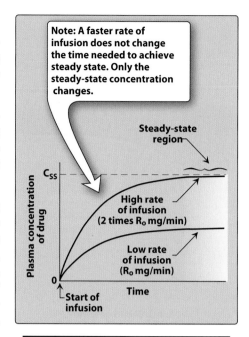

Figure 1.21
Effect of infusion rate on the steady-state concentration of drug in the plasma. R_o = rate of drug infusion; C_{ss} = steady-state concentration.

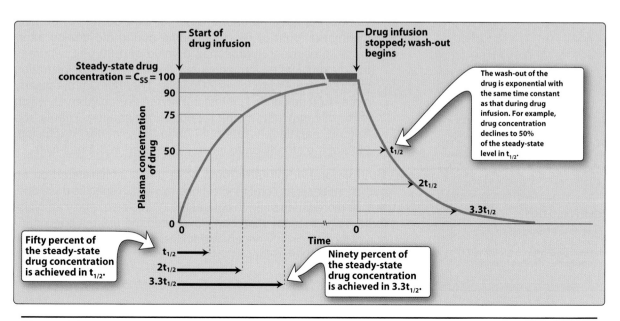

Figure 1.22
Rate of attainment of steady-state concentration of a drug in the plasma after intravenous infusion.

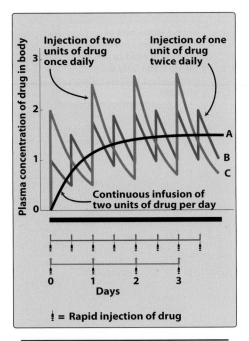

Figure 1.23
Predicted plasma concentrations of a drug given by infusion **(A)**, twice-daily injection **(B)**, or once-daily injection **(C)**. Model assumes rapid mixing in a single body compartment and a half-life of 12 hours.

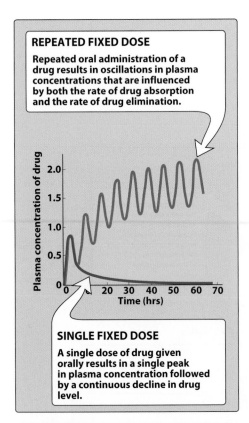

Figure 1.24
Predicted plasma concentrations of a drug given by repeated oral administrations.

only by factors that affect half-life. The rate of approach to steady state is not affected by the rate of infusion. When the infusion is stopped, the plasma concentration of a drug declines (washes out) to zero with the same time course observed in approaching steady state (Figure 1.22).

B. Fixed-dose/fixed-time regimens

Administration of a drug by fixed doses rather than by continuous infusion is often more convenient. However, fixed doses of IV or oral medications given at fixed intervals result in time-dependent fluctuations in the circulating level of drug, which contrasts with the smooth ascent of drug concentration with continuous infusion.

1. **Multiple IV injections:** When a drug is given repeatedly at regular intervals, the plasma concentration increases until a steady state is reached (Figure 1.23). Because most drugs are given at intervals shorter than 5 half-lives and are eliminated exponentially with time, some drug from the first dose remains in the body when the second dose is administered, some from the second dose remains when the third dose is given, and so forth. Therefore, the drug accumulates until, within the dosing interval, the rate of drug elimination equals the rate of drug administration and a steady state is achieved.

   a. **Effect of dosing frequency:** With repeated administration at regular intervals, the plasma concentration of a drug oscillates about a mean. Using smaller doses at shorter intervals reduces the amplitude of fluctuations in drug concentration. However, the dosing frequency changes neither the magnitude of C_{ss} nor the rate of achieving C_{ss}.

   b. **Example of achievement of steady state using different dosage regimens:** Curve B of Figure 1.23 shows the amount of drug in the body when 1 unit of a drug is administered IV and repeated at a dosing interval that corresponds to the half-life of the drug. At the end of the first dosing interval, 0.50 units of drug remain from the first dose when the second dose is administered. At the end of the second dosing interval, 0.75 units are present when the third dose is given. The minimal amount of drug remaining during the dosing interval progressively approaches a value of 1.00 unit, whereas the maximal value immediately following drug administration progressively approaches 2.00 units. Therefore, at the steady state, 1.00 unit of drug is lost during the dosing interval, which is exactly matched by the rate of administration. That is, the "rate in" equals the "rate out." As in the case for IV infusion, 90% of the steady-state value is achieved in 3.3 half-lives.

2. **Multiple oral administrations:** Most drugs administered on an outpatient basis are oral medications taken at a specific dose one, two, or more times daily. In contrast to IV injection, orally administered drugs may be absorbed slowly, and the plasma concentration of the drug is influenced by both the rate of absorption and the rate of elimination (Figure 1.24).

C. Optimization of dose

The goal of drug therapy is to achieve and maintain concentrations within a therapeutic response window while minimizing toxicity and/or adverse effects. With careful titration, most drugs can achieve this goal. If the therapeutic window (see Chapter 2) of the drug is small (for example, *digoxin* or *lithium*), extra caution should be taken in selecting a dosage regimen, and drug levels should be monitored to ensure attainment of the therapeutic range. Drug regimens are administered as a maintenance dose and may require a loading dose if rapid effects are warranted.

1. **Maintenance dose:** Drugs are generally administered to maintain a C_{ss} within the therapeutic window. It takes 4 to 5 half-lives for a drug to achieve C_{ss}. To achieve a given concentration, the rate of administration and the rate of elimination of the drug are important. The dosing rate can be determined by knowing the target concentration in plasma (Cp), clearance (CL) of the drug from the systemic circulation, and the fraction (F) absorbed (bioavailability):

$$\text{Dosing rate} = \frac{(\text{Target } C_{plasma})\,(CL)}{F}$$

2. **Loading dose:** Sometimes rapid obtainment of desired plasma levels is needed (for example, in serious infections or arrhythmias). Therefore, a "loading dose" of drug is administered to achieve the desired plasma level rapidly, followed by a maintenance dose to maintain the steady state (Figure 1.25). In general, the loading dose can be calculated as

Loading dose = $(V_d) \times$ (desired steady-state plasma concentration)/F

Disadvantages of loading doses include increased risk of drug toxicity and a longer time for the plasma concentration to fall if excess levels occur.

3. **Dose adjustment:** The amount of a drug administered for a given condition is estimated based on an "average patient." This approach overlooks interpatient variability in pharmacokinetic parameters such as clearance and V_d, which are quite significant in some cases. Knowledge of pharmacokinetic principles is useful in adjusting dosages to optimize therapy for a given patient. Monitoring drug therapy and correlating it with clinical benefits provides another tool to individualize therapy.

   For drugs with a defined therapeutic range, drug concentrations are measured, and the dosage and frequency are adjusted to obtain the desired levels. When determining a dosage adjustment, V_d can be used to calculate the amount of drug needed to achieve a desired plasma concentration. For example, assume a heart failure patient is not well controlled due to inadequate plasma levels of *digoxin*. Suppose the concentration of *digoxin* in the plasma is C_1 and the desired target concentration is C_2, a higher concentration. The following calculation can be used to determine how much additional *digoxin* should be administered to bring the level from C_1 to C_2.

   $(V_d)(C_1)$ = Amount of drug initially in the body

   $(V_d)(C_2)$ = Amount of drug in the body needed to achieve the desired plasma concentration

   The difference between the two values is the additional dosage needed, which equals $V_d (C_2 - C_1)$.

   Figure 1.26 shows the time course of drug concentration when treatment is started or dosing is changed.

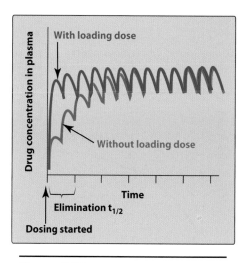

Figure 1.25
Accumulation of drug administered orally without a loading dose and with a single oral loading dose administered at t = 0.

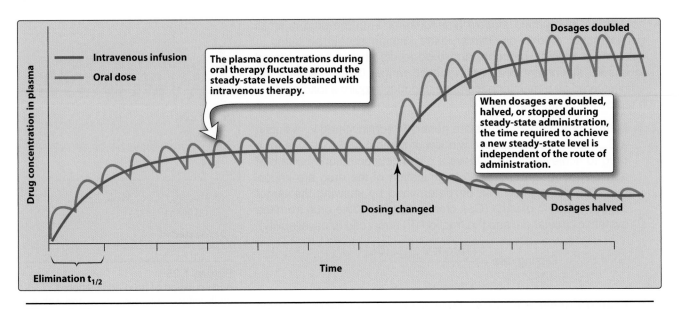

Figure 1.26
Accumulation of drug following sustained administration and following changes in dosing. Oral dosing was at intervals of 50% of $t_{1/2}$.

Study Questions

Choose the ONE best answer.

1.1 An 18-year-old female patient is brought to the emergency department due to drug overdose. Which of the following routes of administration is the most desirable for administering the antidote for the drug overdose?

A. Intramuscular
B. Intravenous
C. Oral
D. Subcutaneous
E. Transdermal

Correct answer = B. The intravenous route of administration is the most desirable because it results in achievement of therapeutic plasma levels of the antidote rapidly.

1.2 Drug A is a weakly basic drug with a pK_a of 7.8. If administered orally, at which of the following sites of absorption will the drug be able to readily pass through the membrane?

A. Mouth (pH approximately 7.0)
B. Stomach (pH of 2.5)
C. Duodenum (pH approximately 6.1)
D. Jejunum (pH approximately 8.0)
E. Ileum (pH approximately 7.0)

Correct answer = D. Because Drug A is a weakly basic drug (pK_a = 7.8), it will be predominantly in the nonionized form in the jejunum (pH of 8.0). For weak bases, the nonionized form will permeate through the cell membrane readily.

1.3 KR2250 is an investigational cholesterol-lowering agent. KR2250 has a high molecular weight and is extensively bound to albumin. KR2250 will have a(n) _____ apparent volume of distribution (V_d).

A. High
B. Low
C. Extremely high
D. Normal

Correct answer = B. Because of its high molecular weight and high protein binding, KR2250 will be effectively trapped within the plasma (vascular) compartment and will have a low apparent volume of distribution.

1.4 A 40-year-old male patient (70 kg) was recently diagnosed with infection involving methicillin-resistant *S. aureus*. He received 2000 mg of vancomycin as an IV loading dose. The peak plasma concentration of vancomycin was 28.5 mg/L. The apparent volume of distribution is:

A. 1 L/kg
B. 7 L/kg
C. 10 L/kg
D. 14 L/kg
E. 70 L/kg

> Correct answer = A. V_d = dose/C = 2000 mg/28.5 mg/L = 70.1 L. Because the patient is 70 kg, the apparent volume of distribution in L/kg will be approximately 1 L/kg (70.1 L/70 kg).

1.5 A 55-year-old woman is brought to the emergency department because of seizures. She has a history of renal disease and currently undergoes dialysis. She receives an intravenous infusion of antiseizure Drug X. Which of the following is likely to be observed with use of Drug X in this patient?

	Half-life	Dosage
A.	↑	↑
B.	↓	↓
C.	↑	↔
D.	↑	↓
E.	↔	↔

> Correct answer = D. Because the patient has a renal disorder, she may not be able to excrete the drug effectively. Therefore, the half-life of Drug X will be prolonged. As the half-life is prolonged, the dosage must be reduced so the patient will not have serious toxic effects of Drug X.

1.6 A 68-year-old woman is brought to the emergency department for treatment of a myocardial infarction. She is currently taking clopidogrel (antiplatelet agent) and aspirin daily, as well as omeprazole (potent CYP inhibitor) for heartburn. Which of the following is the most likely contributor to her myocardial infarction today?

A. Reduced antiplatelet activity of clopidogrel due to aspirin
B. Reduced antiplatelet activity of clopidogrel due to omeprazole
C. Hypersensitivity reaction due to clopidogrel
D. Increased antiplatelet activity of clopidogrel due to omeprazole
E. Increased antiplatelet activity of clopidogrel due to aspirin

> Correct answer = B. Clopidogrel is a prodrug and requires CYP2C19 activity for conversion to an active metabolite. Because omeprazole is a potent CYP inhibitor, clopidogrel is not converted to the active metabolite, and therefore the antiplatelet activity is reduced, potentially contributing to myocardial infarction.

1.7 Which of the following reactions represents Phase II of drug metabolism?

A. Amidation
B. Hydrolysis
C. Oxidation
D. Reduction
E. Sulfation

> Correct answer = E. Phase II metabolic reactions involve conjugation reactions to make phase I metabolites more polar. Sulfation and glucuronidation are the most common phase II conjugation reactions.

1.8 A pharmacokinetic study of a new antihypertensive drug is being conducted in healthy human volunteers. The half-life of the drug after administration by continuous intravenous infusion is 12 hours. Which of the following best approximates the time for the drug to reach steady state?

A. 24 hours
B. 48 hours
C. 72 hours
D. 120 hours
E. 240 hours

Correct answer = B. A drug will reach steady state in about 4 to 5 half-lives. Therefore, for this drug with a half-life of 12 hours, the approximate time to reach steady state will be 48 hours.

1.9 A 64-year-old female patient (60 kg) is treated with experimental Drug A for type 2 diabetes. Drug A is available as tablets with an oral bioavailability of 90%. If the V_d is 2 L/kg and the desired steady-state plasma concentration is 3.0 mg/L, which of the following is the most appropriate oral loading dose of Drug A?

A. 6 mg
B. 6.66 mg
C. 108 mg
D. 360 mg
E. 400 mg

Correct answer = E. For oral dosing, loading dose = [(V_d) × (desired steady-state plasma concentration)/F]. The V_d in this case is corrected to the patient's weight is 120 L. The F value is 0.9 (because bioavailability is 90%, that is, 90/100 = 0.9). Thus, loading dose = (120 L × 3.0 mg/L)/0.9 = 400 mg.

1.10 A 74-year-old man was admitted to the hospital for treatment of heart failure. He received 160 mcg of digoxin intravenously, and the plasma digoxin level was 0.4 ng/mL. If the desired plasma concentration of digoxin for optimal therapeutic activity in heart failure is 1.2 ng/mL, and the patient has an estimated V_d of 400 L, calculate the additional dose of digoxin needed for this patient to achieve the desired plasma concentration.

A. 128 mcg
B. 160 mcg
C. 320 mcg
D. 480 mcg
E. 640 mcg

Correct answer = C. The additional dosage of digoxin needed to achieve the desired plasma concentration can be calculated using the equation V_d ($C_2 - C_1$). C_1 is the current plasma concentration (0.4 ng/mL) and C_2 is the desired plasma concentration (1.2 ng/mL). Therefore, the additional dosage of digoxin is [400 L × (1.2 − 0.4) ng/mL] = 320 mcg.

Drug–Receptor Interactions and Pharmacodynamics

2

Joanna Peris

I. OVERVIEW

Pharmacodynamics describes the actions of a drug on the body. Most drugs exert effects, both beneficial and harmful, by interacting with specialized target macromolecules called receptors, which are present on or in the cell. The drug–receptor complex initiates alterations in biochemical and/or molecular activity of a cell by a process called signal transduction (Figure 2.1).

II. SIGNAL TRANSDUCTION

Drugs act as signals, and receptors act as signal detectors. A drug is termed an "agonist" if it binds to a site on a receptor protein and activates it to initiate a series of reactions that ultimately result in a specific intracellular response. "Second messenger" or effector molecules are part of the cascade of events that translates agonist binding into a cellular response.

A. The drug–receptor complex

Cells have many different types of receptors, each of which is specific for a particular agonist and produces a unique response. Cardiac cell membranes, for example, contain β-adrenergic receptors that bind and respond to epinephrine or norepinephrine. Cardiac cells also contain muscarinic receptors that bind and respond to acetylcholine. These two receptor populations dynamically interact to control the heart's vital functions.

The magnitude of the cellular response is proportional to the number of drug–receptor complexes. This concept is conceptually similar to the formation of complexes between enzyme and substrate and shares many common features, such as specificity of the receptor for a given agonist. Although much of this chapter centers on the interaction of drugs with specific receptors, it is important to know that not all drugs exert effects by interacting with a receptor. Antacids, for instance, chemically neutralize excess gastric acid, thereby reducing stomach upset.

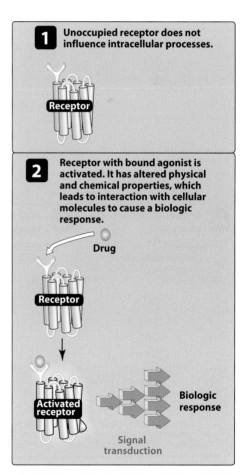

1 Unoccupied receptor does not influence intracellular processes.

Receptor

2 Receptor with bound agonist is activated. It has altered physical and chemical properties, which leads to interaction with cellular molecules to cause a biologic response.

Drug

Receptor

Activated receptor

Biologic response

Signal transduction

Figure 2.1
The recognition of a drug by a receptor triggers a biologic response.

B. Receptor states

Receptors exist in at least two states, inactive (R) and active (R*), that are in reversible equilibrium with one another, usually favoring the inactive state. Binding of agonists causes the equilibrium to shift from R to R* to produce a biologic effect. Antagonists are drugs that bind to the receptor but do not increase the fraction of R*, instead stabilizing the fraction of R. Some drugs (partial agonists) shift the equilibrium from R to R*, but the fraction of R* is less than that caused by an agonist. The magnitude of biological effect is directly related to the fraction of R*. In summary, agonists, antagonists, and partial agonists are examples of molecules or ligands that bind to the activation site on the receptor and can affect the fraction of R*.

C. Major receptor families

A receptor is defined as any biologic molecule to which a drug binds and produces a measurable response. Thus, enzymes, nucleic acids, and structural proteins can act as receptors for drugs or endogenous agonists. However, the richest sources of receptors are membrane-bound proteins that transduce extracellular signals into intracellular responses. These receptors may be divided into four families: 1) ligand-gated ion channels, 2) G protein–coupled receptors, 3) enzyme-linked receptors, and 4) intracellular receptors (Figure 2.2). Generally, hydrophilic ligands interact with receptors that are found on the cell surface (Figure 2.2A, B, C). In contrast, hydrophobic ligands enter cells through the lipid bilayers of the cell membrane to interact with receptors found inside cells (Figure 2.2D).

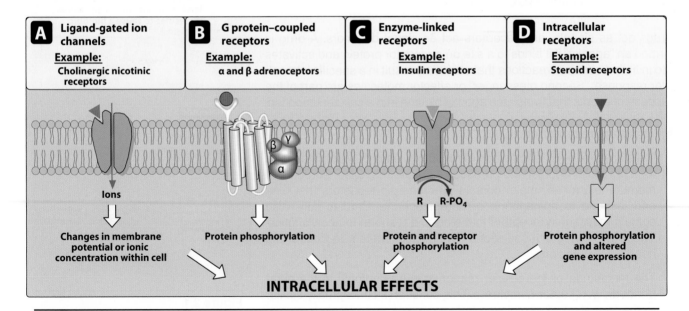

Figure 2.2
Transmembrane signaling mechanisms. **A.** Ligand binds to the extracellular domain of a ligand-gated channel. **B.** Ligand binds to a domain of a transmembrane receptor, which is coupled to a G protein. **C.** Ligand binds to the extracellular domain of a receptor that activates a kinase enzyme. **D.** Lipid-soluble ligand diffuses across the membrane to interact with its intracellular receptor. R = inactive protein.

1. **Transmembrane ligand-gated ion channels:** The extracellular portion of ligand-gated ion channels contains the drug-binding site. This site regulates the opening of the pore through which ions can flow across cell membranes (Figure 2.2A). The channel is usually closed until the receptor is activated by an agonist, which opens the channel for a few milliseconds. Depending on the ion conducted through these channels, these receptors mediate diverse functions, including neurotransmission and muscle contraction. For example, stimulation of the nicotinic receptor by acetylcholine opens a channel that allows sodium influx and potassium outflux across the cell membranes of neurons or muscle cells. This change in ionic concentrations across the membrane generates an action potential in a neuron and contraction in skeletal and cardiac muscle. On the other hand, agonist stimulation of the A subtype of the γ-aminobutyric acid (GABA) receptor increases chloride influx, resulting in hyperpolarization of neurons and less chance of generating an action potential. Drug-binding sites are also found on many voltage-gated ion channels where they can regulate channel function. For example, local anesthetics bind to the voltage-gated sodium channel, inhibiting sodium influx and decreasing neuronal conduction.

2. **Transmembrane G protein–coupled receptors:** The extracellular portion of this receptor contains the ligand-binding site, and the intracellular portion interacts (when activated) with a G protein. There are many kinds of G proteins (for example, G_s, G_i, and G_q), but all types are composed of three protein subunits. The α subunit binds guanosine triphosphate (GTP), and the β and γ subunits anchor the G protein in the cell membrane (Figure 2.3). Binding of an agonist to the receptor increases GTP binding to the α subunit, causing dissociation of the α-GTP complex from the $\beta\gamma$ complex. The α and $\beta\gamma$ subunits are then free to interact with specific cellular effectors, usually an enzyme or an ion channel, that cause further actions within the cell. These responses usually last several seconds to minutes. Often, the activated effectors produce "second messenger" molecules that further activate other effectors in the cell, causing a signal cascade effect.

A common effector, activated by G_s and inhibited by G_i, is adenylyl cyclase, which produces the second messenger cyclic adenosine monophosphate (cAMP). The effector phospholipase C, when activated by G_q, generates two second messengers: inositol 1,4,5-trisphosphate (IP_3) and diacylglycerol (DAG). DAG and cAMP activate specific protein kinases within the cell, leading to a myriad of physiological effects. IP_3 increases intracellular calcium concentration, which in turn activates other protein kinases.

3. **Enzyme-linked receptors:** This family of receptors undergoes conformational changes when activated by a ligand, resulting in

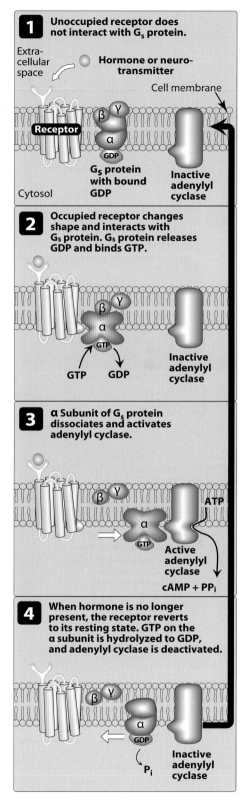

Figure 2.3
The recognition of chemical signals by G protein–coupled membrane receptors affects the activity of adenylyl cyclase. PP_i = inorganic pyrophosphate.

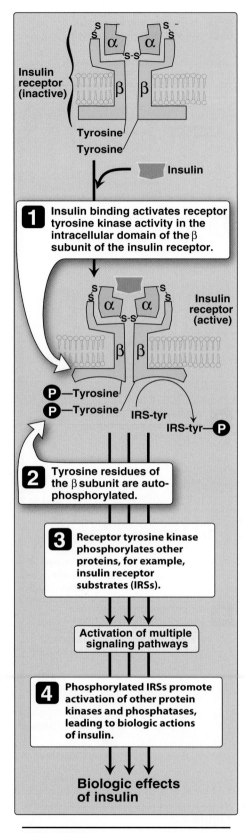

Figure 2.4
Insulin receptor.

increased intracellular enzyme activity (Figure 2.4). This response lasts for minutes to hours. The most common enzyme-linked receptors (for example, growth factors and insulin) possess tyrosine kinase activity. When activated, the receptor phosphorylates tyrosine residues on itself and other specific proteins (Figure 2.4). Phosphorylation can substantially modify the structure of the target protein, thereby acting as a molecular switch. For example, the phosphorylated insulin receptor in turn phosphorylates other proteins that now become active. Thus, enzyme-linked receptors often cause a signal cascade effect like that caused by G protein–coupled receptors.

4. **Intracellular receptors:** The fourth family of receptors differs considerably from the other three in that the receptor is entirely intracellular, and, therefore, the ligand (for example, steroid hormones) must have sufficient lipid solubility to diffuse into the cell to interact with the receptor (Figure 2.5). The primary targets of activated intracellular receptors are transcription factors in the cell nucleus that regulate gene expression. The activation or inactivation of transcription factors alters the transcription of DNA into RNA and subsequently translation of RNA into proteins. The effect of drugs or endogenous ligands that activate intracellular receptors takes hours to days to occur. Other targets of intracellular ligands are structural proteins, enzymes, RNA, and ribosomes. For example, tubulin is the target of antineoplastic agents such as *paclitaxel* (see Chapter 35), the enzyme dihydrofolate reductase is the target of antimicrobials such as *trimethoprim* (see Chapter 31), and the 50S subunit of the bacterial ribosome is the target of macrolide antibiotics such as *erythromycin* (see Chapter 30).

D. Characteristics of signal transduction

Signal transduction has two important features: 1) the ability to amplify small signals and 2) mechanisms to protect the cell from excessive stimulation.

1. **Signal amplification:** A characteristic of G protein–linked and enzyme-linked receptors is the ability to amplify signal intensity and duration via the signal cascade effect. Additionally, activated G proteins persist for a longer duration than does the original agonist–receptor complex. The binding of *albuterol*, for example, may only exist for a few milliseconds, but the subsequent activated G proteins may last for hundreds of milliseconds. Further prolongation and amplification of the initial signal are mediated by the interaction between G proteins and their respective intracellular targets. Because of this amplification, only a fraction of the total receptors for a specific ligand may need to be occupied to elicit a maximal response. Systems that exhibit this behavior are said to have spare receptors. About 99% of insulin receptors are "spare," providing an immense functional reserve that ensures that adequate amounts of glucose enter the cell. On the other hand, only

about 5% to 10% of the total β-adrenoceptors in the heart are spare. Therefore, little functional reserve exists in the failing heart, because most receptors must be occupied to obtain maximum contractility.

2. **Desensitization and down-regulation of receptors:** Repeated or continuous administration of an agonist or antagonist often leads to changes in the responsiveness of the receptor. The receptor may become desensitized due to too much agonist stimulation (Figure 2.6), resulting in a diminished response. This phenomenon, called tachyphylaxis, is often due to phosphorylation that renders receptors unresponsive to the agonist. In addition, receptors may be internalized within the cell, making them unavailable for further agonist interaction (down-regulation). Some receptors, particularly ion channels, require a finite time following stimulation before they can be activated again. During this recovery phase, unresponsive receptors are said to be "refractory." Repeated exposure of a receptor to an antagonist, on the other hand, results in up-regulation of receptors, in which receptor reserves are inserted into the membrane, increasing the number of receptors available. Up-regulation of receptors can make cells more sensitive to agonists and/or more resistant to effects of the antagonist.

III. DOSE–RESPONSE RELATIONSHIPS

Agonist drugs mimic the action of the endogenous ligand for the receptor (for example, *isoproterenol* mimics norepinephrine on β_1 receptors of the heart). The magnitude of the drug effect depends on receptor sensitivity to the drug and the drug concentration at the receptor site, which, in turn, is determined by both the dose of drug administered and by the drug's pharmacokinetic profile, such as rate of absorption, distribution, metabolism, and elimination.

A. Graded dose–response relationship

As the concentration of a drug increases, its pharmacologic effect also gradually increases until all the receptors are occupied (the maximum effect). Plotting the magnitude of response against increasing doses of a drug produces a graded dose–response curve that has the general shape depicted in Figure 2.7A. Two important drug characteristics, potency and efficacy, can be determined by graded dose–response curves.

1. **Potency:** Potency is a measure of the amount of drug necessary to produce an effect. The concentration of drug producing 50% of the maximum effect (EC_{50}) is often used to determine potency. In Figure 2.7, the EC_{50} for Drugs A and B indicate that Drug A is more potent than Drug B, because a lesser amount of Drug A is needed to obtain 50% effect. Therapeutic preparations of drugs reflect their potency. For example, *candesartan* and *irbesartan*

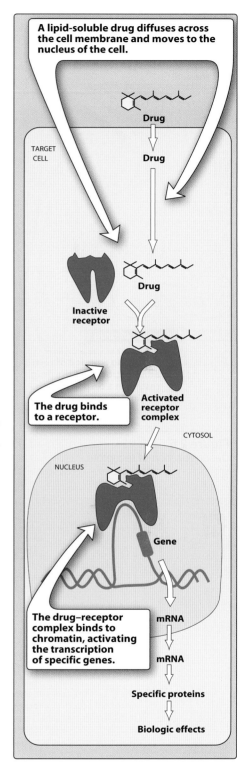

Figure 2.5
Mechanism of intracellular receptors. mRNA = messenger RNA.

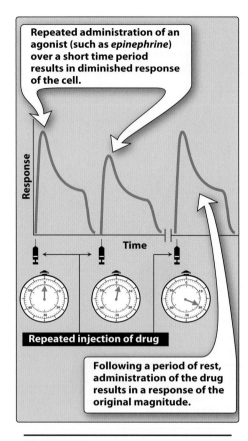

Figure 2.6
Desensitization of receptors.

are angiotensin receptor blockers used to treat hypertension. The therapeutic dose range for *candesartan* is 4 to 32 mg, as compared to 75 to 300 mg for *irbesartan*. Therefore, *candesartan* is more potent than *irbesartan* (it has a lower EC_{50} value). Since the range of drug concentrations that cause from 1% to 99% of maximal response usually spans several orders of magnitude, semilogarithmic plots are used to graph the complete range of doses. As shown in Figure 2.7B, the curves become sigmoidal in shape, which simplifies the interpretation of the dose–response curve.

2. **Efficacy:** Efficacy is the magnitude of response a drug causes when it interacts with a receptor. Efficacy is dependent on the number of drug–receptor complexes formed and the intrinsic activity of the drug (its ability to activate the receptor and cause a cellular response). Maximal efficacy of a drug (E_{max}) assumes that the drug occupies all receptors, and no increase in response is observed in response to higher concentrations of drug. The maximal response differs between full and partial agonists, even when the drug occupies 100% of the receptors. Similarly, even though an antagonist occupies 100% of the receptor sites, no receptor activation results and E_{max} is zero. Efficacy is a more clinically useful characteristic than potency, since a drug with greater efficacy is more therapeutically beneficial than one that is more potent. Figure 2.8 shows the response to drugs of differing potency and efficacy.

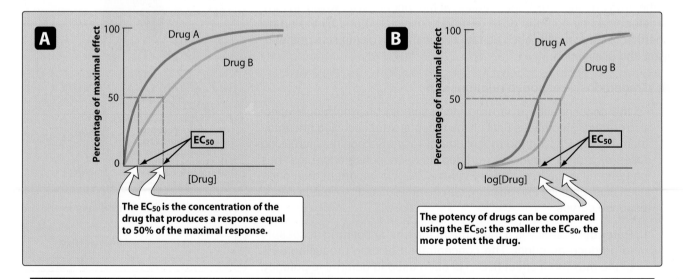

Figure 2.7
The effect of dose on the magnitude of pharmacologic response. **Panel A** is a linear plot. **Panel B** is a semilogarithmic plot of the same data. EC_{50} = drug dose causing 50% of maximal response.

B. Effect of drug concentration on receptor binding

The quantitative relationship between drug concentration and receptor occupancy applies the law of mass action to the kinetics of the binding of drug and receptor molecules:

$$\text{Drug} + \text{Receptor} \rightleftarrows \text{Drug} - \text{receptor complex} \rightarrow \text{Biologic effect}$$

By making the assumption that the binding of one drug molecule does not alter the binding of subsequent molecules and applying the law of mass action, we can mathematically express the relationship between the percentage (or fraction) of bound receptors and the drug concentration:

$$\frac{[DR]}{[R_t]} = \frac{[D]}{K_d + [D]} \quad (1)$$

where [D] = the concentration of free drug, [DR] = the concentration of bound drug, [R_t] = the total number of receptors, and K_d = the equilibrium dissociation constant for the drug from the receptor. The value of K_d can be used to determine the affinity of a drug for its receptor. Affinity describes the strength of the interaction (binding) between a ligand and its receptor. The higher the K_d value, the weaker the interaction and the lower the affinity, and vice versa. Equation (1) defines a curve that has the shapes shown in Figure 2.9 when plotted against drug concentration (Panel A) or log drug concentration (Panel B). As the concentration of free drug increases, the ratio of the concentrations of bound receptors to total receptors approaches unity, thereby producing the maximal effect. Thus, it is not surprising that the curves shown in Figure 2.9 and those representing the relationship between dose and effect (Figure 2.7) are similar.

C. Relationship of drug binding to pharmacologic effect

The law of mass action can be applied to drug concentration and response providing the following assumptions are met: 1) The magnitude of the response is proportional to the amount of receptors occupied by drug, 2) the E_{max} occurs when all receptors are bound, and 3) one molecule of drug binds to only one molecule of receptor. In this case,

$$\frac{[E]}{[E_{max}]} = \frac{[D]}{K_d + [D]} \quad (2)$$

where [E] = the effect of the drug at concentration [D] and [E_{max}] = the maximal effect of the drug.

Thus, it follows that if a specific population of receptors is vital for mediating a physiological effect, the affinity of an agonist for binding to those receptors should be related to the potency of that drug for causing that physiological effect. Many drugs and most neurotransmitters can bind to more than one type of receptor, thereby causing

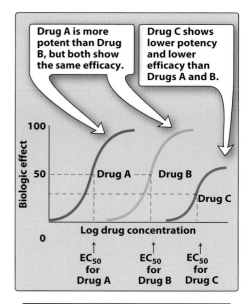

Figure 2.8
Typical dose–response curve for drugs showing differences in potency and efficacy. EC_{50} = drug dose that shows 50% of maximal response.

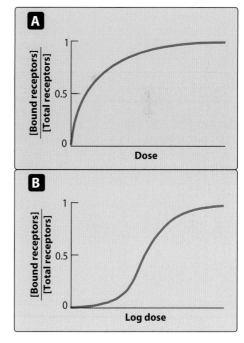

Figure 2.9
The effect of dose on the magnitude of drug binding.

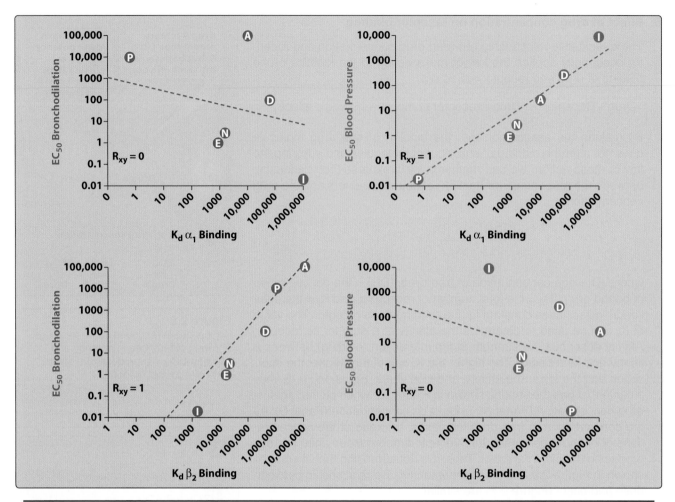

Figure 2.10
Correlation of drug affinity for receptor binding and potency for causing a physiological effect. A positive correlation should exist between the affinity (K_d value) of a drug for binding to a specific receptor subtype and the potency (EC_{50} value) of that drug to cause physiological responses mediated by that receptor population. For example, many drugs have affinity for both α_1 and β_2 adrenergic receptors. The circled letters in the figure represent agonists with varying affinities for α_1 and β_2 receptors. However, from the data provided, it becomes clear that α_1 receptors only mediate changes in blood pressure, while β_2 receptors only mediate changes in bronchodilation.

both desired therapeutic effects and undesired adverse effects. In order to establish a relationship between drug occupation of a particular receptor subtype and the corresponding biological response to that drug, correlation curves of receptor affinity and drug potency are often constructed (Figure 2.10).

IV. INTRINSIC ACTIVITY

As mentioned above, an agonist binds to a receptor and produces a biologic response based on the concentration of the agonist, its affinity for the receptor and, hence, the fraction of occupied receptors. However, the intrinsic activity of a drug further determines its ability to fully or partially activate the receptors. Drugs may be categorized according to their intrinsic activity and resulting E_{max} values.

A. Full agonists

If a drug binds to a receptor and produces a maximal biologic response that mimics the response to the endogenous ligand, it is a full agonist (Figure 2.11). Full agonists bind to a receptor, stabilizing the receptor in its active state and are said to have an intrinsic activity of one. All full agonists for a receptor population should produce the same E_{max}. For example, *phenylephrine* is a full agonist at α_1-adrenoceptors, because it produces the same E_{max} as the endogenous ligand, norepinephrine. Upon binding to α_1-adrenoceptors on vascular smooth muscle, both norepinephrine and *phenylephrine* stabilize the receptor in its active state, thereby increasing G_q activation. Activation of G_q increases intracellular Ca^{2+}, causing interaction of actin and myosin filaments and shortening of the muscle cells. The diameter of the arteriole decreases, causing an increase in resistance to blood flow through the vessel and an increase in blood pressure. Thus, effects of agonists on intracellular molecules, cells, tissues, and intact organisms are all attributable to interaction of the drug with the receptor. For full agonists, the dose–response curves for receptor binding and each of the biological responses should be comparable.

B. Partial agonists

Partial agonists have intrinsic activities greater than zero but less than one (Figure 2.11). Even when all the receptors are occupied, partial agonists cannot produce the same E_{max} as a full agonist. Even so, a partial agonist may have an affinity that is greater than, less than, or equivalent to that of a full agonist. A partial agonist may also act as a partial antagonist of a full agonist (Figure 2.12). As the number of receptors occupied by the partial agonist increases, the number of receptors that can be occupied by the full agonist decreases and therefore E_{max} would decrease until it reached the E_{max} of the partial agonist. This potential of partial agonists to act as both an agonist and antagonist may have therapeutic utility. For example, *aripiprazole*, an atypical antipsychotic, is a partial agonist at selected dopamine receptors. Overactive dopaminergic pathways tend to be inhibited by *aripiprazole*, whereas underactive pathways are stimulated. This might explain the ability of *aripiprazole* to improve symptoms of schizophrenia, with a small risk of causing extrapyramidal adverse effects (see Chapter 11).

C. Inverse agonists

Typically, unbound receptors are inactive and require interaction with an agonist to assume an active conformation. However, some receptors show a spontaneous conversion from R to R* in the absence of an agonist. Inverse agonists, unlike full agonists, stabilize the inactive R form and cause R* to convert to R. This decreases the number of activated receptors to below that observed in the absence of drug (Figure 2.11). Thus, inverse agonists have an intrinsic activity less than zero, reverse the activation state of receptors, and exert the opposite pharmacological effect of agonists.

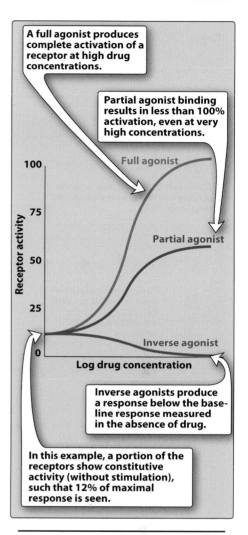

A full agonist produces complete activation of a receptor at high drug concentrations.

Partial agonist binding results in less than 100% activation, even at very high concentrations.

Full agonist

Partial agonist

Inverse agonist

Inverse agonists produce a response below the baseline response measured in the absence of drug.

In this example, a portion of the receptors show constitutive activity (without stimulation), such that 12% of maximal response is seen.

Figure 2.11
Effects of full agonists, partial agonists, and inverse agonists on receptor activity.

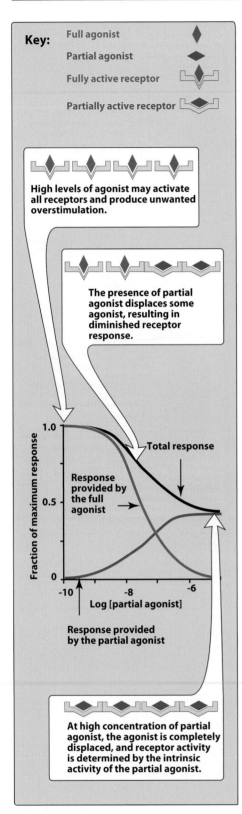

Figure 2.12
Effects of partial agonists.

D. Antagonists

Antagonists bind to a receptor with high affinity but possess zero intrinsic activity. An antagonist has no effect on biological function in the absence of an agonist, but can decrease the effect of an agonist when present. Antagonism may occur either by blocking the drug's ability to bind to the receptor or by blocking its ability to activate the receptor.

1. **Competitive antagonists:** If the antagonist binds to the same site on the receptor as the agonist in a reversible manner, it is "competitive." A competitive antagonist interferes with an agonist binding to its receptor and maintains the receptor in its inactive state. For example, the antihypertensive drug *terazosin* competes with the endogenous ligand norepinephrine at α_1-adrenoceptors, thus decreasing vascular smooth muscle tone and reducing blood pressure. However, increasing the concentration of agonist relative to antagonist can overcome this inhibition. Thus, competitive antagonists characteristically shift the agonist dose–response curve to the right (increased EC_{50}) without affecting E_{max} (Figure 2.13).

2. **Irreversible antagonists:** Irreversible antagonists bind covalently to the active site of the receptor, thereby permanently reducing the number of receptors available to the agonist. An irreversible antagonist causes a downward shift of the E_{max}, with no shift of EC_{50} values (Figure 2.13). In contrast to competitive antagonists, addition of more agonist does not overcome the effect of irreversible antagonists. Thus, irreversible antagonists and allosteric antagonists (see below) are both considered noncompetitive antagonists. A fundamental difference between competitive and noncompetitive antagonists is that competitive antagonists reduce agonist potency (increase EC_{50}) and noncompetitive antagonists reduce agonist efficacy (decrease E_{max}).

3. **Allosteric antagonists:** An allosteric antagonist binds to a site (allosteric site) other than the agonist-binding site and prevents receptor activation by the agonist. This type of antagonist also causes a downward shift of the E_{max} of an agonist, with no change in the EC_{50} value. An example of an allosteric agonist is picrotoxin, which binds to the inside of the GABA-controlled chloride channel. When picrotoxin binds inside the channel, no chloride can pass through the channel, even when GABA fully occupies the receptor.

4. **Functional antagonism:** An antagonist may act at a completely separate receptor, initiating effects that are functionally opposite those of the agonist. A classic example is the functional antagonism by epinephrine to histamine-induced bronchoconstriction. Histamine binds to H_1 histamine receptors on bronchial smooth muscle, causing bronchoconstriction of the bronchial tree. Epinephrine is an agonist at β_2-adrenoceptors on bronchial smooth muscle, which causes the muscles to relax. This functional antagonism is also known as "physiologic antagonism."

V. QUANTAL DOSE–RESPONSE RELATIONSHIPS

Another important dose–response relationship is that between the dose of the drug and the proportion of a population of patients that responds to it. These responses are known as quantal responses, because, for any individual, either the effect occurs or it does not. Graded responses can be transformed to quantal responses by designating a predetermined level of the graded response as the point at which a response occurs or not. For example, a quantal dose–response relationship can be determined in a population for the antihypertensive drug *atenolol*. A positive response is defined as a fall of at least 5 mm Hg in diastolic blood pressure. Quantal dose–response curves are useful for determining doses to which most of the population responds. They have similar shapes as log dose–response curves, and the ED_{50} is the drug dose that causes a therapeutic response in half of the population.

A. Therapeutic index

The therapeutic index (TI) of a drug is the ratio of the dose that produces toxicity in half the population (TD_{50}) to the dose that produces a clinically desired or effective response (ED_{50}) in half the population:

$$TI = TD_{50} / ED_{50}$$

The TI is a measure of a drug's safety, because a larger value indicates a wide margin between doses that are effective and doses that are toxic.

B. Clinical usefulness of the therapeutic index

The TI of a drug is determined using drug trials and accumulated clinical experience. These usually reveal a range of effective doses and a different (sometimes overlapping) range of toxic doses. Although high TI values are required for most drugs, some drugs with low therapeutic indices are routinely used to treat serious diseases. In these cases, the risk of experiencing adverse effects is not as great as the risk of leaving the disease untreated. Figure 2.14 shows the responses to *warfarin*, an oral anticoagulant with a low TI, and *penicillin*, an antimicrobial drug with a large TI.

1. **Warfarin (example of a drug with a small therapeutic index):** As the dose of *warfarin* is increased, a greater fraction of the patients respond (for this drug, the desired response is a two- to threefold increase in the international normalized ratio [INR]) until, eventually, all patients respond (Figure 2.14A). However, at higher doses of *warfarin*, anticoagulation resulting in hemorrhage occurs in a small percent of patients. Agents with a low TI (that is, drugs for which dose is critically important) are those drugs for which bioavailability critically alters the therapeutic effects (see Chapter 1).

2. **Penicillin (example of a drug with a large therapeutic index):** For drugs such as *penicillin* (Figure 2.14B), it is safe and common to give doses in excess of that which is minimally required to achieve a desired response without the risk of adverse effects. In this case, bioavailability does not critically alter the therapeutic or clinical effects.

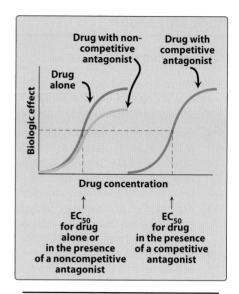

Figure 2.13
Effects of drug antagonists. EC_{50} = drug dose that shows 50% of maximal response.

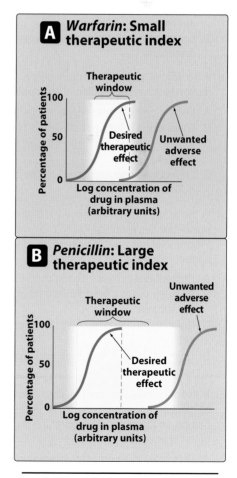

Figure 2.14
Cumulative percentage of patients responding to plasma levels of *warfarin* and *penicillin*.

Study Questions

Choose the ONE best answer.

2.1 Which of the following best describes how a drug that acts as an agonist at the A subtype of GABA receptors affects signal transduction in a neuron?

 A. Activation of this receptor subtype alters transcription of DNA in the nucleus of the neuron.

 B. Activation of this receptor subtype opens ion channels that allow sodium to enter cells and increases the chance of generating an action potential.

 C. Activation of this receptor subtype opens ion channels that allow chloride to enter cells and decreases the chance of generating an action potential.

 D. Activation of this receptor subtype results in G protein activation and increased intracellular second messenger levels.

Correct answer = C. The GABA-A receptor is a ligand-gated ion channel selective for chloride. Agonists for the GABA-A receptor increase opening of channels, resulting in chloride entry into the neuron, hyperpolarization, and decreased action potential events.

2.2 If 1 mg of lorazepam produces the same anxiolytic response as 10 mg of diazepam, which is correct?

 A. Lorazepam is more potent than is diazepam.

 B. Lorazepam is more efficacious than is diazepam.

 C. Lorazepam is a full agonist, and diazepam is a partial agonist.

 D. Lorazepam is a better drug to take for anxiety than is diazepam.

Correct answer = A. A drug that causes the same effect at a lower dose is more potent. B and C are incorrect because without information about the maximal effect of these drugs, no conclusions can be made about efficacy or intrinsic activity. D is incorrect because the maximal response obtained is often more important than the amount of drug needed to achieve it.

2.3 If 10 mg of oxycodone produces a greater analgesic response than does aspirin at any dose, which is correct?

 A. Oxycodone is more efficacious than is aspirin.

 B. Oxycodone is less potent than is aspirin.

 C. Aspirin is a full agonist, and oxycodone is a partial agonist.

 D. Oxycodone and aspirin act on the same drug target.

Correct answer = A. Drugs with greater response at maximally effective concentrations are more efficacious than drugs with a lower maximal response. Choice B is incorrect since no information is given about the half maximal concentrations of either drug. Choices C and D are incorrect since it is not known if both drugs bind to the same receptor population.

2.4 In the presence of propranolol, a higher concentration of epinephrine is required to elicit full antiasthmatic activity. Propranolol has no effect on asthma symptoms. Which is correct regarding these medications?

 A. Epinephrine is less efficacious than is propranolol.

 B. Epinephrine is a full agonist, and propranolol is a partial agonist.

 C. Epinephrine is an agonist, and propranolol is a competitive antagonist.

 D. Epinephrine is an agonist, and propranolol is a noncompetitive antagonist.

Correct answer = C. Since propranolol decreases the effect of epinephrine but the inhibition can be overcome by giving a higher dose of epinephrine, propranolol must be a competitive antagonist. If D were correct, even very high concentrations of epinephrine would not be able to elicit a maximal effect in the presence of propranolol. Since propranolol has no effect by itself, A and B are incorrect.

2.5 In the presence of picrotoxin, diazepam is less efficacious at causing sedation, regardless of the dose. Picrotoxin has no sedative effect, even at the highest dose. Which of the following is correct regarding these agents?

 A. Picrotoxin is a competitive antagonist.

 B. Picrotoxin is a noncompetitive antagonist.

 C. Diazepam is less efficacious than is picrotoxin.

 D. Diazepam is less potent than is picrotoxin.

Correct answer = B. Since picrotoxin decreases the maximal effect of diazepam regardless of the diazepam dose, it is a noncompetitive antagonist. Picrotoxin has no efficacy alone, so C is incorrect. No information is provided about potency of either drug.

2.6 Haloperidol, chlorpromazine, and clozapine are antipsychotic medications that bind to the D2 subtype of dopamine receptors, with a binding affinity of haloperidol > chlorpromazine > clozapine. Which statement would have to be correct to conclude that the mechanism of antipsychotic effects for these drugs is via binding to D2 receptors?

A. Haloperidol should have the lowest potency of the three antipsychotic drugs.

B. D2 receptor binding should also be related to the potency of these drugs in causing Parkinson's-like adverse effects.

C. A positive correlation should exist between the affinity of these drugs to bind to D2 receptors and their potency for antipsychotic actions.

D. Clozapine would have to be more potent than chlorpromazine for decreasing psychosis.

> Correct answer = C. To conclude that the mechanism of antipsychotic effect for these drugs is via binding to D2 receptors, there should be a positive correlation between the affinity of the drugs for D2 receptors and their potency for antipsychotic actions. Haloperidol should have the highest antipsychotic potency and clozapine the lowest. There is no guarantee the therapeutic effects and adverse effects are mediated by the same receptor population; therefore, a different correlation may exist for the adverse effects and D2 receptor affinity.

2.7 If there were spare β_1-adrenergic receptors on cardiac muscle cells, which statement would be correct?

A. The number of spare β_1-adrenergic receptors determines the size of the maximum effect of the agonist epinephrine.

B. Spare β_1 adrenergic receptors make the cardiac tissue less sensitive to epinephrine.

C. A maximal effect of epinephrine is seen when only a portion of β_1 adrenergic receptors are occupied.

D. Spare receptors are active even in the absence of epinephrine.

> Correct answer = C. Only a fraction of the total receptors need to be bound to elicit a maximum cellular response when spare receptors are present. The other choices do not accurately describe the effects of having spare receptors.

2.8 Which of the following up-regulates postsynaptic α_1-adrenergic receptors?

A. Daily use of amphetamine that causes release of norepinephrine

B. A disease that causes an increase in the activity of norepinephrine neurons

C. Daily use of phenylephrine, an α_1 receptor agonist

D. Daily use of prazosin, an α_1 receptor antagonist

> Correct answer = D. Up-regulation of receptors occurs when receptor activation is lower than normal, such as when the receptor is continuously exposed to an antagonist for that receptor. Down-regulation of receptors occurs when receptor activation is greater than normal because of continuous exposure to an agonist, as described in A, B, and C.

2.9 Methylphenidate helps patients with attention deficit hyperactivity disorder (ADHD) maintain attention and perform better at school or work, with an ED_{50} of 10 mg. However, methylphenidate can also cause significant nausea at higher doses (TD_{50} = 30 mg). Which is correct regarding methylphenidate?

A. The therapeutic index of methylphenidate is 3.

B. The therapeutic index of methylphenidate is 0.3.

C. Methylphenidate is more potent at causing nausea than treating ADHD.

D. Methylphenidate is more efficacious at causing nausea than treating ADHD.

> Correct answer = A. Therapeutic index is calculated by dividing TD_{50} by ED_{50} (30/10), making B incorrect. C is incorrect because methylphenidate is more potent at treating ADHD (it takes a lower dose) than causing nausea. D. No information about efficacy is provided.

2.10 Which is correct concerning the safety of using warfarin (with a small therapeutic index) versus penicillin (with a large therapeutic index)?

   A. Warfarin is a safer drug because it has a low therapeutic index.
   B. Warfarin treatment has a high chance of resulting in dangerous adverse effects if bioavailability is altered.
   C. The high therapeutic index makes penicillin a safe drug for all patients.
   D. Penicillin treatment has a high chance of causing dangerous adverse effects if bioavailability is altered.

Correct answer = B. Agents with a low TI (that is, drugs for which dose is critically important) are those drugs for which bioavailability critically alters the therapeutic and adverse effects. A is incorrect, because a drug with a low TI is not generally considered to be safe. C is incorrect because a high TI does not ensure safety across the entire patient population. D is incorrect because the high TI makes it unlikely that bioavailability alters the incidence of therapeutic or adverse effects.

The Autonomic Nervous System

Rajan Radhakrishnan

3

I. OVERVIEW

The autonomic nervous system (ANS), along with the endocrine system, coordinates the regulation and integration of bodily functions. The endocrine system sends signals to target tissues by varying the levels of blood-borne hormones. By contrast, the nervous system exerts effects by the rapid transmission of electrical impulses over nerve fibers that terminate at effector cells, which specifically respond to the release of neuromediator substances. Drugs that produce their primary therapeutic effect by mimicking or altering the functions of the ANS are called autonomic drugs and are discussed in the following four chapters. The autonomic agents act either by stimulating portions of the ANS or by blocking the action of the autonomic nerves. This chapter outlines the fundamental physiology of the ANS and describes the role of neurotransmitters in the communication between extracellular events and chemical changes within the cell.

II. INTRODUCTION TO THE NERVOUS SYSTEM

The nervous system is divided into two anatomical divisions: the central nervous system (CNS), which is composed of the brain and spinal cord, and the peripheral nervous system, which includes neurons located outside the brain and spinal cord—that is, any nerves that enter or leave the CNS (Figure 3.1). The peripheral nervous system is subdivided into the efferent and afferent divisions. The efferent neurons carry signals away from the brain and spinal cord to the peripheral tissues, and the afferent neurons bring information from the periphery to the CNS. Afferent neurons provide sensory input to modulate the function of the efferent division through reflex arcs or neural pathways that mediate a reflex action.

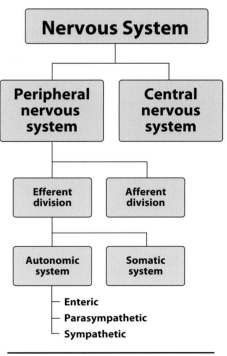

Figure 3.1
Organization of the nervous system.

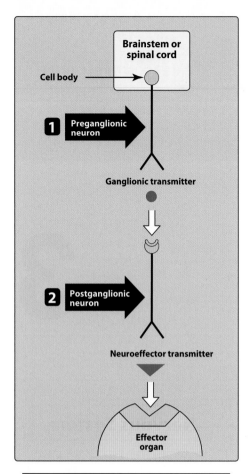

Figure 3.2
Efferent neurons of the autonomic
nervous system.

A. Functional divisions within the nervous system

The efferent portion of the peripheral nervous system is further divided into two major functional subdivisions: the somatic nervous system and the ANS (Figure 3.1). The somatic efferent neurons are involved in the voluntary control of functions such as contraction of the skeletal muscles essential for locomotion. The ANS, conversely, regulates the everyday requirements of vital bodily functions without the conscious participation of the mind. Because of the involuntary nature of the ANS as well as its functions, it is also known as the visceral, vegetative, or involuntary nervous system. It is composed of efferent neurons that innervate visceral smooth muscle, cardiac muscle, vasculature, and the exocrine glands, thereby controlling digestion, cardiac output, blood flow, and glandular secretions.

B. Anatomy of the ANS

1. **Efferent neurons:** The ANS carries nerve impulses from the CNS to the effector organs through two types of efferent neurons: the preganglionic neurons and the postganglionic neurons (Figure 3.2). The cell body of the first nerve cell, the preganglionic neuron, is located within the CNS. The preganglionic neurons emerge from the brainstem or spinal cord and make a synaptic connection in ganglia (an aggregation of nerve cell bodies located in the peripheral nervous system). The ganglia function as relay stations between the preganglionic neuron and the second nerve cell, the postganglionic neuron. The cell body of the postganglionic neuron originates in the ganglion. It is generally nonmyelinated and terminates on effector organs, such as visceral smooth muscle, cardiac muscle, and the exocrine glands.

2. **Afferent neurons:** The afferent neurons (fibers) of the ANS are important in the reflex regulation of this system (for example, by sensing pressure in the carotid sinus and aortic arch) and in signaling the CNS to influence the efferent branch of the system to respond.

3. **Sympathetic neurons:** The efferent ANS is divided into the sympathetic and the parasympathetic nervous systems, as well as the enteric nervous system (Figure 3.1). Anatomically, the sympathetic and the parasympathetic neurons originate in the CNS and emerge from two different spinal cord regions (Figure 3.3). The preganglionic neurons of the sympathetic system come from the thoracic and lumbar regions (T1 to L2) of the spinal cord, and they synapse in two cord-like chains of ganglia that run close to and in parallel on each side of the spinal cord. The preganglionic neurons are short in comparison to the postganglionic ones. Axons of the postganglionic neuron extend from the ganglia to tissues they innervate and regulate (see Chapter 6). In most cases, the preganglionic nerve endings of the sympathetic nervous system are highly branched, enabling one preganglionic neuron to interact with many postganglionic neurons. This arrangement enables activation of numerous effector organs at the same time. [Note: The adrenal medulla, like the sympathetic ganglia, receives preganglionic fibers from the sympathetic system. The adrenal medulla, in response to stimulation by the ganglionic neurotransmitter acetylcholine, secretes epinephrine (adrenaline), and lesser amounts of norepinephrine, directly into the blood.]

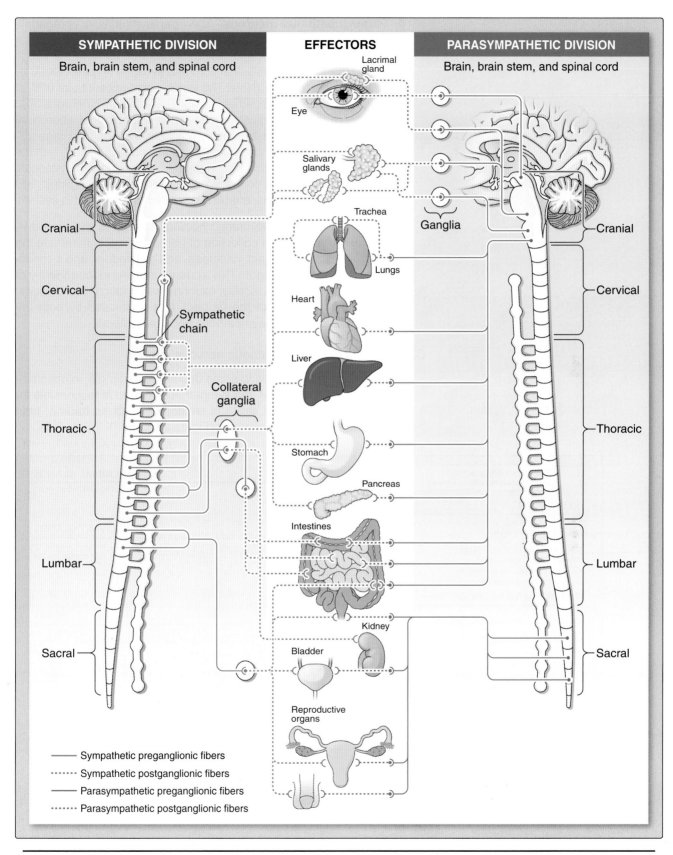

SYMPATHETIC DIVISION
Brain, brain stem, and spinal cord

EFFECTORS

PARASYMPATHETIC DIVISION
Brain, brain stem, and spinal cord

Cranial

Cervical

Sympathetic chain

Collateral ganglia

Thoracic

Lumbar

Sacral

Lacrimal gland

Eye

Salivary glands

Trachea

Ganglia

Lungs

Heart

Liver

Stomach

Pancreas

Intestines

Kidney

Bladder

Reproductive organs

Cranial

Cervical

Thoracic

Lumbar

Sacral

—— Sympathetic preganglionic fibers
······ Sympathetic postganglionic fibers
—— Parasympathetic preganglionic fibers
······ Parasympathetic postganglionic fibers

Figure 3.3
Autonomic nervous system.

4. **Parasympathetic neurons:** The parasympathetic preganglionic fibers arise from cranial nerves III (oculomotor), VII (facial), IX (glossopharyngeal), and X (vagus), as well as from the sacral region (S2 to S4) of the spinal cord and synapse in ganglia near or on the effector organs. [Note: The vagus nerve accounts for 90% of preganglionic parasympathetic fibers. Postganglionic neurons from this nerve innervate most organs in the thoracic and abdominal cavity.] Thus, in contrast to the sympathetic system, the preganglionic fibers are long, and the postganglionic ones are short, with the ganglia close to or within the organ innervated. In most instances, there is a one-to-one connection between the preganglionic and postganglionic neurons, enabling discrete response of this system.

5. **Enteric neurons:** The enteric nervous system is the third division of the ANS. It is a collection of nerve fibers that innervate the gastrointestinal (GI) tract, pancreas, and gallbladder, and it constitutes the "brain of the gut." This system functions independently of the CNS and controls motility, exocrine and endocrine secretions, and microcirculation of the GI tract. It is modulated by both the sympathetic and parasympathetic nervous systems.

C. Functions of the sympathetic nervous system

Although continually active to some degree (for example, in maintaining tone of vascular beds), the sympathetic division is responsible for adjusting in response to stressful situations, such as trauma, fear, hypoglycemia, cold, and exercise (Figure 3.4).

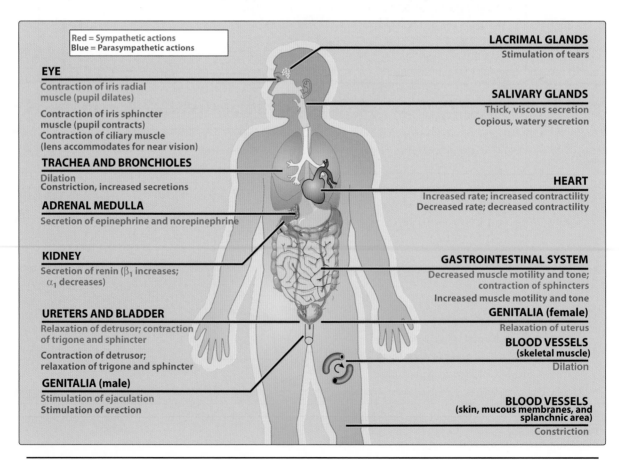

Figure 3.4
Actions of sympathetic and parasympathetic nervous systems on effector organs.

1. **Effects of stimulation of the sympathetic division:** The effect of sympathetic stimulation is an increase in heart rate and blood pressure, mobilization of energy stores, and increase in blood flow to skeletal muscles and the heart while diverting flow from the skin and internal organs. Sympathetic stimulation results in dilation of the pupils and bronchioles (Figure 3.4). It also reduces GI motility and affects function of the bladder and sexual organs.

2. **Fight or flight response:** The changes experienced by the body during emergencies are referred to as the "fight or flight" response (Figure 3.5). These reactions are triggered both by direct sympathetic activation of effector organs and by stimulation of the adrenal medulla to release epinephrine and lesser amounts of norepinephrine. Hormones released by the adrenal medulla directly enter the bloodstream and promote responses in effector organs that contain adrenergic receptors (see Chapter 6). The sympathetic nervous system tends to function as a unit and often discharges as a complete system, for example, during severe exercise or in reactions to fear (Figure 3.5). This system, with its diffuse distribution of postganglionic fibers, is involved in a wide array of physiologic activities. Although it is not essential for survival, it is essential in preparing the body to handle uncertain situations and unexpected stimuli.

D. Functions of the parasympathetic nervous system

The parasympathetic division is involved with maintaining homeostasis within the body. It is required for life, since it maintains essential bodily functions, such as digestion and elimination. The parasympathetic division usually acts to oppose or balance the actions of the sympathetic division and generally predominates the sympathetic system in "rest-and-digest" situations. Unlike the sympathetic system, the parasympathetic system never discharges as a complete system. If it did, it would produce massive, undesirable, and unpleasant symptoms, such as involuntary urination and defecation. Instead, parasympathetic fibers innervating specific organs such as the gut, heart, or eye are activated separately, and the system affects these organs individually.

E. Role of the CNS in the control of autonomic functions

Although the ANS is a motor system, it does require sensory input from peripheral structures to provide information on the current state of the body. This feedback is provided by streams of afferent impulses, originating in the viscera and other autonomically innervated structures that travel to integrating centers in the CNS, such as the hypothalamus, medulla oblongata, and spinal cord. These centers respond to stimuli by sending out efferent reflex impulses via the ANS.

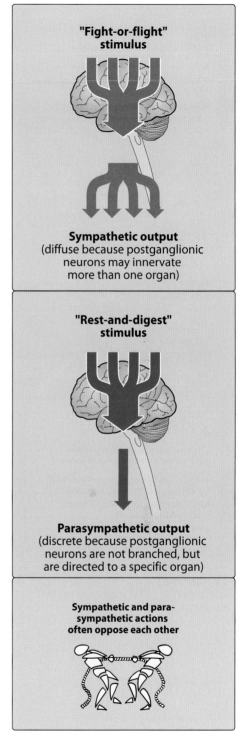

"Fight-or-flight" stimulus

Sympathetic output (diffuse because postganglionic neurons may innervate more than one organ)

"Rest-and-digest" stimulus

Parasympathetic output (discrete because postganglionic neurons are not branched, but are directed to a specific organ)

Sympathetic and parasympathetic actions often oppose each other

Figure 3.5
Sympathetic and parasympathetic actions are elicited by different stimuli.

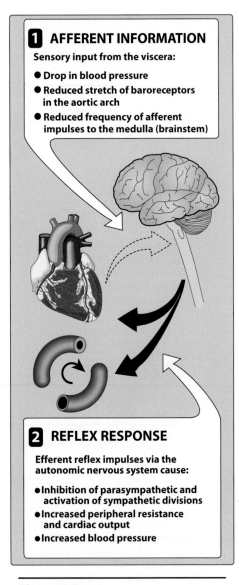

Figure 3.6
Baroreceptor reflex arc response to a decrease in blood pressure.

1. **Reflex arcs:** Most of the afferent impulses are involuntarily translated into reflex responses. For example, a fall in blood pressure causes pressure-sensitive neurons (baroreceptors in the heart, vena cava, aortic arch, and carotid sinuses) to send fewer impulses to cardiovascular centers in the brain. This prompts a reflex response of increased sympathetic output to the heart and vasculature and decreased parasympathetic output to the heart, which results in a compensatory rise in blood pressure and heart rate (Figure 3.6). [Note: In each case, the reflex arcs of the ANS comprise a sensory (afferent) arm and a motor (efferent or effector) arm.]

2. **Emotions and the ANS:** Stimuli that evoke strong feelings, such as rage, fear, and pleasure, can modify activities of the ANS.

F. Innervation by the ANS

1. **Dual innervation:** Most organs are innervated by both divisions of the ANS. Thus, vagal parasympathetic innervation slows the heart rate, and sympathetic innervation increases heart rate. Despite this dual innervation, one system usually predominates in controlling the activity of a given organ. For example, the vagus nerve is the predominant factor for controlling heart rate. The dual innervation of organs is dynamic, and fine-tuned continually to maintain homeostasis.

2. **Sympathetic innervation:** Although most tissues receive dual innervation, some effector organs, such as the adrenal medulla, kidney, pilomotor muscles, and sweat glands, receive innervation only from the sympathetic system.

G. Somatic nervous system

The efferent somatic nervous system differs from the ANS in that a single myelinated motor neuron, originating in the CNS, travels directly to skeletal muscle without the mediation of ganglia. As noted earlier, the somatic nervous system is under voluntary control, whereas the ANS is involuntary. Responses in the somatic division are generally faster than those in the ANS.

H. Summary of differences between sympathetic, parasympathetic, and motor nerves

Major differences in the anatomical arrangement of neurons lead to variations of the functions in each division (Figure 3.7). The sympathetic nervous system is widely distributed, innervating practically all effector systems in the body. By contrast, the distribution of the parasympathetic division is more limited. The sympathetic preganglionic fibers have a much broader influence than the parasympathetic fibers and synapse with a larger number of postganglionic fibers. This type of organization permits a diffuse discharge of the sympathetic nervous system. The parasympathetic division is more circumscribed, with mostly one-to-one interactions, and the ganglia are also close to, or within, organs they innervate. This limits the amount of branching that can be done by this division. [A notable exception is found in

	SYMPATHETIC	PARASYMPATHETIC
Sites of origin	Thoracic and lumbar region of the spinal cord (thoracolumbar)	Brain and sacral area of the spinal cord (craniosacral)
Length of fibers	Short preganglionic Long postganglionic	Long preganglionic Short postganglionic
Location of ganglia	Close to the spinal cord	Within or near effector organs
Preganglionic fiber branching	Extensive	Minimal
Distribution	Wide	Limited
Type of response	Diffuse	Discrete

Figure 3.7
Characteristics of the sympathetic and parasympathetic nervous systems.

the myenteric plexus (major nerve supply to the GI tract), where one preganglionic neuron has been shown to interact with 8000 or more postganglionic fibers.] The anatomical arrangement of the parasympathetic system results in the distinct functions of this division. The somatic nervous system innervates skeletal muscles. One somatic motor neuron axon is highly branched, and each branch innervates a single muscle fiber. Thus, one somatic motor neuron may innervate 100 muscle fibers. This arrangement leads to the formation of a motor unit. The lack of ganglia and the myelination of the motor nerves enable a fast response by the somatic nervous system.

III. CHEMICAL SIGNALING BETWEEN CELLS

Neurotransmission in the ANS is an example of chemical signaling between cells. In addition to neurotransmission, other types of chemical signaling include the secretion of hormones and the release of local mediators (Figure 3.8).

A. Hormones

Specialized endocrine cells secrete hormones into the bloodstream, where they travel throughout the body, exerting effects on broadly distributed target cells (see Chapters 23 through 26).

B. Local mediators

Most cells secrete chemicals that act locally on cells in the immediate environment. Because these chemical signals are rapidly destroyed or removed, they do not enter the blood and are not distributed throughout the body. Histamine (see Chapter 37) and prostaglandins are examples of local mediators.

C. Neurotransmitters

Communication between nerve cells, and between nerve cells and effector organs, occurs through the release of specific chemical signals (neurotransmitters) from the nerve terminals. The release is

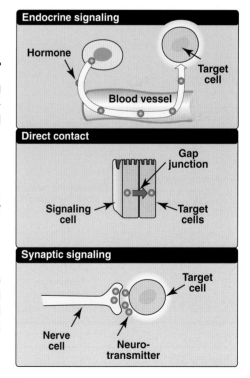

Figure 3.8
Some commonly used mechanisms for transmission of regulatory signals between cells.

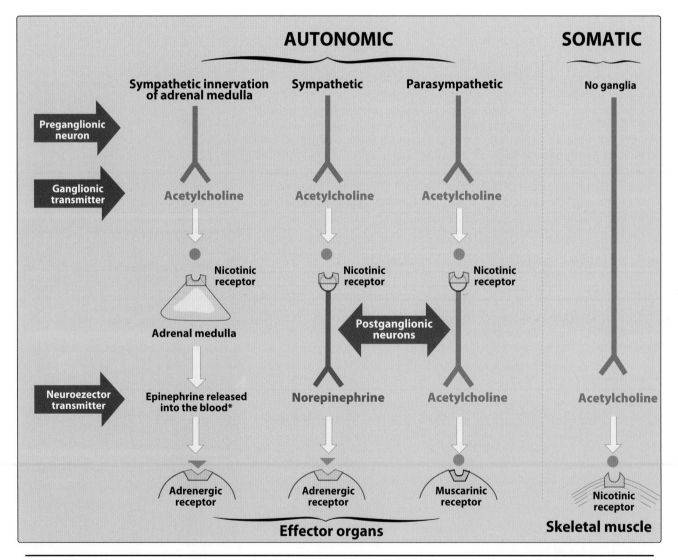

triggered by arrival of the action potential at the nerve ending, leading to depolarization. An increase in intracellular Ca^{2+} initiates fusion of synaptic vesicles with the presynaptic membrane and release of their contents. The neurotransmitters rapidly diffuse across the synaptic cleft, or space (synapse), between neurons and combine with specific receptors on the postsynaptic (target) cell.

1. **Membrane receptors:** All neurotransmitters, and most hormones and local mediators, are too hydrophilic to penetrate the lipid bilayers of target cell plasma membranes. Instead, their signal is mediated by binding to specific receptors on the cell surface of target organs. [Note: A receptor is defined as a recognition site for a sub-

Figure 3.9
Summary of the neurotransmitters released, types of receptors, and types of neurons within the autonomic and somatic nervous systems. Cholinergic neurons are shown in *red* and adrenergic neurons in *blue*. [Note: This schematic diagram does not show that the parasympathetic ganglia are close to or on the surface of the effector organs and that the postganglionic fibers are usually shorter than the preganglionic fibers. By contrast, the ganglia of the sympathetic nervous system are close to the spinal cord. The postganglionic fibers are long, allowing extensive branching to innervate more than one organ system. This allows the sympathetic nervous system to discharge as a unit.] *Epinephrine 80% and norepinephrine 20% released from adrenal medulla.

stance. It has a binding specificity and is coupled to processes that eventually evoke a response. Most receptors are proteins (see Chapter 2).]

2. **Types of neurotransmitters:** Although over 50 signal molecules in the nervous system have been identified, norepinephrine (and the closely related epinephrine), acetylcholine, dopamine, serotonin, histamine, glutamate, and γ-aminobutyric acid are most commonly involved in the actions of therapeutically useful drugs. Each of these chemical signals binds to a specific family of receptors. Acetylcholine and norepinephrine are the primary chemical signals in the ANS, whereas a wide variety of neurotransmitters function in the CNS.

3. **Acetylcholine:** The autonomic nerve fibers can be divided into two groups based on the type of neurotransmitter released. If transmission is mediated by acetylcholine, the neuron is termed cholinergic (Figure 3.9 and Chapters 4 and 5). Acetylcholine mediates the transmission of nerve impulses across autonomic ganglia in both the sympathetic and parasympathetic nervous systems. It is the neurotransmitter at the adrenal medulla. Transmission from the autonomic postganglionic nerves to the effector organs in the parasympathetic system, and a few sympathetic system organs, also involves the release of acetylcholine. In the somatic nervous system, transmission at the neuromuscular junction (the junction of nerve fibers and voluntary muscles) is also cholinergic (Figure 3.9).

4. **Norepinephrine and epinephrine:** When norepinephrine is the neurotransmitter, the fiber is termed adrenergic (Figure 3.9 and Chapters 6 and 7). In the sympathetic system, norepinephrine mediates the transmission of nerve impulses from autonomic postganglionic nerves to effector organs. Epinephrine secreted by the adrenal medulla (not sympathetic neurons) also acts as a chemical messenger in the effector organs. [Note: A few sympathetic fibers, such as those involved in sweating, are cholinergic, and, for simplicity, they are not shown in Figure 3.9.]

IV. SIGNAL TRANSDUCTION IN THE EFFECTOR CELL

The binding of chemical signals to receptors activates enzymatic processes within the cell membrane that ultimately results in a cellular response, such as the phosphorylation of intracellular proteins or changes in the conductivity of ion channels (see Chapter 2). A neurotransmitter can be thought of as a signal and a receptor as a signal detector and transducer. The receptors in the ANS effector cells are classified as adrenergic or cholinergic based on the neurotransmitters or hormones that bind to them. Epinephrine and norepinephrine bind to adrenergic receptors, and acetylcholine binds to cholinergic receptors. Cholinergic receptors are further classified as nicotinic or muscarinic. Some receptors, such as the postsynaptic cholinergic nicotinic receptors in skeletal muscle cells, are directly linked to membrane ion channels and are known as ionotropic receptors. Binding of neurotransmitter to ionotropic receptors directly affects ion permeability (Figure 3.10A).

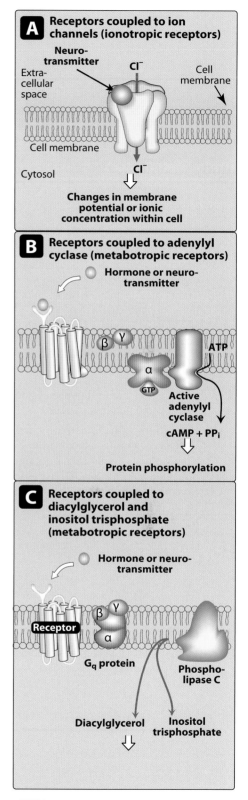

Figure 3.10
Three mechanisms whereby binding of a neurotransmitter leads to a cellular effect.

All adrenergic receptors and cholinergic muscarinic receptors are G protein–coupled receptors (metabotropic receptors). Metabotropic receptors mediate the effects of ligands by activating a second messenger system inside the cell. The two most widely recognized second messengers are the adenylyl cyclase system and the calcium/phosphatidylinositol system (Figure 3.10B, C).

Study Questions

Choose the ONE best answer.

3.1 Which is correct regarding the sympathetic nervous system?

A. It generally mediates body functions in "rest-and-digest" mode.

B. The neurotransmitter at the sympathetic ganglion is norepinephrine (NE).

C. The neurotransmitter at the sympathetic ganglion is acetylcholine (ACh).

D. Sympathetic neurons release ACh in the effector organs.

> Correct answer = C. The neurotransmitter at the sympathetic and parasympathetic ganglia is acetylcholine. The sympathetic system generally mediates body functions in "fight or flight" mode, and the parasympathetic system generally mediates body functions in "rest-and-digest" mode. Sympathetic neurons release NE, and parasympathetic neurons release ACh in the effector cells.

3.2 Why does the somatic nervous system enable a faster response compared to the ANS?

A. Somatic motor neurons have ganglia where neurotransmission is mediated by ACh.

B. Somatic motor neurons have ganglia where neurotransmission is mediated by NE.

C. Somatic motor neurons are not myelinated.

D. Somatic motor neurons are myelinated and do not have ganglia.

> Correct answer = D. Somatic motor neurons are myelinated and have no ganglia. This enables faster transmission in the somatic neurons.

3.3 Which physiological change occurs when the parasympathetic system is activated?

A. Increase in heart rate

B. Inhibition of lacrimation (tears)

C. Dilation of the pupil (mydriasis)

D. Increase in gastric motility

> Correct answer = D. Activation of the parasympathetic system causes an increase in gastric motility, increase in fluid secretions, reduction in heart rate, and constriction of the pupil. In the "rest-and-digest" mode, the parasympathetic system is more active, which helps with digestion.

3.4 Which physiological change is expected when the sympathetic system is inhibited using a pharmacological agent?

A. Reduction in heart rate

B. Increase in blood pressure

C. Decrease in fluid secretions

D. Constriction of blood vessels

> Correct answer = A. Activation of the sympathetic system causes an increase in heart rate, increase in blood pressure, reduction or thickening of fluid secretions, and constriction of blood vessels. Therefore, inhibition of the sympathetic system should theoretically cause a reduction in heart rate, decrease in blood pressure, increase in fluid secretions, and relaxation of blood vessels.

3.5 Which is correct regarding activation of receptors on the effector organs in the ANS?

A. Acetylcholine activates muscarinic receptors.

B. Acetylcholine activates adrenergic receptors.

C. Epinephrine activates nicotinic receptors.

D. Norepinephrine activates muscarinic receptors.

> Correct answer = A. Acetylcholine is the neurotransmitter in the cholinergic system, and it activates both muscarinic and nicotinic cholinergic receptors, not adrenergic receptors. Norepinephrine and epinephrine activate adrenergic receptors, not muscarinic receptors.

3.6 Which statement concerning the parasympathetic nervous system is correct?

 A. The parasympathetic system often discharges as a single, functional system.
 B. The parasympathetic division is involved in near vision, movement of food, and urination.
 C. The postganglionic fibers of the parasympathetic division are long, compared to those of the sympathetic nervous system.
 D. The parasympathetic system controls the secretion of the adrenal medulla.

Correct answer = B. The parasympathetic nervous system maintains essential bodily functions, such as vision, movement of food, and urination. It uses acetylcholine, not norepinephrine, as a neurotransmitter, and it discharges as discrete fibers that are activated separately. The postganglionic fibers of the parasympathetic system are short compared to those of the sympathetic division. The adrenal medulla is under the control of the sympathetic system.

3.7 Which is correct regarding neurotransmitters and neurotransmission?

 A. Neurotransmitters are released from the presynaptic nerve terminals.
 B. Arrival of an action potential in the postsynaptic cell triggers release of neurotransmitter.
 C. Intracellular calcium levels drop in the neuron before the release of neurotransmitter.
 D. Serotonin and dopamine are the primary neurotransmitters in the ANS.

Correct answer = A. Neurotransmitters are released from presynaptic neurons, triggered by the arrival of an action potential in the presynaptic neuron (not in the postsynaptic cell). When an action potential arrives in the presynaptic neuron, calcium enters the presynaptic neuron and calcium levels increase in the neuron before neurotransmitter is released. The main neurotransmitters in the ANS are norepinephrine and acetylcholine.

3.8 An elderly man is brought to the emergency room after ingesting a large quantity of prazosin tablets, a drug that blocks α_1 adrenergic receptors, which mediate effects of epinephrine and norepinephrine on the blood vessels and urinary bladder. Which symptom is most likely to be seen in this patient?

 A. Reduced heart rate (bradycardia)
 B. Dilation of blood vessels (vasorelaxation)
 C. Increased blood pressure
 D. Reduction in urinary frequency

Correct answer = B. Activation of α_1 receptors causes vasoconstriction, reduction in urinary frequency, and an increase in blood pressure, without a direct effect on the heart rate. It may cause reflex tachycardia (increase in heart rate) in some patients. Thus blockade of α_1 receptors could theoretically cause dilation of blood vessels, reduction in blood pressure, and increase in urinary frequency. It should not cause a reduction in heart rate.

3.9 Which statement is correct regarding the autonomic nervous system?

 A. Afferent neurons carry impulses from the central nervous system (CNS) to the effector organs.
 B. Preganglionic neurons of the sympathetic system arise from the cranial nerves, as well as from the sacral region.
 C. When there is a sudden drop in blood pressure, the baroreceptors send signals to the brain to activate the parasympathetic system.
 D. The heart receives both sympathetic and parasympathetic innervation.

Correct answer = D. The heart receives both sympathetic and parasympathetic innervation. Activation of sympathetic neurons increases the heart rate and force of contraction, and activation of parasympathetic neurons reduces the heart rate and force of contraction (slightly). Afferent neurons carry impulses from the periphery to the CNS, and efferent neurons carry signals away from the CNS. Preganglionic neurons of the sympathetic system arise from thoracic and lumbar regions of the spinal cord, whereas the preganglionic neurons of the parasympathetic system arise from cranial nerves and the sacral region. When there is a sudden drop in blood pressure, the sympathetic system is activated, not the parasympathetic system.

3.10 Which is correct regarding membrane receptors and signal transduction?

 A. ANS neurotransmitters bind to membrane receptors on the effector cells, which leads to intracellular events.
 B. Cholinergic muscarinic receptors are ionotropic receptors.
 C. Cholinergic nicotinic receptors are metabotropic receptors.
 D. Metabotropic receptors activate ion channels directly.

Correct answer = A. Neurotransmitters generally bind to membrane receptors on the postsynaptic effector cells and cause cellular effects. Acetylcholine (ACh) binds to cholinergic muscarinic receptors and activates the second messenger pathway in effector cells, which in turn causes cellular events. Receptors that are coupled to second messenger systems are known as metabotropic receptors. Metabotropic receptors do not directly activate ion channels. ACh also binds to cholinergic nicotinic receptors and activates ion channels on the effector cells. The receptors that directly activate ion channels are known as ionotropic receptors.

Cholinergic Agonists

4

Rajan Radhakrishnan

I. OVERVIEW

Drugs affecting the autonomic nervous system (ANS) are divided into two groups according to the type of neuron involved in the mechanism of action. The cholinergic drugs, which are described in this and the following chapter, act on receptors activated by acetylcholine (ACh), whereas the adrenergic drugs (Chapters 6 and 7) act on receptors stimulated by norepinephrine or epinephrine. Cholinergic and adrenergic drugs act by either stimulating or blocking receptors of the ANS. Figure 4.1 summarizes cholinergic agonists discussed in this chapter.

II. THE CHOLINERGIC NEURON

The preganglionic fibers terminating in the adrenal medulla, the autonomic ganglia (both parasympathetic and sympathetic), and the postganglionic fibers of the parasympathetic division use ACh as a neurotransmitter (Figure 4.2). The postganglionic sympathetic division of sweat glands also uses ACh. In addition, cholinergic neurons innervate the muscles of the somatic system and play an important role in the central nervous system (CNS).

A. Neurotransmission at cholinergic neurons

Neurotransmission in cholinergic neurons involves six sequential steps: 1) synthesis of ACh, 2) storage, 3) release, 4) binding of ACh to the receptor, 5) degradation of ACh in the synaptic cleft (the space between the nerve endings and adjacent receptors on nerves or effector organs), and 6) recycling of choline (Figure 4.3).

1. **Synthesis of acetylcholine:** Choline is transported from the extracellular fluid into the cytoplasm of the cholinergic neuron by an energy-dependent carrier system that cotransports sodium and can be inhibited by the drug *hemicholinium*. [Note: Choline has a quaternary nitrogen and carries a permanent positive charge and, thus, cannot diffuse through the membrane.] The uptake of choline is the rate-limiting step in ACh synthesis. Choline acetyltransferase catalyzes the reaction of choline with acetyl coenzyme A (CoA) to form ACh (an ester) in the cytosol.

DIRECT ACTING
Acetylcholine MIOCHOL-E
Bethanechol URECHOLINE
Carbachol MIOSTAT, ISOPTO CARBACHOL
Cevimeline EVOXAC
Methacholine PROVOCHOLINE
Nicotine NICORETTE
Pilocarpine SALAGEN, ISOPTO CARPINE
INDIRECT ACTING (reversible)
Donepezil ARICEPT
Edrophonium ENLON
Galantamine RAZADYNE
Neostigmine BLOXIVERZ
Physostigmine GENERIC ONLY
Pyridostigmine MESTINON
Rivastigmine EXELON
INDIRECT ACTING (irreversible)
Echothiophate PHOSPHOLINE IODIDE
REACTIVATION OF ACETYLCHOLINESTERASE
Pralidoxime PROTOPAM

Figure 4.1
Summary of cholinergic agonists.

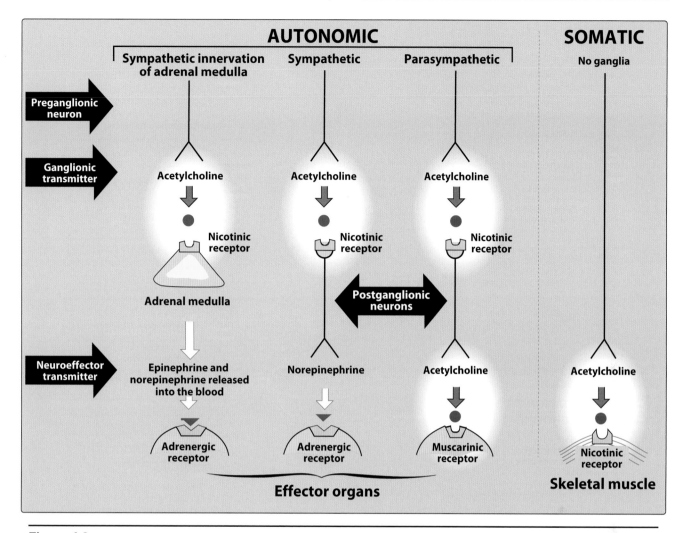

Figure 4.2
Sites of actions of cholinergic agonists in the autonomic and somatic nervous systems.

2. **Storage of acetylcholine in vesicles:** ACh is packaged and stored into presynaptic vesicles by an active transport process. The mature vesicle contains not only ACh but also adenosine triphosphate (ATP) and proteoglycan. Cotransmission from autonomic neurons is the rule rather than the exception. This means that most synaptic vesicles contain the primary neurotransmitter (here, ACh) as well as a cotransmitter (here, ATP) that increases or decreases the effect of the primary neurotransmitter.

3. **Release of acetylcholine:** When an action potential propagated by voltage-sensitive sodium channels arrives at a nerve ending, voltage-sensitive calcium channels on the presynaptic membrane open, causing an increase in the concentration of intracellular calcium. Elevated calcium levels promote the fusion of synaptic vesicles with the cell membrane and the release of contents into the synaptic space. This release can be blocked by botulinum toxin. In contrast, the toxin in black widow spider venom causes all the ACh stored in synaptic vesicles to empty into the synaptic gap.

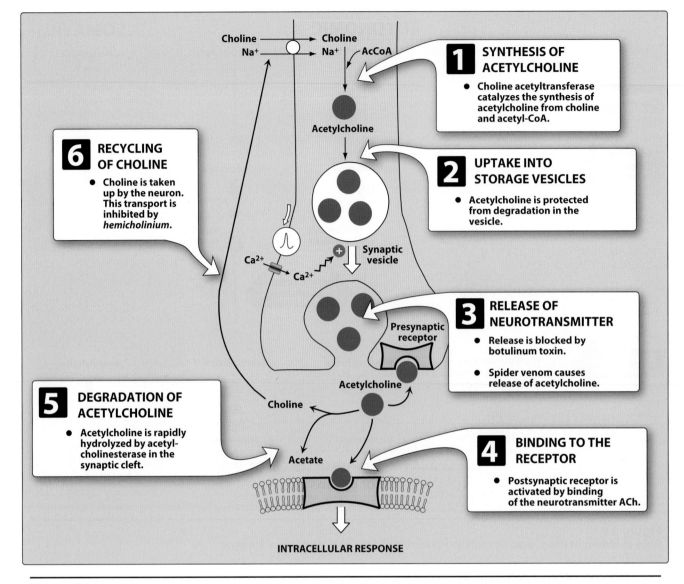

Figure 4.3
Synthesis and release of acetylcholine from the cholinergic neuron. AcCoA = acetyl coenzyme A.

4. **Binding to the receptor:** ACh released from the synaptic vesicles diffuses across the synaptic space and binds to postsynaptic receptors on the target cell, to presynaptic receptors on the membrane of the neuron that released ACh, or to other targeted presynaptic receptors. The postsynaptic cholinergic receptors on the surface of effector organs are divided into two classes: muscarinic and nicotinic (Figure 4.2). Binding to a receptor leads to a biologic response within the cell, such as the initiation of a nerve impulse in a postganglionic fiber or activation of specific enzymes in effector cells, as mediated by second messenger molecules.

5. **Degradation of acetylcholine:** The signal at the postjunctional effector site is rapidly terminated, because acetylcholinesterase (AChE) cleaves ACh to choline and acetate in the synaptic cleft.

6. **Recycling of choline:** Choline may be recaptured by a sodium-coupled, high-affinity uptake system that transports the molecule back into the neuron. There, it is available to be acetylated into ACh.

III. CHOLINERGIC RECEPTORS (CHOLINOCEPTORS)

Two families of cholinoceptors, designated muscarinic and nicotinic receptors, can be distinguished from each other on the basis of their different affinities for agents that mimic the action of ACh (cholinomimetic agents).

A. Muscarinic receptors

Muscarinic receptors belong to the class of G-protein–coupled receptors (metabotropic receptors). These receptors, in addition to binding ACh, also recognize muscarine, an alkaloid in certain poisonous mushrooms. By contrast, the muscarinic receptors show only a weak affinity for *nicotine*, an alkaloid found in tobacco and other plants (Figure 4.4A). There are five subclasses of muscarinic receptors; however, only M_1, M_2, and M_3 receptors have been functionally characterized.

1. **Location of muscarinic receptors:** These receptors are found on the autonomic effector organs, such as the heart, smooth muscle, brain, and exocrine glands. Although all five subtypes are found on neurons, M_1 receptors are also found on gastric parietal cells, M_2 receptors on cardiac cells and smooth muscle, and M_3 receptors on the bladder, exocrine glands, and smooth muscle. [Note: Drugs with muscarinic actions preferentially stimulate muscarinic receptors on these tissues, but at high concentration, they may show some activity at nicotinic receptors.]

2. **Mechanism of acetylcholine signal transduction:** A number of different molecular mechanisms transmit the signal generated by ACh occupation of the receptor. For example, when M_1 or M_3 receptors are activated, the receptor undergoes a conformational change and interacts with a G-protein that activates phospholipase C. This ultimately leads to production of second messengers inositol-1,4,5-trisphosphate (IP_3) and diacylglycerol (DAG). IP_3 causes an increase in intracellular Ca^{2+}. Calcium can then interact to stimulate or inhibit enzymes or to cause hyperpolarization, secretion, or contraction. DAG activates protein kinase C, an enzyme that phosphorylates numerous proteins within the cell. In contrast, activation of the M_2 subtype on the cardiac muscle stimulates a G-protein that inhibits adenylyl cyclase and increases K^+ conductance. The heart responds with a decrease in rate and force of contraction.

3. **Muscarinic agonists:** *Pilocarpine* is a nonselective muscarinic agonist used to treat xerostomia and glaucoma. Attempts are currently underway to develop muscarinic agents that are directed against specific receptor subtypes.

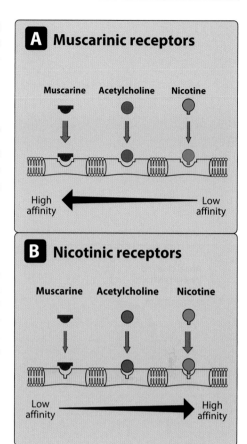

Figure 4.4
Types of cholinergic receptors.

B. Nicotinic receptors

These receptors, in addition to binding ACh, also recognize *nicotine* but show only a weak affinity for muscarine (Figure 4.4B). The nicotinic receptor is composed of five subunits, and it functions as a ligand-gated ion channel (ionotropic receptor). Binding of two ACh molecules elicits a conformational change that allows the entry of sodium ions, resulting in the depolarization of the effector cell. *Nicotine* at low concentration stimulates the receptor, whereas *nicotine* at high concentration blocks the receptor. Nicotinic receptors are located in the CNS, the adrenal medulla, autonomic ganglia, and the neuro-muscular junction (NMJ) in skeletal muscles. Those at the NMJ are sometimes designated N_M, and the others, N_N. The nicotinic receptors of autonomic ganglia differ from those of the NMJ. For example, ganglionic receptors are selectively blocked by *mecamylamine*, whereas NMJ receptors are specifically blocked by *atracurium*.

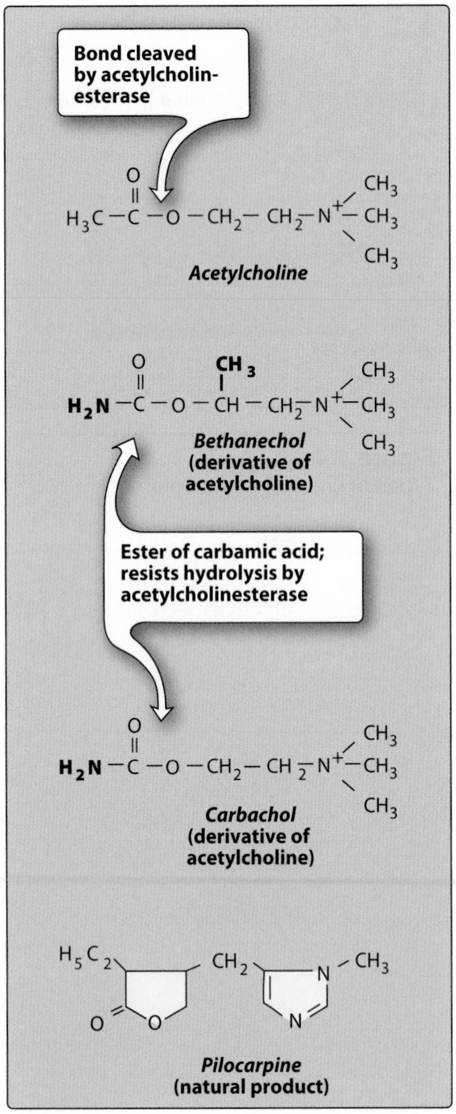

IV. DIRECT-ACTING CHOLINERGIC AGONISTS

Cholinergic agonists mimic the effects of ACh by binding directly to cholinoceptors (muscarinic or nicotinic). These agents may be broadly classified into two groups: 1) choline esters, which include endogenous ACh and synthetic esters of choline, such as *carbachol* and *bethanechol*, and 2) naturally occurring alkaloids, such as *nicotine* and *pilocarpine* (Figure 4.5). All direct-acting cholinergic drugs have a longer duration of action than ACh. The more therapeutically useful drugs (*pilocarpine* and *bethanechol*) preferentially bind to muscarinic receptors and are sometimes referred to as muscarinic agents. However, as a group, the direct-acting agonists show little specificity in their actions, which limits clinical usefulness.

A. Acetylcholine

Acetylcholine [ah-see-teel-KOE-leen] is a quaternary ammonium compound that cannot penetrate membranes. Although it is the neurotransmitter of parasympathetic and somatic nerves as well as autonomic ganglia, it lacks therapeutic importance because of its multiplicity of actions (leading to diffuse effects) and its rapid inactivation by the cholinesterases. ACh has both muscarinic and nicotinic activity. Its actions include the following:

1. **Decrease in heart rate and cardiac output:** The actions of ACh on the heart mimic the effects of vagal stimulation. For example, if injected intravenously, ACh produces a brief decrease in cardiac rate (bradycardia) and cardiac output, mainly because of a reduction in the rate of firing at the sinoatrial (SA) node. [Note: Normal vagal activity regulates the heart by the release of ACh at the SA node.]

2. **Decrease in blood pressure:** Injection of ACh causes vasodilation and lowering of blood pressure by an indirect mechanism of action. ACh activates M_3 receptors found on endothelial cells lining the smooth muscles of blood vessels. This results in the production

Figure 4.5
Comparison of the structures of some cholinergic agonists.

of nitric oxide from arginine. Nitric oxide then diffuses to vascular smooth muscle cells to stimulate protein kinase G production, leading to hyperpolarization and smooth muscle relaxation via phosphodiesterase-3 inhibition. In the absence of administered cholinergic agents, the vascular cholinergic receptors have no known function, because ACh is never released into the blood in significant quantities. *Atropine* blocks these muscarinic receptors and prevents ACh from producing vasodilation.

3. **Other actions:** In the gastrointestinal (GI) tract, acetylcholine increases salivary secretion, increases gastric acid secretion, and stimulates intestinal secretions and motility. It also enhances bronchiolar secretions and causes bronchoconstriction. [Note: *Methacholine*, a direct-acting cholinergic agonist, is used to assist in the diagnosis of asthma due to its bronchoconstricting properties.] In the genitourinary tract, ACh increases the tone of the detrusor muscle, causing urination. In the eye, ACh is involved in stimulation of ciliary muscle contraction for near vision and in the constriction of the pupillae sphincter muscle, causing miosis (marked constriction of the pupil). ACh (1% solution) is instilled into the anterior chamber of the eye to produce miosis during ophthalmic surgery.

B. Bethanechol

Bethanechol [be-THAN-e-kole] is an unsubstituted carbamoyl ester, structurally related to ACh (Figure 4.5). It is not hydrolyzed by AChE due to the esterification of carbamic acid, although it is inactivated through hydrolysis by other esterases. It lacks nicotinic actions (due to addition of the methyl group), but does have strong muscarinic activity. Its major actions are on the smooth musculature of the bladder and GI tract. It has about a 1-hour duration of action.

1. **Actions:** *Bethanechol* directly stimulates muscarinic receptors, causing increased intestinal motility and tone. It also stimulates the detrusor muscle of the bladder, whereas the trigone and sphincter muscles are relaxed. These effects stimulate urination.

2. **Therapeutic uses:** In urologic treatment, *bethanechol* is used to stimulate the atonic bladder, particularly in postpartum or postoperative, nonobstructive urinary retention. *Bethanechol* may also be used to treat neurogenic atony as well as megacolon.

3. **Adverse effects:** *Bethanechol* can cause generalized cholinergic stimulation (Figure 4.6), with sweating, salivation, flushing, decreased blood pressure (with reflex tachycardia), nausea, abdominal pain, diarrhea, and bronchospasm. *Atropine sulfate* may be administered to overcome severe cardiovascular or bronchoconstrictor responses to this agent.

C. Carbachol (carbamylcholine)

Carbachol [KAR-ba-kole] has both muscarinic and nicotinic actions. Like *bethanechol*, *carbachol* is an ester of carbamic acid (Figure 4.5) and a poor substrate for AChE. It is biotransformed by other esterases, but at a much slower rate.

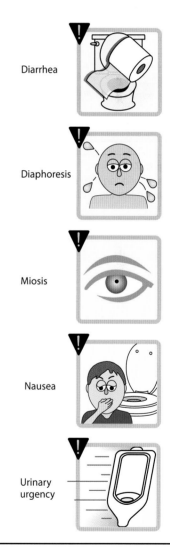

Diarrhea

Diaphoresis

Miosis

Nausea

Urinary urgency

Figure 4.6
Some adverse effects observed with cholinergic agonists.

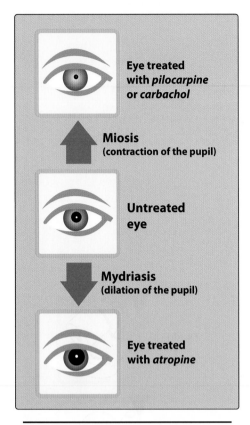

Figure 4.7
Actions of *pilocarpine*, *carbachol*, and *atropine* on the iris and ciliary muscle of the eye.

1. **Actions:** *Carbachol* has profound effects on both the cardiovascular and GI systems because of its ganglion-stimulating activity, and it may first stimulate and then depress these systems. It can cause release of epinephrine from the adrenal medulla by its nicotinic action. Locally instilled into the eye, it mimics the effects of ACh, causing miosis and a spasm of accommodation in which the ciliary muscle of the eye remains in a constant state of contraction. The vision becomes fixed at some particular distance, making it impossible to focus (Figure 4.7). [Note the opposing effects of *atropine*, a muscarinic blocker, on the eye.]

2. **Therapeutic uses:** Because of its high potency, receptor nonselectivity, and relatively long duration of action, *carbachol* is rarely used. Intraocular use provides miosis for eye surgery and lowers intraocular pressure in the treatment of glaucoma.

3. **Adverse effects:** With ophthalmologic use, few adverse effects occur due to lack of systemic penetration (quaternary amine).

D. Pilocarpine

The alkaloid *pilocarpine* [pye-loe-KAR-peen] is a tertiary amine and is stable to hydrolysis by AChE (Figure 4.5). Compared with ACh and its derivatives, it is far less potent but is uncharged and can penetrate the CNS at therapeutic doses. *Pilocarpine* exhibits muscarinic activity and is used primarily in ophthalmology.

1. **Actions:** Applied topically to the eye, *pilocarpine* produces rapid miosis, contraction of the ciliary muscle, and spasm of accommodation. *Pilocarpine* is one of the most potent stimulators of secretions such as sweat, tears, and saliva, but its use for producing these effects has been limited due to its lack of selectivity.

2. **Therapeutic uses:** *Pilocarpine* is used to treat glaucoma and is the drug of choice for emergency lowering of intraocular pressure of both open-angle and angle-closure glaucoma. *Pilocarpine* is extremely effective in opening the trabecular meshwork around the Schlemm canal, causing an immediate drop in intraocular pressure because of the increased drainage of aqueous humor. This action occurs within a few minutes, lasts 4 to 8 hours, and can be repeated. [Note: Topical carbonic anhydrase inhibitors, such as *dorzolamide* and β-adrenergic blockers such as *timolol*, are effective in treating glaucoma but are not used for emergency lowering of intraocular pressure.] The miotic action of *pilocarpine* is also useful in reversing mydriasis due to *atropine*.

   The drug is beneficial in promoting salivation in patients with xerostomia resulting from irradiation of the head and neck. Sjögren syndrome, which is characterized by dry mouth and lack of tears, is treated with oral *pilocarpine* tablets and *cevimeline*, a cholinergic drug that also has the drawback of being nonspecific.

3. **Adverse effects:** *Pilocarpine* can cause blurred vision, night blindness, and brow ache. Poisoning with this agent is characterized by exaggeration of various parasympathetic effects, including

profuse sweating (diaphoresis) and salivation. The effects are similar to those produced by consumption of mushrooms of the genus *Inocybe*, which contain muscarine. Parenteral *atropine*, at doses that can cross the blood–brain barrier, is administered to counteract the toxicity of *pilocarpine*.

V. INDIRECT-ACTING CHOLINERGIC AGONISTS: ANTICHOLINESTERASE AGENTS (REVERSIBLE)

AChE is an enzyme that specifically cleaves ACh to acetate and choline and, thus, terminates its actions. It is located both pre- and postsynaptically in the nerve terminal where it is membrane bound. Inhibitors of AChE (anticholinesterase agents or cholinesterase inhibitors) indirectly provide cholinergic action by preventing the degradation of ACh. This results in an accumulation of ACh in the synaptic space (Figure 4.8). Therefore, these drugs can provoke a response at all cholinoceptors, including both muscarinic and nicotinic receptors of the ANS, as well as at the NMJ and in the brain. The reversible AChE inhibitors can be broadly classified as short-acting or intermediate-acting agents.

A. Edrophonium

Edrophonium [ed-row-FOE-nee-um] is the prototype short-acting AChE inhibitor. *Edrophonium* binds reversibly to the active center of AChE, preventing hydrolysis of ACh. It has a short duration of action of 10 to 20 minutes due to rapid renal elimination. *Edrophonium* is a quaternary amine, and its actions are limited to the periphery. It is used in the diagnosis of myasthenia gravis, an autoimmune disease caused by antibodies to the nicotinic receptor at the NMJ. This causes the degradation of the nicotinic receptors, making fewer receptors available for interaction with ACh. Intravenous injection of *edrophonium* leads to a rapid increase in muscle strength in patients with myasthenia gravis. Care must be taken, because excess drug may provoke a cholinergic crisis (*atropine* is the antidote). *Edrophonium* may also be used to assess cholinesterase inhibitor therapy, for differentiating cholinergic and myasthenic crises, and for reversing the effects of nondepolarizing neuromuscular blockers (NMBs) after surgery. Due to the availability of other agents, *edrophonium* use has become limited.

B. Physostigmine

Physostigmine [fi-zoe-STIG-meen] is a nitrogenous carbamic acid ester found naturally in plants and is a tertiary amine. It is a substrate for AChE, and it forms a relatively stable carbamoylated intermediate with the enzyme, which then becomes reversibly inactivated. The result is potentiation of cholinergic activity throughout the body.

1. **Actions:** *Physostigmine* has a wide range of effects and stimulates not only the muscarinic and nicotinic sites of the ANS, but also the nicotinic receptors of the NMJ. Muscarinic stimulation can cause contraction of GI smooth muscles, miosis,

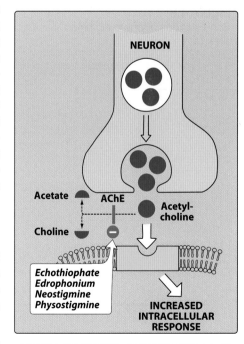

Figure 4.8
Mechanisms of action of indirect cholinergic agonists. AChE = acetylcholinesterase.

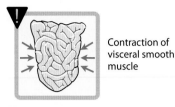
Contraction of visceral smooth muscle

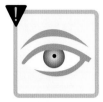
Miosis

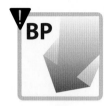
Hypotension

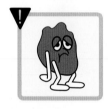
Bradycardia

Figure 4.9
Some actions of *physostigmine*.

bradycardia, and hypotension (Figure 4.9). Nicotinic stimulation can cause skeletal muscle twitches, fasciculations, and skeletal muscle paralysis (at higher doses). Its duration of action is about 30 minutes to 2 hours, and it is considered an intermediate-acting agent. *Physostigmine* can enter and stimulate the cholinergic sites in the CNS.

2. **Therapeutic uses:** *Physostigmine* is used in the treatment of overdoses of drugs with anticholinergic actions, such as *atropine*, and to reverse the effects of NMBs.

3. **Adverse effects:** High doses of *physostigmine* may lead to convulsions. Bradycardia and a fall in cardiac output may also occur. Inhibition of AChE at the NMJ causes the accumulation of ACh and, ultimately through continuous depolarization, results in paralysis of skeletal muscle. However, these effects are rarely seen with therapeutic doses.

C. Neostigmine

Neostigmine [nee-oh-STIG-meen] is a synthetic compound that is also a carbamic acid ester, and it reversibly inhibits AChE in a manner similar to *physostigmine*.

1. **Actions:** Unlike *physostigmine*, *neostigmine* has a quaternary nitrogen. Therefore, it is more polar, is absorbed poorly from the GI tract, and does not enter the CNS. Its effect on skeletal muscle is greater than *physostigmine*, and it can stimulate contractility before it paralyzes. *Neostigmine* has an intermediate duration of action, usually 30 minutes to 2 hours.

2. **Therapeutic uses:** It is used to stimulate the bladder and GI tract and as an antidote for competitive neuromuscular-blocking agents. *Neostigmine* is also used to manage symptoms of myasthenia gravis.

3. **Adverse effects:** Adverse effects of *neostigmine* include those of generalized cholinergic stimulation, such as salivation, flushing, decreased blood pressure, nausea, abdominal pain, diarrhea, and bronchospasm. *Neostigmine* does not cause CNS side effects and is not used to overcome toxicity of central-acting antimuscarinic agents such as *atropine*. *Neostigmine* is contraindicated when intestinal or urinary bladder obstruction is present.

D. Pyridostigmine

Pyridostigmine [peer-id-oh-STIG-meen] is another cholinesterase inhibitor used in the chronic management of myasthenia gravis. Its duration of action is intermediate (3 to 6 hours) but longer than that of *neostigmine*. Adverse effects are similar to those of *neostigmine*.

E. Tacrine, donepezil, rivastigmine, and galantamine

Patients with Alzheimer disease have a deficiency of cholinergic neurons and therefore lower levels of ACh in the CNS. This observation led to the development of anticholinesterases as possible remedies for the loss of cognitive function. *Tacrine* [TAK-reen], the first agent in this category, has been replaced by others because of its hepato-toxicity. Despite the ability of *donepezil* [doe-NEP-e-zil], *rivastigmine* [ri-va-STIG-meen], and *galantamine* [ga-LAN-ta-meen] to delay the progression of Alzheimer disease, none can stop its progression. GI distress is their primary adverse effect (see Chapter 8).

VI. INDIRECT-ACTING CHOLINERGIC AGONISTS: ANTICHOLINESTERASE AGENTS (IRREVERSIBLE)

A number of synthetic organophosphate compounds have the ability to bind covalently to AChE. The result is a long-lasting increase in ACh at all sites where it is released. Many of these drugs are extremely toxic and were developed by the military as nerve agents. Related compounds, such as *parathion* and *malathion*, are used as insecticides.

A. Echothiophate

1. **Mechanism of action:** *Echothiophate* [ek-oe-THI-oh-fate] is an organophosphate that covalently binds via its phosphate group at the active site of AChE (Figure 4.10). Once this occurs, the enzyme is permanently inactivated, and restoration of AChE activity requires the synthesis of new enzyme molecules. Following covalent modification of AChE, the phosphorylated enzyme slowly releases one of its ethyl groups. The loss of an alkyl group, which is called aging, makes it impossible for chemical reactivators, such as *pralidoxime*, to break the bond between the remaining drug and the enzyme.

2. **Actions:** Actions include generalized cholinergic stimulation, paralysis of motor function (causing breathing difficulties), and convulsions. *Echothiophate* produces intense miosis and, thus, has found therapeutic use. Intraocular pressure falls from the facilitation of outflow of aqueous humor. *Atropine* in high dosages can reverse many of the peripheral and some of the central muscarinic effects of *echothiophate*.

3. **Therapeutic uses:** A topical ophthalmic solution of the drug is available for the treatment of open-angle glaucoma. However, *echothiophate* is rarely used due to its side effect profile, which includes the risk of cataracts. Figure 4.11 summarizes actions of some cholinergic agonists.

VII. TOXICOLOGY OF ANTICHOLINESTERASE AGENTS

Irreversible AChE inhibitors (mostly organophosphate compounds) are commonly used as agricultural insecticides in the United States, which has led to numerous cases of accidental poisoning with these agents. In addition, they are frequently used for suicidal and homicidal purposes. Organophosphate nerve gases such as sarin are used as agents of warfare and chemical terrorism. Toxicity with these agents is manifested as nicotinic and muscarinic signs and symptoms (cholinergic crisis). Depending on the agent, the effects can be peripheral or can affect the whole body.

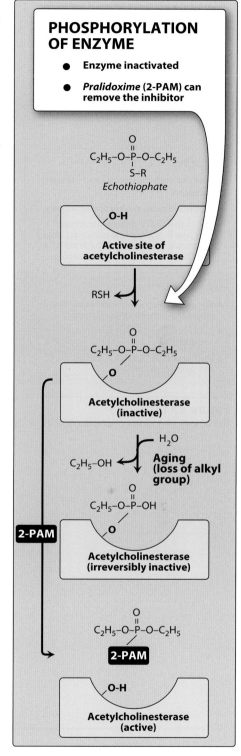

PHOSPHORYLATION OF ENZYME

● **Enzyme inactivated**

● *Pralidoxime* (2-PAM) can remove the inhibitor

Figure 4.10
Covalent modification of acetylcholinesterase by *echothiophate*. Also shown is the reactivation of the enzyme with *pralidoxime* (2-PAM). R = $(CH_3)_3N^+-CH_2-CH_2-$; RSH = $(CH_3)_3N^+-CH_2-CH_2-S-H$.

Bethanechol	Physostigmine	Rivastigmine, galantamine, donepezil
• Used in treatment of urinary retention • Binds preferentially at muscarinic receptors	• Increases intestinal and bladder motility • Reverses CNS and cardiac effects of tricyclic antidepressants • Reverses CNS effects of *atropine* • Uncharged, tertiary amine that can penetrate the CNS	• Used as first-line treatments for Alzheimer disease, though confers modest benefit • Have not been shown to reduce healthcare costs or delay institutionalization • Can be used with *memantine* (*N*-methyl-D-aspartate antagonist) in moderate to severe disease
Carbachol	Neostigmine	Echothiophate
• Binds to both muscarinic and nicotinic receptors • Produces miosis during ocular surgery • Used topically to reduce intraocular pressure in open-angle or narrow-angle glaucoma, particularly in patients who have become tolerant to *pilocarpine*	• Prevents postoperative abdominal distention and urinary retention • Used in treatment of myasthenia gravis • Used as an antidote for competitive neuromuscular blockers • Has intermediate duration of action (0.5 to 2 h)	• Used in treatment of open-angle glaucoma • Has long duration of action (100 h)
Pilocarpine	Edrophonium	Acetylcholine
• Reduces intraocular pressure in open-angle and narrow-angle glaucoma • Binds preferentially at muscarinic receptors • Uncharged, tertiary amine that can penetrate the CNS	• Used for diagnosis of myasthenia gravis • Used as an antidote for competitive neuromuscular blockers • Has short duration of action (10 to 20 min)	• Used to produce miosis in ophthalmic surgery

Figure 4.11
Summary of actions of some cholinergic agonists. CNS = central nervous system.

A. Reactivation of acetylcholinesterase

Pralidoxime [pral-i-DOX-eem] (2-PAM) can reactivate inhibited AChE (Figure 4.10). However, it is unable to penetrate into the CNS and therefore is not useful in treating the CNS effects of organophosphates. The presence of a charged group allows it to approach an anionic site on the enzyme, where it essentially displaces the phosphate group of the organophosphate and regenerates the enzyme. If given before aging of the alkylated enzyme occurs, it can reverse both muscarinic and nicotinic peripheral effects of organophosphates, but not the CNS effects. With the newer nerve agents that produce aging of the enzyme complex within seconds, *pralidoxime* is less effective. In addition, it cannot overcome toxicity of reversible AChE inhibitors (for example, *physostigmine*).

B. Other treatments

Atropine is administered to prevent muscarinic side effects of these agents. Such effects include increased bronchial and salivary secretion, bronchoconstriction, and bradycardia. *Diazepam* is also administered to reduce the persistent convulsion caused by these agents. General supportive measures, such as maintenance of patent airway, oxygen supply, and artificial respiration, may be necessary as well.

STUDY QUESTIONS

Choose the ONE best answer.

4.1 Botulinum toxin blocks the release of acetylcholine from cholinergic nerve terminals. Which is a possible effect of botulinum toxin?

A. Skeletal muscle paralysis
B. Improvement of myasthenia gravis symptoms
C. Increased salivation
D. Reduced heart rate

Correct answer = A. Acetylcholine released by cholinergic neurons acts on nicotinic receptors in the skeletal muscle cells to cause contraction. Therefore, blockade of ACh release causes skeletal muscle paralysis. Myasthenia gravis is an autoimmune disease where antibodies are produced against nicotinic receptors and inactivate nicotinic receptors. A reduction in ACh release therefore worsens (not improves) the symptoms of this condition. Reduction in ACh release by botulinum toxin causes reduction in secretions including saliva (not increase in salivation), causing dry mouth and an increase (not reduction) in heart rate due to reduced vagal activity.

4.2 A patient develops urinary retention after an abdominal surgery. Urinary obstruction was ruled out in this patient. Which strategy would be helpful in promoting urination?

A. Activating nicotinic receptors
B. Inhibiting the release of acetylcholine
C. Inhibiting cholinesterase enzyme
D. Blocking muscarinic receptors

Correct answer = C. Activation of muscarinic receptors in the detrusor muscle of the urinary bladder can promote urination in patients where the tone of detrusor muscle is low. Inhibiting cholinesterase enzyme increases the levels of acetylcholine, and acetylcholine can increase the tone of the detrusor muscle. There are no nicotinic receptors in the detrusor muscle; therefore, activation of nicotinic receptors is not helpful. Inhibiting the release of acetylcholine or blocking muscarinic receptors worsens urinary retention.

4.3 Which of the following drugs could theoretically improve asthma symptoms?

A. Bethanechol
B. Pilocarpine
C. Pyridostigmine
D. Atropine

Correct answer = D. Muscarinic agonists and drugs that increase acetylcholine levels cause constriction of bronchial smooth muscles and could exacerbate asthma symptoms. Bethanechol and pilocarpine are muscarinic agonists, and pyridostigmine is a cholinesterase inhibitor that increases levels of acetylcholine. Atropine is a muscarinic antagonist and therefore does not exacerbate asthma. Theoretically, it should relieve symptoms of asthma (not used clinically for this purpose).

4.4 If an ophthalmologist wants to dilate the pupils for an eye examination, which drug/class of drugs is theoretically useful?

A. Muscarinic receptor activator (agonist)
B. Muscarinic receptor inhibitor (antagonist)
C. Pilocarpine
D. Neostigmine

Correct answer = B. Muscarinic agonists (for example, pilocarpine) contract the circular smooth muscles in the iris sphincter and constrict the pupil (miosis). Anticholinesterases (for example, neostigmine, physostigmine) also cause miosis by increasing the level of ACh. Muscarinic antagonists, on the other hand, relax the circular smooth muscles in the iris sphincter and cause dilation of the pupil (mydriasis).

4.5 In Alzheimer disease, there is a deficiency of cholinergic neuronal function in the brain. Theoretically, which strategy is useful in treating symptoms of Alzheimer disease?

A. Inhibiting cholinergic receptors in the brain
B. Inhibiting the release of acetylcholine in the brain.
C. Inhibiting the acetylcholinesterase enzyme in the brain
D. Activating the acetylcholinesterase enzyme in the brain

Correct answer = C. Because there is already a deficiency in brain cholinergic function in Alzheimer disease, inhibiting cholinergic receptors or inhibiting the release of ACh worsens the condition. Activating the acetylcholinesterase enzyme increases the degradation of ACh, which also worsens the condition. However, inhibiting the acetylcholinesterase enzyme helps to increase the levels of ACh in the brain and thereby relieve the symptoms of Alzheimer disease.

4.6 An elderly female who lives in a farmhouse was brought to the emergency room in serious condition after ingesting a liquid from an unlabeled bottle found near her bed, apparently in a suicide attempt. She presented with diarrhea, frequent urination, convulsions, breathing difficulties, constricted pupils (miosis), and excessive salivation. Which of the following is correct regarding this patient?

A. She most likely consumed an organophosphate pesticide.
B. The symptoms are consistent with sympathetic activation.
C. Her symptoms can be treated using an anticholinesterase agent.
D. Her symptoms can be treated using a cholinergic agonist.

Correct answer = A. The symptoms are consistent with that of cholinergic crisis. Since the elderly female lives on a farm and the symptoms are consistent with a cholinergic crisis (usually caused by cholinesterase inhibitors), it may be assumed that she has consumed an organophosphate pesticide (irreversible cholinesterase inhibitor). Assuming that the symptoms are caused by organophosphate poisoning, administering an anticholinesterase agent or a cholinergic agonist will worsen the condition. The symptoms are not consistent with that of sympathetic activation, as sympathetic activation will cause symptoms opposite to that of cholinergic crisis seen in this patient.

4.7 A patient who received a nondepolarizing neuromuscular blocker (NMB) for skeletal muscle relaxation during surgery is experiencing mild skeletal muscle paralysis after the surgery. Which drug could reverse this effect of NMBs?

A. Pilocarpine
B. Bethanechol
C. Neostigmine
D. Atropine

Correct answer = C. Neuromuscular blockers act by blocking nicotinic receptors on the skeletal muscles. Increasing the levels of ACh in the neuromuscular junctions can reverse the effects of NMBs. Therefore, neostigmine, a cholinesterase inhibitor, could reverse the effects of NMBs. Pilocarpine and bethanechol are preferentially muscarinic agonists and have no effects on the nicotinic receptors. Atropine is a muscarinic antagonist and has no effects on nicotinic receptors.

4.8 A 60-year-old female who had a cancerous growth in the neck region underwent radiation therapy. Her salivary secretion was reduced due to radiation and she suffers from dry mouth (xerostomia). Which drug would be most useful in treating xerostomia in this patient?

A. Acetylcholine
B. Pilocarpine
C. Echothiophate
D. Atropine

Correct answer = B. Salivary secretion may be enhanced by activating muscarinic receptors in the salivary glands. This can be achieved in theory by using a muscarinic agonist or an anticholinesterase agent. Pilocarpine is a muscarinic agonist administered orally for this purpose. Acetylcholine has similar effects as that of pilocarpine; however, it cannot be used therapeutically as it is rapidly destroyed by cholinesterase in the body. Echothiophate is an irreversible cholinesterase inhibitor, but it cannot be used therapeutically because of its toxic effects. Atropine is a muscarinic antagonist and worsens dry mouth.

4.9 A 40-year-old male presents to his family physician with drooping eyelids, difficulty chewing and swallowing, and muscle fatigue even on mild exertion. Which agent could be used to diagnose myasthenia gravis in this patient?

A. Atropine
B. Edrophonium
C. Pralidoxime
D. Echothiophate

Correct answer = B. The function of nicotinic receptors in skeletal muscles is diminished in myasthenia gravis due to the development of antibodies to nicotinic receptors (auto-immune disease). Any drug that increases levels of ACh in the neuromuscular junction can improve symptoms in myasthenia gravis. Thus, edrophonium, a reversible cholinesterase inhibitor with a short duration of action can temporarily improve skeletal muscle weakness in myasthenia gravis, serving as a diagnostic tool. Atropine is a muscarinic antagonist and has no role in skeletal muscle function. Pralidoxime is a drug that is used to reverse the binding of irreversible cholinesterase inhibitors with cholinesterase enzyme and helps to reactivate cholinesterase enzyme. Hence, pralidoxime will not be useful in improving skeletal muscle function in myasthenia gravis.

4.10 Atropa belladonna is a plant that contains atropine (a muscarinic antagonist). Which of the following drugs or classes of drugs will be most useful in treating poisoning with belladonna?

A. Malathion
B. Physostigmine
C. Muscarinic antagonists
D. Nicotinic antagonists

Correct answer = B. Atropine is a competitive muscarinic receptor antagonist that causes anticholinergic effects. Muscarinic agonists or any other drugs that increase the levels of ACh are able to counteract effects of atropine. Thus, anticholinesterases such as malathion and physostigmine can counteract the effects of atropine, in theory. However, since malathion is an irreversible inhibitor of acetylcholinesterase, it is not used for systemic treatment in patients. Muscarinic antagonists worsen the toxicity of atropine. Nicotinic antagonists can worsen the toxicity by acting on parasympathetic ganglionic receptors and thus reducing the release of ACh.

Cholinergic Antagonists

5

Rajan Radhakrishnan and Carinda Feild

I. OVERVIEW

Cholinergic antagonist is a general term for agents that bind to cholinoceptors (muscarinic or nicotinic) and prevent the effects of acetylcholine (ACh) and other cholinergic agonists. The most clinically useful of these agents are selective blockers of muscarinic receptors. They are commonly known as anticholinergic agents (a misnomer, as they antagonize only muscarinic receptors), antimuscarinic agents (more accurate terminology), or parasympatholytics. The effects of parasympathetic innervation are thus, interrupted by these agents, and the actions of sympathetic innervation are left unopposed. A second group of drugs, the ganglionic blockers, shows a preference for nicotinic receptors of the sympathetic and parasympathetic ganglia. Clinically, they are the least important cholinergic antagonists. A third family of compounds, the neuromuscular blocking agents (mostly nicotinic antagonists), interfere with transmission of efferent impulses to skeletal muscles. These drugs are used as skeletal muscle relaxants in surgical anesthesia and as agents to facilitate intubation in surgical and critical care patients. Figure 5.1 summarizes the cholinergic antagonists discussed in this chapter.

II. ANTIMUSCARINIC AGENTS

Commonly known as anticholinergic drugs, these agents (for example, *atropine* and *scopolamine*) block muscarinic receptors (Figure 5.2), causing inhibition of muscarinic functions. In addition, these drugs block the few exceptional sympathetic neurons that are cholinergic, such as those innervating the salivary and sweat glands. Because they do not block nicotinic receptors, the anticholinergic drugs (more precisely, antimuscarinic drugs) have little or no action at skeletal neuromuscular junctions (NMJs) or autonomic ganglia. The anticholinergic drugs are beneficial in a variety of clinical situations. [Note: A number of antihistamines and antidepressants (mainly tricyclic antidepressants) also have antimuscarinic activity.]

ANTIMUSCARINIC AGENTS
Aclidinium TUDORZA
Atropine GENERIC ONLY
Benztropine COGENTIN
Cyclopentolate AKPENTOLATE, CYCLOGYL
Darifenacin ENABLEX
Fesoterodine TOVIAZ
Glycopyrrolate ROBINUL, SEEBRI
Hyoscyamine LEVSIN, OSCIMIN, SYMAX
Ipratropium ATROVENT HFA
Oxybutynin DITROPAN, GELNIQUE, OXYTROL
Scopolamine TRANSDERM SCŌP
Solifenacin VESICARE
Tiotropium SPIRIVA RESPIMAT
Tolterodine DETROL
Trihexyphenidyl GENERIC ONLY
Tropicamide MYDRIACYL, TROPICACYL
Trospium GENERIC ONLY

GANGLIONIC BLOCKERS
Nicotine NICODERM, NICORETTE, NICOTROL

NEUROMUSCULAR BLOCKERS
Cisatracurium NIMBEX
Mivacurium MIVACRON
Pancuronium GENERIC ONLY
Rocuronium GENERIC ONLY
Succinylcholine ANECTINE, QUELICIN
Vecuronium GENERIC ONLY

Figure 5.1
Summary of selected cholinergic antagonists.

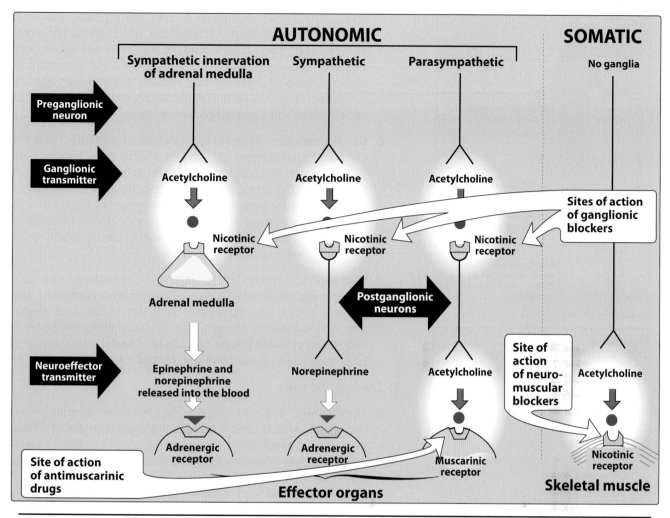

Figure 5.2
Sites of action of cholinergic antagonists.

A. Atropine

Atropine [A-troe-peen] is a tertiary amine extracted from belladonna alkaloid. It has a high affinity for muscarinic receptors and binds competitively to prevent ACh from binding (Figure 5.3). *Atropine* acts both centrally and peripherally. General actions last about 4 hours; however, effects of topical administration in the eye may persist for days. Neuroeffector organs have varying sensitivity to *atropine*. The greatest inhibitory effects are seen in bronchial tissue, salivary and sweat glands, and the heart.

1. *Actions*

a. Eye: *Atropine* blocks muscarinic activity in the eye, resulting in mydriasis (dilation of the pupil), unresponsiveness to light, and cycloplegia (inability to focus for near vision). In patients with angle-closure glaucoma, intraocular pressure may rise dangerously.

b. Gastrointestinal (GI): *Atropine* (as the active isomer, *L-hyoscyamine* [hi-oh-SYE-uh-meen]) can be used as an antispasmodic to reduce activity of the GI tract. *Atropine*

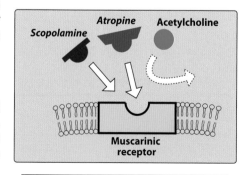

Figure 5.3
Competition of *atropine* and *scopolamine* with *acetylcholine* for the muscarinic receptor.

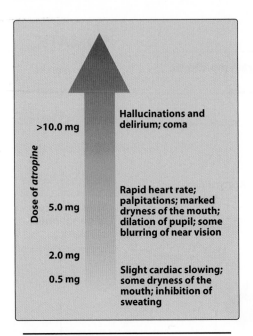

Figure 5.4
Dose-dependent effects of *atropine*.

and *scopolamine* (discussed below) are probably the most potent antispasmodic drugs available. Although gastric motility is reduced, hydrochloric acid production is not significantly affected. Thus, *atropine* is not effective for the treatment of ulcers. Doses of *atropine* that reduce spasms also reduce saliva secretion, ocular accommodation, and urination. These effects decrease compliance with *atropine*.

c. **Cardiovascular:** *Atropine* produces divergent effects on the cardiovascular system, depending on the dose (Figure 5.4). At low doses, the predominant effect is a slight decrease in heart rate. This effect results from blockade of M_1 receptors on the inhibitory prejunctional (or presynaptic) neurons, thus permitting increased ACh release. Higher doses of *atropine* cause a progressive increase in heart rate by blocking M_2 receptors on the sinoatrial node.

d. **Secretions:** *Atropine* blocks muscarinic receptors in the salivary glands, producing dryness of the mouth (xerostomia). The salivary glands are exquisitely sensitive to *atropine*. Sweat and lacrimal glands are similarly affected. [Note: Inhibition of secretions of sweat glands can cause elevated body temperature, which can be dangerous in children and the elderly.]

2. **Therapeutic uses**

   a. **Ophthalmic:** Topical *atropine* exerts both mydriatic and cycloplegic effects, and it permits the measurement of refractive errors without interference by the accommodative capacity of the eye. Shorter-acting antimuscarinics (*cyclopentolate* [sye-kloe-PEN-toe-late] and *tropicamide* [troe-PIK-a-mide]) have largely replaced *atropine* due to prolonged mydriasis observed with *atropine* (7 to 14 days vs. 6 to 24 hours with other agents). [Note: *Phenylephrine* or similar α-adrenergic drugs are preferred for pupillary dilation if cycloplegia is not required.]

   b. **Antispasmodic:** *Atropine* is used as an antispasmodic agent to relax the GI tract.

   c. **Cardiovascular:** Injectable *atropine* is used to treat bradycardia of varying etiologies.

   d. **Antisecretory:** *Atropine* is sometimes used as an antisecretory agent to block secretions in the respiratory tract prior to surgery. [Note: *Glycopyrrolate* (see below) is also used for this indication.]

   e. **Antidote for cholinergic agonists:** *Atropine* is used for the treatment of organophosphate (insecticides, nerve gases) poisoning, of overdose of clinically used anticholinesterases such as *physostigmine*, and in some types of mushroom poisoning (certain mushrooms contain cholinergic substances that block cholinesterases). Massive doses of injectable *atropine* may be required over a long period to counteract the poisons. The ability of *atropine* to enter the central nervous system (CNS) is of particular importance in treating central toxic effects of anticholinesterases.

3. **Pharmacokinetics:** *Atropine* is readily absorbed, partially metabolized by the liver, and eliminated primarily in urine. It has a half-life of about 4 hours.

4. **Adverse effects:** Depending on the dose, *atropine* may cause dry mouth, blurred vision, "sandy eyes," tachycardia, urinary retention, and constipation. Effects on the CNS include restlessness, confusion, hallucinations, and delirium, which may progress to depression, collapse of the circulatory and respiratory systems, and death. Low doses of cholinesterase inhibitors, such as *physostigmine*, may be used to overcome *atropine* toxicity. *Atropine* may also induce troublesome urinary retention. The drug may be dangerous in children, because they are sensitive to its effects, particularly to rapid increases in body temperature.

Figure 5.5
Scopolamine is an effective agent for motion sickness.

B. *Scopolamine*

Scopolamine [skoe-POL-a-meen], another tertiary amine plant alkaloid, produces peripheral effects similar to those of *atropine*. However, *scopolamine* has greater action on the CNS (unlike *atropine*, CNS effects are observed at therapeutic doses) and a longer duration of action as compared to *atropine*. It has some special actions as indicated below.

1. **Actions:** *Scopolamine* is one of the most effective drugs available for motion sickness (Figure 5.5). It also has the unusual effect of blocking short-term memory. In contrast to *atropine*, *scopolamine* produces sedation, but at higher doses, it can produce excitement. *Scopolamine* may produce euphoria and is susceptible to abuse.

2. **Therapeutic uses:** *Scopolamine* is used for the prevention of motion sickness and postoperative nausea and vomiting. For motion sickness, it is available as a topical patch that provides effects for up to 3 days. [Note: As with all drugs used for motion sickness, it is much more effective prophylactically than for treating motion sickness once it occurs.]

3. **Pharmacokinetics and adverse effects:** These aspects are similar to those of *atropine*, with the exception of longer half-life.

C. *Aclidinium, glycopyrrolate, ipratropium,* and *tiotropium*

Ipratropium [i-pra-TROE-pee-um] and *tiotropium* [TYE-oh-TROE-pee-um] are quaternary derivatives of *atropine*, and *glycopyrrolate* [glye-koe-PYE-roe-late] and *aclidinium* [a-kli-DIN-ee-um] are synthetic quaternary compounds. *Ipratropium* is classified as a short-acting muscarinic antagonist (SAMA), while *glycopyrrolate, tiotropium,* and *aclidinium* are classified as long-acting muscarinic antagonists (LAMAs) based on the duration of action. These agents are approved as bronchodilators for maintenance treatment of bronchospasm associated with chronic obstructive pulmonary disease (COPD). *Ipratropium* and *tiotropium* are also used in the acute management of bronchospasm in asthma and chronic management of asthma, respectively (see Chapter 39). All of these agents are delivered via inhalation. Because of the positive charge, these drugs do not enter the systemic circulation or the CNS, restricting effects to the pulmonary system.

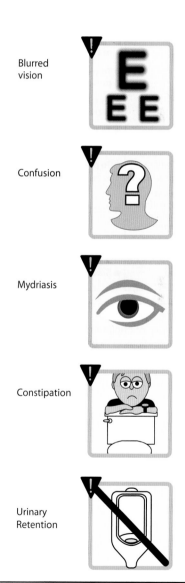

Blurred vision

Confusion

Mydriasis

Constipation

Urinary Retention

Figure 5.6
Adverse effects commonly observed with muscarinic antagonists.

Drug	Therapeutic uses
Muscarinic blockers	
Trihexyphenidyl Benztropine	● Treatment of Parkinson disease ● Management of antipsychotic-induced extrapyramidal effects
Darifenacin Fesoterodine Oxybutynin Solifenacin Tolterodine Trospium	● Treatment of overactive urinary bladder
*Cyclopentolate Tropicamide Atropine**	● In ophthalmology, to produce mydriasis and cycloplegia prior to refraction
*Atropine**	● To treat spastic disorders of the GI tract ● To treat organophosphate poisoning ● To suppress respiratory secretions prior to surgery ● To treat bradycardia
Scopolamine	● To prevent motion sickness
Aclidinium Glycopyrrolate Ipratropium Tiotropium	● Treatment of COPD
Ganglionic blockers	
Nicotine	● Smoking cessation

Figure 5.7
Summary of cholinergic antagonists.
*Contraindicated in angle-closure glaucoma. GI = gastrointestinal; COPD = chronic obstructive pulmonary disease.

D. *Tropicamide* and *cyclopentolate*

These agents are used as ophthalmic solutions for mydriasis and cycloplegia. Their duration of action is shorter than that of *atropine*. *Tropicamide* produces mydriasis for 6 hours and *cyclopentolate* for 24 hours.

E. *Benztropine* and *trihexyphenidyl*

Benztropine and *trihexyphenidyl* are useful as adjuncts with other antiparkinson agents to treat Parkinson disease (see Chapter 8) and other types of parkinsonian syndromes, including antipsychotic-induced extrapyramidal symptoms.

F. *Oxybutynin* and other antimuscarinic agents for overactive bladder

Oxybutynin [ox-i-BYOO-ti-nin], *darifenacin* [dar-e-FEN-a-sin], *fesoterodine* [fes-oh-TER-oh-deen], *solifenacin* [sol-ee-FEN-a-sin], *tolterodine* [tol-TER-oh-deen], and *trospium* [TROSE-pee-um] are synthetic *atropine*-like drugs with antimuscarinic actions.

1. **Actions:** By competitively blocking muscarinic (M_3) receptors in the bladder, intravesical pressure is lowered, bladder capacity is increased, and the frequency of bladder contractions is reduced. Antimuscarinic actions at M_3 receptors in the GI tract, salivary glands, CNS, and eye may cause adverse effects. *Darifenacin* and *solifenacin* are relatively more selective M_3 muscarinic receptor antagonists; however, the other drugs are mainly nonselective muscarinic antagonists, and binding to other muscarinic receptor subtypes may contribute to adverse effects.

2. **Therapeutic uses:** These agents are used for management of overactive bladder and urinary incontinence. *Oxybutynin* is also used in patients with neurogenic bladder.

3. **Pharmacokinetics:** All of the agents are available in oral dosage forms. Most agents have a long half-life, which allows once-daily administration. [Note: Immediate-release *oxybutynin* and *tolterodine* must be dosed two or more times daily; however, extended-release formulations of these agents allow for once-daily dosing.] *Oxybutynin* is also available in a transdermal patch and topical gel formulation. These drugs are hepatically metabolized by the cytochrome P450 system (primarily CYP 3A4 and 2D6), with the exception of *trospium*, which is thought to undergo ester hydrolysis.

4. **Adverse effects:** Side effects include dry mouth, constipation, and blurred vision, which limit tolerability of these agents. Extended-release formulations and the transdermal patch have a lower incidence of adverse effects and may be better tolerated. *Trospium* is a quaternary compound that minimally crosses the blood–brain barrier and has fewer CNS effects than do other agents, making it a preferred choice in treating overactive bladder in patients with dementia. Important characteristics of the muscarinic antagonists are summarized in Figures 5.6 and 5.7.

III. GANGLIONIC BLOCKERS

Ganglionic blockers specifically act on the nicotinic receptors of both parasympathetic and sympathetic autonomic ganglia. Some also block the ion channels of the autonomic ganglia. These drugs show no selectivity toward the parasympathetic or sympathetic ganglia and are not effective as neuromuscular antagonists. Thus, these drugs block the entire output of the autonomic nervous system at the nicotinic receptor. Except for *nicotine*, the other drugs mentioned in this category are nondepolarizing, competitive antagonists. The responses of the nondepolarizing blockers are complex and mostly unpredictable. Therefore, ganglionic blockade is rarely used therapeutically, but often serves as a tool in experimental pharmacology.

A. *Nicotine*

A component of cigarette smoke, *nicotine* [NIK-oh-teen] is a poison with many undesirable actions. It is without therapeutic benefit and is deleterious to health. Depending on the dose, *nicotine* depolarizes autonomic ganglia, resulting first in stimulation and then in paralysis of all ganglia. The stimulatory effects are complex and result from increased release of neurotransmitters (Figure 5.8), due to effects on both sympathetic and parasympathetic ganglia (see Chapter 15 for a full discussion of *nicotine*).

IV. NEUROMUSCULAR BLOCKING AGENTS

These drugs block cholinergic transmission between motor nerve endings and the nicotinic receptors on skeletal muscle (Figure 5.2). They possess some chemical similarities to ACh and act either as antagonists (nondepolarizing) or as agonists (depolarizing) at the receptors on the endplate of the NMJ. Neuromuscular blockers (NMBs) are clinically useful to facilitate rapid intubation when needed due to respiratory failure (rapid sequence intubation). During surgery, they are used to facilitate endotracheal intubation and provide complete muscle relaxation at lower anesthetic doses. This increases the safety of anesthesia by allowing patients to recover quickly and completely. NMBs should not substitute for inadequate anesthesia. NMBs are also used in the intensive care unit (ICU) as adjuvant therapy to facilitate intubation and mechanical ventilation in critically ill patients.

A. Nondepolarizing (competitive) blockers

The first known NMB was *curare* [kyoo-RAH-ree], which Amazon hunters used to paralyze prey. The development of *tubocurarine* [too-boe-kyoo-AR-een] followed, but it has been replaced by agents with fewer adverse effects, such as *cisatracurium* [cis-a-trah-CURE-ih-um], *mivacurium* [mi-vah-KYOO-ree-um], *pancuronium* [pan-kure-OH-nee-um], *rocuronium* [roe-kyoor-OH-nee-um], and *vecuronium* [ve-KYOO-roe-nee-um].

1. Mechanism of action

a. At low doses: NMBs competitively block ACh at the nicotinic receptors (Figure 5.9). They compete with ACh at the receptor without stimulating it, thus preventing depolarization of the

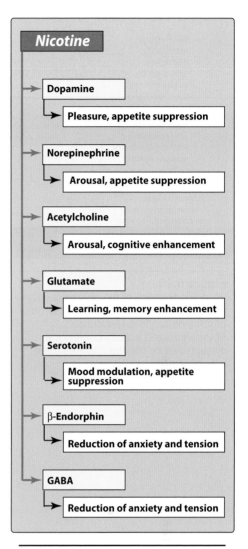

Figure 5.8
Neurochemical effects of *nicotine*. GABA = γ-aminobutyric acid.

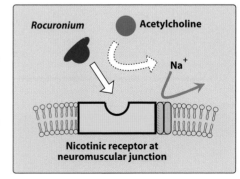

Figure 5.9
Mechanism of action of competitive neuromuscular blocking drugs.

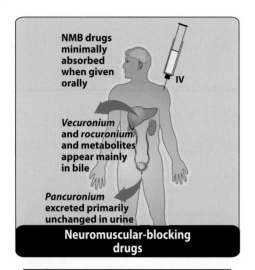

NMB drugs minimally absorbed when given orally

IV

Vecuronium and *rocuronium* and metabolites appear mainly in bile

Pancuronium excreted primarily unchanged in urine

Neuromuscular-blocking drugs

Figure 5.10
Pharmacokinetics of the neuromuscular blocking drugs. *Cisatracurium* undergoes organ-independent elimination. *Mivacurium* and *succinylcholine* are metabolized by plasma cholinesterase. IV = intravenous.

muscle cell membrane and inhibiting muscular contraction. Their competitive action can be overcome by administration of cholinesterase inhibitors, such as *neostigmine* and *edrophonium*, which increase the concentration of ACh in the NMJ. Clinicians employ this strategy to shorten the duration of neuromuscular blockade. In addition, at low doses the muscle responds to direct electrical stimulation from a peripheral nerve stimulator to varying degrees, allowing for monitoring of the extent of neuromuscular blockade.

b. **At high doses:** Nondepolarizing agents can block the ion channels of the motor end plate. This leads to further weakening of neuromuscular transmission, reducing the ability of cholinesterase inhibitors to reverse the actions of the nondepolarizing blockers. With complete blockade, the muscle does not respond to direct electrical stimulation.

2. **Actions:** Muscles have differing sensitivity to blockade by competitive agents. Small, rapidly contracting muscles of the face and eye are most susceptible and are paralyzed first, followed by the fingers, limbs, neck, and trunk muscles. Next, the intercostal muscles are affected and, lastly, the diaphragm. The muscles recover in the reverse manner. [Note: *Sugammadex* is a selective relaxant-binding agent that terminates the action of both *rocuronium* and *vecuronium* and can be used to speed recovery (see Chapter 13).]

3. **Pharmacokinetics:** All NMBs are injected intravenously or occasionally intramuscularly. These agents possess two or more quaternary amines in their bulky ring structure that prevent absorption from the gut. They penetrate membranes very poorly and do not enter cells or cross the blood–brain barrier. Drug action is terminated in a variety of ways (Figure 5.10). *Pancuronium* is excreted unchanged in urine. *Cisatracurium* undergoes organ-independent metabolism (via Hofmann elimination) to laudanosine, which is further metabolized and renally excreted. The amino steroid drugs *vecuronium* and *rocuronium* are deacetylated in the liver and excreted unchanged in bile. *Mivacurium* is eliminated by plasma cholinesterase. The choice of agent depends on the desired onset and duration of muscle relaxation and the route of elimination. Characteristics of the neuromuscular-blocking drugs are shown in Figure 5.11.

4. **Adverse effects:** In general, these agents are safe with minimal side effects. The adverse effects of the specific NMBs are shown in Figure 5.11.

5. **Drug interactions**

a. **Cholinesterase inhibitors:** Drugs such as *neostigmine*, *physostigmine*, *pyridostigmine*, and *edrophonium* can overcome the action of nondepolarizing NMBs. However, with increased dosage, cholinesterase inhibitors can cause a depolarizing block due to elevated ACh concentrations at the end plate membrane. If the NMB has entered the ion channel (is bound to the receptor), cholinesterase inhibitors are not as effective in overcoming blockade.

b. Halogenated hydrocarbon anesthetics: Drugs such as *desflurane* act to enhance neuromuscular blockade by exerting a stabilizing action at the NMJ. These agents sensitize the NMJ to the effects of NMBs.

c. Aminoglycoside antibiotics: Drugs such as *gentamicin* and *tobramycin* inhibit ACh release from cholinergic nerves by competing with calcium ions. They synergize with competitive blockers, enhancing neuromuscular blockade.

d. Calcium channel blockers: These agents may increase the neuromuscular blockade of competitive blockers.

B. Depolarizing agents

Depolarizing blocking agents work by depolarizing the plasma membrane of the muscle fiber, similar to the action of ACh. However, these agents are more resistant to degradation by acetylcholinesterase (AChE) and can more persistently depolarize the muscle fibers. *Succinylcholine* [suk-sin-il-KOE-leen] is the only depolarizing muscle relaxant in use today.

1. Mechanism of action: *Succinylcholine* attaches to the nicotinic receptor and acts like ACh to depolarize the junction (Figure 5.12). Unlike ACh, which is instantly destroyed by AChE, the depolarizing agent persists at high concentrations in the synaptic cleft, remaining attached to the receptor for a longer time and providing sustained depolarization of the muscle cell. [Note: The duration of action is dependent on diffusion from the motor end plate and hydrolysis by plasma cholinesterase (also called butyrylcholinesterase or pseudocholinesterase). Genetic variants in which plasma cholinesterase levels are low or absent lead to prolonged neuromuscular paralysis.] The depolarizing agent first causes opening of the sodium channel associated with nicotinic receptors, which results in depolarization of the receptor (phase I). This leads to a transient twitching of the muscle (fasciculations). Continued binding of the depolarizing agent renders the receptor incapable of transmitting further impulses. With time, continuous depolarization gives way to gradual repolarization as the sodium channel closes or is blocked. This causes a resistance to depolarization (phase II) and flaccid paralysis.

2. Actions: As with the competitive blockers, the respiratory muscles are paralyzed last. *Succinylcholine* initially produces brief muscle fasciculations that cause muscle soreness. This may be prevented by administering a small dose of nondepolarizing NMB prior to *succinylcholine*. Normally, the duration of action of *succinylcholine* is extremely short, due to rapid hydrolysis by plasma

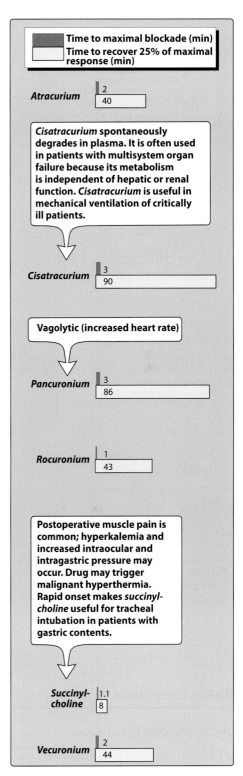

Figure 5.11
Characteristics of neuromuscular blocking drugs.

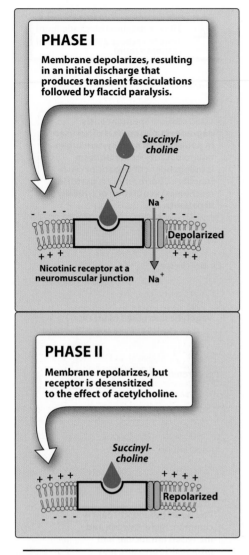

PHASE I

Membrane depolarizes, resulting in an initial discharge that produces transient fasciculations followed by flaccid paralysis.

Succinyl-
choline

Na⁺

Depolarized

Nicotinic receptor at a neuromuscular junction   Na⁺

PHASE II

Membrane repolarizes, but receptor is desensitized to the effect of acetylcholine.

Succinyl-
choline

Repolarized

Figure 5.12
Mechanism of action of depolarizing neuromuscular blocking drugs.

cholinesterase. However, *succinylcholine* that reaches the NMJ is not metabolized, allowing the agent to bind to nicotinic receptors, and redistribution to plasma is necessary for metabolism.

3. **Therapeutic uses:** Because of its rapid onset of action, *succinylcholine* is useful when rapid endotracheal intubation is required. It is also used during electroconvulsive shock treatment.

4. **Pharmacokinetics:** *Succinylcholine* is injected intravenously. Its brief duration of action results from redistribution and rapid hydrolysis by plasma cholinesterase. Drug effects rapidly disappear upon discontinuation.

5. **Adverse effects**

   a. **Hyperthermia:** *Succinylcholine* can potentially induce malignant hyperthermia in susceptible patients (see Chapter 13).

   b. **Apnea:** Administration of *succinylcholine* to a patient who is deficient in plasma cholinesterase or has an atypical form of the enzyme can lead to prolonged apnea due to paralysis of the diaphragm. The rapid release of potassium may also contribute to prolonged apnea in patients with electrolyte imbalances. In patients with electrolyte imbalances receiving *digoxin* or diuretics (such as heart failure patients) *succinylcholine* should be used cautiously or not at all.

   c. **Hyperkalemia:** *Succinylcholine* increases potassium release from intracellular stores. This may be particularly dangerous in burn patients and patients with massive tissue damage in which potassium has been rapidly lost or in patients with renal failure.

Study Questions

Choose the ONE best answer.

5.1 During an ophthalmic surgical procedure, the surgeon wanted to constrict the pupil using a miotic drug. However, he accidentally used another drug that caused dilation of the pupil (mydriasis). Which drug was most likely used?

   A. Acetylcholine
   B. Pilocarpine
   C. Tropicamide
   D. Bethanechol

Correct answer = C. Muscarinic agonists such as ACh, pilocarpine, and bethanechol contract the circular muscles of iris sphincter and cause constriction of the pupil (miosis), whereas muscarinic antagonists such as tropicamide prevent contraction of the circular muscles of the iris and cause dilation of the pupil (mydriasis).

5.2 Sarin is a nerve gas that is an organophosphate cholinesterase inhibitor. Which agent could be used as an antidote to sarin poisoning?

A. Pilocarpine
B. Carbachol
C. Atropine
D. Physostigmine

Correct answer = C. Sarin is an organophosphate cholinesterase inhibitor. It causes an increase in ACh levels in tissues that leads to cholinergic crisis through activation of muscarinic and nicotinic receptors. Most symptoms of cholinergic crisis are mediated by muscarinic receptors and, therefore, the muscarinic antagonist atropine is used as an antidote for sarin poisoning. Cholinergic agonists such as pilocarpine, carbachol, and physostigmine (indirect agonists) worsen symptoms of sarin poisoning.

5.3 A patient with Alzheimer disease needs treatment for overactive bladder (OAB). Which drug is the best choice for this patient?

A. Darifenacin
B. Solifenacin
C. Tolterodine
D. Trospium

Correct answer = D. All of agents for OAB except trospium cross the blood–brain barrier to various degrees and could worsen dementia symptoms in Alzheimer disease. Trospium is a quaternary ammonium compound that minimally crosses the blood–brain barrier.

5.4 A patient with asthma was prescribed a β_2 agonist for acute relief of bronchospasm, but did not respond to treatment. Which drug is the most likely next option for this patient?

A. Benztropine
B. Ipratropium
C. Oxybutynin
D. Physostigmine

Correct answer = B. Major receptors present in the bronchial tissues are muscarinic and adrenergic β_2 receptors. Muscarinic activation causes bronchoconstriction, and β_2 receptor activation causes bronchodilation. Therefore, direct or indirect (physostigmine) muscarinic agonists worsen bronchospasm. Ipratropium is a muscarinic antagonist that can relax bronchial smooth muscles and relieve bronchospasm in patients who are not responsive to β_2 agonists. Benztropine is used in the treatment of Parkinson disease or relief of extrapyramidal symptoms from antipsychotics. Oxybutynin is used for overactive bladder.

5.5 A 50-year-old male who is noncompliant with medications was recently diagnosed with chronic obstructive pulmonary disease (COPD). His physician would like to prescribe an inhaled anticholinergic that is dosed once or twice daily. Which drug is most appropriate for this patient?

A. Atropine
B. Ipratropium
C. Tiotropium
D. Trospium

Correct answer = C. The physician should prescribe a long-acting muscarinic antagonist (LAMA) so that the patient has to inhale the medication only 1 or 2 times daily. Tiotropium is a LAMA, whereas ipratropium is a short-acting muscarinic antagonist (SAMA). Atropine and trospium are muscarinic antagonists, but are not indicated for pulmonary conditions such as asthma or COPD and are not available as inhaled formulations.

5.6 Which is the most effective drug for motion sickness for a person planning to go on a cruise?

A. Atropine
B. Fesoterodine
C. Scopolamine
D. Tropicamide

Correct answer = C. All muscarinic antagonists (anticholinergic drugs) listed are theoretically useful as antimotion sickness drugs; however, scopolamine is the most effective in preventing motion sickness. Tropicamide mostly has ophthalmic uses, and fesoterodine is used for overactive bladder.

5.7 Which is correct regarding ganglion-blocking drugs?

A. Blockade of sympathetic ganglia could result in reduced blood pressure.
B. Blockade of parasympathetic ganglia could result in reduced heart rate.
C. Nicotine is a nondepolarizing ganglion blocker.
D. Atropine is a nondepolarizing ganglion blocker.

Correct answer = A. Selective blockade (in theory) of the sympathetic ganglion causes reduction in norepinephrine release and, therefore, reduction in heart rate and blood pressure. Selective blockade (in theory) of the parasympathetic ganglion causes reduction in ACh release and an increase in heart rate. Receptors at both sympathetic and parasympathetic ganglia are of the nicotinic type. Nicotine is an agonist at nicotinic receptors and produces a depolarizing block in the ganglia. Atropine is a muscarinic antagonist and has no effect on the nicotinic receptors found in the ganglia.

5.8 Which drug is useful in treating sinus bradycardia?

   A. Atropine
   B. Cisatracurium
   C. Neostigmine
   D. Succinylcholine

Correct answer = A. Sinus bradycardia is a condition where the heart rate is below normal and most often caused by increased vagal tone (increased release of ACh in the sino-atrial [SA] node that acts on muscarinic receptors to reduce heart rate). A muscarinic antagonist such as atropine is useful in this situation to bring the heart rate back to normal. Succinylcholine and cisatracurium are nicotinic antagonists and have no effect on muscarinic receptors in the SA node. Neostigmine is a cholinesterase inhibitor and can worsen bradycardia by increasing the level of ACh in the SA node.

5.9 An ICU patient with severe lung injury requires a neuro-muscular blocking agent to assist in his ventilator management. He has liver disease and is currently in renal failure. Which neuromuscular blocker is the best choice for this patient?

   A. Cisatracurium
   B. Pancuronium
   C. Vecuronium
   D. Rocuronium

Correct answer = A. Pancuronium is renally eliminated and the patient has renal failure. Vecuronium and rocuronium are hepatically metabolized and the patient has liver disease. Cisatracurium is cleared by organ-independent metabolism (Hofmann elimination).

5.10 Where would you expect to see the first return of function in skeletal muscles following discontinuation of a nondepolarizing neuromuscular blocking agent?

   A. Arms
   B. Diaphragm
   C. Fingers
   D. Pupils

Correct answer = B. Following administration of a neuro-muscular blocker, the facial muscles are impacted first, but the pupils are not controlled by skeletal muscle and are not affected. The fingers and arms would be next, with the diaphragm function lost last. Function returns in the opposite order, so function of the diaphragm returns first.

Adrenergic Agonists

Rajan Radhakrishnan

I. OVERVIEW

The adrenergic drugs affect receptors that are stimulated by norepinephrine (noradrenaline) or epinephrine (adrenaline). These receptors are known as adrenergic receptors or adrenoceptors. Drugs that activate adrenergic receptors are termed sympathomimetics, and drugs that block activation of adrenergic receptors are termed sympatholytics. Some sympathomimetics directly activate adrenergic receptors (direct-acting agonists), while others act indirectly by enhancing release or blocking reuptake of norepinephrine (indirect-acting agonists). This chapter describes agents that either directly or indirectly stimulate adrenoceptors (Figure 6.1). Sympatholytic drugs are discussed in Chapter 7.

II. THE ADRENERGIC NEURON

Adrenergic neurons release norepinephrine as the primary neurotransmitter. These neurons are found in the central nervous system (CNS) and in the sympathetic nervous system, where they serve as links between ganglia and the effector organs. Adrenergic drugs act on adrenergic receptors, located either presynaptically on the neuron or postsynaptically on the effector organ (Figure 6.2).

A. Neurotransmission at adrenergic neurons

Neurotransmission in adrenergic neurons closely resembles that described for the cholinergic neurons (see Chapter 4), except that norepinephrine is the neurotransmitter instead of acetylcholine. Neurotransmission involves the following steps: synthesis, storage, release, and receptor binding of norepinephrine, followed by removal of the neurotransmitter from the synaptic gap (Figure 6.3).

1. **Synthesis of norepinephrine:** Tyrosine is transported by a carrier into the adrenergic neuron, where it is hydroxylated to dihydroxyphenylalanine (DOPA) by tyrosine hydroxylase. This is the rate-limiting step in the formation of norepinephrine. DOPA is then decarboxylated by the enzyme aromatic L-amino acid decarboxylase to form dopamine in the presynaptic neuron.

DIRECT-ACTING AGENTS
Albuterol ACCUNEB, PROAIR, VENTOLIN
Arformoterol BROVANA
Clonidine CATAPRES, DURACLON
Dobutamine* GENERIC ONLY
Dopamine* GENERIC ONLY
Epinephrine* ADRENALIN, EPIPEN
Fenoldopam CORLOPAM
Formoterol FORADIL, PERFOROMIST
Guanfacine INTUNIV, TENEX
Indacaterol ARCAPTA
Isoproterenol* ISUPREL
Metaproterenol GENERIC ONLY
Midodrine GENERIC ONLY
Mirabegron MYRBETRIQ
Norepinephrine* LEVOPHED
Oxymetazoline AFRIN, VISINE
Phenylephrine NEO-SYNEPHRINE, SUDAFED PE
Salmeterol SEREVENT
Terbutaline GENERIC ONLY

INDIRECT-ACTING AGENTS
Amphetamine ADDERALL
Cocaine GENERIC ONLY

DIRECT AND INDIRECT ACTING (mixed action) AGENTS
Ephedrine AKOVAZ
Pseudoephedrine SUDAFED

Figure 6.1
Summary of adrenergic agonists. Agents marked with an *asterisk* (*) are catecholamines.

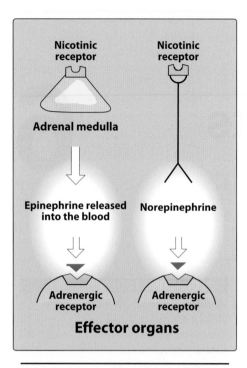

Figure 6.2
Sites of actions of adrenergic agonists.

2. **Storage of norepinephrine in vesicles:** Dopamine is then transported into synaptic vesicles by an amine transporter system. This carrier system is blocked by *reserpine* (see Chapter 7). Next, *dopamine* is hydroxylated to form norepinephrine by the enzyme dopamine β-hydroxylase.

3. **Release of norepinephrine:** An action potential arriving at the nerve junction triggers an influx of calcium ions from the extracellular fluid into the cytoplasm of the neuron. The increase in calcium causes synaptic vesicles to fuse with the cell membrane and to undergo exocytosis and expel their contents into the synapse. Drugs such as *guanethidine* block this release.

4. **Binding to receptors:** Norepinephrine released from the synaptic vesicles diffuses into the synaptic space and binds to postsynaptic receptors on the effector organ or to presynaptic receptors on the nerve ending. Binding of norepinephrine to receptors triggers a cascade of events within the cell, resulting in the formation of intracellular second messengers that act as links (transducers) in the communication between the neurotransmitter and the action generated within the effector cell. Adrenergic receptors use both the cyclic adenosine monophosphate (cAMP) second messenger system and the phosphatidylinositol cycle to transduce the signal into an effect. Norepinephrine also binds to presynaptic receptors (mainly α_2 subtype) that modulate the release of the neurotransmitter.

5. **Removal of norepinephrine:** Norepinephrine may 1) diffuse out of the synaptic space and enter the systemic circulation, 2) be metabolized to inactive metabolites by catechol-O-methyltransferase (COMT) in the synaptic space, or 3) undergo reuptake back into the neuron. The reuptake by the neuronal membrane involves a sodium–chloride (Na^+/Cl^-)–dependent norepinephrine transporter that can be inhibited by tricyclic antidepressants (TCAs), such as *imipramine*; by serotonin–norepinephrine reuptake inhibitors such as *duloxetine*; or by *cocaine*. Reuptake of norepinephrine into the presynaptic neuron is the primary mechanism for termination of its effects.

6. **Potential fates of recaptured norepinephrine:** Once norepinephrine reenters the adrenergic neuron, it may be taken up into synaptic vesicles via the amine transporter system and be sequestered for release by another action potential, or it may persist in a protected pool in the cytoplasm. Alternatively, norepinephrine can be oxidized by monoamine oxidase (MAO) present in neuronal mitochondria.

B. Adrenergic receptors (adrenoceptors)

In the sympathetic nervous system, several classes of adrenoceptors can be distinguished pharmacologically. Two main families of receptors, designated α and β, are classified based on response to the adrenergic agonists *epinephrine*, *norepinephrine*, and *isoproterenol*. Both the α and β receptor types have a number of specific receptor subtypes. Alterations in the primary structure of the receptors influence their affinity for various agents.

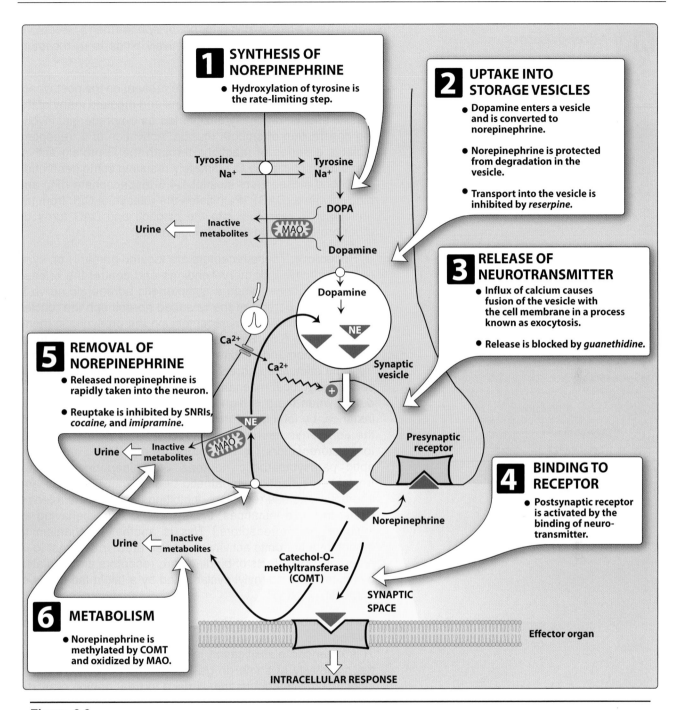

Figure 6.3
Synthesis and release of norepinephrine from the adrenergic neuron. DOPA = dihydroxyphenylalanine; MAO = monoamine oxidase; NE = norepinephrine; SNRI = serotonin–norepinephrine reuptake inhibitor.

1. **α-Adrenoceptors:** The α-adrenoceptors show a weak response to the synthetic agonist *isoproterenol*, but they are responsive to the naturally occurring catecholamines *epinephrine* and *norepinephrine* (Figure 6.4). For α receptors, the rank order of potency and affinity is *epinephrine ≥ norepinephrine >> isoproterenol*. The α-adrenoceptors are divided into two subtypes, α_1 and α_2, based on their affinities for α agonists and antagonists. For example, α_1

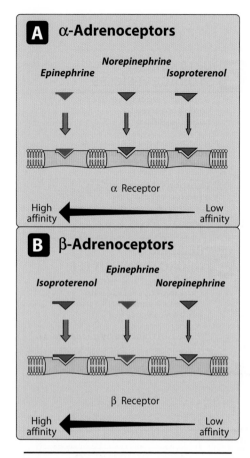

Figure 6.4
Types of adrenergic receptors.

receptors have a higher affinity for *phenylephrine* than α_2 receptors. Conversely, the drug *clonidine* selectively binds to α_2 receptors and has less effect on α_1 receptors.

a. **α_1 Receptors:** These receptors are present on the postsynaptic membrane of the effector organs and mediate many of the classic effects, originally designated as α-adrenergic, involving constriction of smooth muscle. Activation of α_1 receptors initiates a series of reactions through the G-protein activation of phospholipase C, ultimately resulting in the generation of second messengers inositol-1,4,5-trisphosphate (IP_3) and diacylglycerol (DAG). IP_3 initiates the release of Ca^{2+} from the endoplasmic reticulum into the cytosol, and DAG turns on other proteins within the cell (Figure 6.5).

b. **α_2 Receptors:** These receptors are located primarily on sympathetic presynaptic nerve endings and control the release of norepinephrine. When a sympathetic adrenergic nerve is stimulated, a portion of the released norepinephrine "circles back" and reacts with α_2 receptors on the presynaptic membrane (Figure 6.5). Stimulation of α_2 receptors causes feedback inhibition and inhibits further release of norepinephrine from the stimulated adrenergic neuron. This inhibitory action serves as a local mechanism for modulating norepinephrine output when there is high sympathetic activity. [Note: In this instance, by inhibiting further output of norepinephrine from the adrenergic neuron, these receptors are acting as inhibitory autoreceptors.] α_2 Receptors are also found on presynaptic parasympathetic neurons. Norepinephrine released from a presynaptic sympathetic neuron can diffuse to and interact with these receptors, inhibiting acetylcholine release. [Note: In these instances, these receptors are behaving as inhibitory heteroreceptors.] This is another mechanism to modulate autonomic activity in a given area. In contrast to α_1 receptors, the effects of binding at α_2 receptors are mediated by inhibition of adenylyl cyclase and by a fall in the levels of intracellular cAMP.

c. **Further subdivisions:** The α_1 and α_2 receptors are further divided into α_{1A}, α_{1B}, α_{1C}, and α_{1D} and into α_{2A}, α_{2B}, and α_{2C}. This extended classification is necessary for understanding the selectivity of some drugs. For example, *tamsulosin* is a selective α_{1A} antagonist that is used to treat benign prostatic hyperplasia. The drug has fewer cardiovascular side effects because it targets α_{1A} subtype receptors found primarily in the urinary tract and prostate gland and does not affect the α_{1B} subtype found in the blood vessels.

2. **β-Adrenoceptors:** Responses of β receptors differ from those of α receptors and are characterized by a strong response to *isoproterenol*, with less sensitivity to *epinephrine* and *norepinephrine* (Figure 6.4). For β receptors, the rank order of potency is *isoproterenol > epinephrine > norepinephrine.* The β-adrenoceptors can be subdivided into three major subgroups, β_1, β_2, and β_3, based on their affinities for adrenergic agonists and antagonists. β_1 receptors have approximately equal affinities for *epinephrine* and *norepinephrine*, whereas β_2 receptors have a higher affinity for *epinephrine* than

for *norepinephrine*. Thus, tissues with a predominance of β_2 receptors (such as the vasculature of skeletal muscle) are particularly responsive to the effects of circulating epinephrine released by the adrenal medulla. Binding of a neurotransmitter at any of the three types of β receptors results in activation of adenylyl cyclase and increased concentrations of cAMP within the cell.

3. **Distribution of receptors:** Adrenergically innervated organs and tissues usually have a predominant type of receptor. For example, tissues such as the vasculature of skeletal muscle have both α_1 and β_2 receptors, but the β_2 receptors predominate. Other tissues may have one type of receptor almost exclusively. For example, the heart contains predominantly β_1 receptors.

4. **Characteristic responses mediated by adrenoceptors:** It is useful to organize the physiologic responses to adrenergic stimulation according to receptor type, because many drugs preferentially stimulate or block one type of receptor. Figure 6.6 summarizes the most prominent effects mediated by the adrenoceptors. As a generalization, stimulation of α_1 receptors characteristically produces vasoconstriction (particularly in skin and abdominal viscera) and an increase in total peripheral resistance and blood pressure. Stimulation of β_1 receptors characteristically causes cardiac stimulation (increase in heart rate and contractility), whereas stimulation of β_2 receptors produces vasodilation (in skeletal muscle vascular beds) and smooth muscle relaxation. β_3 Receptors are involved in lipolysis (along with β_1), and also have effects on the detrusor muscle of the bladder.

5. **Desensitization of receptors:** Prolonged exposure to the catecholamines reduces the responsiveness of these receptors, a phenomenon known as desensitization. Three mechanisms have been suggested to explain this phenomenon: 1) sequestration of the receptors so that they are unavailable for interaction with the ligand; 2) down-regulation, that is, a disappearance of the receptors either by destruction or by decreased synthesis; and 3) an inability to couple to G-protein, because the receptor has been phosphorylated on the cytoplasmic side.

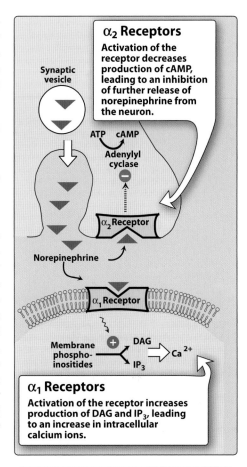

Figure 6.5
Second messengers mediate the effects of α receptors. DAG = diacylglycerol; IP_3 = inositol trisphosphate; ATP = adenosine triphosphate; cAMP = cyclic adenosine monophosphate.

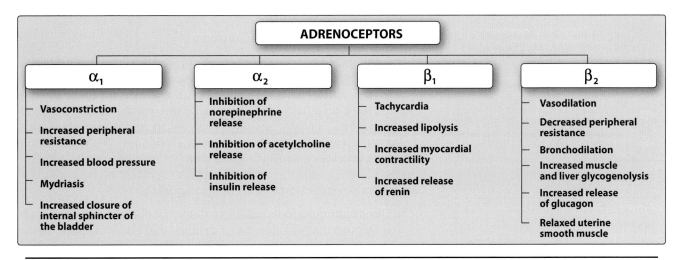

Figure 6.6
Major effects mediated by α- and β-adrenoceptors.

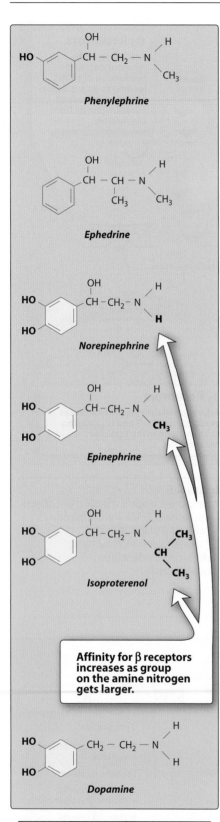

Figure 6.7
Structures of several important adrenergic agonists. Drugs containing the catechol ring are shown in *yellow*.

III. CHARACTERISTICS OF ADRENERGIC AGONISTS

Most adrenergic drugs are derivatives of β-phenylethylamine (Figure 6.7). Substitutions on the benzene ring or on the ethylamine side chains produce a variety of compounds with varying abilities to differentiate between α and β receptors and to penetrate the CNS. Two important structural features of these drugs are 1) the number and location of OH substitutions on the benzene ring and 2) the nature of the substituent on the amino nitrogen.

A. Catecholamines

Sympathomimetic amines that contain the 3,4-dihydroxybenzene group (such as *epinephrine*, *norepinephrine*, *isoproterenol*, and *dopamine*) are called catecholamines. These compounds share the following properties:

1. **High potency:** Catecholamines show the highest potency in directly activating α or β receptors.

2. **Rapid inactivation:** Catecholamines are metabolized by COMT postsynaptically and by MAO intraneuronally, by COMT and MAO in the gut wall, and by MAO in the liver. Thus, catecholamines have only a brief period of action when given parenterally, and they are inactivated (ineffective) when administered orally.

3. **Poor penetration into the CNS:** Catecholamines are polar and, therefore, do not readily penetrate into the CNS. Nevertheless, most catecholamines have some clinical effects (anxiety, tremor, and headaches) that are attributable to action on the CNS.

B. Noncatecholamines

Compounds lacking the catechol hydroxyl groups have longer half-lives, because they are not inactivated by COMT. These include *phenylephrine*, *ephedrine*, and *amphetamine* (Figure 6.7). These agents are poor substrates for MAO (an important route of metabolism) and, thus, show a prolonged duration of action. Increased lipid solubility of many of the noncatecholamines (due to lack of polar hydroxyl groups) permits greater access to the CNS.

C. Substitutions on the amine nitrogen

The nature of the substituent on the amine nitrogen is important in determining β selectivity of the adrenergic agonist. For example, *epinephrine*, with a –CH₃ substituent on the amine nitrogen, is more potent at β receptors than *norepinephrine*, which has an unsubstituted amine. Similarly, *isoproterenol*, which has an isopropyl substituent –CH(CH₃)₂ on the amine nitrogen (Figure 6.7), is a strong β agonist with little α activity (Figure 6.4).

D. Mechanism of action of adrenergic agonists

1. **Direct-acting agonists:** These drugs act directly on α or β receptors, producing effects similar to those that occur following stimulation of sympathetic nerves or release of *epinephrine* from the

adrenal medulla (Figure 6.8). Examples of direct-acting agonists include *epinephrine*, *norepinephrine*, *isoproterenol*, *dopamine*, and *phenylephrine*.

2. **Indirect-acting agonists:** These agents may block the reuptake of *norepinephrine* or cause the release of *norepinephrine* from the cytoplasmic pools or vesicles of the adrenergic neuron (Figure 6.8). The *norepinephrine* then traverses the synapse and binds to α or β receptors. Examples of reuptake inhibitors and agents that cause *norepinephrine* release include *cocaine* and *amphetamine*, respectively.

3. **Mixed-action agonists:** *Ephedrine* and its stereoisomer, *pseudoephedrine*, both stimulate adrenoceptors directly and enhance release of *norepinephrine* from the adrenergic neuron (Figure 6.8).

IV. DIRECT-ACTING ADRENERGIC AGONISTS

Direct-acting agonists bind to adrenergic receptors on effector organs without interacting with the presynaptic neuron. As a group, these agents are widely used in clinical practice.

A. Epinephrine

Epinephrine [ep-i-NEF-rin] is one of the four catecholamines (*epinephrine*, *norepinephrine*, *dopamine*, and *dobutamine*) commonly used in therapy. The first three are naturally occurring neurotransmitters, and the latter is a synthetic compound. In the adrenal medulla, *norepinephrine* is methylated to yield *epinephrine*, which is stored in chromaffin cells along with *norepinephrine*. On stimulation, the adrenal medulla releases about 80% *epinephrine* and 20% *norepinephrine* directly into the circulation. *Epinephrine* interacts with both α and β receptors. At low doses, β effects (vasodilation) on the vascular system predominate, whereas at high doses, α effects (vasoconstriction) are the strongest.

1. **Actions**

    a. **Cardiovascular:** The major actions of *epinephrine* are on the cardiovascular system. *Epinephrine* strengthens the contractility of the myocardium (positive inotrope: β_1 action) and increases its rate of contraction (positive chronotrope: β_1 action). Therefore, cardiac output increases. These effects increase oxygen demands on the myocardium. *Epinephrine* activates β_1 receptors on the kidney to cause renin release. Renin is an enzyme involved in the production of angiotensin II, a potent vasoconstrictor. *Epinephrine* constricts arterioles in the skin, mucous membranes, and viscera (α effects), and it dilates vessels going to the liver and skeletal muscle (β_2 effects). These combined effects result in a decrease in renal blood flow. Therefore, the cumulative effect is an increase in systolic blood pressure, coupled with a

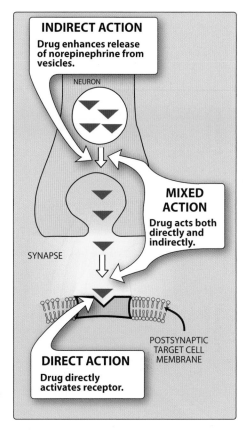

Figure 6.8
Sites of action of direct-, indirect-, and mixed-acting adrenergic agonists.

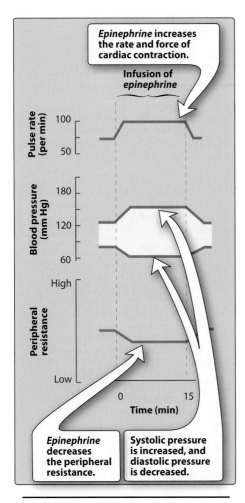

Figure 6.9
Cardiovascular effects of intravenous infusion of low doses of *epinephrine*.

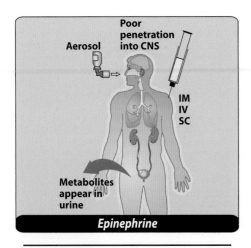

Figure 6.10
Pharmacokinetics of *epinephrine*.
CNS = central nervous system.

slight decrease in diastolic pressure due to β_2 receptor–mediated vasodilation in the skeletal muscle vascular bed (Figure 6.9).

b. Respiratory: *Epinephrine* causes powerful bronchodilation by acting directly on bronchial smooth muscle (β_2 action). It also inhibits the release of allergy mediators such as histamine from mast cells.

c. Hyperglycemia: *Epinephrine* has a significant hyperglycemic effect because of increased glycogenolysis in the liver (β_2 effect), increased release of glucagon (β_2 effect), and a decreased release of *insulin* (α_2 effect).

d. Lipolysis: *Epinephrine* initiates lipolysis through agonist activity on the β receptors of adipose tissue. Increased levels of cAMP stimulate a hormone-sensitive lipase, which hydrolyzes triglycerides to free fatty acids and glycerol.

2. Therapeutic uses

a. Bronchospasm: *Epinephrine* is the primary drug used in the emergency treatment of respiratory conditions when bronchoconstriction has resulted in diminished respiratory function. Thus, in treatment of anaphylactic shock, *epinephrine* is the drug of choice and can be lifesaving in this setting. Within a few minutes after subcutaneous administration, respiratory function greatly improves.

b. Anaphylactic shock: *Epinephrine* is the drug of choice for the treatment of type I hypersensitivity reactions (including anaphylaxis) in response to allergens.

c. Cardiac arrest: *Epinephrine* may be used to restore cardiac rhythm in patients with cardiac arrest.

d. Local anesthesia: Local anesthetic solutions may contain low concentrations (for example, 1:100,000 parts) of *epinephrine*. *Epinephrine* greatly increases the duration of local anesthesia by producing vasoconstriction at the site of injection. *Epinephrine* also reduces systemic absorption of the local anesthetic and promotes local hemostasis.

e. Intraocular surgery: *Epinephrine* is used in the induction and maintenance of mydriasis during intraocular surgery.

3. Pharmacokinetics: *Epinephrine* has a rapid onset but a brief duration of action (due to rapid degradation). The preferred route for anaphylaxis in the outpatient setting is intramuscular (anterior thigh) due to rapid absorption. In emergencies, *epinephrine* is given intravenously (IV) for the most rapid onset of action. It may also be given subcutaneously, by endotracheal tube, or by inhalation (Figure 6.10). It is rapidly metabolized by MAO and COMT, and the metabolites metanephrine and vanillylmandelic acid are excreted in urine.

4. Adverse effects: *Epinephrine* can produce adverse CNS effects that include anxiety, fear, tension, headache, and tremor. It can trigger cardiac arrhythmias, particularly if the patient is receiving *digoxin*. *Epinephrine* can also induce pulmonary edema due to increased afterload caused by vasoconstrictive properties of the drug. Patients with hyperthyroidism may have an increased production of adrenergic receptors in the vasculature, leading to an enhanced response to *epinephrine*, and the dose must be reduced in these individuals. Inhalation anesthetics also sensitize the heart to the effects of *epinephrine*, which may lead to tachycardia. *Epinephrine* increases the release of endogenous stores of glucose. In diabetic patients, dosages of *insulin* may have to be increased. Nonselective β-blockers prevent vasodilatory effects of *epinephrine* on β₂ receptors, leaving α receptor stimulation unopposed. This may lead to increased peripheral resistance and increased blood pressure.

B. Norepinephrine

Because *norepinephrine* [nor-ep-ih-NEF-rin] is the neurotransmitter in the adrenergic neurons, it should, theoretically, stimulate all types of adrenergic receptors. However, when administered in therapeutic doses, the α-adrenergic receptor is most affected.

1. Cardiovascular actions

a. Vasoconstriction: *Norepinephrine* causes a rise in peripheral resistance due to intense vasoconstriction of most vascular beds, including the kidney (α₁ effect). Both systolic and diastolic blood pressures increase (Figure 6.11). [Note: *Norepinephrine* causes greater vasoconstriction than *epinephrine*, because it does not induce compensatory vasodilation via β₂ receptors on blood vessels supplying skeletal muscles. The weak β₂ activity of *norepinephrine* also explains why it is not useful in the treatment of bronchospasm or anaphylaxis.]

b. Baroreceptor reflex: *Norepinephrine* increases blood pressure, and this stimulates the baroreceptors, inducing a rise in vagal activity. The increased vagal activity produces a reflex bradycardia, which is sufficient to counteract the local actions of *norepinephrine* on the heart, although the reflex compensation does not affect the positive inotropic effects of the drug (Figure 6.11). When *atropine*, which blocks the transmission of vagal effects, is given before *norepinephrine*, stimulation of the heart by *norepinephrine* is evident as tachycardia.

2. Therapeutic uses: *Norepinephrine* is used to treat shock (for example, septic shock), because it increases vascular resistance and, therefore, increases blood pressure. It has no other clinically significant uses.

3. Pharmacokinetics: *Norepinephrine* is given IV for rapid onset of action. The duration of action is 1 to 2 minutes, following the end of the infusion. It is rapidly metabolized by MAO and COMT, and inactive metabolites are excreted in the urine.

4. Adverse effects: These are similar to *epinephrine*. In addition, *norepinephrine* is a potent vasoconstrictor and may cause blanching and sloughing of skin along an injected vein. If extravasation (leakage of drug from the vessel into tissues surrounding the injection site) occurs, it can cause tissue necrosis. It should not be administered in peripheral veins, if possible. Impaired circulation

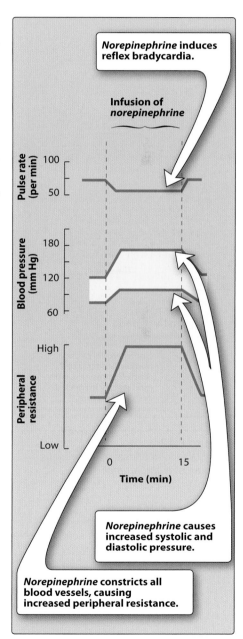

Figure 6.11
Cardiovascular effects of intravenous infusion of *norepinephrine*.

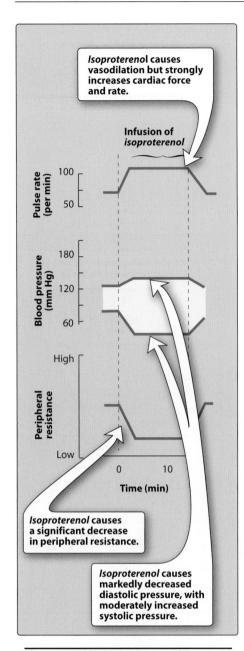

Isoproterenol causes vasodilation but strongly increases cardiac force and rate.

Infusion of isoproterenol

Isoproterenol causes a significant decrease in peripheral resistance.

Isoproterenol causes markedly decreased diastolic pressure, with moderately increased systolic pressure.

Figure 6.12
Cardiovascular effects of intravenous infusion of *isoproterenol*.

from *norepinephrine* may be treated with the α receptor antagonist *phentolamine*. Alternatives to *phentolamine* include intradermal *terbutaline* and topical *nitroglycerin*.

C. Isoproterenol

Isoproterenol [eye-soe-proe-TER-e-nole] is a direct-acting synthetic catecholamine that stimulates both β_1- and β_2-adrenergic receptors. Its nonselectivity is a disadvantage and the reason why it is rarely used therapeutically. Its action on α receptors is insignificant. *Isoproterenol* produces intense stimulation of the heart (β_1 effect), increasing heart rate, contractility, and cardiac output (Figure 6.12). It is as active as *epinephrine* in this action. *Isoproterenol* also dilates the arterioles of skeletal muscle (β_2 effect), resulting in decreased peripheral resistance. Because of its cardiac stimulatory action, it may increase systolic blood pressure slightly, but it greatly reduces mean arterial and diastolic blood pressures (Figure 6.12). *Isoproterenol* is also a potent bronchodilator (β_2 effect). The adverse effects of *isoproterenol* are similar to the β receptor–related side effects of *epinephrine*.

D. Dopamine

Dopamine [DOE-pa-meen], the immediate metabolic precursor of *norepinephrine*, occurs naturally in the CNS in the basal ganglia, where it functions as a neurotransmitter, as well as in the adrenal medulla. *Dopamine* can activate α- and β-adrenergic receptors. For example, at higher doses, it causes vasoconstriction by activating α_1 receptors, whereas at lower doses, it stimulates β_1 cardiac receptors. In addition, D_1 and D_2 dopaminergic receptors, distinct from the α- and β-adrenergic receptors, occur in the peripheral mesenteric and renal vascular beds, where binding of *dopamine* produces vasodilation. D_2 receptors are also found on presynaptic adrenergic neurons, where their activation interferes with *norepinephrine* release.

1. Actions

a. Cardiovascular: *Dopamine* exerts a stimulatory effect on the β_1 receptors of the heart, having both positive inotropic and chronotropic effects (Figure 6.13). At very high doses, *dopamine* activates α_1 receptors on the vasculature, resulting in vasoconstriction.

b. Renal and visceral: *Dopamine* dilates renal and splanchnic arterioles by activating dopaminergic receptors, thereby increasing blood flow to the kidneys and other viscera (Figure 6.13). These receptors are not affected by α- or β-blocking drugs, and in the past, low-dose ("renal-dose") *dopamine* was often used in the prevention or treatment of acute renal failure. However, more recent data suggest there is limited clinical utility in the renal protective effects of *dopamine*.

2. Therapeutic uses: *Dopamine* can be used for cardiogenic and septic shock and is given by continuous infusion. It raises blood pressure by stimulating the β_1 receptors on the heart to increase cardiac output, and α_1 receptors on blood vessels to increase total peripheral resistance. It enhances perfusion to the kidney and splanchnic areas, as described above. Increased blood flow to the kidney enhances

the glomerular filtration rate and causes diuresis. By contrast, *norepinephrine* can diminish blood supply to the kidney and may reduce renal function. *Dopamine* is also used to treat hypotension, severe heart failure, and bradycardia unresponsive to other treatments.

3. **Adverse effects:** An overdose of *dopamine* produces the same effects as sympathetic stimulation. *Dopamine* is rapidly metabolized by MAO or COMT, and its adverse effects (nausea, hypertension, and arrhythmias) are, therefore, short lived.

E. Fenoldopam

Fenoldopam [fen-OL-de-pam] is an agonist of peripheral *dopamine* D_1 receptors. It is used as a rapid-acting vasodilator to treat severe hypertension in hospitalized patients, acting on coronary arteries, kidney arterioles, and mesenteric arteries. *Fenoldopam* is a racemic mixture, and the R-isomer is the active component. It undergoes extensive first-pass metabolism and has a 10-minute elimination half-life after IV infusion. Headache, flushing, dizziness, nausea, vomiting, and tachycardia (due to vasodilation) may occur with this agent.

F. Dobutamine

Dobutamine [doe-BYOO-ta-meen] is a synthetic, direct-acting catecholamine that is primarily a β_1 receptor agonist with minor β_2 and α_1 effects. It increases heart rate and cardiac output with few vascular effects. *Dobutamine* is used to increase cardiac output in acute heart failure (see Chapter 18), as well as for inotropic support after cardiac surgery. The drug increases cardiac output and does not elevate oxygen demands of the myocardium as much as other sympathomimetic drugs. *Dobutamine* should be used with caution in atrial fibrillation, because it increases atrioventricular (AV) conduction. Other adverse effects are similar to *epinephrine*. Tolerance may develop with prolonged use.

G. Oxymetazoline

Oxymetazoline [OX-ee-mee-TAZ-ih-leen] is a direct-acting synthetic adrenergic agonist that stimulates both α_1- and α_2-adrenergic receptors. *Oxymetazoline* is found in many over-the-counter nasal spray decongestants, as well as in ophthalmic drops for the relief of redness of the eyes associated with swimming, colds, and contact lenses. *Oxymetazoline* directly stimulates α receptors on blood vessels supplying the nasal mucosa and conjunctiva, thereby producing vasoconstriction and decreasing congestion. It is absorbed in the systemic circulation regardless of the route of administration and may produce nervousness, headaches, and trouble sleeping. Local irritation and sneezing may occur with intranasal administration. Use for greater than 3 days is not recommended, as rebound congestion and dependence may occur.

H. Phenylephrine

Phenylephrine [fen-ill-EF-reen] is a direct-acting, synthetic adrenergic drug that binds primarily to α_1 receptors. *Phenylephrine* is a vasoconstrictor that raises both systolic and diastolic blood pressures. It has no effect on the heart itself but, rather, induces reflex bradycardia

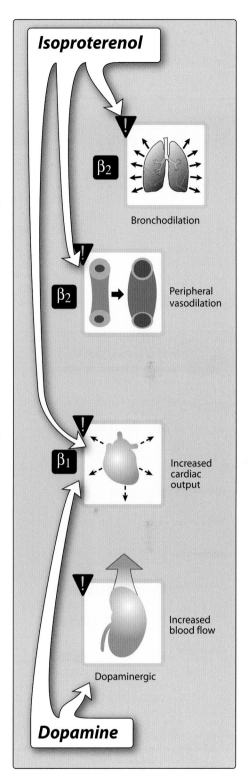

Figure 6.13
Clinically important actions of *isoproterenol* and *dopamine*.

when given parenterally, making it useful in the treatment of paroxysmal supraventricular tachycardia. The drug is used to treat hypotension in hospitalized or surgical patients (especially those with a rapid heart rate). Large doses can cause hypertensive headache and cardiac irregularities. *Phenylephrine* acts as a nasal decongestant when applied topically or taken orally. Although data suggest it may not be as effective, *phenylephrine* has replaced *pseudoephedrine* in many oral decongestants, since *pseudoephedrine* has been misused to make *methamphetamine*. *Phenylephrine* is also used in ophthalmic solutions for mydriasis.

I. Midodrine

Midodrine, a prodrug, is metabolized to the pharmacologically active desglymidodrine. It is a selective α_1 agonist, which acts in the periphery to increase arterial and venous tone. *Midodrine* is indicated for the treatment of orthostatic hypotension. The drug should be given three times daily, with doses at 3- or 4-hour intervals. To avoid supine hypertension, doses within 4 hours of bedtime are not recommended.

J. Clonidine

Clonidine [KLOE-ni-deen] is an α_2 agonist used for the treatment of hypertension. It can also be used to minimize symptoms of withdrawal from opiates, tobacco smoking, and benzodiazepines. Both *clonidine* and the α_2 agonist *guanfacine* [GWAHN-fa-seen] may be used in the management of attention deficit hyperactivity disorder. *Clonidine* acts centrally on presynaptic α_2 receptors to produce inhibition of sympathetic vasomotor centers, decreasing sympathetic outflow to the periphery. The most common side effects of *clonidine* are lethargy, sedation, constipation, and xerostomia. Abrupt discontinuation must be avoided to prevent rebound hypertension. *Clonidine* and another α_2 agonist *methyldopa* are discussed with antihypertensives in Chapter 16.

K. Albuterol, metaproterenol, and terbutaline

Albuterol [al-BYOO-ter-ole], *metaproterenol* [MET-a-proe-TER-e-nol], and *terbutaline* [ter-BYOO-te-leen] are short-acting β_2 agonists (SABAs) used primarily as bronchodilators and administered by a metered-dose inhaler (Figure 6.14). *Albuterol* is the SABA of choice for the management of acute asthma symptoms, because it is more selective for β_2 receptors than *metaproterenol*. Inhaled *terbutaline* is no longer available in the United States, but is still used in other countries. Injectable *terbutaline* is used off-label as a uterine relaxant to suppress premature labor, and use for this indication should not exceed 72 hours. One of the most common side effects of these agents is tremor, but patients tend to develop tolerance to this effect. Other side effects include restlessness, apprehension, and anxiety. When these drugs are administered orally, they may cause tachycardia or arrhythmia (due to β_1 receptor activation), especially in patients with underlying cardiac disease. Monoamine oxidase inhibitors (MAOIs) also increase the risk of adverse cardiovascular effects, and concomitant use should be avoided.

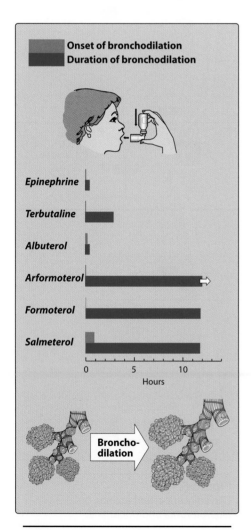

Figure 6.14
Onset and duration of bronchodilation effects of inhaled adrenergic agonists.

L. Salmeterol, formoterol, and indacaterol

Salmeterol [sal-ME-ter-ole], *formoterol* [for-MOH-ter-ole], *arformoterol* (the [R,R]-enantiomer of *formoterol*), and *indacaterol* [IN-da-KA-ter-ol] are long-acting β_2 selective agonists (LABAs) used for the management of respiratory disorders such as asthma and chronic obstructive pulmonary disease (see Chapter 39). A single dose by a metered-dose inhalation device, such as a dry powder inhaler, provides sustained bronchodilation over 12 hours, compared with less than 3 hours for *albuterol*. Unlike *formoterol*, however, *salmeterol* has a somewhat delayed onset of action (Figure 6.14). LABAs are not recommended as monotherapy for the treatment of asthma, because they have been shown to increase the risk of asthma-related deaths; however, these agents are highly efficacious when combined with an asthma controller medication such as an inhaled corticosteroid.

M. Mirabegron

Mirabegron [mir-a-BEG-ron] is a β_3 agonist that relaxes the detrusor smooth muscle and increases bladder capacity. It is used for patients with overactive bladder. *Mirabegron* may increase blood pressure and should not be used in patients with uncontrolled hypertension. It increases levels of *digoxin* and inhibits the CYP2D6 isozyme, which may enhance the effects of other medications metabolized by this pathway (for example, *metoprolol*).

V. INDIRECT-ACTING ADRENERGIC AGONISTS

Indirect-acting adrenergic agonists cause the release, inhibit the reuptake, or inhibit the degradation of epinephrine or norepinephrine (Figure 6.8). They potentiate the effects of epinephrine or norepinephrine produced endogenously, but do not directly affect postsynaptic receptors.

A. Amphetamine

The marked central stimulatory action of *amphetamine* [am-FET-a-meen] is often mistaken by drug abusers as its only action. However, the drug can also increase blood pressure significantly by α_1 agonist action on the vasculature, as well as β_1 stimulatory effects on the heart. Its actions are mediated primarily through an increase in nonvesicular release of catecholamines such as dopamine and norepinephrine from nerve terminals. Thus, *amphetamine* is an indirect-acting adrenergic drug. The actions and therapeutic uses of *amphetamine* and its derivatives are discussed with CNS stimulants (see Chapter 15).

B. Tyramine

Tyramine [TIE-ra-meen] is not a clinically useful drug, but it is important because it is found in fermented foods, such as aged cheese and Chianti wine. It is a normal by-product of tyrosine metabolism. Normally, it is oxidized by MAO in the gastrointestinal tract, but if the patient is taking MAOIs, it can precipitate serious vasopressor episodes. Like *amphetamines*, *tyramine* can enter the nerve terminal and displace stored norepinephrine. The released catecholamine then acts on adrenoceptors.

C. Cocaine

Cocaine [koe-KANE] is unique among local anesthetics in having the ability to block the sodium–chloride (Na^+/Cl^-)–dependent norepinephrine transporter required for cellular uptake of norepinephrine into the adrenergic neuron. Consequently, norepinephrine accumulates in the synaptic space, resulting in enhanced sympathetic activity and potentiation of the actions of epinephrine and norepinephrine. Therefore, small doses of the catecholamines produce greatly magnified effects in an individual taking *cocaine*. In addition, the duration of action of epinephrine and norepinephrine is increased. Like *amphetamines*, it can increase blood pressure by α_1 agonist actions and β stimulatory effects. *Cocaine* as a drug of abuse is discussed in Chapter 45.

VI. MIXED-ACTION ADRENERGIC AGONISTS

Ephedrine [eh-FED-rin] and *pseudoephedrine* [soo-doe-eh-FED-rin] are mixed-action adrenergic agents. They not only enhance release of stored norepinephrine from nerve endings (Figure 6.8) but also directly stimulate both α and β receptors. Thus, a wide variety of adrenergic actions ensue that are similar to those of *epinephrine*, although less potent. *Ephedrine* and *pseudoephedrine* are not catecholamines and are poor substrates for COMT and MAO. Therefore, these drugs have a long duration of action. *Ephedrine* and *pseudoephedrine* have excellent absorption after oral administration and penetrate the CNS, but *pseudoephedrine* has fewer CNS effects. *Ephedrine* is eliminated largely unchanged in urine, and *pseudoephedrine* undergoes incomplete hepatic metabolism before elimination in urine. *Ephedrine* raises systolic and diastolic blood pressures by vasoconstriction and cardiac stimulation and it is indicated in anesthesia-induced hypotension. *Ephedrine* produces bronchodilation, but it is less potent and slower acting than *epinephrine* or *isoproterenol*. It was previously used to prevent asthma attacks but has been replaced by more effective medications. *Ephedrine* produces a mild stimulation of the CNS. This increases alertness, decreases fatigue, and prevents sleep. It also improves athletic performance. [Note: The clinical use of *ephedrine* is declining because of the availability of better, more potent agents that cause fewer adverse effects. *Ephedrine*-containing herbal supplements (mainly ephedra-containing products) have been banned by the U.S. Food and Drug Administration because of life-threatening cardiovascular reactions.] Oral *pseudoephedrine* is primarily used to treat nasal and sinus congestion. *Pseudoephedrine* has been illegally used to produce *methamphetamine*. Therefore, products containing *pseudoephedrine* have certain restrictions and must be kept behind the sales counter in the United States. Important characteristics of the adrenergic agonists are summarized in Figures 6.15 to 6.17.

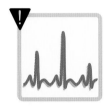
Arrhythmias

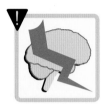
Headache

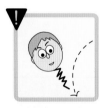
Hyperactivity

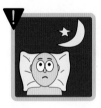
Insomnia

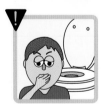
Nausea

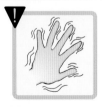
Tremors

Figure 6.15
Some adverse effects observed with adrenergic agonists.

TISSUE	RECEPTOR TYPE	ACTION	OPPOSING ACTIONS
Heart			
• Sinus and AV	β₁	↑ Automaticity	Cholinergic receptors
• Conduction pathway	β₁	↑ Conduction velocity, automaticity	Cholinergic receptors
• Myofibrils	β₁	↑ Contractility, automaticity	
Vascular smooth muscle	β₂	Vasodilation	α-Adrenergic receptors
Bronchial smooth muscle	β₂	Bronchodilation	Cholinergic receptors
Kidneys	β₁	↑ Renin release	α₁-Adrenergic receptors
Liver	β₂, α₁	↑ Glycogenolysis and gluconeogenesis	—
Adipose tissue	β₁, β₃	↑ Lipolysis	α₂-Adrenergic receptors
Skeletal muscle	β₂	↑ Increased contractility Potassium uptake; glycogenolysis Dilates arteries to skeletal muscle Tremor	—
Eye-ciliary muscle	β₂	Relaxation	Cholinergic receptors
GI tract	β₂	↓ Motility	Cholinergic receptors
Gall bladder	β₂	Relaxation	Cholinergic receptors
Urinary bladder detrusor muscle	β₂, β₃	Relaxation	Cholinergic receptors
Uterus	β₂	Relaxation	Oxytocin

Figure 6.16
Summary of β-adrenergic receptors. AV = atrioventricular; GI = gastrointestinal.

	DRUG	RECEPTOR SPECIFICITY	THERAPEUTIC USES
	Epinephrine	α_1, α_2 β_1, β_2	Anaphylactic shock Cardiac arrest In local anesthetics to increase duration of action
	Norepinephrine	α_1, α_2 β_1	Treatment of shock
	Isoproterenol	β_1, β_2	As a cardiac stimulant
	Dopamine	Dopaminergic α_1, β_1	Treatment of shock Treatment of congestive heart failure Raise blood pressure
	Dobutamine	β_1	Treatment of acute heart failure
	Oxymetazoline	α_1	As a nasal decongestant For relief of eye redness
	Phenylephrine	α_1	As a nasal decongestant Raise blood pressure Treatment of paroxysmal supraventricular tachycardia
	Clonidine	α_2	Treatment of hypertension
	Albuterol Metaproterenol Terbutaline	β_2	Treatment of bronchospasm (short-acting)
	Arformoterol Formoterol Indacaterol Salmeterol	β_2	Treatment of bronchospasm (long-acting)
	Amphetamine	α, β, CNS	As a CNS stimulant in treatment of children with ADHD, narcolepsy, and for appetite control
	Ephedrine Pseudoephedrine	α, β, CNS	Raise blood pressure As a nasal decongestant

CATECHOLAMINES
- Rapid onset of action
- Brief duration of action
- Not administered orally
- Do not penetrate the blood-brain barrier

NONCATECHOL-AMINES

Compared to catecholamines:
- Longer duration of action
- All can be administered orally or via inhalation

Figure 6.17
Summary of the therapeutic uses of adrenergic agonists. ADHD = attention deficit hyperactivity disorder; CNS = central nervous system.

Study Questions

Choose the ONE best answer.

6.1 Which of the following is correct regarding adrenergic neurotransmission?

A. Norepinephrine is the major neurotransmitter released from sympathetic nerve terminals.

B. Norepinephrine is mainly released from the adrenal glands.

C. Tricyclic antidepressants and cocaine prevent the release of norepinephrine from the nerve terminals.

D. Monoamine oxidase (MAO) converts dopamine to norepinephrine in the nerve terminal.

Correct answer = A. Norepinephrine (NE) is the major neurotransmitter released from sympathetic nerve terminals. Epinephrine, not norepinephrine, is mainly released from the adrenal glands. Tricyclic antidepressants (TCAs) and cocaine inhibit the reuptake of norepinephrine into the sympathetic nerve terminals, but they do not prevent the release of NE. Dopamine is converted to norepinephrine by dopamine β-hydroxylase, not by MAO.

6.2 Which of the following adrenergic drugs is used in the treatment of overactive bladder?

A. Epinephrine
B. Dobutamine
C. Phenylephrine
D. Mirabegron

Correct answer = D. Detrusor muscles in the urinary bladder wall have β_3 receptors. Stimulation of these receptors relaxes the urinary bladder wall and relieves overactive bladder. Mirabegron is a β_3 agonist and therefore used in treating overactive bladder. None of the other drugs listed have β_3 agonist activity.

6.3 Which of the following classes of adrenergic agents has utility in the management of hypertension?

A. α_1 Agonist
B. α_2 Agonist
C. β_1 Agonist
D. β_3 Agonist

Correct answer = B. α_2 Agonists activate α_2 receptors located in the presynaptic terminal of sympathetic neurons and cause a reduction in the release of norepinephrine from sympathetic nerve terminals. This leads to a reduction in blood pressure. α_2 Agonists such as clonidine and methyldopa are therefore used as antihypertensive agents. α_1 Agonists cause vasoconstriction, and β_1 agonists cause increased cardiac output and renin release, so these agents may increase blood pressure. β_3 Agonists are not used in the management of hypertension.

6.4 Which of the following is correct regarding responses mediated by adrenergic receptors?

A. Stimulation of α_1 receptors increases blood pressure.

B. Stimulation of sympathetic presynaptic α_2 receptors increases norepinephrine release.

C. Stimulation of β_2 receptors increases heart rate (tachycardia).

D. Stimulation of β_2 receptors causes bronchoconstriction.

Correct answer = A. Stimulation of α_1 receptors, mostly found in the blood vessels, causes vasoconstriction and an increase in blood pressure. Stimulation of α_2 receptors on the sympathetic presynaptic terminal reduces the release of norepinephrine. β_2 receptors are not found in the heart, so activation of β_2 receptors does not affect heart rate. Stimulation of β_2 receptors found in the bronchial tissues causes bronchodilation, not bronchoconstriction.

6.5 An asthma patient was given a nonselective β agonist to relieve bronchoconstriction. Which adverse effect would you expect in this patient?

A. Bradycardia
B. Tachycardia
C. Hypotension (reduction in blood pressure)
D. Worsening bronchoconstriction

Correct answer = B. A nonselective β agonist activates both β_1 and β_2 receptors. β_1 Activation causes an increase in heart rate (tachycardia), contractility, and subsequent increase in blood pressure. It relieves bronchoconstriction because of the β_2 receptor activation.

6.6 A 22-year-old male is brought to the emergency room with suspected cocaine overdose. Which of the following symptoms is most likely in this patient?

A. Hypertension
B. Bronchoconstriction
C. Bradycardia
D. Miosis (constriction of pupil)

Correct answer = A. Cocaine is an indirect adrenergic agonist that prevents the reuptake of norepinephrine into the nerve terminals, thus increasing the levels of NE in the synaptic cleft. The increase in NE leads to an increase in blood pressure (hypertension), tachycardia (not bradycardia), mydriasis (not miosis), and other symptoms of sympathetic overactivity.

6.7 A 12-year-old boy with a peanut allergy is brought to the emergency room after accidental consumption of peanuts. He is in anaphylactic shock. Which of the following drugs is most appropriate to treat this patient?

A. Norepinephrine
B. Phenylephrine
C. Dobutamine
D. Epinephrine

Correct answer = D. Norepinephrine has more α agonistic effects and activates mainly α_1, α_2, and β_1 receptors. Epinephrine has more β agonistic effects and activates mainly α_1, α_2, β_1, and β_2 receptors. Phenylephrine has predominantly α effects and activates mainly α_1 receptors. Dobutamine mainly activates β_1 receptors and has no significant effects on β_2 receptors. Thus, epinephrine is the drug of choice in anaphylactic shock that can both stimulate the heart (β_1 activation) and dilate bronchioles (β_2 activation).

6.8 An elderly patient is brought to the emergency room with a blood pressure of 76/60 mm Hg, tachycardia, and low cardiac output. He is diagnosed with acute heart failure. Which of the following drugs is most appropriate to improve his cardiac function?

A. Epinephrine
B. Fenoldopam
C. Dobutamine
D. Isoproterenol

Correct answer = C. Among the choices, the ideal drug to increase contractility in acute heart failure is dobutamine, since it is a selective β_1-adrenergic agonist. Fenoldopam is a dopamine agonist used to treat severe hypertension. The other drugs are nonselective adrenergic agonists that could cause unwanted side effects.

6.9 Which of the following adrenergic agonists is commonly present in nasal sprays available over-the-counter (OTC) to treat nasal congestion?

A. Clonidine
B. Albuterol
C. Oxymetazoline
D. Formoterol

Correct answer = C. Drugs with selective α_1 agonistic activity are commonly used as nasal decongestants because of their ability to cause vasoconstriction in the nasal vessels. Oxymetazoline is an α_1 agonist and therefore the preferred drug among the choices as a nasal decongestant. Clonidine is an α_2 agonist, albuterol is a β_2 agonist, and formoterol is a long-acting β_2 agonist.

6.10 A patient who has hypertension and mild asthma attacks bought a herbal remedy for asthma online. He does not take any prescription medications for asthma, but takes a β_1-selective blocker for hypertension. The herbal remedy relieves the asthma attacks, but his blood pressure seems to increase despite the β-blocker therapy. Which of the following drugs is most likely present in the herbal remedy?

A. Phenylephrine
B. Norepinephrine
C. Ephedrine
D. Salmeterol

Correct answer = C. Both ephedrine and salmeterol can relieve asthma symptoms, as they activate β_2 receptors in the bronchioles and cause bronchodilation. However, salmeterol is a selective β_2 agonist and should not increase blood pressure. By contrast, ephedrine stimulates the release of norepinephrine and acts as a direct agonist at α- and β-adrenergic receptors, thus causing an increase in blood pressure. Phenylephrine (a nonselective α agonist) does not cause bronchodilation, so it would not relieve asthma symptoms. Norepinephrine is a nonselective adrenergic agonist that does not have any stimulatory effects on β_2 receptors. In addition, norepinephrine is not active when given orally.

Adrenergic Antagonists

7

Rajan Radhakrishnan and Sandhya Jinesh

I. OVERVIEW

The adrenergic antagonists (also called adrenergic blockers or sympatholytics) bind to adrenoceptors but do not trigger the usual receptor-mediated intracellular effects. These drugs act by either reversibly or irreversibly attaching to the adrenoceptors, thus preventing activation by endogenous or exogenous agonists. Like the agonists, the adrenergic antagonists are classified according to their relative affinities for α or β receptors in the sympathetic nervous system. Numerous adrenergic antagonists have important roles in clinical medicine, primarily to treat diseases associated with the cardiovascular system. [Note: Antagonists that block dopamine receptors are most important in the central nervous system (CNS) and are, therefore, considered in that section.] The adrenergic antagonists discussed in this chapter are summarized in Figure 7.1.

II. α-ADRENERGIC BLOCKING AGENTS

α-Adrenergic blocking agents antagonize the subtype(s) of α-adrenergic receptors (α_1 or α_2), depending on the specificity of the agent for the receptor subtype(s). Drugs that block α_1-adrenoceptors profoundly affect blood pressure. Because normal sympathetic control of the vasculature occurs in large part through agonist actions on α_1-adrenergic receptors, blockade of these receptors reduces the sympathetic tone of the blood vessels, resulting in decreased peripheral vascular resistance. This lowered blood pressure induces reflex tachycardia. The magnitude of the response depends on the sympathetic tone of the individual when the agent is given. Selective α_2-adrenergic blockers have limited clinical utility.

A. Phenoxybenzamine

Phenoxybenzamine [fen-ox-ee-BEN-za-meen] is a nonselective, noncompetitive blocker of α_1- and α_2-adrenergic receptors.

1. Actions

    a. Cardiovascular effects: The drug prevents α_1 receptor vasoconstriction of peripheral blood vessels caused by endogenous catecholamines, which leads to decreased peripheral resistance and resultant reflex tachycardia. However, by blocking

α BLOCKERS
Alfuzosin UROXATRAL
Doxazosin CARDURA
Phenoxybenzamine DIBENZYLINE
Phentolamine GENERIC ONLY
Prazosin MINIPRESS
Silodosin RAPAFLO
Tamsulosin FLOMAX
Terazosin GENERIC ONLY
Yohimbine YOCON

β BLOCKERS
Acebutolol GENERIC ONLY
Atenolol TENORMIN
Betaxolol BETOPTIC-S
Bisoprolol GENERIC ONLY
Carteolol GENERIC ONLY
Carvedilol COREG, COREG CR
Esmolol BREVIBLOC
Labetalol GENERIC ONLY
Levobunolol BETAGAN
Metipranolol GENERIC ONLY
Metoprolol LOPRESSOR, TOPROL-XL
Nadolol CORGARD
Nebivolol BYSTOLIC
Pindolol GENERIC ONLY
Propranolol INDERAL LA, INNOPRAN XL
Timolol BETIMOL, ISTALOL, TIMOPTIC

DRUGS AFFECTING NEURO-TRANSMITTER UPTAKE OR RELEASE
Reserpine GENERIC ONLY

Figure 7.1
Summary of blocking agents and drugs affecting neurotransmitter uptake or release.

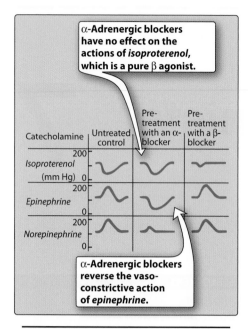

Figure 7.2
Summary of effects of adrenergic blockers on the changes in blood pressure induced by *isoproterenol*, *epinephrine*, and *norepinephrine*.

presynaptic α_2 receptors on the sympathetic nerve terminals in the heart, *phenoxybenzamine* causes an increase in the release of norepinephrine, which in turn increases heart rate and cardiac output (mediated by β_1 receptors). This may also lead to cardiac arrhythmias and anginal pain. Thus, the drug has been unsuccessful in maintaining lowered blood pressure in hypertension, and it is no longer used for this purpose.

b. Epinephrine reversal: All α-adrenergic blockers reverse the α agonist actions of *epinephrine*. For example, the vasoconstrictive action of *epinephrine* is interrupted, but vasodilation of other vascular beds caused by stimulation of β_2 receptors is not blocked. Therefore, in the presence of *phenoxybenzamine*, the systemic blood pressure decreases in response to *epinephrine* (Figure 7.2). [Note: The actions of *norepinephrine* are not reversed but are diminished because *norepinephrine* lacks significant β agonist action on the vasculature.] *Phenoxybenzamine* has no effect on the actions of *isoproterenol*, which is a pure β agonist (Figure 7.2).

2. Therapeutic uses: *Phenoxybenzamine* is used in the treatment of sweating and hypertension associated with pheochromocytoma, a catecholamine-secreting tumor of cells derived from the adrenal medulla. *Phenoxybenzamine* is sometimes effective in treating Raynaud disease and frostbite.

3. Adverse effects: *Phenoxybenzamine* can cause postural hypotension, nasal stuffiness, nausea, and vomiting. It may inhibit ejaculation. It may also induce reflex tachycardia, which is mediated by the baroreceptor reflex. *Phenoxybenzamine* should be used with caution in patients with cerebrovascular or cardiovascular disease.

B. Phentolamine

In contrast to *phenoxybenzamine*, *phentolamine* [fen-TOLE-a-meen] produces a competitive block of α_1 and α_2 receptors. Effects last for approximately 4 hours after a single injection. Pharmacological effects of *phentolamine* are very similar to those of *phenoxybenzamine*. It is used for the diagnosis and short-term management of pheochromocytoma. It is also used locally to prevent dermal necrosis following extravasation of *norepinephrine*. *Phentolamine* is useful to treat hypertensive crisis due to abrupt withdrawal of *clonidine* or ingestion of tyramine-containing foods in patients taking monoamine oxidase inhibitors.

C. Prazosin, terazosin, and doxazosin

Prazosin [PRAY-zoe-sin], *terazosin* [ter-AY-zoe-sin], and *doxazosin* [dox-AY-zoe-sin] are selective competitive blockers of the α_1 receptor. In contrast to *phenoxybenzamine* and *phentolamine*, they are useful in the treatment of hypertension. [Note: *Tamsulosin* [tam-SUE-loh-sin], *alfuzosin* [al-FYOO-zoe-sin], and *silodosin* [sye-LOE-doe-sin] are examples of other selective α_1 antagonists indicated for the treatment of benign prostatic hyperplasia (see Chapter 41).] Metabolism leads to inactive products that are excreted in urine except for those of *doxazosin*, which appear in feces. *Doxazosin* is the longest acting of these drugs.

1. **Mechanism of action:** These agents decrease peripheral vascular resistance and lower blood pressure by causing relaxation of both arterial and venous smooth muscle. Unlike *phenoxybenzamine* and *phentolamine*, these drugs cause minimal changes in cardiac output, renal blood flow, and glomerular filtration rate. *Tamsulosin*, *alfuzosin*, and *silodosin* have less pronounced effects on blood pressure because they are less selective for α_{1B} receptors found in the blood vessels and more selective for α_{1A} receptors in the prostate and bladder. Blockade of the α_{1A} receptors decreases tone in the smooth muscle of the bladder neck and prostate and improves urine flow.

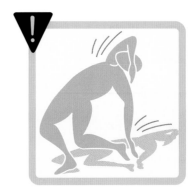

Figure 7.3
First dose of α_1 receptor blocker may produce an orthostatic hypotensive response that can result in syncope (fainting).

2. **Therapeutic uses:** Individuals with elevated blood pressure treated with one of these drugs do not become tolerant to its action. However, the first dose of these drugs may produce an exaggerated orthostatic hypotensive response (Figure 7.3) that can result in syncope (fainting). This action, termed a "first-dose" effect, may be minimized by adjusting the first dose to one-third or one-fourth of the normal dose and by giving the drug at bedtime. These drugs may cause modest improvement in lipid profiles and glucose metabolism in hypertensive patients. Because of inferior cardiovascular outcomes as compared to other antihypertensives, α_1 antagonists are not used as monotherapy for the treatment of hypertension (see Chapter 16).

3. **Adverse effects:** α_1-Blockers such as *prazosin* and *doxazosin* may cause dizziness, a lack of energy, nasal congestion, headache, drowsiness, and orthostatic hypotension (although to a lesser degree than that observed with *phenoxybenzamine* and *phentolamine*). An additive antihypertensive effect occurs when α_1 antagonists are given with vasodilators such as nitrates or PDE-5 inhibitors (for example, *sildenafil*), thereby necessitating cautious dose titration and use at the lowest possible doses. These agents may cause "floppy iris syndrome," a condition in which the iris billows in response to intraoperative eye surgery. Figure 7.4 summarizes some adverse effects observed with α-blockers.

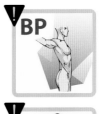

Orthostatic hypotension

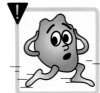

Tachycardia

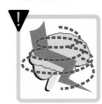

Dizziness and headache

Sexual dysfunction

D. Yohimbine

Yohimbine [yo-HIM-bean] is a selective competitive α_2-blocker that works at the level of the CNS to increase sympathetic outflow to the periphery. It is found as a component of the bark of the yohimbe tree (*Pausinystalia yohimbe*) and has been used as a sexual stimulant and in the treatment of erectile dysfunction. Its use in the treatment of these disorders is not recommended due to lack of demonstrated efficacy.

III. β-ADRENERGIC BLOCKING AGENTS

All of the clinically available β-blockers are competitive antagonists. Nonselective β-blockers act at both β_1 and β_2 receptors, whereas cardioselective β antagonists primarily block β_1 receptors. [Note: There are no clinically useful β_2 selective antagonists.] These drugs also differ in

Figure 7.4
Some adverse effects commonly observed with α-adrenergic blocking agents.

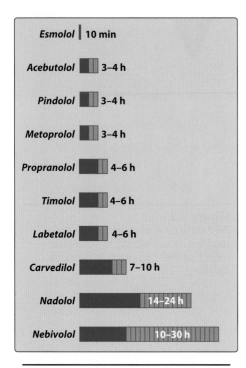

Figure 7.5
Elimination half-lives for some
β-blockers.

intrinsic sympathomimetic activity (ISA), CNS effects, blockade of sympathetic receptors, vasodilation, and pharmacokinetics (Figure 7.5). Although all β-blockers lower blood pressure, they do not induce postural hypotension, because the α-adrenoceptors remain functional. Therefore, normal sympathetic control of the vasculature is maintained. β-Blockers are effective in treating systemic as well as portal hypertension, angina, cardiac arrhythmias, myocardial infarction, heart failure, hyperthyroidism, and glaucoma. They are also used for the prophylaxis of migraine headaches. [Note: The names of all β-blockers end in "-olol" except for *labetalol* and *carvedilol*.]

A. Propranolol: a nonselective β antagonist

Propranolol [proe-PRAN-oh-lole] is the prototype β-adrenergic antagonist and blocks both β_1 and β_2 receptors with equal affinity. Sustained-release preparations for once-a-day dosing are available. Nonselective β-blockers, including *propranolol*, have the ability to block the actions of *isoproterenol* (β_1, β_2 agonist) on the cardiovascular system. Thus, in the presence of a β-blocker, *isoproterenol* does not produce cardiac stimulation (β_1 mediated) or reductions in mean arterial pressure and diastolic pressure (β_2 mediated; Figure 7.2). [Note: In the presence of a nonselective β-blocker, *epinephrine* no longer lowers diastolic blood pressure or stimulates the heart, but its vasoconstrictive action (mediated by α receptors) remains unimpaired. The actions of *norepinephrine* on the cardiovascular system are mediated primarily by α receptors and are, therefore, mostly unaffected.]

1. Actions

   a. Cardiovascular: *Propranolol* diminishes cardiac output, having both negative inotropic and chronotropic effects (Figure 7.6). It directly depresses sinoatrial and atrioventricular nodal activity. The resulting bradycardia usually limits the dose of the drug. During exercise or stress, when the sympathetic nervous system is activated, β-blockers attenuate the expected increase in heart rate. Cardiac output, workload, and oxygen consumption are decreased by blockade of β_1 receptors, and these effects are useful in the treatment of angina (see Chapter 20). The β-blockers are effective in attenuating supraventricular cardiac arrhythmias, but generally are not effective against ventricular arrhythmias (except those induced by exercise).

   b. Peripheral vasoconstriction: Nonselective blockade of β receptors prevents β_2-mediated vasodilation in skeletal muscles, increasing peripheral vascular resistance (Figure 7.6). The reduction in cardiac output produced by all β-blockers leads to decreased blood pressure, which triggers a reflex peripheral vasoconstriction that is reflected in reduced blood flow to the periphery. In patients with hypertension, total peripheral resistance returns to normal or decreases with long-term use of *propranolol* as a result of down regulation of the β receptors. There is a gradual reduction of both systolic and diastolic blood pressures in hypertensive patients.

   c. Bronchoconstriction: Blocking β_2 receptors in the lungs of susceptible patients causes contraction of the bronchiolar smooth muscle (Figure 7.6). This can precipitate an exacerbation in patients with chronic obstructive pulmonary disease (COPD) or asthma. Therefore, β-blockers, particularly nonselective ones, are contraindicated in patients with asthma and should be avoided in COPD.

d. Disturbances in glucose metabolism: β-Blockade leads to decreased glycogenolysis and decreased glucagon secretion. Therefore, if *propranolol* is given to a diabetic patient receiving *insulin*, careful monitoring of blood glucose is essential, because pronounced hypoglycemia may occur after *insulin* injection. β-Blockers also attenuate the normal physiologic response to hypoglycemia. [Note: Diaphoresis with hypoglycemia still occurs, as this is mediated through the neurotransmitter acetylcholine.]

2. Therapeutic uses

a. Hypertension: *Propranolol* does not reduce blood pressure in people with normal blood pressure. *Propranolol* lowers blood pressure in hypertension by several different mechanisms of action. Decreased cardiac output is the primary mechanism, but inhibition of renin release from the kidney, decrease in total peripheral resistance with long-term use, and decreased sympathetic outflow from the CNS also contribute to the antihypertensive effects (see Chapter 16).

b. Angina pectoris: *Propranolol* decreases the oxygen requirement of heart muscle and, therefore, is effective in reducing chest pain on exertion that is common in angina. *Propranolol* is therefore useful in the management of chronic stable angina.

c. Myocardial infarction: *Propranolol* and other β-blockers have a protective effect on the myocardium. Thus, patients who have had one myocardial infarction seem to be protected against a second heart attack by prophylactic use of β-blockers. In addition, administration of a β-blocker immediately following a myocardial infarction reduces infarct size and early mortality. The mechanism for these effects may be a reduction in the actions of circulating catecholamines that increase the oxygen demand in an already ischemic heart muscle. *Propranolol* also reduces the incidence of sudden arrhythmic death after myocardial infarction.

d. Migraine: *Propranolol* is effective in reducing migraine episodes when used prophylactically (see Chapter 37). It is one of the more useful β-blockers for this indication, due to its lipophilic nature that allows it to penetrate the CNS. [Note: For the acute management of migraine, serotonin agonists such as *sumatriptan* are used, as well as other drugs.]

e. Hyperthyroidism: *Propranolol* and other β-blockers are effective in blunting the widespread sympathetic stimulation that occurs in hyperthyroidism. In acute hyperthyroidism (thyroid storm), β-blockers may be lifesaving in protecting against serious cardiac arrhythmias.

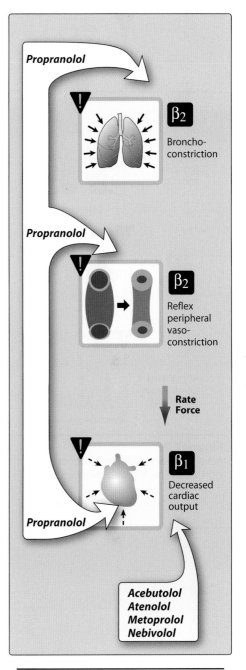

Figure 7.6
Actions of *propranolol* and other β-blockers.

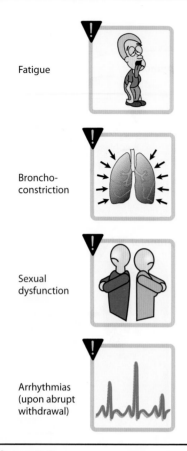

Fatigue

Broncho-
constriction

Sexual
dysfunction

Arrhythmias
(upon abrupt
withdrawal)

Figure 7.7
Adverse effects commonly observed in
individuals treated with *propranolol*.

3. **Pharmacokinetics:** After oral administration, *propranolol* is almost completely absorbed. It is subject to first-pass effect, and only about 25% of an administered dose reaches the circulation. The volume of distribution of *propranolol* is quite large (4 L/kg), and the drug readily crosses the blood–brain barrier due to its high lipophilicity. *Propranolol* is extensively metabolized, and most metabolites are excreted in the urine.

4. **Adverse effects**

   a. **Bronchoconstriction:** *Propranolol* has the potential to cause significant bronchoconstriction due to blockade of β_2 receptors (Figure 7.7). Death by asphyxiation has been reported for patients with asthma who inadvertently received the drug. Therefore, *propranolol* is contraindicated in patients with COPD or asthma.

   b. **Arrhythmias:** Treatment with β-blockers must never be stopped abruptly because of the risk of precipitating cardiac arrhythmias, which may be severe. The β-blockers must be tapered off gradually over a period of at least a few weeks. Long-term treatment with a β antagonist leads to up-regulation of the β receptor. On suspension of therapy, the increased receptors can precipitate worsened angina or hypertension through action of endogenous catecholamines on the up-regulated β receptors.

   c. **Sexual impairment:** Impaired sexual activity has been reported in male patients taking *propranolol*. The reasons for this are not clear and may be independent of β receptor blockade. However, β-blockers do not affect ejaculation (mediated by α receptors).

   d. **Metabolic disturbances:** β-Blockade leads to decreased glycogenolysis and decreased glucagon secretion. Fasting hypoglycemia may occur. In addition, β-blockers can prevent the counterregulatory effects of catecholamines during hypoglycemia. Thus, the perception of symptoms of hypoglycemia such as tremor, tachycardia, and nervousness are blunted by β-blockers. A major role of β receptors is to mobilize energy molecules such as free fatty acids. [Note: Lipases in fat cells are activated mainly by β receptor stimulation, leading to the metabolism of triglycerides into free fatty acids.] Patients administered nonselective β-blockers may have increased triglycerides and reduced high-density lipoprotein ("good" cholesterol) through β-blockade. These effects on the serum lipid profile may be less pronounced with the use of β_1-selective antagonists such as *metoprolol*.

   e. **CNS effects:** *Propranolol* has numerous CNS-mediated effects, including depression, dizziness, lethargy, fatigue, weakness, visual disturbances, hallucinations, short-term memory loss, emotional lability, vivid dreams (including nightmares), and depression. Fewer CNS effects may be seen with more hydrophilic β-blockers (for example, *atenolol*) because they do not cross the blood–brain barrier as readily.

f. Drug interactions: Drugs that interfere with, or inhibit, the metabolism of *propranolol*, such as *cimetidine*, *fluoxetine*, *paroxetine*, and *ritonavir*, may potentiate its antihypertensive effects. Conversely, those that stimulate or induce its metabolism, such as barbiturates, *phenytoin*, and *rifampin*, can decrease its effects. Nonselective β-blockers such as *propranolol* may prevent the rescue effects of *epinephrine* in anaphylaxis.

B. Nadolol and timolol: nonselective β antagonists

Nadolol [NAH-doh-lole] and *timolol* [TIM-o-lole] also block β_1- and β_2-adrenoceptors and are more potent than *propranolol*. *Nadolol* has a very long duration of action (Figure 7.5). *Timolol* reduces the production of aqueous humor in the eye. It is used topically in the treatment of chronic open-angle glaucoma.

1. **Treatment of glaucoma:** β-Blockers, such as topically applied *timolol*, are effective in diminishing intraocular pressure in glaucoma (Figure 7.8). This occurs by decreasing the secretion of aqueous humor by the ciliary body. *Carteolol* [kar-TEE-oh-lol], *levobunolol* [lee-voe-BYOO-noe-lole], and *metipranolol* [met-i-PRAN-oh-lol] are nonselective β antagonists, whereas *betaxolol* [be-TAKS-oh-lol] is a β_1-selective agent. Unlike the cholinergic drugs, these agents neither affect the ability of the eye to focus for near vision nor change pupil size. When administered intraocularly, the onset is about 30 minutes, and the effects last for 12 to 24 hours. The β-blockers are only used for chronic management of glaucoma. In an acute attack of glaucoma, *pilocarpine* is still the drug of choice for emergency lowering of intraocular pressure. Other agents used in the treatment of glaucoma are summarized in Figure 7.8.

CLASS OF DRUG	DRUG NAMES	MECHANISM OF ACTION	SIDE EFFECTS
β-Adrenergic antagonists (topical)	*Betaxolol, carteolol, levobunolol, metipranolol, timolol*	Decrease of aqueous humor production	Ocular irritation; contraindicated in patients with asthma, obstructive airway disease, bradycardia, and congestive heart failure.
α-Adrenergic agonists (topical)	*Apraclonidine, brimonidine*	Decrease of aqueous humor production and increase of aqueous outflow	Red eye and ocular irritation, allergic reactions, malaise, and headache.
Cholinergic agonists (topical)	*Pilocarpine, carbachol*	Increase of aqueous outflow	Eye or brow pain, increased myopia, and decreased vision.
Prostaglandin-like analogues (topical)	*Latanoprost, travoprost, bimatoprost*	Increase of aqueous humor outflow	Red eye and ocular irritation, increased iris pigmentation, and excessive hair growth of eye lashes.
Carbonic anhydrase inhibitors (topical and systemic)	*Dorzolamide* and *brinzolamide* (topical), *acetazolamide*, and *methazolamide* (oral)	Decrease of aqueous humor production	Transient myopia, nausea, diarrhea, loss of appetite and taste, and renal stones (oral drugs).

Figure 7.8
Classes of drugs used to treat glaucoma.

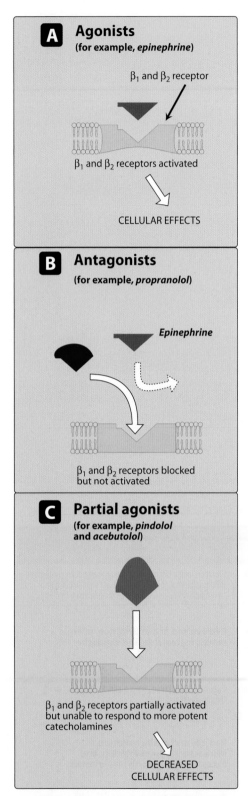

A **Agonists**
(for example, *epinephrine*)

β₁ and β₂ receptor

β₁ and β₂ receptors activated

CELLULAR EFFECTS

B **Antagonists**
(for example, *propranolol*)

Epinephrine

β₁ and β₂ receptors blocked
but not activated

C **Partial agonists**
(for example, *pindolol*
and *acebutolol*)

β₁ and β₂ receptors partially activated
but unable to respond to more potent
catecholamines

DECREASED
CELLULAR EFFECTS

Figure 7.9
Comparison of agonists, antagonists,
and partial agonists of β-adrenoceptors.

C. Acebutolol, atenolol, betaxolol, bisoprolol, esmolol, metoprolol, and nebivolol: selective β₁ antagonists

Drugs that preferentially block the β₁ receptors minimize the unwanted bronchoconstriction (β₂ effect) seen with use of nonselective agents in asthma patients. Cardioselective β-blockers, such as *acebutolol* [a-se-BYOO-toe-lole], *atenolol* [a-TEN-oh-lole], and *metoprolol* [me-TOE-proe-lole], antagonize β₁ receptors at doses 50- to 100-fold less than those required to block β₂ receptors. This cardioselectivity is most pronounced at low doses and is lost at high doses. [Note: Because β₁ selectivity of these agents is lost at high doses, they may antagonize β₂ receptors.]

1. **Actions:** These drugs lower blood pressure in hypertension and increase exercise tolerance in angina (Figure 7.6). *Esmolol* [EZ-moe-lole] has a very short half-life (Figure 7.5) due to metabolism of an ester linkage. It is only available intravenously and is used to control blood pressure or heart rhythm in critically ill patients and those undergoing surgery or diagnostic procedures. In addition to its cardioselective β-blockade, *nebivolol* [ne-BIV-oh-lole] releases nitric oxide from endothelial cells and causes vasodilation. In contrast to *propranolol*, the cardioselective β-blockers have fewer effects on pulmonary function, peripheral resistance, and carbohydrate metabolism. Nevertheless, asthma patients treated with these agents must be carefully monitored to make certain that respiratory activity is not compromised. Because these drugs have less effect on peripheral vascular β₂ receptors, coldness of extremities (Raynaud phenomenon), a common side effect of β-blockers, is less frequent.

2. **Therapeutic uses:** The cardioselective β-blockers are useful in hypertensive patients with impaired pulmonary function. These agents are also first-line therapy for chronic stable angina. *Bisoprolol* and the extended-release formulation of *metoprolol* are indicated for the management of chronic heart failure.

D. Acebutolol and pindolol: antagonists with partial agonist activity

1. **Actions**

   a. **Cardiovascular:** *Acebutolol* (β₁-selective antagonist) and *pindolol* (nonselective β-blocker) [PIN-doe-lole] are not pure antagonists. These drugs can also weakly stimulate both β₁ and β₂ receptors (Figure 7.9) and are said to have ISA. These partial agonists stimulate the β receptor to which they are bound, yet they inhibit stimulation by the more potent endogenous catecholamines, epinephrine and norepinephrine. The result of these opposing actions is a diminished effect on reduction of cardiac rate and cardiac output compared to that of β-blockers without ISA.

   b. **Decreased metabolic effects:** β-Blockers with ISA minimize the disturbances of lipid and carbohydrate metabolism that are seen with other β-blockers. For example, these agents do not decrease plasma HDL levels.

2. **Therapeutic use:** β-Blockers with ISA are effective in hypertensive patients with moderate bradycardia, because a further decrease in heart rate is less pronounced with these drugs. [Note:

β-blockers with ISA are not used for stable angina or arrhythmias due to their partial agonist effect.] Overall, β-blockers with ISA are infrequently used in clinical practice. Figure 7.10 summarizes some of the indications for β-blockers.

E. Labetalol and carvedilol: antagonists of both α- and β-adrenoceptors

1. **Actions:** *Labetalol* [lah-BET-a-lole] and *carvedilol* [CAR-ve-dil-ol] are nonselective β-blockers with concurrent α_1-blocking actions that produce peripheral vasodilation, thereby reducing blood pressure. They contrast with the other β-blockers that produce initial peripheral vasoconstriction, and these agents are, therefore, useful in treating hypertensive patients for whom increased peripheral vascular resistance is undesirable. *Carvedilol* also decreases lipid peroxidation and vascular wall thickening, effects that have benefit in heart failure.

2. **Therapeutic use in hypertension and heart failure:** *Labetalol* is used as an alternative to *methyldopa* in the treatment of pregnancy-induced hypertension. Intravenous *labetalol* is also used to treat hypertensive emergencies, because it can rapidly lower blood pressure (see Chapter 16). β-Blockers should not be given to patients with an acute exacerbation of heart failure, as they can worsen the condition. However, *carvedilol* as well as *metoprolol* and *bisoprolol* are beneficial in patients with stable chronic heart failure. These agents work by blocking the effects of sympathetic stimulation on the heart, which causes worsening heart failure over time (see Chapter 18).

3. **Adverse effects:** Orthostatic hypotension and dizziness are associated with α_1-blockade. Figure 7.11 summarizes the receptor specificities and uses of the β-adrenergic antagonists.

IV. DRUGS AFFECTING NEUROTRANSMITTER RELEASE OR UPTAKE

Some agents act on the adrenergic neuron, either to interfere with neurotransmitter release from storage vesicles or to alter the uptake of the neurotransmitter into the adrenergic neuron. However, due to the advent of newer and more effective agents with fewer side effects, these agents are seldom used therapeutically. *Reserpine* [re-SER-peen] is one of the remaining agents in this category.

Reserpine, a plant alkaloid, blocks the Mg^{2+}/adenosine triphosphate–dependent transport of biogenic amines (norepinephrine, dopamine, and serotonin) from the cytoplasm into storage vesicles in the adrenergic nerve terminals in all body tissues. This causes the ultimate depletion of biogenic amines. Sympathetic function, in general, is impaired because of decreased release of norepinephrine. *Reserpine* has a slow onset, a long duration of action, and effects that persist for many days after discontinuation. It has been used for the management of hypertension but has largely been replaced with newer agents with better side effect profiles and fewer drug interactions. It is also indicated in agitated psychotic states such as schizophrenia to relieve symptoms.

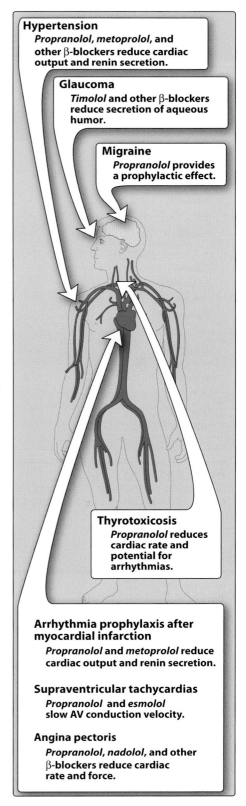

Hypertension
Propranolol, metoprolol, and other β-blockers reduce cardiac output and renin secretion.

Glaucoma
Timolol and other β-blockers reduce secretion of aqueous humor.

Migraine
Propranolol provides a prophylactic effect.

Thyrotoxicosis
Propranolol reduces cardiac rate and potential for arrhythmias.

Arrhythmia prophylaxis after myocardial infarction
Propranolol and *metoprolol* reduce cardiac output and renin secretion.

Supraventricular tachycardias
Propranolol and *esmolol* slow AV conduction velocity.

Angina pectoris
Propranolol, nadolol, and other β-blockers reduce cardiac rate and force.

Figure 7.10
Some clinical applications of β-blockers. AV = atrioventricular.

DRUG	RECEPTOR SPECIFICITY	THERAPEUTIC USES
Propranolol	β_1, β_2	**Hypertension** **Migraine** **Hyperthyroidism** **Angina pectoris** **Myocardial infarction**
Nadolol *Pindolol*[1]	β_1, β_2	**Hypertension**
Timolol	β_1, β_2	**Glaucoma, hypertension**
Atenolol *Bisoprolol*[2] *Esmolol* *Metoprolol*[2]	β_1	**Hypertension** **Angina** **Myocardial infarction** **Atrial fibrillation**
Acebutolol[1]	β_1	**Hypertension**
Nebivolol	β_1, NO ↑	**Hypertension**
Carvedilol[2] *Labetalol*	$\alpha_1, \beta_1, \beta_2$	**Hypertension**

Figure 7.11
Summary of β-adrenergic antagonists. NO = nitric oxide. [1]*Acebutolol* and *pindolol* are partial agonists, as well. [2]*Bisoprolol*, *metoprolol*, and *carvedilol* are also used for the treatment of heart failure.

Study Questions

Choose the ONE best answer.

7.1 A 60-year-old patient started a new antihypertensive medication. His blood pressure is well controlled, but he complains of fatigue, drowsiness, and fainting when he gets up from the bed (orthostatic hypotension). Which of the following drugs is he most likely taking?

A. Metoprolol
B. Propranolol
C. Prazosin
D. Alfuzosin

Correct answer = C. Because they block α_1-mediated vaso-constriction, α-blockers (prazosin) are more likely to cause orthostatic hypotension, as compared to β-blockers (metoprolol, propranolol). Alfuzosin is a more selective antagonist for α_{1A} receptors in the prostate and bladder and is less likely to cause hypotension than prazosin.

7.2 A 30-year-old male patient was brought to the ER with amphetamine overdose. He presented with high blood pressure and arrhythmias. Which drug is the most appropriate to treat the cardiovascular symptoms of amphetamine overdose in this patient?

A. Metoprolol
B. Prazosin
C. Labetalol
D. Nebivolol

Correct answer = C. Amphetamine is an indirect adrenergic agonist that mainly enhances the release of norepinephrine from peripheral sympathetic neurons. Therefore, it activates all types of adrenergic receptors (that is, α and β receptors) and causes an increase in blood pressure. Since both α and β receptors are activated indirectly by amphetamine, α-blockers (prazosin) or β-blockers (metoprolol, nebivolol) alone cannot relieve the cardiovascular effects of amphetamine poisoning. Labetalol blocks both α_1 and beta receptors and can minimize the cardiovascular effects of amphetamine overdose.

7.3 A new antihypertensive drug was tested in an animal model of hypertension. The drug when given alone reduces blood pressure in the animal. Norepinephrine when given in the presence of this drug did not cause any significant change in blood pressure or heart rate in the animal. The mechanism of action of the new drug is similar to which of the following agents?

A. Doxazosin
B. Clonidine
C. Atenolol
D. Carvedilol

Correct answer = D. Norepinephrine activates both α_1 and β_1 receptors and causes an increase in heart rate and blood pressure. A drug that prevents the increase in blood pressure caused by norepinephrine should be similar to carvedilol that antagonizes both α_1 and β_1 receptors. Doxazosin is an α_1 antagonist, clonidine is an α_2 agonist, and atenolol is a β antagonist, and these drugs cannot completely prevent the cardiovascular effects of norepinephrine.

7.4 A β-blocker was prescribed for hypertension in a patient with asthma. After a week of treatment, the asthma attacks got worse, and the patient was asked to stop taking the β-blocker. Which β-blocker would you suggest as an alternative that is less likely to worsen the asthma?

A. Propranolol
B. Metoprolol
C. Labetalol
D. Carvedilol

Correct answer = B. The patient was most likely given a nonselective β-blocker (antagonizes both β_1 and β_2 receptors) that made the asthma worse due to β_2 antagonism. An alternative is to prescribe a cardioselective (antagonizes only β_1) β-blocker that does not antagonize β_2 receptors in the bronchioles. Metoprolol is a cardioselective β-blocker. Propranolol, labetalol, and carvedilol are nonselective β-blockers and could worsen the asthma.

7.5 A 70-year-old male is treated with doxazosin for overflow incontinence due to his enlarged prostate. He complains of dizzy spells while getting up from bed at night. Which drug would you suggest as an alternative that may not cause dizziness?

A. Propranolol
B. Phentolamine
C. Tamsulosin
D. Terazosin

Correct answer = C. Dizziness in this elderly patient could be due to orthostatic hypotension caused by doxazosin. Tamsulosin is an α_1 antagonist that is more selective to the α_1 receptor subtype (α_{1A}) present in the prostate and less selective to the α_1 receptor subtype (α_{1B}) present in the blood vessels. Therefore, tamsulosin should not affect blood pressure significantly and may not cause dizziness. Terazosin and phentolamine antagonize both these subtypes and cause significant hypotension as a side effect. Propranolol is a nonselective beta-blocker that is not indicated in overflow incontinence.

7.6 A 50-year-old male was in anaphylactic shock after being stung by a hornet. The medical team tried to reverse the bronchoconstriction and hypotension using epinephrine; however, the patient did not fully respond to the treatment. The patient's wife mentioned that he is taking a prescription medication for blood pressure. Which medication is he most likely taking that contributed to a reduced response to epinephrine?

A. Doxazosin
B. Propranolol
C. Metoprolol
D. Acebutolol

Correct answer = B. Epinephrine reverses hypotension by activating β_1 receptors and relieves bronchoconstriction by activating β_2 receptors in anaphylaxis. Since epinephrine was not effective in reversing hypotension or bronchoconstriction in this patient, it could be assumed that the patient was on a nonselective β-blocker (propranolol). Doxazosin (α_1-blocker), metoprolol, or acebutolol (both β_1-selective blockers) would not have completely prevented the effects of epinephrine.

7.7 Which of the following is correct regarding α-adrenergic blockers?

A. α-Adrenergic blockers are used in the treatment of hypotension in anaphylactic shock.
B. α-Adrenergic blockers are used in the treatment of benign prostatic hyperplasia (BPH).
C. α-Adrenergic blockers may cause bradycardia.
D. α-Adrenergic blockers reduce the frequency of urination.

Correct answer = B. α-Adrenergic blockers are used in the treatment of BPH because of their relaxant effect on prostate smooth muscles. Being antihypertensive agents, they are not useful in treating hypotension in anaphylaxis. α-Adrenergic blockers generally cause reflex tachycardia (not bradycardia) due to the significant drop in blood pressure caused by them. They increase (not reduce) the frequency of urination by relaxing the internal sphincter of the urinary bladder, which is controlled by α_1 receptors.

7.8 Which of the following is correct regarding β-blockers?

A. Treatment with β-blockers should not be stopped abruptly.
B. Propranolol is a cardioselective β-blocker.
C. Cardioselective β-blockers worsen asthma.
D. β-Blockers decrease peripheral resistance by causing vasorelaxation.

Correct answer = A. If β-blocker therapy is stopped abruptly, that could cause angina and rebound hypertension. This could be due to the up-regulation of β receptors in the body. β-Blockers do not cause direct vasorelaxation. Therefore, they do not decrease peripheral resistance with short-term use. Propranolol is a nonselective β-blocker (not cardioselective). Cardioselective β-blockers antagonize only $β_1$ receptors and do not worsen asthma, as they do not antagonize $β_2$ receptors.

7.9 Which of the following drugs is commonly used topically in the treatment of glaucoma?

A. Esmolol
B. Timolol
C. Silodosin
D. Yohimbine

Correct answer = B. β-Blockers reduce the formation of aqueous humor in the eye and therefore reduce intraocular pressure, thus relieving glaucoma. Timolol is a nonselective β-blocker that is commonly used topically to treat glaucoma. Esmolol is a short-acting β-blocker that is used intravenously for hypertension or arrhythmias. Silodosin is an $α_1$ antagonist used for BPH, and yohimbine is a $α_2$ antagonist used for sexual dysfunction.

7.10 Which of the following drugs has the highest potential to worsen orthostatic hypotension when given together with prazosin?

A. Propranolol
B. Atenolol
C. Nebivolol
D. Labetalol

Correct answer = D. Labetalol is a nonselective β-blocker with $α_1$-blocking activity. Prazosin causes orthostatic hypotension due to its $α_1$-blockade, which could be enhanced by adding labetalol. Propranolol, atenolol and nebivolol do not have $α_1$-blocking effects.

Drugs for Neurodegenerative Diseases

Jose A. Rey

8

I. OVERVIEW

Most drugs that affect the central nervous system (CNS) act by altering some step in the neurotransmission process. Drugs affecting the CNS may act presynaptically by influencing the production, storage, release, or termination of action of neurotransmitters. Other agents may activate or block postsynaptic receptors. This chapter provides an overview of the CNS, with a focus on those neurotransmitters that are involved in the actions of the clinically useful CNS drugs. These concepts are useful in understanding the etiology and treatment strategies for the neurodegenerative disorders that respond to drug therapy: Parkinson disease, Alzheimer disease, multiple sclerosis (MS), and amyotrophic lateral sclerosis (ALS) (Figure 8.1).

II. NEUROTRANSMISSION IN THE CNS

The basic functioning of neurons in the CNS is similar to that of the autonomic nervous system (ANS) described in Chapter 3. For example, transmission of information in both the CNS and in the periphery involves the

ANTI-PARKINSON DRUGS
Amantadine GOCOVRI
Apomorphine APOKYN
Benztropine COGENTIN
Bromocriptine PARLODEL
Carbidopa LODOSYN
Entacapone COMTAN
Levodopa (w/ Carbidopa) SINEMET
Levodopa (w/ Carbidopa+ Entacapone) STALEVO
Pramipexole MIRAPEX
Rasagiline AZILECT
Ropinirole REQUIP
Rotigotine NEUPRO
Safinamide XADAGO
Selegiline (Deprenyl) ELDEPRYL, ZELAPAR
Tolcapone TASMAR
Trihexyphenidyl GENERIC ONLY

ANTI-ALZHEIMER DRUGS
Donepezil ARICEPT
Galantamine RAZADYNE
Memantine NAMENDA
Rivastigmine EXELON

Figure 8.1
Summary of agents used in the treatment of Parkinson disease, Alzheimer disease, multiple sclerosis, and amyotrophic lateral sclerosis. (Figure continues on next page)

103

ANTI-MULTIPLE SCLEROSIS DRUGS

*Alemtuzumab*LEMTRADA
Azathioprine AZASAN, IMURAN
*Cyclophosphamide*GENERIC ONLY
*Daclizumab*ZINBRYTA
*Dalfampridine*AMPYRA
*Dexamethasone*DECADRON
*Dimethyl fumarate*TECFIDERA
*Fingolimod*GILENYA
*Glatiramer*COPAXONE
Interferon β_{1a} AVONEX, REBIF
Interferon β_{1b} BETASERON, EXTAVIA
*Natalizumab*TYSABRI
*Ocrelizumab*OCREVUS
*Prednisone*DELTASONE
*Teriflunomide*AUBAGIO

ANTI-ALS DRUGS

*Edaravone*RADICAVA
*Riluzole*RILUTEK

Figure 8.1 (continued)
Summary of agents used in the treatment of Parkinson disease, Alzheimer disease, multiple sclerosis, and amyotrophic lateral sclerosis.

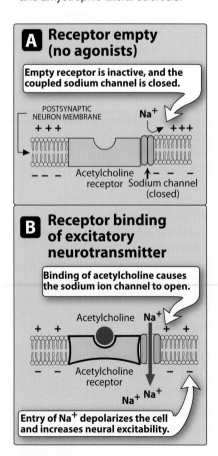

A **Receptor empty (no agonists)**

Empty receptor is inactive, and the coupled sodium channel is closed.

POSTSYNAPTIC NEURON MEMBRANE
+ + +   Na$^+$ + + +
Acetylcholine   – – –
receptor   Sodium channel
(closed)

B **Receptor binding of excitatory neurotransmitter**

Binding of acetylcholine causes the sodium ion channel to open.

Acetylcholine Na$^+$
+ +   + +
– –   Acetylcholine   – –
receptor
Na$^+$ Na$^+$
Na$^+$

Entry of Na$^+$ depolarizes the cell and increases neural excitability.

Figure 8.2
Binding of the excitatory neurotransmitter, acetylcholine, causes depolarization of the neuron.

release of neurotransmitters that diffuse across the synaptic cleft to bind to specific receptors on the postsynaptic neuron. In both systems, the recognition of the neurotransmitter by the membrane receptor of the postsynaptic neuron triggers intracellular changes. However, several major differences exist between neurons in the peripheral ANS and those in the CNS. The circuitry of the CNS is more complex than that of the ANS, and the number of synapses in the CNS is far greater. The CNS, unlike the peripheral ANS, contains networks of inhibitory neurons that are constantly active in modulating the rate of neuronal transmission. In addition, the CNS communicates through the use of multiple neurotransmitters, whereas the ANS uses only two primary neurotransmitters, acetylcholine, and norepinephrine.

III. SYNAPTIC POTENTIALS

In the CNS, receptors in most synapses are coupled to ion channels. Binding of the neurotransmitter to the postsynaptic membrane receptors results in a rapid but transient opening of ion channels. Open channels allow specific ions inside and outside the cell membrane to flow down their concentration gradients. The resulting change in the ionic composition across the membrane of the neuron alters the postsynaptic potential, producing either depolarization or hyperpolarization of the postsynaptic membrane, depending on the specific ions and the direction of their movement.

A. Excitatory pathways

Neurotransmitters can be classified as either excitatory or inhibitory, depending on the nature of the action they elicit. Stimulation of excitatory neurons causes a movement of ions that results in a depolarization of the postsynaptic membrane. These excitatory postsynaptic potentials (EPSP) are generated by the following: 1) Stimulation of an excitatory neuron causes the release of neurotransmitters, such as glutamate or acetylcholine, which bind to receptors on the postsynaptic cell membrane. This causes a transient increase in the permeability of sodium (Na$^+$) ions. 2) The influx of Na$^+$ causes a weak depolarization, or EPSP, that moves the postsynaptic potential toward its firing threshold. 3) If the number of stimulated excitatory neurons increases, more excitatory neurotransmitter is released. This ultimately causes the EPSP depolarization of the postsynaptic cell to pass a threshold, thereby generating an all-or-none action potential. [Note: The generation of a nerve impulse typically reflects the activation of synaptic receptors by thousands of excitatory neurotransmitter molecules released from many nerve fibers.] Figure 8.2 shows an example of an excitatory pathway.

B. Inhibitory pathways

Stimulation of inhibitory neurons causes movement of ions that results in a hyperpolarization of the postsynaptic membrane. These inhibitory postsynaptic potentials (IPSP) are generated by the following: 1) Stimulation of inhibitory neurons releases neurotransmitters, such as γ-aminobutyric acid (GABA) or glycine, which bind to receptors on the postsynaptic cell membrane. This causes a transient increase in the permeability of specific ions, such as potassium (K$^+$) and chloride (Cl$^-$). 2) The influx of Cl$^-$ and efflux of K$^+$ cause a weak hyperpolarization, or IPSP, that moves the postsynaptic potential away from its firing threshold. This diminishes the generation of action potentials. Figure 8.3 shows an example of an inhibitory pathway.

C. Combined effects of the EPSP and IPSP

Most neurons in the CNS receive both EPSP and IPSP input. Thus, several different types of neurotransmitters may act on the same neuron, but each binds to its own specific receptor. The overall action is the summation of the individual actions of the various neurotransmitters on the neuron. The neurotransmitters are not uniformly distributed in the CNS but are localized in specific clusters of neurons, the axons of which may synapse with specific regions of the brain. Many neuronal tracts, thus, seem to be chemically coded, and this may offer greater opportunity for selective pharmacological modulation of certain neuronal pathways.

IV. NEURODEGENERATIVE DISEASES

Neurodegenerative diseases of the CNS include Parkinson disease, Alzheimer disease, MS, and ALS. These devastating illnesses are characterized by the progressive loss of selected neurons in discrete brain areas, resulting in characteristic disorders of movement, cognition, or both.

V. OVERVIEW OF PARKINSON DISEASE

Parkinsonism is a progressive neurological disorder of muscle movement, characterized by tremors, muscular rigidity, bradykinesia, and postural and gait abnormalities. Most cases involve people over the age of 65, among whom the incidence is about 1 in 100 individuals.

A. Etiology

The cause of Parkinson disease is unknown for most patients. The disease is correlated with destruction of dopaminergic neurons in the substantia nigra with a consequent reduction of dopamine actions in the corpus striatum, parts of the basal ganglia system that are involved in motor control.

1. **Substantia nigra:** The substantia nigra, part of the extrapyramidal system, is the source of dopaminergic neurons (shown in *red* in Figure 8.4) that terminate in the neostriatum. Each dopaminergic neuron makes thousands of synaptic contacts within the neostriatum and therefore modulates the activity of a large number of cells. These dopaminergic projections from the substantia nigra fire tonically rather than in response to specific muscular movements or sensory input. Thus, the dopaminergic system appears to serve as a tonic, sustaining influence on motor activity, rather than participating in specific movements.

2. **Neostriatum:** Normally, the neostriatum is connected to the substantia nigra by neurons (shown in *orange* in Figure 8.4) that secrete the inhibitory transmitter GABA at their termini. In turn, cells of the substantia nigra send neurons back to the neostriatum, secreting the inhibitory transmitter dopamine at their termini. This mutual inhibitory pathway normally maintains a degree of inhibition

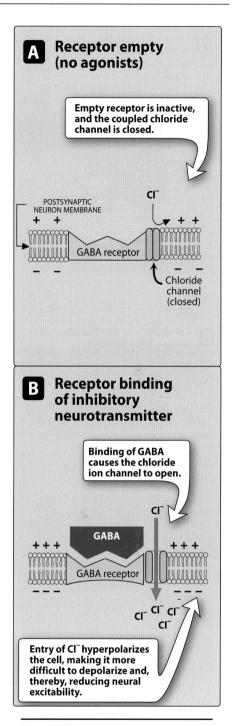

A **Receptor empty (no agonists)**

Empty receptor is inactive, and the coupled chloride channel is closed.

POSTSYNAPTIC NEURON MEMBRANE

GABA receptor

Cl⁻

Chloride channel (closed)

B **Receptor binding of inhibitory neurotransmitter**

Binding of GABA causes the chloride ion channel to open.

Cl⁻

GABA

GABA receptor

Cl⁻ Cl⁻ Cl⁻
Cl⁻

Entry of Cl⁻ hyperpolarizes the cell, making it more difficult to depolarize and, thereby, reducing neural excitability.

Figure 8.3
Binding of the inhibitory neurotransmitter, γ-aminobutyric acid (GABA), causes hyperpolarization of the neuron.

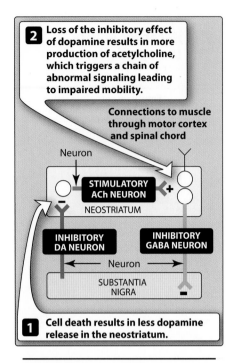

2 Loss of the inhibitory effect of dopamine results in more production of acetylcholine, which triggers a chain of abnormal signaling leading to impaired mobility.

Connections to muscle through motor cortex and spinal chord

Neuron

STIMULATORY ACh NEURON

NEOSTRIATUM

INHIBITORY DA NEURON

INHIBITORY GABA NEURON

Neuron

SUBSTANTIA NIGRA

1 Cell death results in less dopamine release in the neostriatum.

Figure 8.4
Role of substantia nigra in Parkinson disease. ACh = acetylcholine; DA = dopamine; GABA = γ-aminobutyric acid.

of both areas. In Parkinson disease, destruction of cells in the substantia nigra results in the degeneration of the nerve terminals that secrete dopamine in the neostriatum. Thus, the normal inhibitory influence of dopamine on cholinergic neurons in the neostriatum is significantly diminished, resulting in overproduction, or a relative overactivity, of acetylcholine by the stimulatory neurons (shown in *green* in Figure 8.4). This triggers a chain of abnormal signaling, resulting in loss of the control of muscle movements.

3. **Secondary parkinsonism:** Drugs such as the phenothiazines and *haloperidol*, whose major pharmacologic action is blockade of dopamine receptors in the brain, may produce parkinsonian symptoms (also called pseudoparkinsonism). These drugs should be used with caution in patients with Parkinson disease.

B. Strategy of treatment

In addition to an abundance of inhibitory dopaminergic neurons, the neostriatum is also rich in excitatory cholinergic neurons that oppose the action of dopamine (Figure 8.4). Many of the symptoms of parkinsonism reflect an imbalance between the excitatory cholinergic neurons and the greatly diminished number of inhibitory dopaminergic neurons. Therapy is aimed at restoring dopamine in the basal ganglia and antagonizing the excitatory effect of cholinergic neurons, thus reestablishing the correct dopamine/acetylcholine balance.

VI. DRUGS USED IN PARKINSON DISEASE

Many currently available drugs aim to maintain CNS dopamine levels, or signaling, as constant as possible. These agents offer temporary relief from the symptoms of the disorder, but they do not arrest or reverse the neuronal degeneration caused by the disease.

A. Levodopa and carbidopa

Levodopa [lee-voe-DOE-pa] is a metabolic precursor of dopamine (Figure 8.5). It restores dopaminergic neurotransmission in the neostriatum by enhancing the synthesis of dopamine in the surviving neurons of the substantia nigra. In early disease, the number of residual dopaminergic neurons in the substantia nigra (typically about 20% of normal) is adequate for conversion of *levodopa* to dopamine. Thus, in new patients, the therapeutic response to *levodopa* is consistent, and the patient rarely complains that the drug effects "wear off." Unfortunately, with time, the number of neurons decreases, and fewer cells are capable of converting exogenously administered *levodopa* to dopamine. Consequently, motor control fluctuation develops. Relief provided by *levodopa* is only symptomatic, and it lasts only while the drug is present in the body.

1. **Mechanism of action**

   a. **Levodopa:** Dopamine does not cross the blood–brain barrier, but its immediate precursor, *levodopa*, is actively transported into the CNS and converted to dopamine (Figure 8.5). *Levodopa* must be administered with *carbidopa* [kar-bi-DOE-pa]. Without

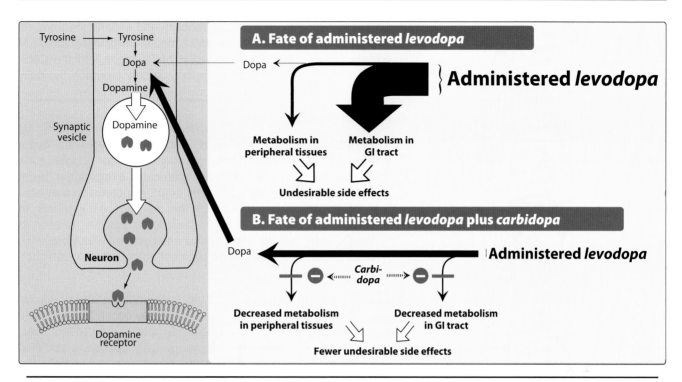

Figure 8.5
Synthesis of dopamine from *levodopa* in the absence and presence of *carbidopa*, an inhibitor of dopamine decarboxylase in the peripheral tissues. (GI = gastrointestinal.)

carbidopa, much of the drug is decarboxylated to dopamine in the periphery, resulting in diminished effect, nausea, vomiting, cardiac arrhythmias, and hypotension.

b. Carbidopa: *Carbidopa*, a dopamine decarboxylase inhibitor, diminishes the metabolism of *levodopa* in the periphery, thereby increasing the availability of *levodopa* to the CNS. The addition of *carbidopa* lowers the dose of *levodopa* needed by four- to five-fold and, consequently, decreases the severity of adverse effects arising from peripherally formed dopamine.

2. Therapeutic uses: *Levodopa* in combination with *carbidopa* is an efficacious drug regimen for the treatment of Parkinson disease. It decreases rigidity, tremors, and other symptoms of parkinsonism. In approximately two-thirds of patients with Parkinson disease, *levodopa–carbidopa* substantially reduces the severity of symptoms for the first few years of treatment. Patients typically experience a decline in response during the 3rd to 5th year of therapy. Withdrawal from the drug must be gradual.

3. Absorption and metabolism: The drug is absorbed rapidly from the small intestine (when empty of food). *Levodopa* has an extremely short half-life (1 to 2 hours), which causes fluctuations in plasma concentration. This may produce fluctuations in motor response, which generally correlate with the plasma concentration of *levodopa*, or perhaps give rise to the more troublesome "on–off" phenomenon, in which the motor fluctuations are not related to plasma levels in a simple way. Motor fluctuations may cause the

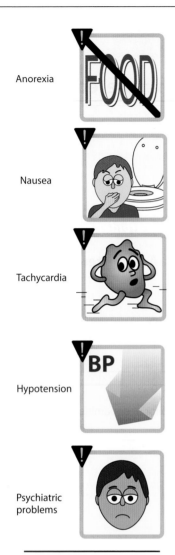

Anorexia

Nausea

Tachycardia

Hypotension

Psychiatric problems

Figure 8.6
Adverse effects of *levodopa*.

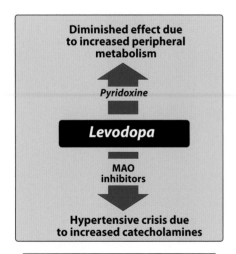

Diminished effect due to increased peripheral metabolism

Pyridoxine

Levodopa

MAO inhibitors

Hypertensive crisis due to increased catecholamines

Figure 8.7
Some drug interactions observed with *levodopa*. MAO = monoamine oxidase.

patient to suddenly lose normal mobility and experience tremors, cramps, and immobility. Ingestion of meals, particularly if high in protein, interferes with the transport of *levodopa* into the CNS. Thus, *levodopa* should be taken on an empty stomach, typically 30 minutes before a meal.

4. Adverse effects

a. **Peripheral effects:** Anorexia, nausea, and vomiting occur because of stimulation of the chemoreceptor trigger zone (Figure 8.6). Tachycardia and ventricular extrasystole result from dopaminergic action on the heart. Hypotension may also develop. Adrenergic action on the iris causes mydriasis. In some individuals, blood dyscrasias and a positive reaction to the Coombs test are seen. Saliva and urine may turn brownish color because of the melanin pigment produced from catecholamine oxidation.

b. **CNS effects:** Visual and auditory hallucinations and abnormal involuntary movements (dyskinesias) may occur. These effects are the opposite of parkinsonian symptoms and reflect overactivity of dopamine in the basal ganglia. *Levodopa* can also cause mood changes, depression, psychosis, and anxiety.

5. Interactions: The vitamin pyridoxine (B_6) increases the peripheral breakdown of *levodopa* and diminishes its effectiveness (Figure 8.7). Concomitant administration of *levodopa* and nonselective monoamine oxidase inhibitors (MAOIs), such as *phenelzine*, can produce a hypertensive crisis caused by enhanced catecholamine production. Therefore, concomitant administration of these agents is contraindicated. In many psychotic patients, *levodopa* exacerbates symptoms, possibly through the buildup of central catecholamines. Cardiac patients should be carefully monitored for the possible development of arrhythmias. Antipsychotic drugs are generally contraindicated in Parkinson disease, because they potently block dopamine receptors and may augment parkinsonian symptoms. However, low doses of atypical antipsychotics, such as *quetiapine* or *clozapine*, are sometimes used to treat *levodopa*-induced psychotic symptoms.

B. Selegiline, rasagiline, and safinamide

Selegiline [seh-LEDGE-ah-leen], also called *deprenyl* [DE-pre-nill], selectively inhibits monoamine oxidase (MAO) type B, the enzyme that metabolizes dopamine. It does not inhibit MAO type A (metabolizes norepinephrine and serotonin) unless given above recommended doses, where it loses its selectivity. By decreasing the metabolism of dopamine, *selegiline* increases dopamine levels in the brain (Figure 8.8). When *selegiline* is administered with *levodopa*, it enhances the actions of *levodopa* and substantially reduces the required dose. Unlike nonselective MAOIs, *selegiline* at recommended doses has little potential for causing hypertensive crises. However, the drug loses selectivity at high doses, and there is a risk for severe hypertension. *Selegiline* is metabolized to *methamphetamine* and *amphetamine*, whose stimulating properties may produce insomnia if the drug is administered later than mid-afternoon.

Rasagiline [ra-SA-gi-leen], an irreversible and selective inhibitor of brain MAO type B, has five times the potency of *selegiline*. Unlike *selegiline*, *rasagiline* is not metabolized to an *amphetamine*-like substance. *Safinamide* [sa-FIN-a-mide] is also a selective inhibitor of MAO type B indicated for use as an adjunct to *levodopa–carbidopa*.

C. Catechol-*O*-methyltransferase inhibitors

Normally, the methylation of *levodopa* by catechol-*O*-methyltransferase (COMT) to 3-*O*-methyldopa is a minor pathway for *levodopa* metabolism. However, when peripheral dopamine decarboxylase activity is inhibited by *carbidopa*, a significant concentration of 3-*O*-methyldopa is formed that competes with *levodopa* for active transport into the CNS (Figure 8.9). *Entacapone* [en-TAK-a-pone] and *tolcapone* [TOLE-ka-pone] selectively and reversibly inhibit COMT. Inhibition of COMT by these agents leads to decreased plasma concentrations of 3-*O*-methyldopa, increased central uptake of *levodopa*, and greater concentrations of brain dopamine. Both of these agents reduce the symptoms of "wearing-off" phenomena seen in patients on *levodopa–carbidopa*. The two drugs differ primarily in their pharmacokinetic and adverse effect profiles.

1. **Pharmacokinetics:** Oral absorption of both drugs occurs readily and is not influenced by food. They are extensively bound to plasma albumin, with a limited volume of distribution. *Tolcapone* has a relatively long duration of action (probably due to its affinity for the enzyme) compared to *entacapone*, which requires more frequent dosing. Both drugs are extensively metabolized and eliminated in feces and urine. The dosage may need to be adjusted in patients with moderate or severe cirrhosis.

2. **Adverse effects:** Both drugs exhibit adverse effects that are observed in patients taking *levodopa–carbidopa*, including diarrhea, postural hypotension, nausea, anorexia, dyskinesias, hallucinations, and sleep disorders. Most seriously, fulminating hepatic necrosis is associated with *tolcapone* use. Therefore, it should be used, along

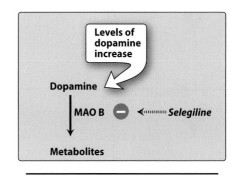

Figure 8.8
Action of *selegiline* (*deprenyl*) in dopamine metabolism. (MAO B = monoamine oxidase type B.)

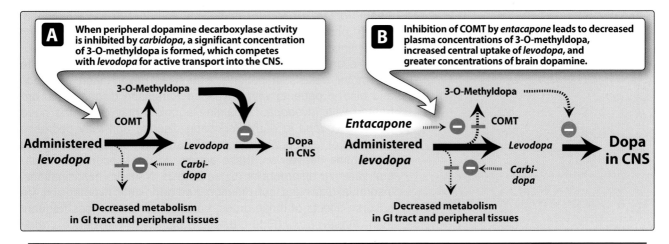

Figure 8.9
Effect of *entacapone* on dopa concentration in the central nervous system (CNS). COMT = catechol-*O*-methyltransferase.

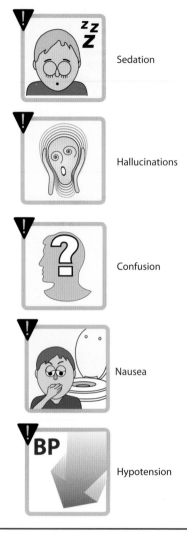

Figure 8.10
Some adverse effects of dopamine agonists.

with appropriate hepatic function monitoring, only in patients in whom other modalities have failed. *Entacapone* does not exhibit this toxicity and has largely replaced *tolcapone* in clinical practice.

D. Dopamine receptor agonists

This group of antiparkinsonian compounds includes *bromocriptine* [broe-moe-KRIP-teen], an ergot derivative, and the nonergot drugs, *ropinirole* [roe-PIN-i-role], *pramipexole* [pra-mi-PEX-ole], *rotigotine* [ro-TIG-oh-teen], and *apomorphine* [A-poe-more-feen]. These agents have a longer duration of action than that of *levodopa* and are effective in patients exhibiting fluctuations in response to *levodopa*. Initial therapy with these drugs is associated with less risk of developing dyskinesias and motor fluctuations as compared to patients started on *levodopa*. *Bromocriptine*, *pramipexole*, and *ropinirole* are effective in patients with Parkinson disease complicated by motor fluctuations and dyskinesias. However, these drugs are ineffective in patients who have not responded to *levodopa*. *Apomorphine* is an injectable dopamine agonist that is used in severe and advanced stages of the disease to supplement oral medications. Adverse effects severely limit the utility of the dopamine agonists (Figure 8.10).

1. **Bromocriptine:** The actions of the ergot derivative *bromocriptine* are similar to those of *levodopa*, except that hallucinations, confusion, delirium, nausea, and orthostatic hypotension are more common, whereas dyskinesia is less prominent. In psychiatric illness, *bromocriptine* may cause the mental condition to worsen. It should be used with caution in patients with a history of myocardial infarction or peripheral vascular disease due to the risk of vasospasm. Because *bromocriptine* is an ergot derivative, it has the potential to cause pulmonary and retroperitoneal fibrosis.

2. **Apomorphine, pramipexole, ropinirole, and rotigotine:** These are nonergot dopamine agonists that are approved for the treatment of Parkinson disease. *Ropinirole* is also indicated for the treatment of restless legs syndrome. *Pramipexole* and *ropinirole* are orally active agents. *Apomorphine* and *rotigotine* are available in injectable and transdermal delivery systems, respectively. *Apomorphine* is used for acute management of the hypomobility "off" phenomenon in advanced Parkinson disease. *Rotigotine* is administered as a once-daily transdermal patch that provides even drug levels over 24 hours. These agents alleviate the motor deficits in patients who have never taken *levodopa* and also in patients with advanced Parkinson disease who are treated with *levodopa*. Dopamine agonists may delay the need to use *levodopa* in early Parkinson disease and may decrease the dose of *levodopa* in advanced Parkinson disease. Unlike the ergotamine derivatives, these agents do not exacerbate peripheral vascular disorders or cause fibrosis. Nausea, hallucinations, insomnia, dizziness, constipation, and orthostatic hypotension are adverse effects of these drugs, but dyskinesias are less frequent than with *levodopa* (Figure 8.11). *Pramipexole* is mainly excreted unchanged in the urine, and dosage adjustments are needed in renal dysfunction. The fluoroquinolone antibiotics and other inhibitors of the cytochrome P450 (CYP450) 1A2 isoenzyme (for example, *fluvoxamine*) may inhibit the metabolism of *ropinirole*,

requiring an adjustment in *ropinirole* dosage. Figure 8.12 summarizes some properties of dopamine agonists.

E. Amantadine

It was accidentally discovered that the antiviral drug *amantadine* [a-MAN-ta-deen] has an antiparkinsonian action. *Amantadine* has several effects on a number of neurotransmitters implicated in parkinsonism, including increasing the release of dopamine, blocking cholinergic receptors, and inhibiting the *N*-methyl-D-aspartate (NMDA) type of glutamate receptors. The drug may cause restlessness, agitation, confusion, and hallucinations, and, at high doses, it may induce acute toxic psychosis. Orthostatic hypotension, urinary retention, peripheral edema, and dry mouth also may occur. *Amantadine* is less efficacious than *levodopa*, and tolerance develops more readily. However, *amantadine* has fewer adverse effects.

F. Antimuscarinic agents

The antimuscarinic agents are much less efficacious than *levodopa* and play only an adjuvant role in antiparkinsonism therapy. The actions of *benztropine* [BENZ-troe-peen] and *trihexyphenidyl* [tri-hex-ee-FEN-i-dill] are similar, although individual patients may respond more favorably to one drug or the other. Blockade of cholinergic transmission produces effects similar to augmentation of dopaminergic transmission, since it helps to correct the imbalance in the dopamine/acetylcholine activity (Figure 8.4). These agents can induce mood changes and confusion, and produce xerostomia, constipation, and visual problems typical of muscarinic blockers (see Chapter 5). They interfere with gastrointestinal peristalsis and are contraindicated in patients with glaucoma, prostatic hyperplasia, or pyloric stenosis.

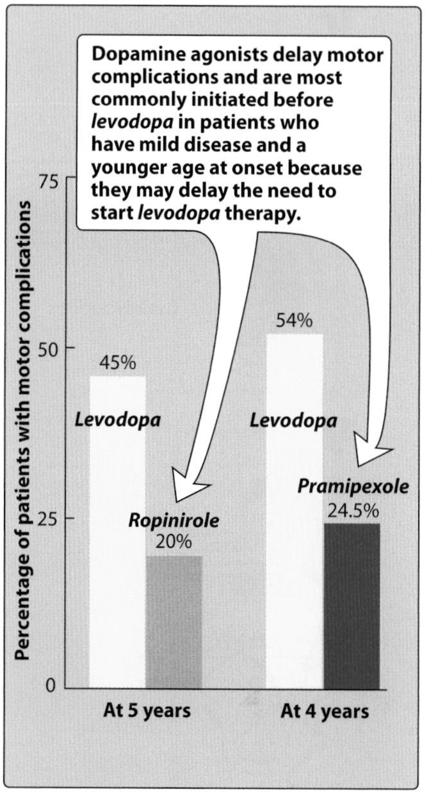

Dopamine agonists delay motor complications and are most commonly initiated before *levodopa* in patients who have mild disease and a younger age at onset because they may delay the need to start *levodopa* therapy.

Figure 8.11
Motor complications in patients treated with *levodopa* or dopamine agonists.

VII. DRUGS USED IN ALZHEIMER DISEASE

Dementia of the Alzheimer type has three distinguishing features: 1) accumulation of senile plaques (β-amyloid accumulations), 2) formation of numerous neurofibrillary tangles, and 3) loss of cortical neurons, particularly cholinergic neurons. Current therapies aim to either improve cholinergic transmission within the CNS or prevent excitotoxic actions resulting from overstimulation of NMDA-glutamate receptors in selected areas of the brain. Pharmacologic intervention for Alzheimer disease is

Characteristic	Pramipexole	Ropinirole	Rotigotine
Bioavailability	>90%	55%	45%
V_d	7 L/kg	7.5 L/kg	84 L/kg
Half-life	8 h[1]	6 h	7 h[3]
Metabolism	Negligible	Extensive	Extensive
Elimination	Renal	Renal[2]	Renal[2]

Figure 8.12
Pharmacokinetic properties of dopamine agonists *pramipexole*, *ropinirole*, and *rotigotine*. V_d = volume of distribution. [1]Increases to 12 hours in patients older than 65 years. [2]Less than 10% excreted unchanged. [3]Administered as a once-daily transdermal patch.

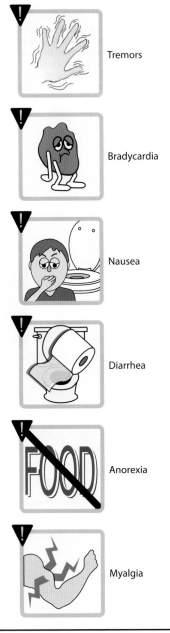

Figure 8.13
Adverse effects of AChE inhibitors.

only palliative and provides modest short-term benefit. None of the available therapeutic agents alter the underlying neurodegenerative process.

A. Acetylcholinesterase inhibitors

Numerous studies have linked the progressive loss of cholinergic neurons and, presumably, cholinergic transmission within the cortex to the memory loss that is a hallmark symptom of Alzheimer disease. It is postulated that inhibition of acetylcholinesterase (AChE) within the CNS improves cholinergic transmission, at least at those neurons that are still functioning. The reversible AChE inhibitors approved for the treatment of Alzheimer disease include *donepezil* [doe-NE-peh-zil], *galantamine* [ga-LAN-ta-meen], and *rivastigmine* [ri-va-STIG-meen]. These agents have some selectivity for AChE in the CNS, as compared to the periphery. *Galantamine* may also augment the action of acetylcholine at nicotinic receptors in the CNS. At best, these compounds may provide a modest reduction in the rate of loss of cognitive functioning in Alzheimer patients. *Rivastigmine* is the only agent approved for the management of dementia associated with Parkinson disease and also the only AChE inhibitor available as a transdermal formulation. *Rivastigmine* is hydrolyzed by AChE to a carbamylated metabolite and has no interactions with drugs that alter the activity of CYP450 enzymes. The other agents are substrates for CYP450 and have a potential for such interactions. Common adverse effects include nausea, diarrhea, vomiting, anorexia, tremors, bradycardia, and muscle cramps (Figure 8.13).

B. NMDA receptor antagonist

Stimulation of glutamate receptors in the CNS appears to be critical for the formation of certain memories. However, overstimulation of glutamate receptors, particularly of the NMDA type, may result in excitotoxic effects on neurons and is suggested as a mechanism for neurodegenerative or apoptotic (programmed cell death) processes. Binding of glutamate to the NMDA receptor assists in the opening of an ion channel that allows Ca^{2+} to enter the neuron. Excess intracellular Ca^{2+} can activate a number of processes that ultimately damage neurons and lead to apoptosis. *Memantine* [meh-MAN-teen] is an NMDA receptor antagonist indicated for moderate to severe Alzheimer disease. It acts by blocking the NMDA receptor and limiting Ca^{2+} influx into the neuron, such that toxic intracellular levels are not achieved. *Memantine* is well tolerated, with few dose-dependent adverse events. Expected adverse effects, such as confusion, agitation, and restlessness, are often indistinguishable from the symptoms of Alzheimer disease. Given its different mechanism of action and possible neuroprotective effects, *memantine* is often given in combination with an AChE inhibitor.

VIII. DRUGS USED IN MULTIPLE SCLEROSIS

MS is an autoimmune inflammatory demyelinating disease of the CNS. The course of MS is variable. For some, MS may consist of one or two acute neurologic episodes. In others, it is a chronic, relapsing, or progressive disease that may span 10 to 20 years. Historically, corticosteroids (for example, *dexamethasone* and *prednisone*) have been used to treat acute exacerbations of the disease. Chemotherapeutic agents, such as *cyclophosphamide* and *azathioprine*, have also been used.

A. Disease-modifying therapies

Drugs currently approved for MS are indicated to decrease relapse rates or, in some cases, to prevent accumulation of disability. The major target of these medications is to modify the immune response through inhibition of white blood cell–mediated inflammatory processes that eventually lead to myelin sheath damage and decreased or inappropriate axonal communication between cells.

1. **Interferon β_{1a} and interferon β_{1b}:** The immunomodulatory effects of *interferon* [in-ter-FEER-on] help to diminish the inflammatory responses that lead to demyelination of the axon sheaths. Adverse effects of these medications may include depression, local injection site reactions, increases in hepatic enzymes, and flu-like symptoms.

2. **Glatiramer:** *Glatiramer* [gluh-TEER-a-mur] is a synthetic polypeptide that resembles myelin protein and may act as a decoy to T-cell attack. Some patients experience a postinjection reaction that includes flushing, chest pain, anxiety, and itching. It is usually self-limiting.

3. **Fingolimod:** *Fingolimod* [fin-GO-li-mod] is an oral drug that alters lymphocyte migration, resulting in fewer lymphocytes in the CNS. *Fingolimod* may cause first-dose bradycardia and is associated with an increased risk of infection and macular edema.

4. **Teriflunomide:** *Teriflunomide* [te-ree-FLOO-no-mide] is an oral pyrimidine synthesis inhibitor that leads to a lower concentration of active lymphocytes in the CNS. *Teriflunomide* may cause elevated liver enzymes. It should be avoided in pregnancy.

5. **Dimethyl fumarate:** *Dimethyl fumarate* [dye-METH-il FOO-ma-rate] is an oral agent that may alter the cellular response to oxidative stress to reduce disease progression. Flushing and abdominal pain are the most common adverse events.

6. **Monoclonal antibodies:** *Alemtuzumab* [AL-em-TOOZ-ue-mab], *daclizumab* [dah-KLIH-zyoo-mab], *natalizumab* [na-ta-LIZ-oo-mab], and *ocrelizumab* [OK-re-LIZ-ue-mab] are monoclonal antibodies indicated for the treatment of MS. *Ocrelizumab* is the first agent to be approved for primary progressive forms of the disease. These agents can be associated with significant toxicities, such as progressive multifocal leukoencephalopathy with *natalizumab*, serious infections with *daclizumab* and *alemtuzumab*, and autoimmune disorders with *alemtuzumab*. As such, these agents may be reserved for patients who have failed other therapies.

B. Symptomatic treatment

Many different classes of drugs are used to manage symptoms of MS such as spasticity, constipation, bladder dysfunction, and depression. *Dalfampridine* [DAL-fam-pre-deen], an oral potassium channel blocker, improves walking speeds in patients with MS. It is the first drug approved for this use.

IX. DRUGS USED IN AMYOTROPHIC LATERAL SCLEROSIS

ALS is characterized by progressive degeneration of motor neurons, resulting in the inability to initiate or control muscle movement. *Riluzole* [RIL-ue-zole] and *edaravone* [e-DAR-a-vone] are indicated for the management of ALS. *Riluzole*, an oral NMDA receptor antagonist, is believed to act by inhibiting glutamate release and blocking sodium channels. *Riluzole* may improve survival time in patients suffering from ALS. *Edaravone* is an intravenous free radical scavenger and antioxidant that may slow the progression of ALS.

Study Questions

Choose the ONE best answer.

8.1 A 75-year-old man with moderate Parkinson disease is no longer responding to anticholinergic treatment for his tremors and bradykinesia. Which combination of antiparkinsonian drugs is an appropriate treatment plan?

A. Amantadine, carbidopa, and entacapone

B. Levodopa, carbidopa, and entacapone

C. Pramipexole, carbidopa, and entacapone

D. Ropinirole, carbidopa, and selegiline

Correct answer = B. To reduce the dose of levodopa and its peripheral side effects, the peripheral decarboxylase inhibitor, carbidopa, is coadministered. As a result of this combination, more levodopa is available for metabolism by catechol-*O*-methyltransferase (COMT) to 3-*O*-methyldopa, which competes with levodopa for the active transport processes into the CNS. By administering entacapone (an inhibitor of COMT), the competing product is not formed, and more levodopa enters the brain. The other choices are not appropriate because neither peripheral decarboxylase, nor COMT, nor monoamine oxidase metabolizes amantadine or the direct-acting dopamine agonists ropinirole and pramipexole; thus carbidopa and entacapone should only be given with levodopa, otherwise they are not contributing to the clinical response of the patient.

8.2 Peripheral adverse effects of levodopa, including nausea, hypotension, and cardiac arrhythmias, can be diminished by including which drug in the therapy?

A. Amantadine

B. Ropinirole

C. Carbidopa

D. Entacapone

Correct answer = C. Carbidopa inhibits the peripheral decarboxylation of levodopa to dopamine, thereby diminishing the gastrointestinal and cardiovascular side effects of levodopa. The other agents listed do not ameliorate adverse effects of levodopa.

8.3 Which antiparkinsonian drug may cause vasospasm?

A. Amantadine

B. Bromocriptine

C. Entacapone

D. Ropinirole

Correct answer = B. Bromocriptine is a dopamine receptor agonist that may cause vasospasm. It is contraindicated in patients with peripheral vascular disease. Ropinirole directly stimulates dopamine receptors, but it does not cause vasospasm. The other drugs do not act directly on dopamine receptors.

8.4 Modest improvement in the memory of patients with Alzheimer disease may occur with drugs that increase transmission at which receptor?

A. Adrenergic

B. Cholinergic

C. Dopaminergic

D. Serotonergic

Correct answer = B. AChE inhibitors, such as galantamine, increase cholinergic transmission in the CNS and may cause a modest delay in the progression of Alzheimer disease. Increased transmission at the other types of receptors listed does not result in improved memory.

8.5 A 70-year-old woman with moderate to severe dementia of the Alzheimer type has been treated with an acetylcholinesterase inhibitor for 6 months at maximum dosing with minimal effect. Which medication is a glutamate receptor antagonist that could provide added benefit for management of her moderate to severe symptoms of Alzheimer disease?

A. Rivastigmine
B. Pramipexole
C. Memantine
D. Galantamine

> Correct answer = C. When combined with an acetylcholinesterase inhibitor, memantine has modest efficacy in keeping patients with Alzheimer disease at or above baseline for at least 6 months and may delay disease progression. It is currently not approved for mild cognitive impairment or mild AD.

8.6 An 80-year-old male patient with moderate Alzheimer disease had a short trial of an oral medication for Alzheimer disease and experienced frequent nausea, along with difficulty swallowing the medication. Which agent is best for management of Alzheimer disease in this patient?

A. Rivastigmine
B. Donepezil
C. Memantine
D. Rotigotine

> Correct answer = A. Rivastigmine is the only agent available as a transdermal delivery system (patch) for the treatment of Alzheimer disease. It may also be used for dementia associated with Parkinson disease. Daily use of the rivastigmine patch provides steady drug levels to treat Alzheimer disease, with a possible reduced incidence of nausea. Rotigotine is available as a transdermal delivery system; however, it is indicated for Parkinson disease and not for Alzheimer disease.

8.7 Which medication would benefit a 55-year-old female patient recently diagnosed with amyotrophic lateral sclerosis (ALS)?

A. Pramipexole
B. Galantamine
C. Riluzole
D. Glatiramer

> Correct answer = C. Riluzole is approved for the debilitating and lethal illness of ALS. It is used to, ideally, delay the progression and need for ventilator support in severe patients. It is believed to work by decreasing the release of glutamate from the presynaptic terminal.

8.8 A 48-year-old woman with relapsing multiple sclerosis has had intolerable adverse reactions to interferon beta (depression) and dimethyl fumarate (angioedema) and now requires an alternative treatment option. Which medication is most appropriate for this patient?

A. Riluzole
B. Rotigotine
C. Teriflunomide
D. Galantamine

> Correct answer = C. Teriflunomide is believed to exert its disease modifying and anti-inflammatory effects by inhibiting the enzyme dihydroorotate dehydrogenase to reduce pyrimidine synthesis. Teriflunomide may provide an alternative treatment option with a different side effect profile compared to the prior two attempted treatments. The other agents are not indicated for the treatment of multiple sclerosis.

8.9 Which agent may cause tremors as an adverse effect and, thus, should be used with caution in patients with Parkinson disease, even though it is also indicated for the treatment of dementia associated with Parkinson disease?

A. Benztropine
B. Rotigotine
C. Rivastigmine
D. Dimethyl fumarate

> Correct answer = C. Though rivastigmine is an acetylcholinesterase inhibitor, which can cause tremors as an adverse effect, its use is not contraindicated in patients with Parkinson disease, as this agent is also the only medication approved for dementia associated with Parkinson disease. It should be used with caution, as it may worsen the parkinsonian-related tremors. A risk–benefit discussion should occur with the patient and the caregiver before rivastigmine is used.

8.10 A 50-year-old male patient with secondary progressive multiple sclerosis reports continued difficulty walking and the distance that he can walk before being overcome by fatigue. Which agent may be beneficial to improve walking speed and disability in this patient?

A. Dalfampridine
B. Donepezil
C. Riluzole
D. Bromocriptine

> Correct answer = A. Dalfampridine is a potassium channel blocker that exerts its therapeutic effect in multiple sclerosis via potassium channel blockade and has been proven to improve walking speed and disability in patients with multiple sclerosis. It is the only agent that is indicated to improve walking speed in patients with MS. The other agents are not indicated for the treatment of multiple sclerosis.

Anxiolytic and Hypnotic Drugs

Jose A. Rey

9

I. OVERVIEW

Disorders involving anxiety are among the most common mental disorders. Anxiety is an unpleasant state of tension, apprehension, or uneasiness (a fear that arises from either a known or an unknown source). The physical symptoms of severe anxiety are similar to those of fear (such as tachycardia, sweating, trembling, and palpitations) and involve sympathetic activation. Episodes of mild anxiety are common life experiences and do not warrant treatment. However, severe, chronic, debilitating anxiety may be treated with antianxiety drugs (sometimes called anxiolytics) and/or some form of psychotherapy. Because many antianxiety drugs also cause some sedation, they may be used clinically as both anxiolytic and hypnotic (sleep-inducing) agents. Figure 9.1 summarizes the anxiolytic and hypnotic agents. Some antidepressants are also indicated for certain anxiety disorders; however, they are discussed with the antidepressants (see Chapter 10).

II. BENZODIAZEPINES

Benzodiazepines are widely used anxiolytic drugs. They have largely replaced barbiturates and *meprobamate* in the treatment of anxiety and insomnia, because benzodiazepines are generally considered to be safer and more effective (Figure 9.2). Though benzodiazepines are commonly used, they are not necessarily the best choice for anxiety or insomnia. Certain antidepressants with anxiolytic action, such as the selective serotonin reuptake inhibitors (SSRIs), are preferred in many cases, and nonbenzodiazepine hypnotics and antihistamines may be preferable for insomnia.

A. Mechanism of action

The targets for benzodiazepine actions are the γ-aminobutyric acid (GABA$_A$) receptors. [Note: GABA is the major inhibitory neurotransmitter in the central nervous system (CNS).] The GABA$_A$ receptors are composed of a combination of five α, β, and γ subunits that span the postsynaptic membrane (Figure 9.3). For each subunit, many subtypes exist (for example, there are six subtypes of the α subunit). Binding of GABA to its receptor triggers an opening of the central ion channel, allowing chloride through the pore. The influx of

BENZODIAZEPINES
Alprazolam XANAX
Chlordiazepoxide LIBRIUM
Clonazepam KLONOPIN
Clorazepate TRANXENE
Diazepam VALIUM, DIASTAT
Estazolam GENERIC ONLY
Flurazepam GENERIC ONLY
Lorazepam ATIVAN
Midazolam GENERIC ONLY
Oxazepam GENERIC ONLY
Quazepam DORAL
Temazepam RESTORIL
Triazolam HALCION
BENZODIAZEPINE ANTAGONIST
Flumazenil GENERIC ONLY
OTHER ANXIOLYTIC DRUGS
Antidepressants VARIOUS (SEE CHAPTER 10)
Buspirone GENERIC ONLY
Meprobamate GENERIC ONLY
BARBITURATES
Amobarbital AMYTAL
Pentobarbital NEMBUTAL
Phenobarbital GENERIC ONLY
Secobarbital SECONAL
OTHER HYPNOTIC AGENTS
Antihistamines VARIOUS (SEE CHAPTER 37)
Doxepin SILENOR
Eszopiclone LUNESTA
Ramelteon ROZEREM
Suvorexant BELSOMRA
Tasimelteon HETLIOZ
Zaleplon SONATA
Zolpidem AMBIEN, INTERMEZZO, ZOLPIMIST

Figure 9.1
Summary of anxiolytic and hypnotic drugs.

chloride ions causes hyperpolarization of the neuron and decreases neurotransmission by inhibiting the formation of action potentials. Benzodiazepines modulate GABA effects by binding to a specific, high-affinity site (distinct from the GABA-binding site) located at the interface of the α subunit and the γ subunit on the $GABA_A$ receptor (Figure 9.3). Benzodiazepines increase the frequency of channel openings produced by GABA. The clinical effects of individual benzodiazepines correlate well with the binding affinity of each drug for the GABA receptor–chloride ion channel complex.

B. Actions

All benzodiazepines exhibit the following actions to some extent:

1. **Reduction of anxiety:** At low doses, the benzodiazepines are anxiolytic. They are thought to reduce anxiety by selectively enhancing GABAergic transmission in neurons having the α_2 subunit in their $GABA_A$ receptors, thereby inhibiting neuronal circuits in the limbic system of the brain.

2. **Sedative/hypnotic:** All benzodiazepines have sedative and calming properties, and some can produce hypnosis (artificially produced sleep) at higher doses. The hypnotic effects are mediated by the α_1-$GABA_A$ receptors.

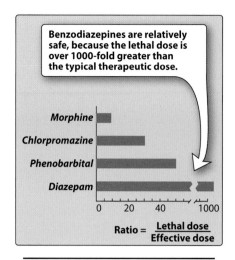

Figure 9.2
Ratio of lethal dose to effective dose for *morphine* (an opioid, see Chapter 14), *chlorpromazine* (an antipsychotic, see Chapter 11), and the anxiolytic, hypnotic drugs, *phenobarbital* and *diazepam*.

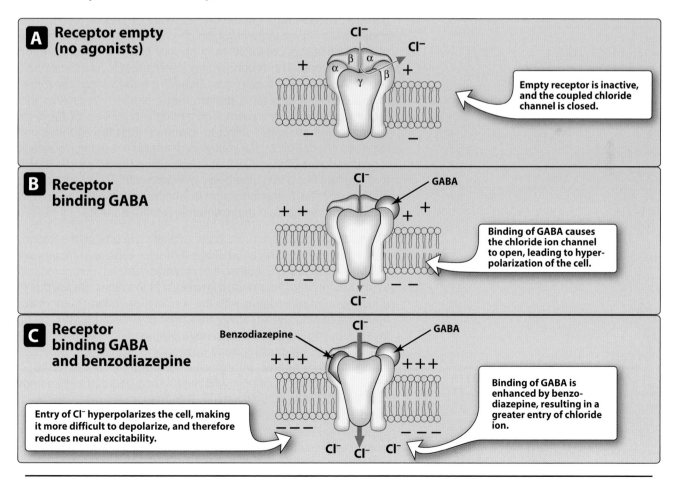

Figure 9.3
Schematic diagram of benzodiazepine–GABA–chloride ion channel complex. GABA = γ-aminobutyric acid.

3. **Anterograde amnesia:** Temporary impairment of memory with the use of the benzodiazepines is also mediated by the α_1-GABA$_A$ receptors. The ability to learn and form new memories is also impaired.

4. **Anticonvulsant:** This effect is partially, although not completely, mediated by α_1-GABA$_A$ receptors.

5. **Muscle relaxant:** At high doses, the benzodiazepines relax the spasticity of skeletal muscle, probably by increasing presynaptic inhibition in the spinal cord, where the α_2-GABA$_A$ receptors are largely located. [Note: *Baclofen* [BAK-loe-fen] is a muscle relaxant that is believed to affect GABA receptors at the level of the spinal cord.]

C. Therapeutic uses

The individual benzodiazepines show small differences in their relative anxiolytic, anticonvulsant, and sedative properties. However, pharmacokinetic considerations are often important in choosing one benzodiazepine over another.

1. **Anxiety disorders:** Benzodiazepines are effective for the treatment of anxiety associated with panic disorder, generalized anxiety disorder (GAD), social anxiety disorder, performance anxiety, and extreme phobias, such as fear of flying. The benzodiazepines are also useful in treating anxiety related to depression and schizophrenia. These drugs should be reserved for severe anxiety and should not be used to manage the stress of everyday life. Because of their addictive potential, they should only be used for short periods of time. The longer-acting agents, such as *clonazepam* [kloe-NAZ-e-pam], *lorazepam* [lor-AZ-e-pam], and *diazepam* [dye-AZ-e-pam], are often preferred in patients with anxiety that require prolonged treatment. The antianxiety effects of the benzodiazepines are less subject to tolerance than the sedative and hypnotic effects. [Note: Tolerance is decreased responsiveness to repeated doses of the drug that occurs when used for more than 1 to 2 weeks.] For panic disorders, *alprazolam* [al-PRAY-zoe-lam] is effective for short- and long-term treatment, although it may cause withdrawal reactions in approximately 30% of patients.

2. **Sleep disorders:** Benzodiazepine hypnotics decrease the latency to sleep onset and increase stage II of non–rapid eye movement (REM) sleep. Both REM sleep and slow-wave sleep are decreased. In the treatment of insomnia, it is important to balance the sedative effect needed at bedtime with the residual sedation ("hangover") upon awakening. Short-acting *triazolam* [try-AY-zoe-lam] is effective in treating individuals who have problems falling asleep. The risk of withdrawal and rebound insomnia is higher with *triazolam* than with other agents. Intermediate-acting *temazepam* [te-MAZ-e-pam] is useful for patients who experience frequent awakenings and have difficulty staying asleep. *Temazepam* should be administered 1 to 2 hours before the desired bedtime. Long-acting *flurazepam* [flure-AZ-e-pam] is rarely used, due to its extended half-life, which may result in excessive daytime sedation and accumulation of the drug, especially in the elderly. *Estazolam* [eh-STAY-zoe-lam] and *quazepam* [QUAY-ze-pam] are considered intermediate- and long-acting agents, respectively. In general, hypnotics should be used for only a limited time, usually 1 to 3 weeks.

3. **Amnesia:** The shorter-acting agents are often employed as premedication for anxiety-provoking and unpleasant procedures, such as endoscopy, dental procedures, and angioplasty. They cause a form of conscious sedation, allowing the patient to be receptive to instructions during these procedures. *Midazolam* [mi-DAY-zoe-lam] is a benzodiazepine used to facilitate anterograde amnesia while providing sedation prior to anesthesia.

4. **Seizures:** *Clonazepam* is occasionally used as an adjunctive therapy for certain types of seizures, whereas *lorazepam* and *diazepam* are the drugs of choice in terminating status epilepticus (see Chapter 12). Due to cross-tolerance, *chlordiazepoxide* [klor-di-az-e-POX-ide], *clorazepate* [klor-AZ-e-pate], *diazepam*, *lorazepam*, and *oxazepam* [ox-AZ-e-pam] are useful in the acute treatment of alcohol withdrawal and reduce the risk of withdrawal-related seizures.

5. **Muscular disorders:** *Diazepam* is useful in the treatment of skeletal muscle spasms and in treating spasticity from degenerative disorders, such as multiple sclerosis and cerebral palsy.

D. Pharmacokinetics

1. **Absorption and distribution:** The benzodiazepines are lipophilic. They are rapidly and completely absorbed after oral administration, distribute throughout the body, and penetrate into the CNS.

2. **Duration of action:** The half-lives of the benzodiazepines are important clinically, because the duration of action may determine the therapeutic usefulness. The benzodiazepines can be roughly divided into short-, intermediate-, and long-acting groups (Figure 9.4). The longer-acting agents form active metabolites with long half-lives. However, **with some benzodiazepines, the clinical duration of action does not correlate with the actual half-life** (otherwise, a dose of *diazepam* could conceivably be given only every other day, given its long half-life and active metabolites). This may be due to receptor dissociation rates in the CNS and subsequent redistribution to fatty tissues and other areas.

3. **Fate:** Most benzodiazepines, including *chlordiazepoxide* and *diazepam*, are metabolized by the hepatic microsomal system to compounds that are also active. For these benzodiazepines, the apparent half-life of the drug represents the combined actions of the parent drug and its metabolites. The benzodiazepines are excreted in the urine as glucuronides or oxidized metabolites. All benzodiazepines cross the placenta and may depress the CNS of the newborn if given before birth. The benzodiazepines are not recommended for use during pregnancy. Nursing infants may also be exposed to the drugs in breast milk.

E. Dependence

Psychological and physical dependence can develop if high doses of benzodiazepines are given for a prolonged period. All benzodiazepines are controlled substances. Abrupt discontinuation of these agents results in withdrawal symptoms, including confusion, anxiety, agitation, restlessness, insomnia, tension, and (rarely) seizures. Benzodiazepines with a short elimination half-life, such as *triazolam,*

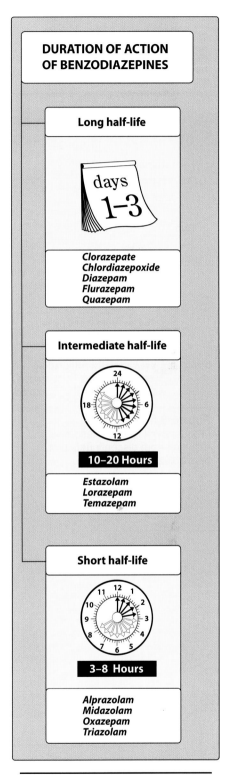

DURATION OF ACTION OF BENZODIAZEPINES

Long half-life

days 1-3

Clorazepate
Chlordiazepoxide
Diazepam
Flurazepam
Quazepam

Intermediate half-life

10–20 Hours

Estazolam
Lorazepam
Temazepam

Short half-life

3–8 Hours

Alprazolam
Midazolam
Oxazepam
Triazolam

Figure 9.4
Comparison of the durations of action of the benzodiazepines.

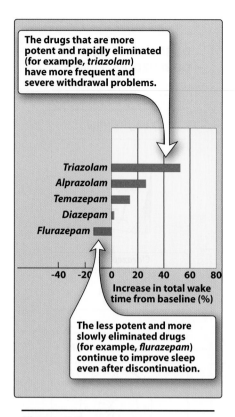

Figure 9.5
Frequency of rebound insomnia resulting from discontinuation of benzodiazepine therapy.

induce more abrupt and severe withdrawal reactions than those seen with drugs that are slowly eliminated such as *flurazepam* (Figure 9.5).

F. Adverse effects

Drowsiness and confusion are the most common adverse effects of the benzodiazepines. Ataxia occurs at high doses and precludes activities that require fine motor coordination, such as driving an automobile. Cognitive impairment (decreased recall and retention of new knowledge) can occur with use of benzodiazepines. Benzodiazepines should be used cautiously in patients with liver disease. Alcohol and other CNS depressants enhance the sedative–hypnotic effects of the benzodiazepines. Benzodiazepines are, however, considerably less dangerous than the older anxiolytic and hypnotic drugs. As a result, a drug overdose is seldom lethal unless other central depressants, such as alcohol or opioids, are taken concurrently.

III. BENZODIAZEPINE ANTAGONIST

Flumazenil [floo-MAZ-eh-nill] is a GABA receptor antagonist that rapidly reverses the effects of benzodiazepines. The drug is available for intravenous (IV) administration only. Onset is rapid, but the duration is short, with a half-life of about 1 hour. Frequent administration may be necessary to maintain reversal of a long-acting benzodiazepine. Administration of *flumazenil* may precipitate withdrawal in dependent patients or cause seizures if a benzodiazepine is used to control seizure activity. Seizures may also result if the patient has a mixed ingestion with tricyclic antidepressants or antipsychotics. Dizziness, nausea, vomiting, and agitation are the most common adverse effects.

IV. OTHER ANXIOLYTIC AGENTS

A. Antidepressants

Many antidepressants are effective in the treatment of chronic anxiety disorders and should be considered as first-line agents, especially in patients with concerns for addiction or dependence. SSRIs (such as *escitalopram* or *paroxetine*) or serotonin/norepinephrine reuptake inhibitors (SNRIs, such as *venlafaxine* or *duloxetine*) may be used alone or prescribed in combination with a benzodiazepine during the

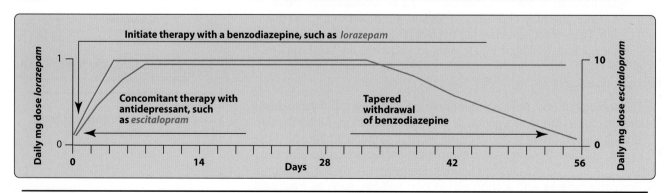

Figure 9.6
Treatment guideline for persistent anxiety.

first week of treatment (Figure 9.6). After 4 to 6 weeks, when the anti-depressant begins to produce an anxiolytic effect, the benzodiazepine dose can be tapered. While only certain SSRIs or SNRIs have been approved for the treatment of anxiety disorders such as GAD, the efficacy of these drugs is most likely a class effect. Long-term use of antidepressants and benzodiazepines for anxiety disorders is often required to maintain ongoing benefit and prevent relapse.

B. Buspirone

Buspirone [byoo-SPYE-rone] is useful for the chronic treatment of GAD and has an efficacy comparable to that of benzodiazepines. It has a slow onset of action and is not effective for short-term or "as-needed" treatment of acute anxiety. The actions of *buspirone* appear to be mediated by serotonin (5-HT$_{1A}$) receptors, although it also displays some affinity for D$_2$ dopamine receptors and 5-HT$_{2A}$ serotonin receptors. Thus, its mode of action differs from that of the benzodiazepines. In addition, *buspirone* lacks the anticonvulsant and muscle-relaxant properties of the benzodiazepines. The frequency of adverse effects is low, with the most common effects being headache, dizziness, nervousness, nausea, and light-headedness. Sedation and psychomotor and cognitive dysfunction are minimal, and dependence is unlikely. *Buspirone* does not potentiate the CNS depression of alcohol. Figure 9.7 compares common adverse effects of *buspirone* and the benzodiazepine *alprazolam*.

V. BARBITURATES

The barbiturates were formerly the mainstay of treatment to sedate patients or to induce and maintain sleep. They have been largely replaced by the benzodiazepines, primarily because barbiturates induce tolerance and physical dependence, are lethal in overdose, and are associated with severe withdrawal symptoms. All barbiturates are controlled substances.

A. Mechanism of action

The sedative–hypnotic action of the barbiturates is due to their interaction with GABA$_A$ receptors, which enhances GABAergic transmission. The binding site of barbiturates on the GABA receptor is distinct from that of the benzodiazepines. Barbiturates potentiate GABA action on chloride entry into the neuron by prolonging the duration of the chloride channel openings. In addition, barbiturates can block excitatory glutamate receptors. These molecular actions lead to decreased neuronal activity.

B. Actions

Barbiturates are classified according to their duration of action (Figure 9.8). Long-acting *phenobarbital* [fee-noe-BAR-bi-tal] has a duration of action greater than a day. *Pentobarbital* [pen-toe-BAR-bi-tal], *secobarbital* [see-koe-BAR-bi-tal], *amobarbital* [am-oh-BAR-bi-tal], and *butalbital* [bu-TAL-bi-tal] are short-acting barbiturates.

1. **Depression of CNS:** At low doses, the barbiturates produce sedation (have a calming effect and reduce excitement). At higher

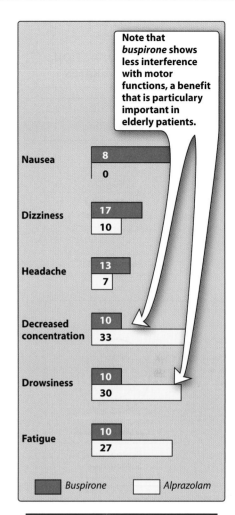

Note that *buspirone* shows less interference with motor functions, a benefit that is particulary important in elderly patients.

	Buspirone	Alprazolam
Nausea	8	0
Dizziness	17	10
Headache	13	7
Decreased concentration	10	33
Drowsiness	10	30
Fatigue	10	27

Figure 9.7
Comparison of common adverse effects of *buspirone* and *alprazolam*. Results are expressed as the percentage of patients showing each symptom.

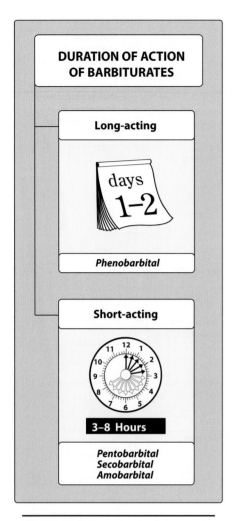

DURATION OF ACTION OF BARBITURATES

Long-acting

days 1-2

Phenobarbital

Short-acting

3–8 Hours

Pentobarbital
Secobarbital
Amobarbital

Figure 9.8
Barbiturates classified according to their durations of action.

doses, the drugs cause hypnosis, followed by anesthesia (loss of feeling or sensation), and, finally, coma and death. Thus, any degree of depression of the CNS is possible, depending on the dose. Barbiturates do not raise the pain threshold and have no analgesic properties. They may even exacerbate pain. Chronic use leads to tolerance.

2. **Respiratory depression:** Barbiturates suppress the hypoxic and chemoreceptor response to CO_2, and overdose is followed by respiratory depression and death.

C. **Therapeutic uses**

1. **Anesthesia:** The ultra–short-acting barbiturates have been historically used intravenously to induce anesthesia but have been replaced by other agents.

2. **Anticonvulsant:** *Phenobarbital* has specific anticonvulsant activity that is distinguished from the nonspecific CNS depression. However, *phenobarbital* can depress cognitive development in children and decrease cognitive performance in adults, and it should be used for seizures only if other therapies have failed. Similarly, *phenobarbital* may be used for the treatment of refractory status epilepticus.

3. **Sedative/hypnotic:** Barbiturates have been used as mild sedatives to relieve anxiety, nervous tension, and insomnia. When used as hypnotics, they suppress REM sleep more than other stages. However, the use of barbiturates for insomnia is no longer generally accepted, given their adverse effects and potential for tolerance. *Butalbital* is commonly used in combination products (with *acetaminophen* and *caffeine* or *aspirin* and *caffeine*) as a sedative to assist in the management of tension or migraine headaches.

D. **Pharmacokinetics**

Barbiturates are well absorbed after oral administration and distribute throughout the body. All barbiturates redistribute from the brain to the splanchnic areas, to skeletal muscle, and, finally, to adipose tissue. Barbiturates readily cross the placenta and can depress the fetus. These agents are metabolized in the liver, and inactive metabolites are excreted in urine.

E. **Adverse effects**

Barbiturates cause drowsiness, impaired concentration, and mental and psychomotor impairment (Figure 9.9). The CNS depressant effects of barbiturates synergize with those of *ethanol*.

Hypnotic doses of barbiturates produce a drug "hangover" that may lead to impaired ability to function normally for many hours after waking. Occasionally, nausea and dizziness occur. Barbiturates induce cytochrome P450 (CYP450) microsomal enzymes in the liver. Therefore, chronic barbiturate administration diminishes the action of many drugs that are metabolized by the CYP450 system. Barbiturates are contraindicated in patients with acute intermittent porphyria. Abrupt withdrawal from barbiturates may cause tremors, anxiety, weakness, restlessness, nausea and vomiting, seizures, delirium, and cardiac arrest. Withdrawal is much more severe than that associated with opioids and can result in death. Death may also result from overdose. Severe depression of respiration and central cardiovascular depression results in a shock-like condition with shallow, infrequent breathing. Treatment includes supportive care and gastric decontamination for recent ingestions.

VI. OTHER HYPNOTIC AGENTS

A. Zolpidem

The hypnotic *zolpidem* [ZOL-pi-dem] is not structurally related to benzodiazepines, but it binds to $GABA_A$ receptors with relative selectivity for those with the α_1 subunit. *Zolpidem* has no anticonvulsant or muscle-relaxing properties at hypnotic doses. It shows few withdrawal effects, exhibits minimal rebound insomnia, and little tolerance occurs with prolonged use. *Zolpidem* is rapidly absorbed after oral administration. It has a rapid onset of action and short elimination half-life (about 2 to 3 hours). The drug provides a hypnotic effect for approximately 5 hours (Figure 9.10). [Note: A lingual spray and an extended-release formulation are also available. A sublingual tablet formulation may be used for middle-of-the-night awakening.] *Zolpidem* undergoes hepatic oxidation by the CYP450 system to inactive products. Thus, drugs such as *rifampin*, which induce this enzyme system, shorten the half-life of *zolpidem*, and drugs that inhibit the CYP3A4 isoenzyme may increase the half-life. Adverse effects of *zolpidem* include headache, dizziness, anterograde amnesia, and next-morning impairment (especially with extended-release formulations). Sleepwalking, sleep-driving, and performing other activities while not fully awake have been reported. Unlike the benzodiazepines, at usual hypnotic doses, the nonbenzodiazepine drugs, *zolpidem*, *zaleplon*, and *eszopiclone*, do not significantly alter the various sleep stages and, hence, are often the preferred hypnotics. All three agents are controlled substances.

B. Zaleplon

Zaleplon [ZAL-e-plon] is an oral nonbenzodiazepine hypnotic similar to *zolpidem*; however, *zaleplon* causes fewer residual effects on psychomotor and cognitive function compared to *zolpidem* or the benzodiazepines. This may be due to its rapid elimination, with a half-life of approximately 1 hour. The drug is metabolized by CYP3A4.

C. Eszopiclone

Eszopiclone [es-ZOE-pi-clone] is an oral nonbenzodiazepine hypnotic that has been shown to be effective for insomnia for up to 6 months. *Eszopiclone* is rapidly absorbed (time to peak, 1 hour), extensively metabolized by oxidation and demethylation via the CYP450 system, and mainly excreted in urine. Elimination half-life is approximately 6 hours. Adverse events with *eszopiclone* include anxiety, dry mouth, headache, peripheral edema, somnolence, and unpleasant taste.

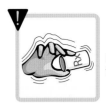
Potential for addiction

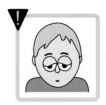
Drowsiness

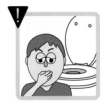
Nausea

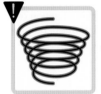
Vertigo

Tremors

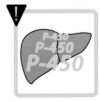
Enzyme induction

Figure 9.9
Adverse effects of barbiturates.

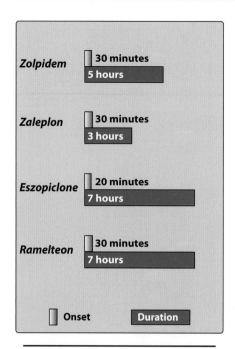

Figure 9.10
Onset and duration of action of the commonly used nonbenzodiazepine hypnotic agents.

D. Melatonin receptor agonists

Ramelteon [ram-EL-tee-on] and *tasimelteon* [tas-i-MEL-tee-on] are selective agonists at the MT$_1$ and MT$_2$ subtypes of melatonin receptors. Melatonin is a hormone secreted by the pineal gland that helps to maintain the circadian rhythm underlying the normal sleep–wake cycle. Stimulation of MT$_1$ and MT$_2$ receptors by *ramelteon* and *tasimelteon* is thought to induce and promote sleep. They have minimal potential for abuse, and no evidence of dependence or withdrawal has been observed. Therefore, *ramelteon* and *tasimelteon* can be administered long-term. *Ramelteon* is indicated for the treatment of insomnia characterized by difficulty falling asleep (increased sleep latency). Common adverse effects of *ramelteon* include dizziness, fatigue, and somnolence. *Ramelteon* may also increase prolactin levels. *Tasimelteon* is indicated for non–24-hour sleep–wake disorder, often experienced by patients who are blind. The most common adverse effects of *tasimelteon* are headache, abnormal dreams, increase in liver function tests, and possible upper respiratory tract infections. CYP450 1A2 and 3A4 are the principle isoenzymes required for metabolism of *ramelteon* and *tasimelteon*, and, thus, drug–drug interactions are possible with inducers or inhibitors of these enzymes.

E. Antihistamines

Antihistamines with sedating properties, such as diphenhydramine, *hydroxyzine*, and *doxylamine*, are effective in treating mild situational insomnia (see Chapter 37). However, they have undesirable adverse effects (such as anticholinergic effects) that make them less useful than the benzodiazepines and the nonbenzodiazepines. Sedative antihistamines are marketed in numerous over-the-counter products.

F. Antidepressants

The use of sedating antidepressants with strong antihistamine profiles has been ongoing for decades. *Doxepin* [DOX-e-pin], an older tricyclic agent with SNRI mechanisms of antidepressant and anxiolytic action, is approved at low doses for the management of insomnia. Other antidepressants, such as *trazodone* [TRAZ-oh-done], *mirtazapine* [mir-TAZ-a-pine], and other older tricyclic antidepressants with strong antihistamine properties are used off-label for the treatment of insomnia (see Chapter 10).

G. Suvorexant

Suvorexant [soo-voe-REX-ant] is an antagonist of the orexin receptor. Orexin is a neuropeptide that promotes wakefulness. Antagonism of the effects of orexin suppresses the wake drive from this neuropeptide. This antagonism may also explain the adverse events that are similar to signs of narcolepsy and cataplexy. The loss of orexin-producing neurons is believed to be an underlying pathology for narcolepsy. Daytime somnolence and increased suicidal ideation are other reported adverse effects. *Suvorexant* is mainly metabolized by CYP450 3A4, and, thus, it may have drug interactions with CYP3A4 inducers or inhibitors.

Figure 9.11 summarizes the therapeutic disadvantages and advantages of some of the anxiolytic and hypnotic drugs.

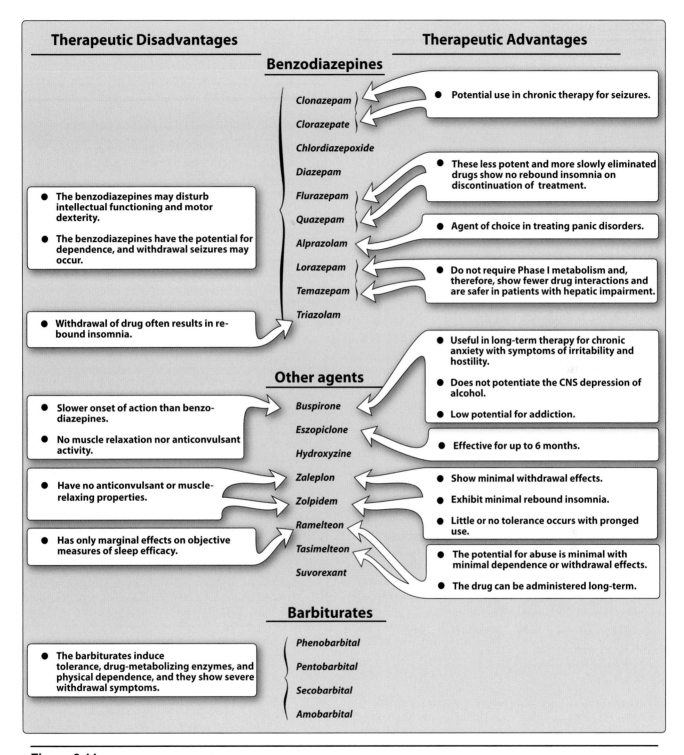

Figure 9.11
Therapeutic disadvantages and advantages of some anxiolytic and hypnotic agents. CNS = central nervous system.

Study Questions

Choose the ONE best answer.

9.1 Which one of the following statements is correct regarding benzodiazepines?

A. Benzodiazepines directly open chloride channels.
B. Benzodiazepines show analgesic actions.
C. Clinical improvement of anxiety requires 2 to 4 weeks of treatment with benzodiazepines.
D. All benzodiazepines have some sedative effects.

Correct answer = D. Although all benzodiazepines can cause sedation, the drugs labeled "benzodiazepines" in Figure 9.1 are promoted for the treatment of sleep disorder. Benzodiazepines enhance the binding of GABA$_A$ to its receptor, which increases the permeability of chloride. The benzodiazepines do not relieve pain but may reduce the anxiety associated with pain. Unlike the tricyclic antidepressants and the monoamine oxidase inhibitors, the benzodiazepines are effective within hours of administration. Benzodiazepines do not produce general anesthesia and therefore are relatively safe drugs with a high therapeutic index.

9.2 Which one of the following is a short-acting hypnotic?

A. Phenobarbital
B. Diazepam
C. Chlordiazepoxide
D. Triazolam

Correct answer = D. Triazolam is a short-acting hypnotic agent. It causes little daytime sedation. The other medications listed are longer acting with longer half-lives.

9.3 Which one of the following statements is correct regarding the anxiolytic and hypnotic agents?

A. Diazepam and phenobarbital induce the cytochrome P450 enzyme system.
B. Phenobarbital is useful in the treatment of acute intermittent porphyria.
C. Phenobarbital induces respiratory depression, which is enhanced by the consumption of ethanol.
D. Buspirone has actions similar to those of benzodiazepines.

Correct answer = C. Barbiturates and ethanol are a potentially lethal combination because of a high risk for respiratory depression. Only phenobarbital strongly induces the synthesis of the hepatic cytochrome P450 drug-metabolizing system. Phenobarbital is contraindicated in the treatment of acute intermittent porphyria. Buspirone lacks the anticonvulsant and muscle-relaxant properties of the benzodiazepines and causes only minimal sedation.

9.4 A 45-year-old man who has been injured in a car accident is brought into the emergency department. His blood alcohol level at admission is 275 mg/dL. Hospital records show a prior hospitalization for alcohol-related seizures. His wife confirms that he has been drinking heavily for 3 weeks. What treatment should be provided to the patient if he goes into withdrawal?

A. No pharmacological treatment is necessary.
B. Lorazepam.
C. Phenytoin.
D. Buspirone.

Correct answer = B. It is important to treat the seizures associated with alcohol withdrawal. Benzodiazepines such as chlordiazepoxide, diazepam, or the shorter-acting lorazepam are effective in controlling this problem. They are less sedating than phenytoin, have fewer adverse effects, and are cross-tolerant with alcohol. Buspirone will not prevent the seizures associated with alcohol withdrawal.

9.5 A 36-year-old male patient reports difficulty falling asleep for the past 2 weeks but needs to be able to wake up at 6 AM for work and doesn't want any daytime sedation. Which medication is best to recommend for the treatment of his insomnia?

A. Temazepam
B. Flurazepam
C. Zaleplon
D. Buspirone

Correct answer = C. Zaleplon has the shortest half-life and duration of action. Buspirone is not effective as a hypnotic agent. Temazepam and flurazepam have a longer duration of action and reduce nighttime awakenings but have a greater risk of daytime sedation or hangover effect compared with zaleplon.

9.6 A 45-year-old woman reports constant daytime anxiety about work and family problems. This is causing difficulties functioning and participating in necessary daily activities. Which of the following agents has a rapid anxiolytic effect and is best for the acute management of her anxiety?

A. Buspirone
B. Venlafaxine
C. Lorazepam
D. Escitalopram

Correct answer = C. The benzodiazepines have same-day, first-dose efficacy for anxiety, whereas the other agents require 2 to 8 weeks for clinically significant improvement in anxiety to occur.

9.7 Which of the following sedative–hypnotic agents utilizes melatonin receptor agonist as the mechanism of action to induce sleep?

A. Zolpidem
B. Eszopiclone
C. Estazolam
D. Tasimelteon

Correct answer = D. Tasimelteon is a melatonin receptor agonist to promote sleep, especially in those individuals with non–24-hour sleep–wake disorder. Zolpidem, eszopiclone, and estazolam all utilize the benzodiazepine receptor.

9.8 A 50-year-old man presents with insomnia not responsive to sleep hygiene interventions. He has a long history of alcohol and opioid abuse. He has been successfully sober for 10 years but is very concerned about future addiction and dependence. Which is most appropriate to address insomnia and minimize the risk for dependence in this patient?

A. Zaleplon
B. Flurazepam
C. Doxepin
D. Zolpidem

Correct answer = C. Only doxepin, a tricyclic agent with significant antihistaminergic properties, is considered to have no risk of addiction or dependence. The other agents are all controlled substances with some risk for addiction or dependence, especially when used for extended periods.

9.9 A 68-year-old female patient is demonstrating signs and symptoms of insomnia, especially difficulty falling asleep. She is afraid of taking a medication that can negatively affect her memory and concentration, as she is still working as a bookkeeper. She has been taking temazepam for the past 4 days and has noticed a memory problem and would like to discontinue this medication. Which medication is most appropriate to treat the insomnia and minimize the risk for cognitive impairment?

A. Diphenhydramine
B. Zolpidem
C. Alprazolam
D. Ramelteon

Correct answer = D. All of these agents, except ramelteon, have been associated with cognitive impairments, including memory impairment. Diphenhydramine likely causes its cognitive problems from its anticholinergic and antihistaminergic effects. Zolpidem and alprazolam are well-known causes of cognitive impairment, including anterograde amnesia. Ramelteon is a noncontrolled hypnotic agent acting as a melatonin receptor agonist. It is not considered to have a risk for cognitive impairment compared with the other agents listed.

9.10 An 18-year-old woman is admitted to the emergency room after an accidental overdose of alprazolam. She is unconscious and not considered a regular user of any medications or illicit drugs. Which treatment could be used to reverse the effect of the alprazolam overdose?

A. Diazepam
B. Ramelteon
C. Flumazenil
D. Naloxone

Correct answer = C. Flumazenil is only indicated to reverse the effects of benzodiazepines via antagonism of the benzodiazepine receptor. It should be used with caution because of a risk of seizures if the patient has been a long-time recipient of benzodiazepines or if the overdose attempt was with mixed drugs. Naloxone is an opioid receptor antagonist. The other agents are not efficacious in reversing effects of benzodiazepines.

Antidepressants

10

Jose A. Rey

I. OVERVIEW

The symptoms of depression are feelings of sadness and hopelessness, as well as the inability to experience pleasure in usual activities, changes in sleep patterns and appetite, loss of energy, and suicidal thoughts. Mania is characterized by the opposite behavior: enthusiasm, anger, rapid thought and speech patterns, extreme self-confidence, and impaired judgment. This chapter provides an overview of drugs used for the treatment of depression and mania.

II. MECHANISM OF ANTIDEPRESSANT DRUGS

Most antidepressant drugs (Figure 10.1) potentiate, either directly or indirectly, the actions of norepinephrine and/or serotonin (5-HT) in the brain. This, along with other evidence, led to the biogenic amine theory, which proposes that depression is due to a deficiency of monoamines, such as norepinephrine and serotonin, at certain key sites in the brain. Conversely, the theory proposes that mania is caused by an overproduction of these neurotransmitters. However, the biogenic amine theory of depression and mania is overly simplistic. It fails to explain the time course for a therapeutic response, which usually occurs over several weeks compared to the immediate pharmacodynamic effects of the agents, which are usually immediate. This suggests that decreased reuptake of neurotransmitters is only an initial effect of the drugs, which may not be directly responsible for the antidepressant effects.

III. SELECTIVE SEROTONIN REUPTAKE INHIBITORS

The selective serotonin reuptake inhibitors (SSRIs) are a group of antidepressant drugs that specifically inhibit serotonin reuptake, having 300- to 3000-fold greater selectivity for the serotonin transporter, as compared to the norepinephrine transporter. This contrasts with the tricyclic antidepressants (TCAs) and serotonin-norepinephrine reuptake inhibitors (SNRIs) that nonselectively inhibit the reuptake of norepinephrine and serotonin (Figure 10.2). Moreover, the SSRIs have little blocking activity at muscarinic, α-adrenergic, and histaminic

SELECTIVE SEROTONIN REUPTAKE INHIBITORS (SSRIs)
Citalopram CELEXA
Escitalopram LEXAPRO
Fluoxetine PROZAC
Fluvoxamine LUVOX
Paroxetine PAXIL
Sertraline ZOLOFT
SEROTONIN-NOREPINEPHRINE REUPTAKE INHIBITORS (SNRIs)
Desvenlafaxine PRISTIQ
Duloxetine CYMBALTA
Levomilnacipran FETZIMA
Venlafaxine EFFEXOR
ATYPICAL ANTIDEPRESSANTS
Bupropion WELLBUTRIN, ZYBAN
Mirtazapine REMERON
Nefazodone GENERIC ONLY
Trazodone GENERIC ONLY
Vilazodone VIIBRYD
Vortioxetine TRINTELLIX
TRICYCLIC ANTIDEPRESSANTS (TCAs)
Amitriptyline GENERIC ONLY
Amoxapine GENERIC ONLY
Clomipramine ANAFRANIL
Desipramine NORPRAMIN
Doxepin SILENOR
Imipramine TOFRANIL
Maprotiline GENERIC ONLY
Nortriptyline PAMELOR
Protriptyline VIVACTIL
Trimipramine SURMONTIL
MONOAMINE OXIDASE INHIBITORS (MAOIs)
Isocarboxazid MARPLAN
Phenelzine NARDIL
Selegiline EMSAM
Tranylcypromine PARNATE

Figure 10.1
Summary of antidepressants.
(Figure continues on next page)

H_1 receptors. Because they have different adverse effects and are relatively safe in overdose, the SSRIs have largely replaced TCAs and monoamine oxidase inhibitors (MAOIs) as the drugs of choice in treating depression. The SSRIs include *fluoxetine* [floo-OX-e-teen] (the prototypic drug), *citalopram* [sye-TAL-oh-pram], *escitalopram* [es-sye-TAL-oh-pram], *fluvoxamine* [floo-VOX-e-meen], *paroxetine* [pa-ROX-e-teen], and *sertraline* [SER-tra-leen]. *Escitalopram* is the pure S-enantiomer of *citalopram*.

A. Actions

The SSRIs block the reuptake of serotonin, leading to increased concentrations of the neurotransmitter in the synaptic cleft. Antidepressants, including SSRIs, typically take at least 2 weeks to produce significant improvement in mood, and maximum benefit may require up to 12 weeks or more (Figure 10.3).

B. Therapeutic uses

The primary indication for SSRIs is depression. A number of other psychiatric disorders also respond favorably to SSRIs, including obsessive–compulsive disorder, panic disorder, generalized anxiety disorder, posttraumatic stress disorder, social anxiety disorder, premenstrual dysphoric disorder, and bulimia nervosa (only *fluoxetine* is approved for bulimia).

C. Pharmacokinetics

All of the SSRIs are well absorbed after oral administration. Peak levels are seen in approximately 2 to 8 hours on average. Food has little effect on absorption (except with *sertraline*, for which food increases its absorption). The majority of SSRIs have plasma half-lives that range between 16 and 36 hours. Metabolism by cytochrome P450 (CYP450)–dependent enzymes and glucuronide or sulfate conjugation occur extensively. *Fluoxetine* differs from the other members of the class by having a much longer half-life (50 hours), and the half-life of its active metabolite *S*-norfluoxetine is quite long, averaging 10 days. *Fluoxetine* and *paroxetine* are potent inhibitors of a CYP450 isoenzyme (CYP2D6). Other CYP450 isoenzymes (CYP2C9/19, CYP3A4, and CYP1A2) are involved with SSRI metabolism and may also be inhibited to various degrees by the SSRIs.

D. Adverse effects

Although the SSRIs are considered to have fewer and less severe adverse effects than the TCAs and MAOIs, the SSRIs are not without adverse effects, such as headache, sweating, anxiety and agitation, hyponatremia, gastrointestinal (GI) effects (nausea, vomiting, and diarrhea), weakness and fatigue, sexual dysfunction, changes in weight, sleep disturbances (insomnia and somnolence), and the above-mentioned potential for drug–drug interactions (Figure 10.4).

1. **Sleep disturbances:** *Paroxetine* and *fluvoxamine* are generally more sedating than activating, and they may be useful in patients

DRUGS USED TO TREAT MANIA and BIPOLAR DISORDER
Carbamazepine TEGRETOL, EQUETRO, CARBATROL
Lamotrigine LAMICTAL
Lithium LITHOBID
Valproic acid DEPAKENE, DEPAKOTE

Figure 10.1 (continued)

DRUG	UPTAKE INHIBITION	
	Norepinephrine	Serotonin
Selective serotonin reuptake inhibitor		
Fluoxetine	0	++++
Serotonin-norepinephrine reuptake inhibitors		
Venlafaxine*	++	++++
Duloxetine	++++	++++
Tricyclic antidepressants		
Imipramine	++++	+++
Nortriptyline	++++	++

Figure 10.2
Relative receptor specificity of some antidepressant drugs. **Venlafaxine* inhibits norepinephrine reuptake only at high doses. ++++ = very strong affinity; +++ = strong affinity; ++ = moderate affinity; + = weak affinity; 0 = little or no affinity.

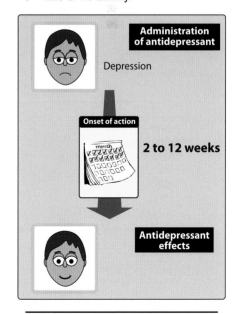

Figure 10.3
Onset of therapeutic effects of the major antidepressant drugs requires several weeks.

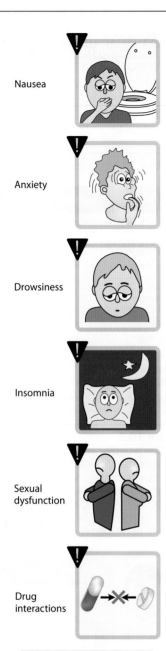

Nausea

Anxiety

Drowsiness

Insomnia

Sexual dysfunction

Drug interactions

Figure 10.4
Some commonly observed adverse effects of selective serotonin reuptake inhibitors.

who have difficulty sleeping. Conversely, patients who are fatigued or complaining of excessive somnolence may benefit from one of the more activating SSRIs, such as *fluoxetine* or *sertraline*.

2. **Sexual dysfunction:** Sexual dysfunction, which may include loss of libido, delayed ejaculation, and anorgasmia, is common with the SSRIs.

3. **Use in children and teenagers:** Antidepressants should be used cautiously in children and teenagers, because of reports of suicidal ideation as a result of SSRI treatment. Pediatric patients should be observed for worsening depression and suicidal thinking with initiation or dosage change of any antidepressant. *Fluoxetine, sertraline*, and *fluvoxamine* are approved for use in children to treat obsessive–compulsive disorder, and *fluoxetine* and *escitalopram* are approved to treat childhood depression.

4. **Overdose:** Overdose with SSRIs does not usually cause cardiac arrhythmias, with the exception of *citalopram*, which may cause QT prolongation. Seizures are a possibility because all antidepressants may lower the seizure threshold. SSRIs have the potential to cause serotonin syndrome, especially when used in the presence of an MAOI or other highly serotonergic drug. Serotonin syndrome may include the symptoms of hyperthermia, muscle rigidity, sweating, myoclonus (clonic muscle twitching), and changes in mental status and vital signs.

5. **Discontinuation syndrome:** SSRIs have the potential to cause a discontinuation syndrome after their abrupt withdrawal, particularly the agents with shorter half-lives and inactive metabolites. *Fluoxetine* has the lowest risk of causing an SSRI discontinuation syndrome due to its longer half-life and active metabolite. Possible signs and symptoms of SSRI discontinuation syndrome include headache, malaise and flu-like symptoms, agitation and irritability, nervousness, and changes in sleep pattern.

IV. SEROTONIN-NOREPINEPHRINE REUPTAKE INHIBITORS

Venlafaxine [VEN-la-fax-een], *desvenlafaxine* [dez-VEN-la-fax-een], *levomilnacipran* [lee-voe-mil-NA-si-pran], and *duloxetine* [doo-LOX-e-teen] inhibit the reuptake of both serotonin and norepinephrine (Figure 10.5) and, thus, are termed SNRIs. Depression is often accompanied by chronic pain, such as backache and muscle aches, for which SSRIs are relatively ineffective. This pain is, in part, modulated by serotonin and norepinephrine pathways in the central nervous system. With dual inhibition of serotonin and norepinephrine reuptake, both the SNRIs and the TCAs may be effective in relieving pain. These agents are also used in the treatment of pain syndromes, such as diabetic peripheral neuropathy, postherpetic neuralgia, fibromyalgia, and low back pain. The SNRIs, unlike the TCAs, have little activity at α-adrenergic, muscarinic, or histamine receptors and, thus, have fewer receptor-mediated adverse effects than the TCAs. The SNRIs may precipitate a discontinuation syndrome if treatment is abruptly stopped.

A. Venlafaxine and desvenlafaxine

Venlafaxine is an inhibitor of serotonin reuptake and, at medium to higher doses, is an inhibitor of norepinephrine reuptake. *Venlafaxine* has minimal inhibition of the CYP450 isoenzymes and is a substrate of the CYP2D6 isoenzyme. *Desvenlafaxine* is the active, demethylated metabolite of *venlafaxine*. The most common side effects of *venlafaxine* are nausea, headache, sexual dysfunction, dizziness, insomnia, sedation, and constipation. At high doses, there may be an increase in blood pressure and heart rate. The clinical activity and adverse effect profile of *desvenlafaxine* are similar to that of *venlafaxine*.

B. Duloxetine

Duloxetine inhibits serotonin and norepinephrine reuptake at all doses. It is extensively metabolized in the liver to inactive metabolites and should be avoided in patients with liver dysfunction. GI side effects are common with *duloxetine*, including nausea, dry mouth, and constipation. Insomnia, dizziness, somnolence, sweating, and sexual dysfunction are also seen. *Duloxetine* may increase blood pressure or heart rate. *Duloxetine* is a moderate inhibitor of CYP2D6 isoenzymes and may increase concentrations of drugs metabolized by this pathway, such as antipsychotics.

C. Levomilnacipran

Levomilnacipran is an enantiomer of *milnacipran* (an older SNRI used for the treatment of depression in Europe and fibromyalgia in the United States). The adverse effect profile of *levomilnacipran* is similar to other SNRIs. It is primarily metabolized by CYP3A4, and, thus, activity may be altered by inducers or inhibitors of this enzyme system.

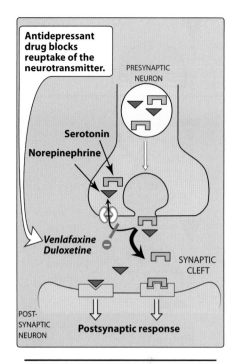

Figure 10.5
Proposed mechanism of action of selective serotonin-norepinephrine reuptake inhibitor antidepressant drugs.

V. ATYPICAL ANTIDEPRESSANTS

The atypical antidepressants are a mixed group of agents that have actions at several different sites. This group includes *bupropion* [byoo-PROE-pee-on], *mirtazapine* [mir-TAZ-a-peen], *nefazodone* [ne-FAZ-oh-done], *trazodone* [TRAZ-oh-done], *vilazodone* [vil-AZ-oh-done], and *vortioxetine* [vor-TEE-ox-e-teen].

A. Bupropion

Bupropion is a weak dopamine and norepinephrine reuptake inhibitor that is used to alleviate the symptoms of depression. *Bupropion* is also useful for decreasing cravings and attenuating withdrawal symptoms of nicotine in patients trying to quit smoking. Side effects may include dry mouth, sweating, nervousness, tremor, and a dose-dependent increased risk for seizures. It has a very low incidence of sexual dysfunction. *Bupropion* is metabolized by the CYP2B6 pathway and has a relatively low risk for drug–drug interactions, given the few agents that inhibit/induce this enzyme. Use of *bupropion* should be avoided in patients at risk for seizures or those who have eating disorders such as bulimia.

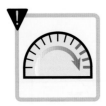

Weight gain

Sedation

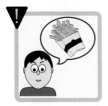

Increased appetite

Figure 10.6
Some commonly observed adverse effects of *mirtazapine*.

B. Mirtazapine

Mirtazapine enhances serotonin and norepinephrine neurotransmission by serving as an antagonist at central presynaptic α_2 receptors. Additionally, some of the antidepressant activity may be related to antagonism at 5-HT$_2$ receptors. It is sedating because of its potent antihistaminic activity, but it does not cause the antimuscarinic side effects of the TCAs or interfere with sexual function like the SSRIs. Sedation, increased appetite, and weight gain frequently occur (Figure 10.6).

C. Nefazodone and trazodone

These drugs are weak inhibitors of serotonin reuptake and are also antagonists at the postsynaptic 5-HT$_{2a}$ receptor. Both agents are sedating, probably because of their potent histamine H$_1$-blocking activity. *Trazodone* is commonly used off-label for the management of insomnia. *Trazodone* has been associated with priapism, and *nefazodone* has been associated with a risk for hepatotoxicity. Both agents also have mild-to-moderate α_1 receptor antagonism, contributing to orthostasis and dizziness.

D. Vilazodone

Vilazodone is a serotonin reuptake inhibitor and a 5-HT$_{1a}$ receptor partial agonist. Although the extent to which the 5-HT$_{1a}$ receptor activity contributes to its therapeutic effects is unknown, this possible mechanism of action renders it unique from that of the SSRIs. The adverse effect profile of *vilazodone* is similar to the SSRIs, including a risk for discontinuation syndrome if abruptly stopped.

E. Vortioxetine

Vortioxetine utilizes a combination of serotonin reuptake inhibition, 5-HT$_{1a}$ agonism, and 5-HT$_3$ and 5-HT$_7$ antagonism as its suggested mechanisms of action to treat depression. It is unclear to what extent the activities other than inhibition of serotonin reuptake influence the overall effects of *vortioxetine*. The common adverse effects include nausea, constipation, and sexual dysfunction, which may be expected due to its serotonergic mechanisms.

VI. TRICYCLIC ANTIDEPRESSANTS

The TCAs inhibit norepinephrine and serotonin reuptake into the presynaptic neuron and, thus, if discovered today, might have been referred to as SNRIs, except for their differences in adverse effects relative to this newer class of antidepressants. The TCAs include the tertiary amines *imipramine* [ee-MIP-ra-meen] (the prototype drug), *amitriptyline* [a-mee-TRIP-ti-leen], *clomipramine* [kloe-MIP-ra-meen], *doxepin* [DOX-e-pin], and *trimipramine* [trye-MIP-ra-meen], and the secondary amines *desipramine* [dess-IP-ra-meen] and *nortriptyline* [nor-TRIP-ti-leen] (the *N*-demethylated metabolites of *imipramine* and *amitriptyline*, respectively) and *protriptyline* [proe-TRIP-ti-leen]. *Maprotiline* [ma-PROE-ti-leen] and *amoxapine* [a-MOX-a-peen] are related "tetracyclic" antidepressant agents and are commonly included in the general class of TCAs.

A. Mechanism of action

1. **Inhibition of neurotransmitter reuptake:** TCAs and *amoxapine* are potent inhibitors of the neuronal reuptake of norepinephrine and serotonin into presynaptic nerve terminals. *Maprotiline* and *desipramine* are relatively selective inhibitors of norepinephrine reuptake.

2. **Blocking of receptors:** TCAs also block serotonergic, α-adrenergic, histaminic, and muscarinic receptors. It is not known if any of these actions produce the therapeutic benefit of the TCAs. However, actions at these receptors are likely responsible for many of their adverse effects. *Amoxapine* also blocks 5-HT$_2$ and dopamine D$_2$ receptors.

B. Actions

The TCAs improve mood, in 50% to 70% of individuals with major depression. The onset of the mood elevation is slow, requiring 2 weeks or longer (Figure 10.3). Patient response can be used to adjust dosage. Tapering of these agents is recommended to minimize discontinuation syndromes and cholinergic rebound effects.

C. Therapeutic uses

The TCAs are effective in treating moderate to severe depression. Some patients with panic disorder also respond to TCAs. *Imipramine* is used as an alternative to *desmopressin* or nonpharmacologic therapies (enuresis alarms) in the treatment of bed-wetting in children. The TCAs, particularly *amitriptyline*, have been used to help prevent migraine headache and treat chronic pain syndromes (for example, neuropathic pain) in a number of conditions for which the cause of pain is unclear. Low doses of TCAs, especially *doxepin*, can be used to treat insomnia.

D. Pharmacokinetics

TCAs are well absorbed upon oral administration. As a result of their variable first-pass metabolism in the liver, TCAs have low and inconsistent bioavailability. These drugs are metabolized by the hepatic microsomal system (and, thus, may be sensitive to agents that induce or inhibit the CYP450 isoenzymes) and conjugated with glucuronic acid. Ultimately, the TCAs are excreted as inactive metabolites via the kidney.

E. Adverse effects

Blockade of muscarinic receptors leads to blurred vision, xerostomia, urinary retention, sinus tachycardia, constipation, and aggravation of angle-closure glaucoma (Figure 10.7). These agents affect cardiac conduction similar to *quinidine* and may precipitate life-threatening arrhythmias in an overdose situation. The TCAs also block α-adrenergic receptors, causing orthostatic hypotension, dizziness, and reflex tachycardia. Sedation is related to the ability of these drugs to block histamine H$_1$ receptors. Weight gain is a common adverse effect of the TCAs. Sexual dysfunction occurs in a minority of patients, and the incidence is lower than that associated with the SSRIs.

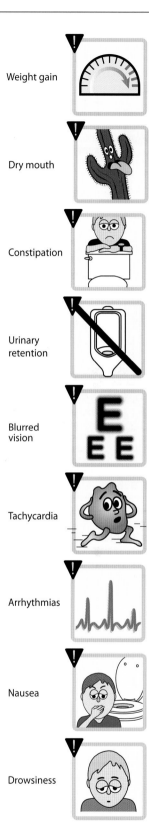

Weight gain

Dry mouth

Constipation

Urinary retention

Blurred vision

Tachycardia

Arrhythmias

Nausea

Drowsiness

Figure 10.7
Some commonly observed adverse effects of tricyclic antidepressants.

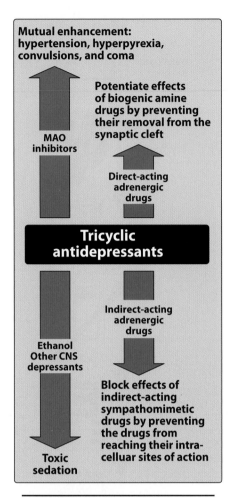

Figure 10.8
Drugs interacting with tricyclic antidepressants. CNS = central nervous system; MAO = monoamine oxidase.

All antidepressants, including TCAs, should be used with caution in patients with bipolar disorder, even during their depressed state, because antidepressants may cause a switch to manic behavior. The TCAs have a narrow therapeutic index (for example, five- to six-fold the maximal daily dose of *imipramine* can be lethal). Depressed patients who are suicidal should be given only limited quantities of these drugs and be monitored closely. Drug interactions with the TCAs are shown in Figure 10.8. The TCAs may exacerbate certain medical conditions, such as benign prostatic hyperplasia, epilepsy, and preexisting arrhythmias.

VII. MONOAMINE OXIDASE INHIBITORS

Monoamine oxidase (MAO) is a mitochondrial enzyme found in nerve and other tissues, such as the gut and liver. In the neuron, MAO functions as a "safety valve" to oxidatively deaminate and inactivate any excess neurotransmitters (for example, norepinephrine, dopamine, and serotonin) that may leak out of synaptic vesicles when the neuron is at rest. The MAOIs may irreversibly or reversibly inactivate the enzyme, permitting neurotransmitters to escape degradation and, therefore, to accumulate within the presynaptic neuron and leak into the synaptic space. The four MAOIs currently available for the treatment of depression include *phenelzine* [FEN-el-zeen], *tranylcypromine* [tran-il-SIP-roe-meen], *isocarboxazid* [eye-soe-car-BOX-ih-zid], and *selegiline* [seh-LEDGE-ah-leen]. [Note: *Selegiline* is also used for the treatment of Parkinson disease. It is the only antidepressant available in a transdermal delivery system.] Use of MAOIs is limited due to the complicated dietary restrictions required while taking these agents.

A. Mechanism of action

Most MAOIs, such as *phenelzine*, form stable complexes with the enzyme, causing irreversible inactivation. This results in increased stores of norepinephrine, serotonin, and dopamine within the neuron and subsequent diffusion of excess neurotransmitter into the synaptic space (Figure 10.9). These drugs inhibit not only MAO in the brain but also MAO in the liver and gut that catalyzes oxidative deamination of drugs and potentially toxic substances, such as tyramine, which is found in certain foods. The MAOIs, therefore, show a high incidence of drug–drug and drug–food interactions. *Selegiline* administered as the transdermal patch may produce less inhibition of gut and hepatic MAO at low doses because it avoids first-pass metabolism.

B. Actions

Although MAO is fully inhibited after several days of treatment, the antidepressant action of the MAOIs, like that of the SSRIs, SNRIs, and TCAs, is delayed several weeks. *Selegiline* and *tranylcypromine* have an amphetamine-like stimulant effect that may produce agitation or insomnia.

C. Therapeutic uses

The MAOIs are indicated for depressed patients who are unresponsive or intolerant of other antidepressants. Because of their risk for drug–drug and drug–food interactions, the MAOIs are considered last-line agents in many treatment settings.

D. Pharmacokinetics

These drugs are well absorbed after oral administration. Enzyme regeneration, when irreversibly inactivated, varies, but it usually occurs several weeks after termination of the drug. Thus, when switching antidepressant agents, a minimum of 2 weeks of delay must be allowed after termination of MAOI therapy and the initiation of another antidepressant from any other class. MAOIs are hepatically metabolized and excreted rapidly in urine.

E. Adverse effects

Severe and often unpredictable side effects, due to drug–food and drug–drug interactions, limit the widespread use of MAOIs. For example, tyramine, which is contained in foods, such as aged cheeses and meats, liver, pickled or smoked fish, and red wines, is normally inactivated by MAO in the gut. Individuals receiving a MAOI are unable to degrade tyramine obtained from the diet. Tyramine causes the release of large amounts of stored catecholamines from nerve terminals, resulting in a hypertensive crisis, with signs and symptoms such as occipital headache, stiff neck, tachycardia, nausea, hypertension, cardiac arrhythmias, seizures, and, possibly, stroke. Patients must, therefore, be educated to avoid tyramine-containing foods. Other possible adverse effects of treatment with MAOIs include drowsiness, orthostatic hypotension, blurred vision, dry mouth, and constipation. SSRIs should not be coadministered with MAOIs due to the risk of serotonin syndrome. Both SSRIs and MAOIs require a washout period of at least 2 weeks before the other type is administered, with the exception of *fluoxetine*, which should be discontinued at least 6 weeks before an MAOI is initiated. In addition, the MAOIs have many other critical drug interactions, and caution is required when administering these agents concurrently with other drugs. Figure 10.10 summarizes the side effects of the antidepressant drugs.

VIII. SEROTONIN–DOPAMINE ANTAGONISTS

While 60% to 80% of patients respond favorably to antidepressants, 20% to 40% experience a partial or poor response to monotherapy. The serotonin–dopamine antagonists (SDAs), or atypical antipsychotics, are occasionally used as adjunctive treatments to antidepressants in partial responders. *Aripiprazole*, *brexpiprazole*, *quetiapine*, and the combination of *fluoxetine* and *olanzapine* are approved for use as adjuncts in major depressive disorder (MDD).

XI. TREATMENT OF MANIA AND BIPOLAR DISORDER

The treatment of bipolar disorder has increased in recent years due to increased recognition of the disorder and also an increase in the number of available medications for the treatment of mania.

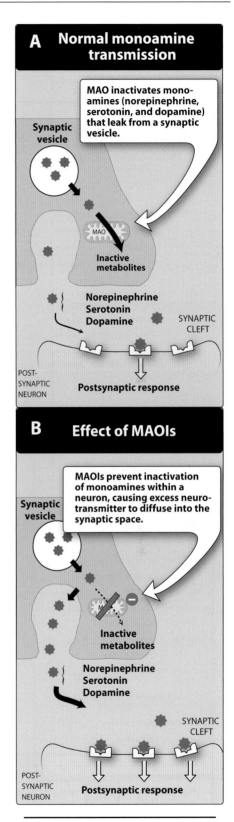

Figure 10.9
Mechanism of action of monoamine oxidase inhibitors (MAOIs).

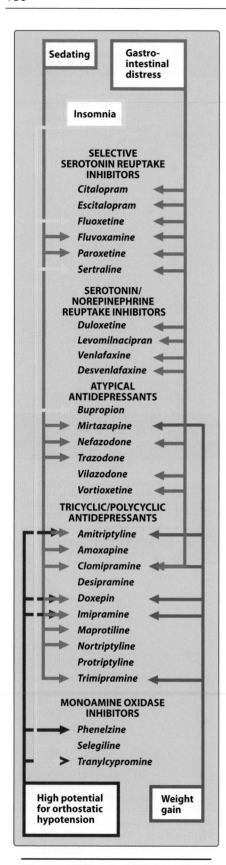

Figure 10.10
Side effects of some drugs used to treat depression.

A. Lithium

Lithium salts are used acutely and prophylactically for managing bipolar patients. *Lithium* is effective in treating 60% to 80% of patients exhibiting mania and hypomania. Although many cellular processes are altered by treatment with *lithium*, the mode of action is unknown. The therapeutic index of *lithium* is extremely low, and *lithium* can be toxic. Common adverse effects may include headache, dry mouth, polydipsia, polyuria, polyphagia, GI distress, fine hand tremor, dizziness, fatigue, dermatologic reactions, and sedation. Adverse effects due to higher plasma levels may indicate toxicity and include ataxia, slurred speech, coarse tremors, confusion, and convulsions. Thyroid function may be decreased and should be monitored. *Lithium* is renally eliminated, and though caution should be used when dosing this drug in renally impaired patients, it may be the best choice in patients with hepatic impairment.

B. Other drugs

Several antiepileptic drugs, including *carbamazepine*, *valproic acid*, and *lamotrigine* (see Chapter 12) are approved as mood stabilizers for bipolar disorder. Other agents that may improve manic symptoms include the older (*chlorpromazine* and *haloperidol*) and newer antipsychotics. The atypical antipsychotics *risperidone*, *olanzapine*, *ziprasidone*, *aripiprazole*, *asenapine*, *cariprazine*, and *quetiapine* (see Chapter 11) are also used for the management of mania. *Quetiapine*, *lurasidone*, and the combination of *olanzapine* and *fluoxetine* have been approved for bipolar depression.

Study Questions

Choose the ONE best answer.

10.1 A 55-year-old teacher was diagnosed with depression. After 6 weeks of therapy with fluoxetine, his symptoms improved, but he complains of sexual dysfunction. Which of the following drugs might be useful for management of depression in this patient?

A. Sertraline
B. Citalopram
C. Mirtazapine
D. Lithium

Correct answer = C. Mirtazapine is largely free from sexual side effects. However, sexual dysfunction commonly occurs with SSRIs (sertraline and citalopram), as well as with TCAs and SNRIs. Lithium is used for the treatment of mania and bipolar disorder.

10.2 A 25-year-old woman has a long history of depressive symptoms accompanied by body aches and pain secondary to a car accident. Which of the following drugs might be useful in this patient?

A. Fluoxetine
B. Sertraline
C. Phenelzine
D. Duloxetine

Correct answer = D. Duloxetine is an SNRI that can be used for depression accompanied by symptoms of pain. SSRIs (fluoxetine and sertraline) and MAOIs (phenelzine) have little activity against pain syndromes.

10.3 A 51-year-old woman with symptoms of major depression also has angle-closure glaucoma. Which antidepressant should be avoided in this patient?

A. Amitriptyline
B. Bupropion
C. Mirtazapine
D. Fluvoxamine

Correct answer = A. Because of its potent antimuscarinic activity, amitriptyline should not be given to patients with glaucoma because of the risk of acute increases in intraocular pressure. The other antidepressants all lack antagonist activity at the muscarinic receptor.

10.4 A 36-year-old man presents with symptoms of compulsive behavior. He realizes that his behavior is interfering with his ability to accomplish his daily tasks but cannot seem to stop himself. Which drug would be most helpful to this patient?

A. Desipramine
B. Paroxetine
C. Amitriptyline
D. Selegiline

Correct answer = B. SSRIs are particularly effective in treating obsessive–compulsive disorder, and paroxetine is approved for this condition. The other drugs are less effective in the treatment of obsessive–compulsive disorder.

10.5 Which antidepressant has, as its two proposed principal mechanisms of action, 5-HT$_{1a}$ receptor partial agonism and 5-HT reuptake inhibition?

A. Fluoxetine
B. Aripiprazole
C. Maprotiline
D. Vilazodone

Correct answer = D. In addition to inhibition of serotonin reuptake, the antidepressant activity of vilazodone may be related to its 5-HT$_{1a}$ receptor agonism. Though aripiprazole is also proposed to have 5-HT$_{1a}$ partial agonism, it is not a serotonin reuptake inhibitor.

10.6 Which antidepressant is the most sedating?

A. Bupropion
B. Duloxetine
C. Doxepin
D. Venlafaxine

Correct answer = C. Doxepin is the most sedating of the list due to its histamine-blocking activity.

10.7 Which mood stabilizer is completely renally eliminated and may be beneficial for patients with hepatic impairment?

A. Valproic acid
B. Carbamazepine
C. Lithium
D. Risperidone

Correct answer = C. Lithium is the only agent for bipolar disorder that does not require hepatic metabolism and, thus, may be dosed without issue in a hepatically impaired patient. However, if the patient had renal impairment, the lithium dosage would have to be adjusted.

10.8 Which antidepressant has, as its two principal mechanisms of action, 5-HT$_{2A}$ receptor antagonism and α_2 receptor antagonism?

A. Fluoxetine
B. Doxepin
C. Maprotiline
D. Mirtazapine

Correct answer = D. Mirtazapine is the only antidepressant with this combination of mechanisms of action that are believed to contribute to its therapeutic effects.

10.9 Which mood-stabilizing agent is most likely to decrease the thyroid function?

A. Carbamazepine
B. Lithium
C. Valproic acid
D. Chlorpromazine

Correct answer = B. Lithium is best known for causing a drug-induced hypothyroidism in patients after long-term use. Though it is possible with other mood stabilizers, lithium has the most reported cases, and thus, thyroid function tests should be performed at baseline and during follow-up to monitor for this possible effect.

10.10 Which antidepressant agent has significant α_1 receptor antagonism and, thus, is a poor choice in an elderly female with depressive symptoms due to a higher risk of falls related to orthostatic hypotension?

A. Venlafaxine
B. Bupropion
C. Escitalopram
D. Amitriptyline

Correct answer = D. Venlafaxine, bupropion, and escitalopram have very little effect on decreasing blood pressure (no α_1 receptor antagonism) and are considered acceptable choices for treatment of depression in the elderly. Amitriptyline is associated with a high risk for orthostasis in the elderly and should be avoided due to its adverse effect profile and risk for falls.

Antipsychotic Drugs

11

Jose A. Rey

I. OVERVIEW

The antipsychotic drugs are used primarily to treat schizophrenia, but they are also effective in other psychotic and manic states. The use of antipsychotic medications involves a difficult trade-off between the benefit of alleviating psychotic symptoms and the risk of a wide variety of adverse effects. Antipsychotic drugs (Figure 11.1) are not curative and do not eliminate chronic thought disorders, but they often decrease the intensity of hallucinations and delusions and permit the person with schizophrenia to function in a supportive environment.

II. SCHIZOPHRENIA

Schizophrenia is a type of chronic psychosis characterized by delusions, hallucinations (often in the form of voices), and disturbances in thought. The onset of illness is often during late adolescence or early adulthood. It occurs in about 1% of the population and is a chronic and disabling disorder. Schizophrenia has a strong genetic component and probably reflects some fundamental developmental and biochemical abnormality, possibly a dysfunction of the mesolimbic or mesocortical dopaminergic neuronal pathways.

III. ANTIPSYCHOTIC DRUGS

The antipsychotic drugs are usually divided into first- and second-generation agents. The first-generation drugs are further classified as "low potency" or "high potency." This classification does not indicate clinical effectiveness of the drugs but rather specifies affinity for the dopamine D_2 receptor, which, in turn, may influence the adverse effect profile of the drug.

A. First-generation antipsychotics

The first-generation antipsychotic drugs (also called conventional) are competitive inhibitors at a variety of receptors, but their antipsychotic effects reflect competitive blockade of dopamine D_2 receptors. First-generation antipsychotics are more likely to be associated with

FIRST-GENERATION ANTIPSYCHOTIC (low potency)
Chlorpromazine GENERIC ONLY
Thioridazine GENERIC ONLY

FIRST-GENERATION ANTIPSYCHOTIC (high potency)
Fluphenazine GENERIC ONLY
Haloperidol HALDOL
Loxapine GENERIC ONLY
Molindone GENERIC ONLY
Perphenazine GENERIC ONLY
Pimozide ORAP
Prochlorperazine COMPRO, PROCOMP
Thiothixene GENERIC ONLY
Trifluoperazine GENERIC ONLY

SECOND-GENERATION ANTIPSYCHOTIC
Aripiprazole ABILIFY, ARISTADA
Asenapine SAPHRIS
Brexpiprazole REXULTI
Cariprazine VRAYLAR
Clozapine CLOZARIL, FAZACLO
Iloperidone FANAPT
Lurasidone LATUDA
Olanzapine ZYPREXA
Paliperidone INVEGA
Pimavanserin NUPLAZID
Quetiapine SEROQUEL
Risperidone RISPERDAL
Ziprasidone GEODON

Figure 11.1
Summary of antipsychotic agents.

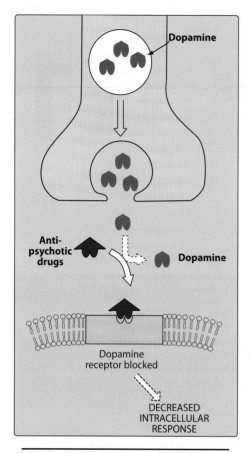

Figure 11.2
Dopamine-blocking actions of antipsychotic drugs.

movement disorders known as extrapyramidal symptoms (EPS), particularly drugs that bind tightly to dopaminergic neuroreceptors, such as *haloperidol* [HAL-oh-PER-i-dol]. Movement disorders are somewhat less likely with medications that bind less potently, such as *chlorpromazine* [klor-PROE-ma-zeen]. No one drug is clinically more effective than another.

B. Second-generation antipsychotic drugs

The second-generation antipsychotic drugs (also called "atypical" antipsychotics) have a lower incidence of EPS than the first-generation agents but are associated with a higher risk of metabolic adverse effects, such as diabetes, hypercholesterolemia, and weight gain. The second-generation drugs owe their unique activity to blockade of both serotonin and dopamine receptors.

1. **Drug selection:** Second-generation agents are generally used as first-line therapy for schizophrenia to minimize the risk of debilitating EPS associated with the first-generation drugs that act primarily at the dopamine D_2 receptor. The second-generation antipsychotics exhibit an efficacy that is equivalent to, and occasionally exceeds, that of the first-generation antipsychotic agents. Differences in therapeutic efficacy among the second-generation drugs have not been established, and individual patient response and comorbid conditions must often be used to guide drug selection.

2. **Refractory patients:** Approximately 10% to 20% of patients with schizophrenia have an insufficient response to first- and second-generation antipsychotics. For these patients, *clozapine* [KLOE-za-peen] has shown to be an effective antipsychotic with a minimal risk of EPS. However, its clinical use is limited to refractory patients because of serious adverse effects. *Clozapine* can produce bone marrow suppression, seizures, and cardiovascular side effects, such as orthostasis. The risk of severe agranulocytosis necessitates frequent monitoring of white blood cell counts.

C. Mechanism of action

1. **Dopamine antagonism:** All of the first-generation and most of the second-generation antipsychotic drugs block D_2 dopamine receptors in the brain and the periphery (Figure 11.2).

2. **Serotonin receptor–blocking activity:** Most of the second-generation agents exert part of their action through inhibition of serotonin receptors (5-HT), particularly 5-HT_{2A} receptors. *Clozapine* has high affinity for D_1, D_4, 5-HT_2, muscarinic, and α-adrenergic receptors, but it is also a weak dopamine D_2 receptor antagonist (Figure 11.3). *Risperidone* [ris-PER-ih-dohn] blocks 5-HT_{2A} receptors to a greater extent than it does D_2 receptors, as does *olanzapine* [oh-LANZ-ah-peen]. The second-generation antipsychotics *aripiprazole* [a-rih-PIP-ra-zole], *brexpiprazole* [brex-PIP-ra-zole], and *cariprazine* [kar-IP-ra-zeen] are partial agonists at D_2 and 5-HT_{1A} receptors, as well as antagonists of 5-HT_{2A} receptors. *Quetiapine* [qwe-TY-uh-peen] is relatively weak at blockade of D_2 and 5-HT_{2A} receptors. Its low risk for EPS may also be related to the relatively short period of time it binds to the

D_2 receptor. *Pimavanserin* [pim-a-VAN-ser-in] appears to act as an inverse agonist and antagonist at the 5-HT_{2A} receptor and the 5-HT_{2C} receptor, with no appreciable affinity for dopamine receptors. *Pimavanserin* is indicated for psychosis associated with Parkinson disease.

D. Actions

The clinical effects of antipsychotic drugs reflect a blockade at dopamine and/or serotonin receptors. However, many antipsychotic agents also block cholinergic, adrenergic, and histaminergic receptors (Figure 11.4). It is unknown what role, if any, these actions have in alleviating the symptoms of psychosis. However, the undesirable adverse effects of antipsychotic drugs often result from pharmacological actions at these other receptors.

1. **Antipsychotic effects:** All antipsychotic drugs can reduce hallucinations and delusions associated with schizophrenia (known as "positive" symptoms) by blocking D_2 receptors in the mesolimbic system of the brain. The "negative" symptoms, such as blunted affect, apathy, and impaired attention, as well as cognitive impairment, are not as responsive to therapy, particularly with the first-generation antipsychotics. Many second-generation agents, such as *clozapine*, can ameliorate the negative symptoms to some extent.

2. **Extrapyramidal effects:** Dystonias (sustained contraction of muscles leading to twisting, distorted postures), Parkinson-like symptoms, akathisia (motor restlessness), and tardive dyskinesia (involuntary movements, usually of the tongue, lips, neck, trunk, and limbs) can occur with both acute and chronic treatment. Blockade of dopamine receptors in the nigrostriatal pathway is believed to cause these unwanted movement symptoms. The second-generation antipsychotics exhibit a lower incidence of EPS.

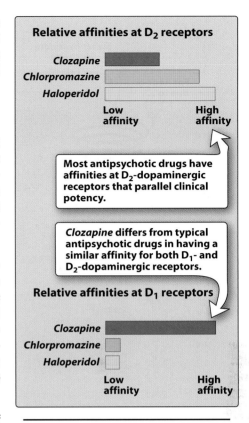

Relative affinities at D_2 receptors

Clozapine
Chlorpromazine
Haloperidol

Low affinity — High affinity

Most antipsychotic drugs have affinities at D_2-dopaminergic receptors that parallel clinical potency.

Clozapine differs from typical antipsychotic drugs in having a similar affinity for both D_1- and D_2-dopaminergic receptors.

Relative affinities at D_1 receptors

Clozapine
Chlorpromazine
Haloperidol

Low affinity — High affinity

Figure 11.3
Relative affinities of *clozapine*, *chlorpromazine*, and *haloperidol* at D_1 and D_2 dopaminergic receptors.

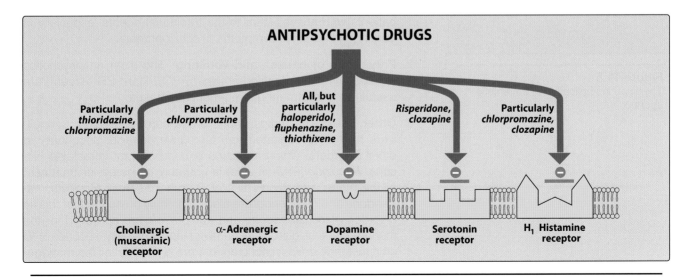

ANTIPSYCHOTIC DRUGS

Particularly *thioridazine*, *chlorpromazine* — Cholinergic (muscarinic) receptor

Particularly *chlorpromazine* — α-Adrenergic receptor

All, but particularly *haloperidol*, *fluphenazine*, *thiothixene* — Dopamine receptor

Risperidone, *clozapine* — Serotonin receptor

Particularly *chlorpromazine*, *clozapine* — H_1 Histamine receptor

Figure 11.4
Antipsychotic drugs block dopaminergic and serotonergic receptors as well as adrenergic, cholinergic, and histamine-binding receptors.

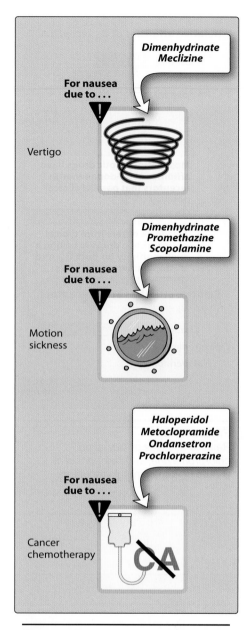

For nausea due to . . .

Vertigo

Dimenhydrinate
Meclizine

For nausea due to . . .

Motion sickness

Dimenhydrinate
Promethazine
Scopolamine

For nausea due to . . .

Cancer chemotherapy

Haloperidol
Metoclopramide
Ondansetron
Prochlorperazine

Figure 11.5
Therapeutic application of antiemetic agents.

3. **Antiemetic effects:** The antipsychotic drugs have antiemetic effects that are mediated by blocking D_2 receptors of the chemoreceptor trigger zone of the medulla (see Chapter 40). Figure 11.5 summarizes the antiemetic uses of antipsychotic agents, as well as other drugs that combat nausea.

4. **Anticholinergic effects:** Some of the antipsychotics, particularly *thioridazine* [THYE-oh-RID-a-zeen], *chlorpromazine*, *clozapine*, and *olanzapine*, produce anticholinergic effects. These effects include blurred vision, dry mouth (the exception is *clozapine*, which increases salivation), confusion, and inhibition of gastrointestinal and urinary tract smooth muscle, leading to constipation and urinary retention. The anticholinergic effects may actually assist in reducing the risk of EPS with these agents.

5. **Other effects:** Blockade of α-adrenergic receptors causes orthostatic hypotension and light-headedness. The antipsychotics also alter temperature-regulating mechanisms and can produce poikilothermia (condition in which body temperature varies with the environment). In the pituitary, antipsychotics that block D_2 receptors may cause an increase in prolactin release. Sedation occurs with those drugs that are potent antagonists of the H_1-histamine receptor, including *chlorpromazine*, *olanzapine*, *quetiapine*, and *clozapine*. Sexual dysfunction may also occur with the antipsychotics due to various receptor-binding characteristics. Weight gain is also a common adverse effect of antipsychotics and is more significant with the second-generation agents.

E. **Therapeutic uses**

1. **Treatment of schizophrenia:** The antipsychotics are the only efficacious pharmacological treatment for schizophrenia. The first-generation antipsychotics are generally most effective in treating the positive symptoms of schizophrenia. The atypical antipsychotics with $5-HT_{2A}$ receptor–blocking activity may be effective in many patients who are resistant to the traditional agents, especially in treating the negative symptoms of schizophrenia.

2. **Prevention of nausea and vomiting:** The older antipsychotics (most commonly, *prochlorperazine* [PROE-klor-PER-a-zeen]) are useful in the treatment of drug-induced nausea.

3. **Other uses:** The antipsychotic drugs can be used as tranquilizers to manage agitated and disruptive behavior secondary to other disorders. *Chlorpromazine* is used to treat intractable hiccups. *Pimozide* [PIM-oh-zide] is primarily indicated for treatment of the motor and phonic tics of Tourette disorder. However, *risperidone* and *haloperidol* are also commonly prescribed for this tic disorder. Also, *risperidone* and *aripiprazole* are approved for the management of disruptive behavior and irritability secondary to autism. Many antipsychotic agents are approved for the management of the manic and mixed symptoms associated with bipolar disorder. *Lurasidone* [loo-RAS-i-done] and *quetiapine* are indicated for the treatment of bipolar depression. *Paliperidone* [pal-ee-PER-i-dohn] is approved for the treatment of schizoaffective

disorder. Some antipsychotics (*aripiprazole*, *brexpiprazole*, and *quetiapine*) are used as adjunctive agents with antidepressants for treatment-refractory depression.

F. Absorption and metabolism

After oral administration, the antipsychotics show variable absorption that is unaffected by food (except for *ziprasidone* [zi-PRAS-i-done], *lurasidone*, and *paliperidone*, the absorption of which is increased with food). These agents readily pass into the brain and have a large volume of distribution. They are metabolized to many different metabolites, usually by the cytochrome P-450 system in the liver, particularly the CYP2D6, CYP1A2, and CYP3A4 isoenzymes. Some metabolites are active and have been developed as pharmacological agents themselves (for example, *paliperidone* is the active metabolite of *risperidone*, and the antidepressant *amoxapine* is the active metabolite of *loxapine*). *Fluphenazine decanoate*, *haloperidol decanoate*, *risperidone microspheres*, *paliperidone palmitate*, *aripiprazole monohydrate*, *aripiprazole lauroxil*, and *olanzapine pamoate* are long-acting injectable (LAI) formulations of antipsychotics. These formulations usually have a therapeutic duration of action of 2 to 4 weeks, with some having a duration of 6 to 12 weeks. Therefore, these LAI formulations are often used to treat outpatients and individuals who are nonadherent with oral medications.

G. Adverse effects

Adverse effects of the antipsychotic drugs can occur in practically all patients and are significant in about 80% (Figure 11.6).

1. **Extrapyramidal effects:** The inhibitory effects of dopaminergic neurons are normally balanced by the excitatory actions of cholinergic neurons in the striatum. Blocking dopamine receptors alters this balance, causing a relative excess of cholinergic influence, which results in extrapyramidal motor effects. The appearance of the movement disorders is generally time- and dose dependent, with dystonias occurring within a few hours to days of treatment, followed by akathisias occurring within days to weeks. Parkinson-like symptoms of bradykinesia, rigidity, and tremor usually occur within weeks to months of initiating treatment. Tardive dyskinesia (see below), which can be irreversible, may occur after months or years of treatment.

   If cholinergic activity is also blocked, a new, more nearly normal balance is restored, and extrapyramidal effects are minimized. This can be achieved by administration of an anticholinergic drug, such as *benztropine* [BENZ-troe-peen]. The therapeutic trade-off is a lower incidence of EPS in exchange for the adverse effect of muscarinic receptor blockade. Akathisia may respond better to β-blockers (for example, *propranolol*) or benzodiazepines, rather than anticholinergic medications.

2. **Tardive dyskinesia:** Long-term treatment with antipsychotics can cause this motor disorder. Patients display involuntary movements, including bilateral and facial jaw movements and "fly-catching" motions of the tongue. A prolonged holiday from antipsychotics may cause the symptoms to diminish or disappear within a few months. However, in many individuals, tardive dyskinesia is

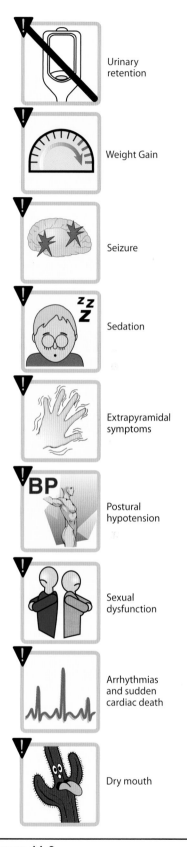

Figure 11.6
Adverse effects observed in individuals treated with antipsychotic drugs.

irreversible and persists after discontinuation of therapy. Tardive dyskinesia is postulated to result from an increased number of dopamine receptors that are synthesized as a compensatory response to long-term dopamine receptor blockade. This makes the neuron supersensitive to the actions of dopamine, and it allows the dopaminergic input to this structure to overpower the cholinergic input, causing excess movement in the patient. Traditional anti-EPS medications may actually worsen this condition. *Valbenazine* [val-BEN-a-zeen] and *deutetrabenazine* [doo-TET-ra-BEN-a-zeen] are inhibitors of the vesicular monoamine transporter, and they are indicated for the management of tardive dyskinesia. These agents cause a decreased uptake of monoamines into synaptic vesicles and depletion of monoamine stores, ideally focused on dopamine, to address the symptoms of tardive dyskinesia.

3. **Neuroleptic malignant syndrome:** This potentially fatal reaction to antipsychotic drugs is characterized by muscle rigidity, fever, altered mental status and stupor, unstable blood pressure, and myoglobinemia. Treatment necessitates discontinuation of the antipsychotic agent and supportive therapy. Administration of *dantrolene* or *bromocriptine* may be helpful.

4. **Other effects:** Drowsiness occurs during the first few weeks of treatment. These agents may also cause confusion. Those antipsychotics with potent antimuscarinic activity often produce dry mouth, urinary retention, constipation, and loss of visual accommodation. Others may block α-adrenergic receptors, resulting in lowered blood pressure and orthostatic hypotension. The antipsychotics depress the hypothalamus, thereby affecting thermoregulation and causing amenorrhea, galactorrhea, gynecomastia, infertility, and erectile dysfunction. Significant weight gain is often a reason for nonadherence. Glucose and lipid profiles should be monitored in patients taking antipsychotics, as the second-generation agents may increase these laboratory parameters and possibly exacerbate preexisting diabetes or hyperlipidemia. Some antipsychotics have been associated with mild to significant QT prolongation. *Thioridazine* has the highest risk, and *ziprasidone* and *iloperidone* [eye-low-PER-ee-dohn] also have cautions with their use due to this effect. Other antipsychotics have a general precaution regarding QT prolongation, even if the risk is relatively low.

5. **Cautions and contraindications:** All antipsychotics may lower the seizure threshold and should be used cautiously in patients with seizure disorders or those with an increased risk for seizures, such as withdrawal from alcohol. These agents also carry the warning of increased risk for mortality when used in elderly patients with dementia-related behavioral disturbances and psychosis. Antipsychotics used in patients with mood disorders should also be monitored for worsening of mood and suicidal ideation or behaviors.

H. Maintenance treatment

Patients who have had two or more psychotic episodes secondary to schizophrenia should receive maintenance therapy for at least 5 years, and some experts prefer indefinite therapy. The rate of relapse may be lower with second-generation drugs (Figure 11.7). Figure 11.8 summarizes the therapeutic uses of some of the antipsychotic drugs.

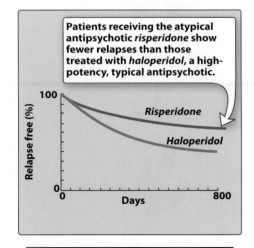

Patients receiving the atypical antipsychotic *risperidone* show fewer relapses than those treated with *haloperidol*, a high-potency, typical antipsychotic.

Figure 11.7
Rates of relapse among patients with schizophrenia after maintenance therapy with either *risperidone* or *haloperidol*.

DRUG	THERAPEUTIC NOTES
First generation	
Chlorpromazine	Moderate to high potential for EPS; moderate to high potential for weight gain, orthostasis, sedation, anti-muscarinic effects.
Fluphenazine	Oral formulation has a high potential for EPS; low potential for weight gain, sedation, and orthostasis; low to moderate potential for antimuscarinic effects; common use is in the LAI formulation administered every 2–3 weeks in patients with schizophrenia and a history of noncompliance with oral antipsychotic regimens.
Haloperidol	High potential for EPS; low potential for anti-adrenergic (orthostasis) or antimuscarinic adverse events; low potential for weight gain or sedation; available in a LAI formulation administered every 4 weeks.
Second generation	
Aripiprazole	Low potential for EPS; low potential for weight gain; low potential for sedation and antimuscarinic effects; also approved for the treatment of bipolar disorder; also approved for autistic disorder in children, and as an adjunctive treatment for major depression; two LAI formulations are available.
Asenapine	Low potential for EPS; low potential for weight gain; low to moderate potential for sedation; low potential for orthostasis; also approved for the treatment of bipolar disorder; available as a sublingual formulation.
Brexpiprazole	Low potential for EPS; low potential for weight gain; low potential for sedation; also approved as an adjunctive treatment for partial response or refractory major depression with an antidepressant.
Cariprazine	Low potential for EPS; low potential for weight gain; possible nausea and gastrointestinal distress; also approved for manic/mixed episodes associated with bipolar disorder.
Clozapine	Very low potential for EPS; risk for blood dyscrasias (for example, agranulocytosis = ~1%); risk for seizures; risk for myocarditis; high potential for the following: sialorrhea, weight gain, antimuscarinic effects, orthostasis, and sedation.
Lurasidone	Low potential for EPS; minimal weight gain; also approved for use in treating depression associated with bipolar disorder; food increases absorption.
Olanzapine	Low potential for EPS; moderate to high potential for weight gain and sedation; low potential for orthostasis; also approved for the treatment of bipolar disorder; available as a LAI formulation administered every 2–4 weeks.
Paliperidone	Low to moderate potential for EPS; low potential for weight gain; low potential for sedation; available as a LAI formulation administered every 4 weeks and as an alternate LAI formulation administered every 12 weeks; also approved for use in schizoaffective disorder.
Quetiapine	Low potential for EPS; moderate potential for weight gain; moderate potential for orthostasis; moderate to high potential for sedation; also approved for the treatment of bipolar disorder and as an adjunctive treatment for major depression.
Risperidone	Low to moderate potential for EPS; low to moderate potential for weight gain; low to moderate potential for orthostasis; low to moderate potential for sedation; also approved for the treatment of bipolar disorder; also approved for autistic disorder in children; available as a LAI formulation administered every 2 weeks.
Ziprasidone	Low potential for extrapyramidal effects; contraindicated in patients with history of cardiac arrhythmias; minimal weight gain. Used in treatment of bipolar depression.

Figure 11.8
Summary of antipsychotic agents commonly used to treat schizophrenia. EPS = extrapyramidal effects; LAI = long-acting injectable.

Study Questions

Choose the ONE best answer.

11.1 An adolescent male is newly diagnosed with schizophrenia. Which antipsychotic agent may have the best chance to improve his apathy and blunted affect?

A. Chlorpromazine
B. Fluphenazine
C. Haloperidol
D. Risperidone

Correct answer = D. Risperidone is the only antipsychotic on the list that has some reported benefit in improving the negative symptoms of schizophrenia. All of the agents have the potential to diminish the hallucinations and delusional thought processes (positive symptoms).

11.2 Which of the following antipsychotics is a partial agonist at the dopamine D_2 receptor?

A. Brexpiprazole
B. Clozapine
C. Haloperidol
D. Risperidone

Correct answer = A. Brexpiprazole is the only agent listed that acts as a partial agonist at D_2 receptors. Theoretically, the drug enhances action at these receptors under low dopamine conditions and blocks activation when dopamine levels are high. All of the other drugs are antagonistic at D_2 receptors.

11.3 A 21-year-old man has recently begun pimozide therapy for Tourette disorder. He has been having "different-appearing tics," such as prolonged contraction of the facial muscles, and he experiences opisthotonos (extrapyramidal spasm of the body in which the head and heels are bent backward and the body is bowed forward). Which of the following drugs would be beneficial in reducing these symptoms?

A. Benztropine
B. Bromocriptine
C. Prochlorperazine
D. Risperidone

Correct answer = A. The patient is experiencing EPS due to pimozide, and a muscarinic antagonist such as benztropine would be effective in reducing the symptoms. The other drugs would have no effect or, in the case of prochlorperazine and risperidone, might increase the adverse symptoms.

11.4 A 28-year-old woman with schizoaffective disorder (combination of mood and psychotic symptoms) reports difficulty falling asleep. Which of the following would be most beneficial in this patient?

A. Olanzapine
B. Haloperidol
C. Paliperidone
D. Ziprasidone

Correct answer = C. Paliperidone is the only agent that is approved for schizoaffective disorder. Olanzapine has significant sedative activity as well as antipsychotic properties and is the drug most likely to alleviate this patient's report of insomnia. Although other antipsychotics may benefit this patient's disorder, paliperidone has the indication for this disorder, and if the underlying disorder is improved, then the symptom of insomnia may also improve without risking other unwanted adverse effects, such as the weight gain associated with olanzapine.

11.5 Which of the following antipsychotic agents is considered to be the most potent and thus have the highest risk of extrapyramidal symptoms?

A. Thioridazine
B. Haloperidol
C. Quetiapine
D. Chlorpromazine

Correct answer = B. Among the older, conventional, or typical antipsychotics on this list, haloperidol is the most potent and would thus be expected to have the highest incidence of EPS. The atypical antipsychotics listed (quetiapine) could be considered low potency based on their common dosing and are considered to have the lowest risk for EPS.

11.6 Which antipsychotic has the most sedative potential and is sometimes, questionably, used as a hypnotic agent in certain clinical settings?

A. Fluphenazine
B. Thiothixene
C. Quetiapine
D. Haloperidol

Correct answer = C. Quetiapine has strong antihistaminergic effects causing sedation and is sometimes used at low doses as a sedative–hypnotic, even though this use is considered off-label. The other antipsychotic agents listed are weaker at blocking the histamine receptor and therefore are not as sedating.

11.7 A 30-year-old male patient is treated with haloperidol for schizophrenia. His psychotic symptoms are well managed with haloperidol; however, he is reporting restlessness, the inability to sit still at the dinner table, and his family notices that he frequently paces the hallway. Which is the best agent to treat this antipsychotic-induced akathisia?

A. Benztropine
B. Dantrolene
C. Bromocriptine
D. Propranolol

Correct answer = D. Propranolol, a β-blocker, is considered the drug of choice for the management of antipsychotic-induced akathisia. Benztropine is more effective for pseudoparkinsonism and acute dystonias. Bromocriptine is more effective for Parkinson-like symptoms, and dantrolene is a muscle relaxant that is best reserved for managing some symptoms of neuroleptic malignant syndrome.

11.8 Which antipsychotic agent is available in an LAI formulation that may be useful for patients with difficulty adhering to therapy?

A. Asenapine

B. Chlorpromazine

C. Clozapine

D. Aripiprazole

Correct answer = D. Aripiprazole is available in two different LAI formulations. The other agents listed do not have LAI formulations. Risperidone, fluphenazine, haloperidol, olanzapine, and paliperidone are other antipsychotics that are available in LAI formulations.

11.9 Which antipsychotic agent is most associated with the possibility of a hematological dyscrasia such as agranulocytosis in a patient being treated for schizophrenia?

A. Chlorpromazine

B. Buspirone

C. Lithium

D. Clozapine

Correct answer = D. Clozapine is the only antipsychotic medication that has a black box warning and a risk of agranulocytosis in approximately 1% of the patients treated. This requires regular monitoring of white blood cell counts. Although other antipsychotics have case reports of blood dyscrasias, clozapine is considered to have the highest risk.

11.10 Which antipsychotic agent has been most associated with significant QT interval prolongation and should be used with caution in patients with preexisting arrhythmias or patients taking other drugs associated with QT prolongation?

A. Thioridazine

B. Risperidone

C. Asenapine

D. Lurasidone

Correct answer = A. Of the antipsychotic drugs listed, thioridazine has the highest risk for causing QT interval prolongation. Although this is a general warning for many antipsychotics, thioridazine has been issued a "black box warning," suggesting that it is associated with the greatest risk.

Drugs for Epilepsy

12

Jeannine M. Conway and Angela K. Birnbaum

I. OVERVIEW

Approximately 10% of the population has at least one seizure in their lifetime. Globally, epilepsy is the fourth most common neurologic disorder after migraine, cerebrovascular disease (stroke), and Alzheimer's disease. Epilepsy is not a single entity but an assortment of different seizure types and syndromes originating from several mechanisms that have in common the sudden, excessive, and synchronous discharge of cerebral neurons. This abnormal electrical activity may result in a variety of events, including loss of consciousness, abnormal movements, atypical or odd behavior, and distorted perceptions that are of limited duration but recur if untreated. The site of origin of abnormal neuronal firing determines the symptoms that occur. For example, if the motor cortex is involved, the patient may experience abnormal movements or a generalized convulsion. Seizures originating in the parietal or occipital lobe may include visual, auditory, and olfactory hallucinations. Medications are the most widely used mode of treatment for patients with epilepsy. In general, seizures can be controlled with one medication in approximately 75% of patients. Patients may require more than one medication in order to optimize seizure control, and some patients may never obtain total seizure control. A summary of antiseizure medications is shown in Figure 12.1.

II. ETIOLOGY OF SEIZURES

Epilepsy can be due to an underlying genetic, structural, or metabolic cause or an unknown etiology. In most cases, epilepsy has no identifiable cause. The neuronal discharge in epilepsy results from firing of a small population of neurons in a specific area of the brain referred to as the "primary focus." Focal areas that are functionally abnormal may be triggered into activity by changes in physiologic factors, such as an alteration in blood gases, pH, electrolytes, and blood glucose and changes in environmental factors, such as sleep deprivation, alcohol intake, and stress. A number of causes, such as illicit drug use, tumor, head injury, hypoglycemia, meningeal infection, and the rapid withdrawal of alcohol from an alcoholic, can precipitate seizures. In cases when the source of a seizure can be determined and corrected, medication may not be necessary. For example, a seizure that is caused by a drug reaction is not epilepsy and

Brivaracetam BRIVIACT
Carbamazepine TEGRETOL
Clobazam ONFI
Clonazepam KLONOPIN
Diazepam VALIUM
Divalproex DEPAKOTE
Eslicarbazepine APTIOM
Ethosuximide ZARONTIN
Felbamate FELBATOL
Fosphenytoin CEREBYX
Gabapentin NEURONTIN
Lacosamide VIMPAT
Lamotrigine LAMICTAL
Levetiracetam KEPPRA
Lorazepam ATIVAN
Oxcarbazepine TRILEPTAL
Perampanel FYCOMPA
Phenobarbital GENERIC ONLY
Phenytoin DILANTIN
Pregabalin LYRICA
Primidone MYSOLINE
Rufinamide BANZEL
Tiagabine GABITRIL
Topiramate TOPAMAX
Vigabatrin SABRIL
Zonisamide ZONEGRAN

Figure 12.1
Summary of agents used in the treatment of epilepsy.

does not require chronic therapy. In other situations, antiseizure medications may be needed when the primary cause of the seizures cannot be corrected. Though multiple specific epilepsy syndromes that include symptoms other than seizures have been classified, a discussion of these syndromes is beyond the scope of this chapter.

III. CLASSIFICATION OF SEIZURES

It is important to correctly classify seizures to determine appropriate treatment. Seizures have been categorized by site of origin, etiology, electrophysiologic correlation, and clinical presentation. Nomenclature developed by the International League Against Epilepsy is considered the standard classification for seizures and epilepsy syndromes (Figure 12.2). Seizures have been classified into two broad groups: focal and generalized.

A. Focal

Focal seizures involve only a portion of one hemisphere of the brain. The symptoms of each seizure type depend on the site of neuronal discharge and on the extent to which the electrical activity spreads to other neurons in the brain. Focal seizures may progress to become bilateral tonic–clonic seizures. Patients may lose consciousness or awareness. This seizure type may begin with a motor or nonmotor activity.

B. Generalized

Generalized seizures may begin locally and then progress to include abnormal electrical discharges throughout both hemispheres of the brain. Primary generalized seizures may be convulsive or nonconvulsive, and the patient usually has an immediate loss of consciousness.

1. **Tonic–clonic:** These seizures result in loss of consciousness, followed by tonic (continuous contraction) and clonic (rapid contraction and relaxation) phases. The seizure may be followed by a period of confusion and exhaustion due to depletion of glucose and energy stores.

2. **Absence:** These seizures involve a brief, abrupt, and self-limiting loss of consciousness. The onset generally occurs in patients at 3 to 5 years of age and lasts until puberty or beyond. The patient stares and exhibits rapid eye blinking, which lasts for 3 to 5 seconds. An absence seizure has a very distinct three-per-second spike and wave discharge seen on electroencephalogram.

3. **Myoclonic:** These seizures consist of short episodes of muscle contractions that may recur for several minutes. They generally occur after wakening and exhibit as brief jerks of the limbs. Myoclonic seizures occur at any age but usually begin around puberty or early adulthood.

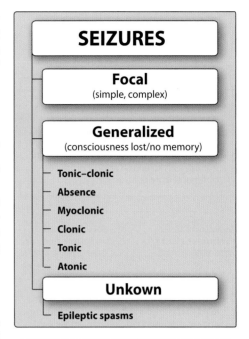

Figure 12.2
Classification of epilepsy.

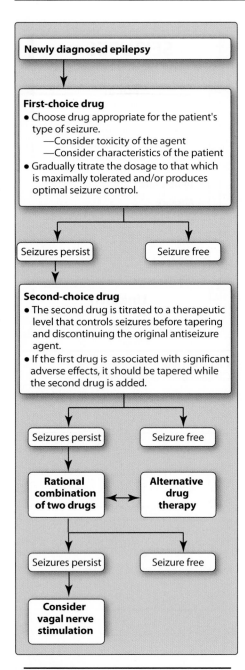

Figure 12.3
Therapeutic strategies for managing newly diagnosed epilepsy.

4. **Clonic:** These seizures consist of short episodes of muscle contractions that may closely resemble myoclonic seizures. Consciousness is more impaired with clonic seizures as compared to myoclonic.

5. **Tonic:** These seizures involve increased tone in the extension muscles and are generally less than 60 seconds.

6. **Atonic:** These seizures are also known as drop attacks and are characterized by a sudden loss of muscle tone.

C. Mechanism of action of antiseizure medications

Drugs reduce seizures through mechanisms such as blocking voltage-gated channels (Na^+ or Ca^{2+}), enhancing inhibitory γ-aminobutyric acid (GABA)ergic impulses and interfering with excitatory glutamate transmission. Some antiseizure medications appear to have multiple targets within the central nervous system (CNS), whereas the mechanism of action for some agents is poorly defined. Antiseizure medications suppress seizures but do not "cure" or "prevent" epilepsy.

IV. DRUG SELECTION

Choice of drug treatment is based on the classification of the seizures, patient-specific variables (for example, age, comorbid medical conditions, lifestyle, and personal preference), and characteristics of the drug (such as cost and drug interactions). For example, focal-onset seizures are treated with a different set of medications than primary generalized seizures, although the list of effective agents overlaps. The toxicity of the agent and characteristics of the patient are major considerations in drug selection. In newly diagnosed patients, monotherapy is instituted with a single agent until seizures are controlled or toxicity occurs (Figure 12.3). Compared with those receiving combination therapy, patients receiving monotherapy exhibit better medication adherence and fewer side effects. If seizures are not controlled with the first medication, monotherapy with an alternate medication or the addition of medications should be considered (Figure 12.4). Failing that, other medical management (vagal nerve stimulation, surgery, etc.) should be considered. Awareness of the antiseizure medications available and their mechanisms of action, pharmacokinetics, potential for drug–drug interactions, and adverse effects is essential for successful treatment of the patient.

V. ANTISEIZURE MEDICATIONS

The Food and Drug Administration has approved many new antiseizure medications in the last few decades. Some of these agents are thought to have potential advantages over older drugs in terms of pharmacokinetics, tolerability, and reduced risk for drug–drug interactions. However, studies have failed to demonstrate that the newer drugs are significantly more

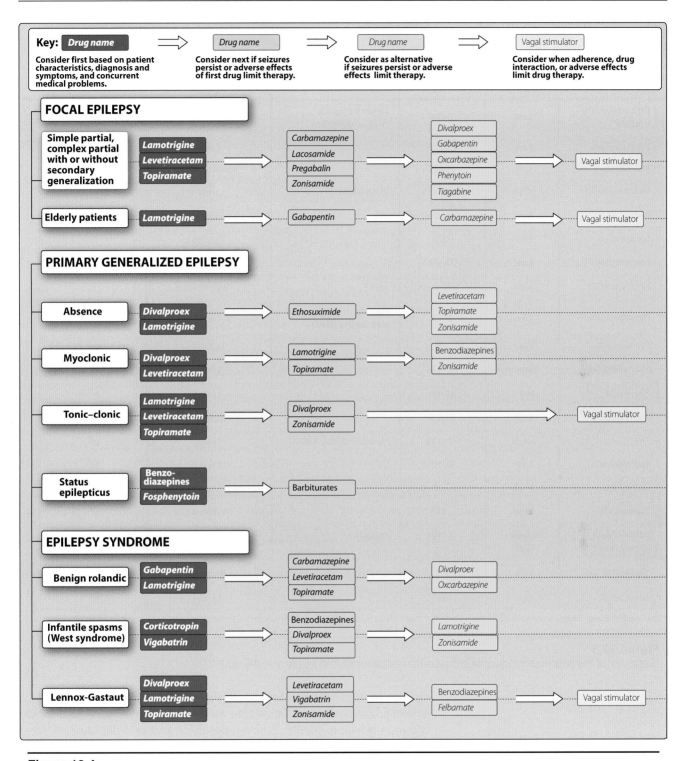

Figure 12.4
Therapeutic indications for the antiseizure agents. Benzodiazepines = *diazepam* and *lorazepam*.

ANTISEIZURE MEDICATION	PROTEIN BINDING*	HALF-LIFE**	ACTIVE METABOLITE	MAJOR ORGAN OF ELIMINATION	DRUG INTERACTIONS
Brivaracetam	Low	9		Liver	✔
Carbamazepine	Moderate	6–15	CBZ-10,11-epoxide	Liver	✔
Eslicarbazepine acetate^	Low	8–24	Eslicarbazepine (S-licarbazepine)	Kidney	✔
Ethosuximide	Low	25–26		Liver	✔
Felbamate	Low	20–23		Kidney/Liver	✔
Fosphenytoin^	High	12–60	phenytoin	Liver	✔
Gabapentin	Low	5–9		Kidney	
Lacosamide	Low	13		Various	
Lamotrigine	Low	25–32		Liver	✔
Levetiracetam	Low	6–8		Hydrolysis	
Oxcarbazepine^	Low	5–13	Monohydroxy metabolite (MHD)	Liver	✔
Perampanel	High	105		Liver	✔
Phenobarbital	Low	72–124		Liver	✔
Phenytoin	High	12–60		Liver	✔
Pregabalin	Low	5–6.5		Kidney	
Primidone	High	72–124	Phenobarbital, PEMA	Liver	✔
Rufinamide	Low	6–10		Liver	✔
Tiagabine	High	7–9		Liver	✔
Topiramate	Low	21		Various	✔
Valproic acid (Divalproex)	Moderate/ High	6–18	Various	Liver	✔
Vigabatrin	Low	7.5		Kidney	✔
Zonisamide	Low	63		Liver	✔

*Low = 60% or less, Moderate = 61%-85%, High = >85%. **Half-life in hours. ^Prodrug. PEMA = phenylethylmalonamide.

Figure 12.5
Summary of the pharmacokinetics of antiseizure medications used as chronic therapy.

efficacious than are the older agents. Figure 12.5 summarizes pharmacokinetic properties of the antiseizure medications, and Figure 12.6 shows common adverse effects. Suicidal behavior and suicidal ideation have been identified as a risk with antiseizure medications. In addition, virtually, all antiseizure medications have been associated with multiorgan hypersensitivity reactions, a rare idiosyncratic reaction characterized by rash, fever, and systemic organ involvement.

A. Benzodiazepines

Benzodiazepines bind to GABA inhibitory receptors to reduce the firing rate. Most benzodiazepines are reserved for emergency or acute seizure treatment due to tolerance. However, clonazepam [kloe-NAY-ze-pam] and clobazam [KLOE-ba-zam] may be prescribed as adjunctive therapy for particular types of seizures. Diazepam [dye-AZ-e-pam] is also available for rectal administration to avoid or interrupt prolonged generalized tonic–clonic seizures or clusters when oral administration is not possible.

B. Brivaracetam

Brivaracetam [briv-a-RA-se-tam] is approved for treatment of focal-onset seizures in adults. It demonstrates high and selective affinity for a synaptic vesicle protein (SV2A); however, the exact mechanism of anti-seizure action is unknown. The drug is well absorbed after oral administration and metabolized by both hydrolysis and CYP2C19 (minor). Comedication with strong CYP-inducing medications may lead to lower plasma concentrations. *Brivaracetam* is a moderate inhibitor of epoxide hydrolase, resulting in increased levels of the active metabolite of *carbamazepine* when the drugs are coadministered.

C. Carbamazepine

Carbamazepine [kar-ba-MAZ-a-peen] blocks sodium channels, thereby possibly inhibiting the generation of repetitive action potentials in the epileptic focus and preventing spread. *Carbamazepine* is effective for treatment of focal seizures, generalized tonic–clonic seizures, trigeminal neuralgia, and bipolar disorder. It induces its own metabolism, resulting in lower total *carbamazepine* blood concentrations at higher doses. *Carbamazepine* is an inducer of the CYP1A2, CYP2C, CYP3A, and UDP glucuronosyltransferase (UGT) enzymes, which increases the clearance of other drugs (Figure 12.7). Hyponatremia may be noted in some patients, especially the elderly, and may necessitate a change in medication. *Carbamazepine* should not be prescribed for patients with absence seizures because it may cause an increase in seizures.

D. Eslicarbazepine

Eslicarbazepine [es-li-kar-BAZ-a-peen] *acetate* is a prodrug that is converted to the active metabolite *eslicarbazepine* (S-licarbazepine) by hydrolysis. S-licarbazepine is the active metabolite of *oxcarbazepine*. It is a voltage-gated sodium channel blocker and is approved for focal seizures in adults. *Eslicarbazepine* exhibits linear pharmacokinetics and is eliminated via glucuronidation. The side effect profile includes dizziness, somnolence, diplopia, and headache. Serious adverse reactions such as rash, psychiatric side effects, and hyponatremia occur rarely.

E. Ethosuximide

Ethosuximide [eth-oh-SUX-i-mide] reduces propagation of abnormal electrical activity in the brain, most likely by inhibiting T-type calcium channels. It is most effective in treating absence seizures.

F. Felbamate

Felbamate [FEL-ba-mate] has a broad spectrum of anticonvulsant action with multiple proposed mechanisms including the blocking of voltage-dependent sodium channels, competing with the glycine-binding site on the *N*-methyl-ᴅ-aspartate (NMDA) glutamate receptor, blocking of calcium channels, and potentiating GABA action. It is an inhibitor of drugs metabolized by CYP2C19 and induces drugs metabolized by CYP3A4. It is reserved for use in refractory epilepsies

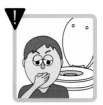
Nausea and vomiting

Sedation

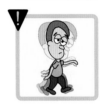
Ataxia

Rash

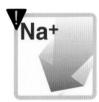
Hyponatremia

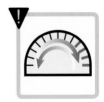
Weight gain or weight loss

Teratogenicity

Osteoporosis

Figure 12.6
Notable adverse effects of antiseizure medications.

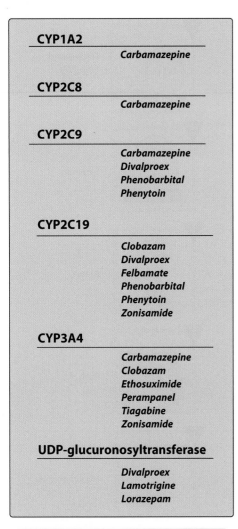

CYP1A2
Carbamazepine

CYP2C8
Carbamazepine

CYP2C9
Carbamazepine
Divalproex
Phenobarbital
Phenytoin

CYP2C19
Clobazam
Divalproex
Felbamate
Phenobarbital
Phenytoin
Zonisamide

CYP3A4
Carbamazepine
Clobazam
Ethosuximide
Perampanel
Tiagabine
Zonisamide

UDP-glucuronosyltransferase
Divalproex
Lamotrigine
Lorazepam

Figure 12.7
CYP metabolism of the antiseizure medications.

(particularly Lennox-Gastaut syndrome) because of the risk of aplastic anemia (about 1:4000) and hepatic failure.

G. Gabapentin

Gabapentin [GA-ba-pen-tin] is an analog of GABA. However, it does not act at GABA receptors, enhance GABA actions or convert to GABA. Although *gabapentin* binds to the α2δ subunit of voltage-gated calcium channels, the precise mechanism of action is not known. It is approved as adjunct therapy for focal seizures and treatment of postherpetic neuralgia. *Gabapentin* exhibits nonlinear pharmacokinetics (see Chapter 1) due to its uptake by a saturable transport system from the gut. *Gabapentin* does not bind to plasma proteins and is excreted unchanged through the kidneys. Reduced dosing is required in renal disease. *Gabapentin* is well tolerated by the elderly population with focal seizures due to its relatively mild adverse effects. It may also be a good choice for the older patient because there are few drug interactions.

H. Lacosamide

Lacosamide [la-KOE-sa-mide] affects voltage-gated sodium channels, resulting in stabilization of hyperexcitable neuronal membranes and inhibition of repetitive neuronal firing. *Lacosamide* binds to collapsin response mediator protein-2 (CRMP-2), a phosphoprotein involved in neuronal differentiation and control of axonal outgrowth. The role of CRMP-2 binding in seizure control is unknown. *Lacosamide* is approved for adjunctive treatment of focal seizures. The most common adverse events that limit treatment include dizziness, headache, and fatigue.

I. Lamotrigine

Lamotrigine [la-MOE-tri-jeen] blocks sodium channels and high voltage–dependent calcium channels. *Lamotrigine* is effective in a wide variety of seizure types, including focal, generalized, absence seizures, and Lennox-Gastaut syndrome. It is also used to treat bipolar disorder. *Lamotrigine* is metabolized primarily to the 2-N-glucuronide metabolite through the UGT1A4 pathway. As with other antiseizure medications, general inducers increase *lamotrigine* clearance leading to lower *lamotrigine* concentrations, whereas *divalproex* results in a significant decrease in *lamotrigine* clearance (higher *lamotrigine* concentrations). *Lamotrigine* dosages should be reduced when adding *valproate* to therapy. Slow titration is necessary with *lamotrigine* (particularly when adding *lamotrigine* to a regimen that includes *valproate*) due to risk of rash, which may progress to a serious, life-threatening reaction.

J. Levetiracetam

Levetiracetam [lee-ve-tye-RA-se-tam] is approved for adjunct therapy of focal-onset, myoclonic, and primary generalized tonic–clonic seizures in adults and children. It demonstrates high affinity for a synaptic vesicle protein (SV2A). The drug is well absorbed after oral administration and is excreted in urine mostly unchanged, resulting in few to no drug interactions. *Levetiracetam* can cause mood alterations that may require a dose reduction or a change of medication.

K. Oxcarbazepine

Oxcarbazepine [ox-kar-BAY-zeh-peen] is a prodrug that is rapidly reduced to the 10-monohydroxy (MHD) metabolite responsible for its anticonvulsant activity. MHD blocks sodium channels and is thought to modulate calcium channels. It is approved for use in adults and children with focal seizures. *Oxcarbazepine* is a less potent inducer of CYP3A4 and UGT than is *carbamazepine*. The adverse effect of hyponatremia limits its use in the elderly.

L. Perampanel

Perampanel [per-AM-pa-nel] is a selective α-amino-3-hydroxy-5-methyl-4-isoxazolepropionic acid antagonist resulting in reduced excitatory activity. *Perampanel* has a long half-life enabling once-daily dosing. It is approved for adjunctive treatment of focal and generalized tonic–clonic seizures. This medication has a warning for serious psychiatric and behavioral reactions including aggression, hostility, irritability, anger, and homicidal ideation.

M. Phenobarbital and primidone

The primary mechanism of action of *phenobarbital* [fee-noe-BAR-bih-tal] is enhancement of the inhibitory effects of GABA-mediated neurons (see Chapter 9). *Primidone* is metabolized to *phenobarbital* (major) and phenylethylmalonamide, both with anticonvulsant activity. *Phenobarbital* is used primarily in the treatment of status epilepticus when other agents fail.

N. Phenytoin and fosphenytoin

Phenytoin [FEN-i-toin] blocks voltage-gated sodium channels by selectively binding to the channel in the inactive state and slowing its rate of recovery. It is effective for treatment of focal and generalized tonic–clonic seizures and in the treatment of status epilepticus. *Phenytoin* induces CYP2C and CYP3A families and the UGT enzyme system. *Phenytoin* exhibits saturable enzyme metabolism resulting in nonlinear pharmacokinetic properties (small increases in the daily dose can produce large increases in plasma concentration, resulting in drug-induced toxicity; Figure 12.8). Depression of the CNS occurs particularly in the cerebellum and vestibular system, causing nystagmus and ataxia. The elderly are highly susceptible to this effect. Gingival hyperplasia may cause the gums to grow over the teeth (Figure 12.9). Long-term use may lead to development of peripheral neuropathies and osteoporosis. Although *phenytoin* is advantageous due to its low cost, the actual cost of therapy may be higher, considering the potential for serious toxicity and adverse effects.

Fosphenytoin [FOS-phen-i-toin] is a prodrug that is rapidly converted to *phenytoin* in the blood within minutes. Whereas *fosphenytoin* may be administered intramuscularly (IM), *phenytoin sodium* should never be given IM, as it causes tissue damage and necrosis. *Fosphenytoin* is the drug of choice and standard of care for IV and IM administration of *phenytoin*.

O. Pregabalin

Pregabalin [pree-GA-ba-lin] binds to the $\alpha_2\delta$ site, an auxiliary subunit of voltage-gated calcium channels in the CNS, inhibiting excitatory neurotransmitter release. The drug has proven effects on focal-onset seizures, diabetic peripheral neuropathy, postherpetic neuralgia, and fibromyalgia. More than 90% of *pregabalin* is eliminated renally. It has

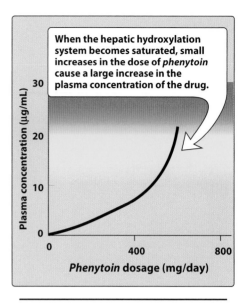

When the hepatic hydroxylation system becomes saturated, small increases in the dose of *phenytoin* cause a large increase in the plasma concentration of the drug.

Figure 12.8
Nonlinear effect of *phenytoin* dosage on the plasma concentration of the drug.

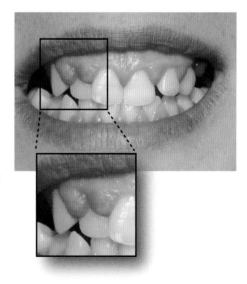

Figure 12.9
Gingival hyperplasia in patient treated with *phenytoin*.

no significant effects on drug metabolism and few drug interactions. Dosage adjustments are needed in renal dysfunction.

P. Rufinamide

Rufinamide [roo-FIN-a-mide] acts at sodium channels. It is approved for the adjunctive treatment of seizures associated with Lennox-Gastaut syndrome in children one year of age and older and in adults. *Rufinamide* is a weak inhibitor of CYP2E1 and a weak inducer of CYP3A4 enzymes. Food increases absorption and peak serum concentrations. Serum concentrations of *rufinamide* are affected by other antiseizure medications. *Carbamazepine* and *phenytoin* can reduce and *valproate* can increase the serum concentrations of *rufinamide*. Adverse effects include the potential for shortened QT intervals. Patients with familial short QT syndrome should not be treated with *rufinamide*.

Q. Tiagabine

Tiagabine [ty-AG-a-been] blocks GABA uptake into presynaptic neurons permitting more GABA to be available for receptor binding and thereby enhancing inhibitory activity. *Tiagabine* is effective as adjunctive treatment in focal seizures. In postmarketing surveillance, seizures have occurred in patients using *tiagabine* who did not have epilepsy. *Tiagabine* should not be used for indications other than epilepsy.

R. Topiramate

Topiramate [toe-PEER-a-mate] has multiple mechanisms of action. It blocks voltage-dependent sodium channels, reduces high-voltage calcium currents (L type), is a carbonic anhydrase inhibitor, and may act at glutamate (NMDA) sites. *Topiramate* is effective for use in focal and primary generalized epilepsy. It is also approved for prevention of migraine. It mildly inhibits CYP2C19 and coadministration with *phenytoin* and *carbamazepine* may reduce serum concentrations of *topiramate*. Adverse effects include somnolence, weight loss, and paresthesias. Renal stones, glaucoma, oligohidrosis (decreased sweating), and hyperthermia have also been reported.

S. Valproic acid and divalproex

Possible mechanisms of action include sodium channel blockade, blockade of GABA transaminase (GABA-T), and action at the T-type calcium channels. These varied mechanisms provide a broad spectrum of activity against seizures. It is effective for the treatment of focal and primary generalized epilepsies. *Valproic acid* [val-PRO-ik A-sid] is available as a free acid. *Divalproex* [dye-val-PRO-ex] *sodium* is a combination of *sodium valproate* [val-PROE-ate] and *valproic acid* that is converted to *valproate* ion in the gastrointestinal tract. It was developed to improve gastrointestinal tolerance of *valproic acid*. All of the available salt forms are equivalent in efficacy (*valproic acid* and *sodium valproate*). Commercial products are available in multiple-salt dosage forms and extended-release formulations. Therefore, the risk for medication errors is high, and it is essential to be familiar with all preparations. *Valproate* inhibits metabolism of the CYP2C9, UGT, and epoxide hydrolase systems (Figure 12.7). Rare hepatotoxicity may cause a rise in liver enzymes, which should be monitored frequently. Use in children under age 2 and women should be avoided if possible.

T. Vigabatrin

Vigabatrin [vye-GA-ba-trin] acts as an irreversible inhibitor of GABA-T. GABA-T is the enzyme responsible for metabolism of GABA. *Vigabatrin* is associated with visual field loss ranging from mild to severe in 30% or more of patients. *Vigabatrin* is only available through physicians and pharmacies that participate in the REMS (risk evaluation and mitigation strategies) program.

U. Zonisamide

Zonisamide [zoe-NIS-a-mide] is a sulfonamide derivative that has a broad spectrum of action. The compound has multiple effects, including blockade of both voltage-gated sodium channels and T-type calcium currents. It has a limited amount of carbonic anhydrase activity. *Zonisamide* is approved for use in patients with focal epilepsy. It is metabolized by the CYP3A4 isozyme and may, to a lesser extent, be affected by CYP3A5 and CYP2C19. In addition to typical CNS adverse effects, *zonisamide* may cause kidney stones. Oligohidrosis has been reported, and patients should be monitored for increased body temperature and decreased sweating. *Zonisamide* is contraindicated in patients with sulfonamide or carbonic anhydrase inhibitor hypersensitivity.

VI. STATUS EPILEPTICUS

In status epilepticus, two or more seizures occur without recovery of full consciousness in between episodes. These may be focal or generalized, convulsive or nonconvulsive. Status epilepticus is life threatening and requires emergency treatment usually consisting of parenteral administration of a fast-acting medication such as a benzodiazepine, followed by a slower-acting medication such as *phenytoin, fosphenytoin, divalproex,* or *levetiracetam.*

VII. WOMEN'S HEALTH AND EPILEPSY

Women of childbearing potential with epilepsy require assessment of their antiseizure medications in regard to contraception and pregnancy planning. Several antiseizure medications increase the metabolism of hormonal contraceptives, potentially rendering them ineffective. These include *phenytoin, phenobarbital, carbamazepine, topiramate, oxcarbazepine, rufinamide,* and *clobazam.* These medications increase the metabolism of contraceptives regardless of the delivery system used (for example, patch, ring, implants, and oral tablets). Pregnancy planning is vital, as many antiseizure medications have the potential to affect fetal development and cause birth defects. All women considering pregnancy should be on high doses (1 to 5 mg) of folic acid prior to conception. *Divalproex* and barbiturates should be avoided. If possible, women already taking *divalproex* should be placed on other therapies before pregnancy and counseled about the potential for birth defects, including cognitive (Figure 12.10) and behavioral abnormalities and neural tube defects. The pharmacokinetics of antiseizure medications and the frequency and severity of seizures may change during pregnancy. Regular monitoring by both an obstetrician and a neurologist is important. All women with epilepsy should be encouraged to register with the Antiepileptic Drug Pregnancy Registry. Figure 12.11 summarizes important characteristics of the antiseizure medications.

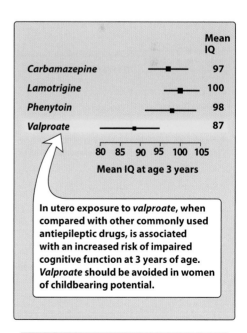

In utero exposure to *valproate*, when compared with other commonly used antiepileptic drugs, is associated with an increased risk of impaired cognitive function at 3 years of age. *Valproate* should be avoided in women of childbearing potential.

Figure 12.10
Cognitive function at 3 years of age after fetal exposure to doses of antiepileptic drugs. The means (*black squares*) and 95% confidence intervals (*horizontal lines*) are given for the children's IQ as a function of the antiepileptic drugs.

DRUG	MECHANISM OF ACTION	ADVERSE EFFECTS AND COMMENTS
Brivaracetam	**Binds SV2A**	Sedation, dizziness, fatigue, and irritability.
Carbamazepine	**Blocks Na+ channels**	Hyponatremia, drowsiness, fatigue, dizziness, and blurred vision. Drug use has also been associated with Stevens-Johnson syndrome. Blood dyscrasias: neutropenia, leukopenia, thrombocytopenia, pancytopenia, and anemias.
Divalproex	**Multiple mechanisms of action**	Weight gain, easy bruising, nausea, tremor, hair loss, GI upset, liver damage, alopecia, and sedation. Hepatic failure, pancreatitis, and teratogenic effects have been observed. Broad spectrum of antiseizure activity.
Eslicarbazepine acetate	**Blocks Na+ channels**	Nausea, rash, hyponatremia, headache, sedation, dizziness, vertigo, ataxia, and diplopia.
Ethosuximide	**Blocks Ca2+ channels**	Drowsiness, hyperactivity, nausea, sedation, GI upset, weight gain, lethargy, SLE, and rash. Blood dyscrasias can occur; periodic CBCs should be done. Abrupt discontinuance of drug may cause seizures.
Felbamate	**Multiple mechanisms of action**	Insomnia, dizziness, headache, ataxia, weight gain, and irritability. Aplastic anemia and hepatic failure. Broad spectrum of antiseizure activity. Requires patient to sign informed consent at dispensing.
Gabapentin	**Unknown**	Mild drowsiness, dizziness, ataxia, weight gain, and diarrhea. Few drug interactions. One hundred percent renal elimination.
Lacosamide	**Multiple mechanisms of action**	Dizziness, fatigue, and headache. Few drug interactions; Schedule V.
Lamotrigine	**Multiple mechanisms of action**	Nausea, drowsiness, dizziness, headache, and diplopia. Rash (Stevens-Johnson syndrome—potentially life threatening). Broad spectrum of antiseizure activity.
Levetiracetam	**Binds SV2A**	Sedation, dizziness, headache, anorexia, fatigue, infections, and behavioral symptoms. Few drug interactions. Broad spectrum of antiseizure activity.
Oxcarbazepine	**Blocks Na+ channels**	Nausea, rash, hyponatremia, headache, sedation, dizziness, vertigo, ataxia, and diplopia.
Perampanel	**Blocks AMPA glutamate receptors**	Serious psychiatric and behavioral reactions, dizziness, somnolence, fatigue, gait disturbance, and falls, long half-life.
Phenytoin	**Blocks Na+ channels**	Gingival hyperplasia, confusion, slurred speech, double vision, ataxia, sedation, dizziness, and hirsutism. Stevens-Johnson syndrome—potentially life threatening. Not recommended for chronic use. Primary treatment for status epilepticus (*fosphenytoin*).
Pregabalin	**Multiple mechanisms of action**	Weight gain, somnolence, dizziness, headache, diplopia, and ataxia. One hundred percent renal elimination; Schedule V.
Rufinamide	**Unknown**	Shortened QT interval. Multiple drug interactions.
Tiagabine	**Blocks GABA uptake**	Sedation, weight gain, fatigue, headache, tremor, dizziness, and anorexia. Multiple drug interactions.
Topiramate	**Multiple mechanisms of action**	Paresthesia, weight loss, nervousness, depression, anorexia, anxiety, tremor, cognitive complaints, headache, and oligohidrosis. Few drug interactions. Broad spectrum of antiseizure activity.
Vigabatrin	**Irreversible binding of GABA-T**	Vision loss, anemia, somnolence, fatigue, peripheral neuropathy, weight gain. Available only through SHARE pharmacies.
Zonisamide	**Multiple mechanisms of action**	Nausea, anorexia, ataxia, confusion, difficulty concentrating, sedation, paresthesia, and oligohidrosis. Broad spectrum of antiseizure activity.

Figure 12.11
Summary of antiseizure drugs. AMPA = α-amino-3-hydroxy-5-methyl-4-isoxazolepropionic acid; CBC = complete blood count; GABA = γ-aminobutyric acid; GABA-T = γ-aminobutyric acid transaminase; GI = gastrointestinal; SLE = systemic lupus erythematosus.

Study Questions

Choose the ONE best answer.

12.1 A 9-year-old boy is sent for neurologic evaluation because of episodes of apparent inattention. Over the past year, the child has experienced episodes during which he develops a blank look on his face and his eyes blink for 15 seconds. He immediately resumes his previous activity. Which best describes seizures in this patient?

A. Focal
B. Tonic–clonic
C. Absence
D. Myoclonic

Correct answer = C. The patient is experiencing episodes of absence seizures where consciousness is impaired briefly. Absence seizures generally begin in children aged 4 to 12 years. Diagnosis includes obtaining an electroencephalogram that shows generalized 3-Hz waves.

12.2 A child is experiencing absence seizures that interrupt his ability to pay attention during school and activities. Which therapy is most appropriate for this patient?

A. Ethosuximide
B. Carbamazepine
C. Diazepam
D. Watchful waiting

Correct answer = A. The patient has had many seizures that interrupt his ability to pay attention during school and activities, so therapy is justified. Carbamazepine may make the seizures more frequent. Diazepam is not indicated for absence seizures.

12.3 Which drug is most useful for the treatment of absence seizures?

A. Topiramate
B. Tiagabine
C. Levetiracetam
D. Lamotrigine

Correct answer = D. Of the drugs listed, lamotrigine has the best data for use in absence seizures and is the best choice. Tiagabine is only used for focal seizures. Topiramate and levetiracetam may be options if lamotrigine does not work.

12.4 A 25-year-old woman with generalized seizures is well controlled on valproate. She indicates that she is interested in becoming pregnant in the next year. With respect to her antiseizure medication, which of the following should be considered?

A. Leave her on her current therapy.
B. Consider switching to lamotrigine.
C. Consider adding a second antiseizure medication.
D. Decrease her valproate dose.

Correct answer = B. Valproate is a poor choice in women of childbearing age and should be avoided if possible. A review of the medication history of this patient is warranted. If she has not tried any other antiseizure medication, then consideration of another antiseizure medication may be beneficial. Studies show that valproate taken during pregnancy can have a detrimental effect on cognitive abilities in children. However, treatment with valproate may not be avoidable as it could be the only choice for some women. In these cases, the lowest effective dose should be used.

12.5 A woman with generalized seizures is well controlled with lamotrigine. She becomes pregnant and begins to have breakthrough seizures. What is most likely happening?

A. Her epilepsy is getting worse.
B. Lamotrigine concentrations are increasing.
C. Lamotrigine concentrations are decreasing.
D. Lamotrigine is no longer efficacious for this patient.

Correct answer = C. Pregnancy alters the pharmacokinetics of lamotrigine. As pregnancy progresses, women can require increased dosages to maintain blood concentrations and seizure control.

12.6 A 42-year-old man undergoes a neurologic evaluation because of episodes of apparent confusion. Over the past year, the man has experienced episodes during which he develops a blank look on his face and fails to respond to questions. Moreover, it appears to take several minutes before the man recovers from the episodes. Which best describes this type of seizure?

A. Focal (aware)
B. Focal (impaired awareness)
C. Tonic–clonic
D. Absence

Correct answer = B. The patient is experiencing episodes of focal seizures with impaired consciousness. Typically, staring is accompanied by impaired consciousness and recall. If asked a question, the patient might respond with an inappropriate or unintelligible answer. Automatic movements are associated with most focal seizures and involve the mouth and face (lip smacking, chewing, tasting, and swallowing movements), upper extremities (fumbling, picking, tapping, or clasping movements), and vocal apparatus (grunts or repetition of words and phrases), as are complex acts (such as walking or mixing foods in a bowl).

12.7 A 52-year-old man has had several focal seizures with impaired consciousness over the last year. Which is the most appropriate initial therapy for this patient?

A. Ethosuximide
B. Levetiracetam
C. Diazepam
D. Carbamazepine plus primidone

Correct answer = B. The patient has had many seizures, and the risks of not starting drug therapy would be substantially greater than the risks of treating his seizures. Because the patient has impaired consciousness during the seizure, he is at risk for injury during an attack. Monotherapy with primary agents is preferred for most patients. The advantages of monotherapy include reduced frequency of adverse effects, absence of interactions between antiepileptic drugs, lower cost, and improved compliance. Ethosuximide and diazepam are not indicated for focal seizures.

12.8 A patient with focal seizures has been treated for 6 months with carbamazepine but, recently, has been experiencing breakthrough seizures on a more frequent basis. You are considering adding a second drug to the antiseizure regimen. Which of the following drugs is least likely to have a pharmacokinetic interaction with carbamazepine?

A. Topiramate
B. Tiagabine
C. Levetiracetam
D. Lamotrigine

Correct answer = C. Of the drugs listed, all of which are approved as adjunct therapy for refractory focal seizures, only levetiracetam does not affect the pharmacokinetics of other antiepileptic drugs, and other drugs do not significantly alter its pharmacokinetics. However, any of the listed drugs could be added depending on the plan and the patient characteristics. Treatment of epilepsy is complex, and diagnosis is based on history and may need to be reevaluated when drug therapy fails or seizures increase.

12.9 Which is a first-line medication for generalized tonic–clonic seizures?

A. Ethosuximide
B. Felbamate
C. Vigabatrin
D. Topiramate

Correct answer = D. Topiramate is a broad-spectrum antiseizure medication that is indicated for primary generalized tonic–clonic seizures. Ethosuximide should only be used for absence seizures. Felbamate is reserved for refractory seizures due to the risk of aplastic anemia and liver failure. Vigabatrin is not indicated for generalized seizures and is associated with visual field defects.

12.10 A 75-year-old woman had a stroke approximately 1 month ago. She is continuing to have small focal seizures where she fails to respond appropriately while talking. Which is the most appropriate treatment for this individual?

A. Phenytoin
B. Oxcarbazepine
C. Levetiracetam
D. Phenobarbital

Correct answer = C. Levetiracetam is renally cleared and prone to very few drug interactions. Elderly patients usually have more comorbidities and take more medications than do younger patients. Oxcarbazepine may cause hyponatremia, which is more symptomatic in the elderly. Phenytoin and phenobarbital have many drug interactions and a side effect profile that may be especially troublesome in the elderly age group, including dizziness that may lead to falls, cognitive issues, and bone health issues.

Anesthetics

Brandon Lopez and Chris Giordano

13

I. OVERVIEW

For patients undergoing surgical or medical procedures, different levels of sedation can provide important benefits to facilitate procedural interventions. These levels of sedation range from anxiolysis to general anesthesia and can create:

- Sedation and reduced anxiety
- Lack of awareness and amnesia
- Skeletal muscle relaxation
- Suppression of undesirable reflexes
- Analgesia

Because no single agent provides all desired objectives, several categories of drugs are combined to produce the optimum level of sedation required (Figure 13.1). Drugs are chosen to provide safe and efficient sedation based on the type and duration of the procedure and patient characteristics, such as organ function, medical conditions, and concurrent medications (Figure 13.2). Preoperative medications provide anxiolysis and analgesia and mitigate unwanted side effects of the anesthetic or the procedure itself. Neuromuscular blockers enable endotracheal intubation and muscle relaxation to facilitate surgery. Potent general anesthetic medications are delivered via inhalation and/or intravenously. Except for *nitrous oxide*, inhaled anesthetics are volatile, halogenated hydrocarbons, while intravenous (IV) anesthetics consist of several chemically unrelated drug classes commonly used to rapidly induce and/or maintain a state of general anesthesia.

II. LEVELS OF SEDATION

The levels of sedation occur in a dose-related continuum, which is variable and depends on individual patient response to various drugs. These "artificial" levels of sedation start with light sedation (anxiolysis) and continue to moderate sedation, then deep sedation, and finally a state of general anesthesia. The hallmarks of escalation from one level to the next are recognized by changes in mentation, hemodynamic stability, and respiratory competency (Figure 13.3). This escalation in levels is often very subtle and unpredictable; therefore, the sedation provider must always be ready to manage the unanticipated next level of sedation.

PREOPERATIVE MEDICATIONS
Analgesics
Antacids
Antiemetics
Benzodiazepines*

ANALGESICS
Acetaminophen TYLENOL, OFIRMEV
Celecoxib CELEBREX
Gabapentin NEURONTIN
Ketamine KETALAR*
Opioids (see Chapter 14)

GENERAL ANESTHETICS: INHALED
Desflurane SUPRANE
Isoflurane FORANE
Nitrous oxide GENERIC ONLY
Sevoflurane ULTANE

GENERAL ANESTHETICS: INTRAVENOUS
Dexmedetomidine PRECEDEX
Etomidate AMIDATE
Methohexital BREVITAL
Propofol DIPRIVAN

NEUROMUSCULAR BLOCKERS (see Chapter 5)
Cisatracurium, mivacurium, pancuronium, rocuronium, succinylcholine, vecuronium

LOCAL ANESTHETICS: AMIDES
Bupivacaine MARCAINE
Lidocaine XYLOCAINE
Mepivacaine CARBOCAINE
Ropivacaine NAROPIN

LOCAL ANESTHETICS: ESTERS
Chloroprocaine NESACAINE
Tetracaine GENERIC ONLY

Figure 13.1
Summary of common drugs used for anesthesia. *Can cause general anesthesia with higher doses. See Chapter 5 for summary of neuromuscular blocking agents.

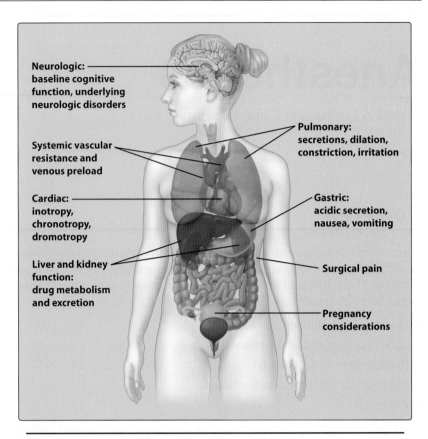

Figure 13.2
Overall considerations when delivering an anesthetic.

III. STAGES OF GENERAL ANESTHESIA

General anesthesia is a reversible state of central nervous system (CNS) depression, causing loss of response to and perception of stimuli. The state of general anesthesia can be divided into three stages: induction, maintenance, and recovery. Induction is the time from administration of a potent anesthetic to development of unconsciousness, while maintenance is the sustained period of general anesthesia. Recovery starts with the discontinuation of the anesthetic and continues until the return of consciousness and protective reflexes. Induction of anesthesia depends on how fast effective concentrations of anesthetic reach the brain. Recovery is essentially the reverse of induction and depends on how fast the anesthetic

	MINIMAL (ANXIOLYSIS)	MODERATE	DEEP	GENERAL
Mentation	Responds normally to verbal stimuli	Responds purposefully to verbal or tactile stimuli	Responds purposefully to repeated verbal or painful stimuli	Unarousable to painful stimuli
Airway competency	Unaffected	Adequate	Intervention may be required	Intervention usually required
Respiratory system	Unaffected	Adequate	May be inadequate	Frequently inadequate
Cardiovascular system	Unaffected	Usually maintained	Usually maintained	May be impaired

Figure 13.3
Anesthetic levels of sedation.

diffuses from the brain. The depth of general anesthesia is the degree to which the CNS is depressed, as evident in electroencephalograms.

A. Induction

General anesthesia in adults is normally induced with an IV agent like *propofol*, producing unconsciousness in 30 to 40 seconds. Often, an IV neuromuscular blocker such as *rocuronium*, *vecuronium*, or *succinylcholine* is administered to facilitate endotracheal intubation by eliciting muscle relaxation. For children without IV access, nonpungent volatile agents, such as *sevoflurane*, are administered via inhalation to induce general anesthesia.

B. Maintenance of anesthesia

After administering the induction drug, vital signs and response to stimuli are vigilantly monitored to balance the amount of drug continuously inhaled or infused to maintain general anesthesia. Maintenance is commonly provided with volatile anesthetics, although total intravenous anesthesia (TIVA) with drugs like *propofol* can be used to maintain general anesthesia. Opioids such as *fentanyl* are used for analgesia along with inhalation agents, because the latter alter consciousness but not perception of pain.

C. Recovery

After cessation of the maintenance anesthetic drug, the patient is evaluated for return of consciousness. For most anesthetic agents, redistribution from the site of action (rather than metabolism of the drug) underlies recovery. Neuromuscular blocking drugs are typically reversed after completion of surgery, unless enough time has elapsed for their metabolism. The patient is monitored to assure full recovery of all normal physiologic functions (spontaneous respiration, blood pressure, heart rate, and all protective reflexes).

IV. INHALATION ANESTHETICS

Inhaled gases are used primarily for maintenance of anesthesia after administration of an IV drug (Figure 13.4). Depth of anesthesia can be rapidly altered by changing the inhaled gas concentration. Inhalational agents have steep dose–response curves with very narrow therapeutic indices, so the difference in concentrations from eliciting general anesthesia to cardiopulmonary collapse is small. No antagonists exist. To minimize waste, inhaled gases are delivered in a recirculation system that contains absorbents to remove carbon dioxide and allow rebreathing of the gas. Recently, there has been greater attention to the anthropogenic emissions of these potent greenhouse gases, which are typically released from hospital rooftops after each procedure.

A. Common features of inhalation anesthetics

Modern inhalation anesthetics are nonflammable, nonexplosive agents, which include *nitrous oxide* and volatile, halogenated hydrocarbons. These agents decrease cerebrovascular resistance, resulting in increased brain perfusion. They cause bronchodilation but also decrease both respiratory drive and hypoxic pulmonary vasoconstriction

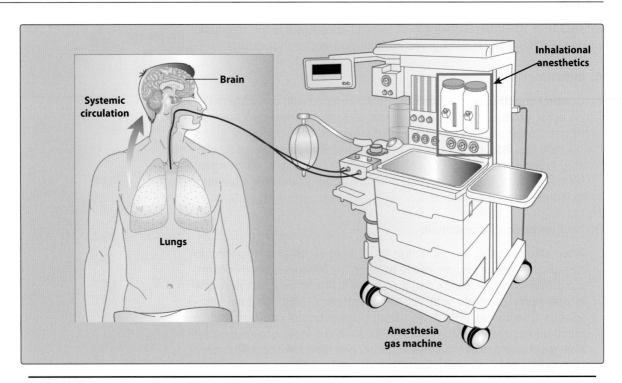

Figure 13.4
Volatile anesthetics delivered to the patient are absorbed via the lungs into the systemic circulation causing dose-dependent CNS depression.

(increased pulmonary vascular resistance in poorly oxygenated regions of the lungs, redirecting blood flow to better oxygenated regions). Movement of these gases from the lungs to various body compartments depends upon their solubility in blood and tissues, as well as on blood flow. The following factors play a role in induction and recovery:

B. Potency

Potency is defined quantitatively as the minimum alveolar concentration (MAC), which is the end-tidal concentration of inhaled anesthetic needed to eliminate movement in 50% of patients exposed to a noxious stimulus. MAC is the median effective dose (ED_{50}) of the anesthetic, expressed as the percentage of gas in a mixture required to achieve that effect. Numerically, MAC is small for potent anesthetics such as *isoflurane* and large for less potent agents such as *nitrous oxide*. Thus, the inverse of MAC is an index of potency (Figure 13.5). *Nitrous oxide* alone cannot produce general anesthesia because any admixture with a survivable oxygen percentage cannot reach its MAC value. The more lipid soluble an anesthetic, the lower the concentration needed to produce anesthesia and, therefore, the higher the potency. Factors that can increase MAC (make the patient more resistant) include hyperthermia, drugs that increase CNS catecholamines, and chronic ethanol abuse. Factors that can decrease MAC (make the patient more sensitive) include increased age, hypothermia, pregnancy, sepsis, acute intoxication, concurrent IV anesthetics, and α_2-adrenergic receptor agonists (*clonidine* and *dexmedetomidine*).

C. Uptake and distribution of inhalation anesthetics

The principal objective of inhalation anesthesia is a constant and optimal brain partial pressure (P_{br}) of inhaled anesthetic (to create a partial

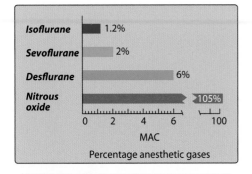

Figure 13.5
Minimal alveolar concentrations (MAC) for anesthetic gases are used to compare pharmacologic effects of different agents (high MAC = low potency).

pressure equilibrium between alveoli [P_{alv}] and brain [P_{br}]). Measuring the P_{alv} is the most practical and feasible way to ascertain the P_{br} for the inhaled anesthetic concentration, but this necessitates adequate time for the two compartments to reach equilibrium. The partial pressure of an anesthetic gas that originates by pulmonary entry is the driving force moving the gas from the alveolar space into the bloodstream (P_a), which transports the drug to the brain and other body compartments. Because gases move from one body compartment to another according to partial pressure gradients, steady state is achieved when the partial pressure in each of these compartments is equivalent to that in the inspired mixture. [Note: At equilibrium, $P_{alv} = P_a = P_{br}$.] The time course for attaining this steady state is determined by the following factors:

1. **Alveolar wash-in:** This refers to replacement of normal lung gases with the inspired anesthetic mixture. The time required for this process is directly proportional to the functional residual capacity of the lung (volume of gas remaining in the lungs at the end of a normal expiration) and inversely proportional to ventilatory rate. It is independent of the physical properties of the gas. As the partial pressure builds within the lung, anesthetic gas transfer from the lung begins.

2. **Anesthetic uptake (removal to peripheral tissues other than the brain):** Uptake is the product of the gas solubility in the blood, cardiac output (CO), and gradient between alveolar and blood anesthetic partial pressures.

   a. **Solubility in blood:** This is determined by a physical property of the anesthetic called the blood:gas partition coefficient (the ratio of the concentration of anesthetic in the liquid [blood] phase to the concentration of anesthetic in the gas phase when the anesthetic is in equilibrium between the two phases; Figure 13.6). For inhaled anesthetics, think of the blood as a pharmacologically inactive reservoir. Drugs with low versus high blood solubility differ in their rate of induction of anesthesia. When an anesthetic gas with low blood solubility such as *nitrous oxide* diffuses from the alveoli into the circulation, little anesthetic dissolves in the blood. Therefore, equilibrium between the inspired anesthetic and arterial blood occurs rapidly with relatively few additional molecules of anesthetic required to raise the arterial anesthetic partial pressure. By contrast, anesthetic gases with high blood solubility, such as *isoflurane*, dissolve more fully in the blood; therefore, greater amounts of gas and longer periods of time are required to raise blood partial pressure. This results in longer periods for induction, recovery, and time to change in depth of anesthesia in response to changes in the drug concentration. The solubility in blood is ranked as follows: *isoflurane > sevoflurane > nitrous oxide > desflurane*.

   b. **Cardiac output:** CO is inversely correlated with induction time for inhaled anesthetics. This counterintuitive phenomenon is explained by the threshold of drug concentration required to alter neuronal activity and the time neurons are exposed to the drug in the passing blood. During low CO, a longer period of time permits a larger concentration of gas to dissolve in the slowly moving bloodstream. Furthermore,

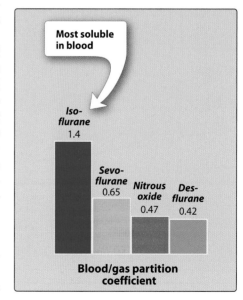

Figure 13.6
Blood/gas partition coefficients for some inhalation anesthetics.

this large bolus of drug has longer contact time to diffuse into neuronal tissue when it traverses the blood–brain barrier. Although a high CO will quickly transport the drug to the brain, a lower concentration of the drug with a shorter exposure time slows down the rate of induction.

c. Alveolar-to-venous partial pressure gradient: This gradient between the alveolar and returning venous gas partial pressure results from the tissue uptake from the arterial delivery. The arterial circulation distributes the anesthetic to various tissues, and tissue uptake is dependent on the tissue blood flow, blood-to-tissue partial pressure difference, and blood-to-tissue solubility coefficient. As venous circulation returns to the lung blood with low or no dissolved anesthetic gas, this high gradient causes gas to move from the alveoli into the blood. If a large alveolar-to-venous partial pressure gradient persists, the peripheral tissue gas uptake must be high, and therefore, the induction time is longer. Over time, as the partial pressure of gas in venous blood approximates the inspired mixture and subsequent alveolar concentration, no further uptake from the lung occurs.

3. **Effect of different tissue types on anesthetic uptake:** The time required for a tissue compartment to reach steady state with the partial pressure of the inspired anesthetic gas is inversely proportional to the blood flow to that tissue (greater flow equals less time to reach equilibrium). Time to steady state is directly proportional to the capacity of that tissue to store anesthetic (greater storage capacity equals longer time to reach equilibrium). Furthermore, capacity is directly proportional to the volume of tissue and the tissue:blood solubility coefficient of the gas. Four major tissue compartments determine the time course of anesthetic uptake:

a. Vessel-rich group (brain, heart, liver, kidney, and endocrine glands): Highly perfused tissues rapidly attain steady state with the partial pressure of anesthetic in the blood.

b. Skeletal muscles: These tissues are moderately perfused with a large storage capacity, which lengthens the time required to achieve steady state.

c. Fat: Fat is poorly perfused but has a very large storage capacity for the highly lipophilic volatile anesthetics. This poor perfusion to a high-capacity compartment drastically prolongs the time required to achieve steady state.

d. Vessel-poor group (bone, ligaments, and cartilage): These are very poorly perfused and have a low capacity to store anesthetic gas. Therefore, these tissues have minimal impact on the time course of anesthetic distribution in the body.

4. **Washout:** When an inhalation anesthetic gas is removed from the inspired admixture, the body becomes the repository of anesthetic gas to be circulated back to the alveolar compartment. The same factors that influence uptake and equilibrium of the inspired anesthetic determine the time course of its exhalation from the body. Thus, *nitrous oxide* exits the body faster than does *isoflurane* (Figure 13.7).

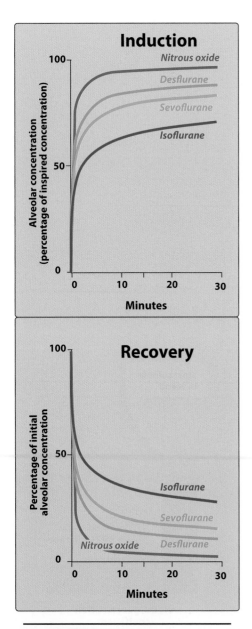

Figure 13.7
Changes in the alveolar blood concentrations of some inhalation anesthetics over time.

D. Mechanism of action

No specific receptor has been identified as the locus to create a state of general anesthesia. The fact that chemically unrelated compounds produce unconsciousness argues against the existence of a single receptor, and it appears that a variety of molecular mechanisms may contribute to the activity of anesthetics. At clinically effective concentrations, general anesthetics increase the sensitivity of the γ-aminobutyric acid (GABA$_A$) receptors to the inhibitory neurotransmitter GABA. This increases chloride ion influx and hyperpolarization of neurons. Postsynaptic neuronal excitability and, thus, CNS activity are diminished (Figure 13.8). Unlike other anesthetics, *nitrous oxide* and *ketamine* do not have actions on GABA$_A$ receptors. Their effects are mediated via inhibition of *N*-methyl-ᴅ-aspartate (NMDA) receptors. [Note: The NMDA receptor is a glutamate receptor, which is the body's main excitatory neurotransmitter.] Receptors other than GABA that are affected by volatile anesthetics include the inhibitory glycine receptors found in the spinal motor neurons. Additionally, inhalation anesthetics block excitatory postsynaptic currents found on nicotinic receptors. However, the mechanisms by which anesthetics perform these modulatory roles are not fully understood.

E. Isoflurane

Isoflurane [eye-so-FLOOR-ane], like other halogenated gases, produces dose-dependent hypotension predominantly from relaxation of systemic vasculature. Hypotension can be treated with a direct-acting vasoconstrictor, such as *phenylephrine* (see Chapter 6). Because it undergoes little metabolism, *isoflurane* is considered nontoxic to the liver and kidney. Its pungent odor stimulates respiratory reflexes (breath holding, salivation, coughing, laryngospasm), so it is not used for inhalation induction. With a higher blood solubility than *desflurane* and *sevoflurane*, *isoflurane* takes longer to reach equilibrium, making it less ideal for short procedures; however, its low cost makes it a good option for longer surgeries.

F. Desflurane

Desflurane [DES-floor-ane] provides very rapid onset and recovery due to low blood solubility. This makes it a popular anesthetic for short procedures. It has a low volatility, which requires administration via a special heated vaporizer. Like *isoflurane*, it decreases vascular resistance and perfuses all major tissues very well. *Desflurane* has significant respiratory irritation like *isoflurane* so it should not be used for inhalation induction. Its degradation is minimal and tissue toxicity is rare. Higher cost occasionally prohibits its use.

G. Sevoflurane

Sevoflurane [see-voe-FLOOR-ane] has low pungency or respiratory irritation. This makes it useful for inhalation induction, especially with pediatric patients who do not tolerate IV placement. It has a rapid onset and recovery due to low blood solubility. *Sevoflurane* has low hepatotoxic potential, but compounds formed from reactions in the anesthesia circuit (soda lime) may be nephrotoxic with very low fresh gas flow that allows longer chemical reaction time.

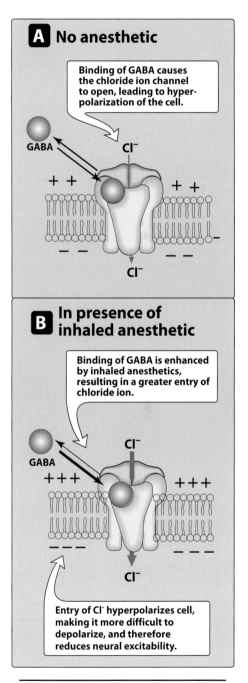

A No anesthetic

Binding of GABA causes the chloride ion channel to open, leading to hyperpolarization of the cell.

GABA   Cl⁻

+ +   + +

Cl⁻

B In presence of inhaled anesthetic

Binding of GABA is enhanced by inhaled anesthetics, resulting in a greater entry of chloride ion.

GABA   Cl⁻

+++   +++

Cl⁻

Entry of Cl⁻ hyperpolarizes cell, making it more difficult to depolarize, and therefore reduces neural excitability.

Figure 13.8
An example of modulation of a ligand-gated membrane channel modulated by inhaled anesthetics. GABA = γ-aminobutyric acid; Cl⁻ = chloride ion.

H. Nitrous oxide

Nitrous oxide [NYE-truss OX-ide] ("laughing gas") is a nonirritating potent sedative that is unable to create a state of general anesthesia. It is frequently used at concentrations of 30% to 50% in combination with oxygen to create moderate sedation, particularly in dentistry. *Nitrous oxide* does not depress respiration, and maintains cardiovascular hemodynamics as well as muscular strength. *Nitrous oxide* can be combined with other inhalational agents to establish general anesthesia, which lowers the required concentration of the combined volatile agent. This gas admixture further reduces many unwanted side effects of the other volatile agent that impact cardiovascular output and cerebral blood flow. *Nitrous oxide* is poorly soluble in blood and other tissues, allowing it to move very rapidly in and out of the body. This can be problematic in closed body compartments because *nitrous oxide* can increase the volume (exacerbating a pneumothorax) or pressure (sinus or middle ear pressure); it replaces nitrogen in various air spaces faster than the nitrogen leaves. Its speed of movement allows *nitrous oxide* to retard oxygen uptake during recovery, thereby causing "diffusion hypoxia." This can be overcome by delivering high concentrations of inspired oxygen during recovery. Some characteristics of the inhalation anesthetics are summarized in Figure 13.9.

I. Malignant hyperthermia

In a very small percentage of susceptible patients, exposure to halogenated hydrocarbon anesthetics (or *succinylcholine*) may induce malignant hyperthermia (MH), a rare life-threatening condition. MH causes a drastic and uncontrolled increase in skeletal muscle oxidative metabolism, overwhelming the body's capacity to supply oxygen, remove carbon dioxide, and regulate temperature, eventually leading to circulatory collapse and death if not treated immediately. Strong evidence indicates that MH is due to an excitation–contraction coupling defect. Burn victims and individuals with muscular dystrophy, myopathy, myotonia, and osteogenesis imperfecta are susceptible to MH-like events and caution should be taken. Susceptibility to MH is often inherited as an autosomal dominant disorder. Should a patient exhibit symptoms of MH, *dantrolene* is given as the anesthetic mixture is withdrawn, and measures are taken to rapidly cool the patient. *Dantrolene* [DAN-troe-leen] blocks release of Ca^{2+} from the sarcoplasmic reticulum of muscle cells, reducing heat production and relaxing muscle tone. It should be available whenever triggering agents are administered. In addition, the patient must be monitored and supported for respiratory, circulatory, and renal problems. Use of *dantrolene* and avoidance of triggering agents such as halogenated anesthetics in susceptible individuals have markedly reduced mortality from MH. A more soluble formulation of *dantrolene* has become commercially available that drastically reduces the constitution time needed to make this drug in emergencies.

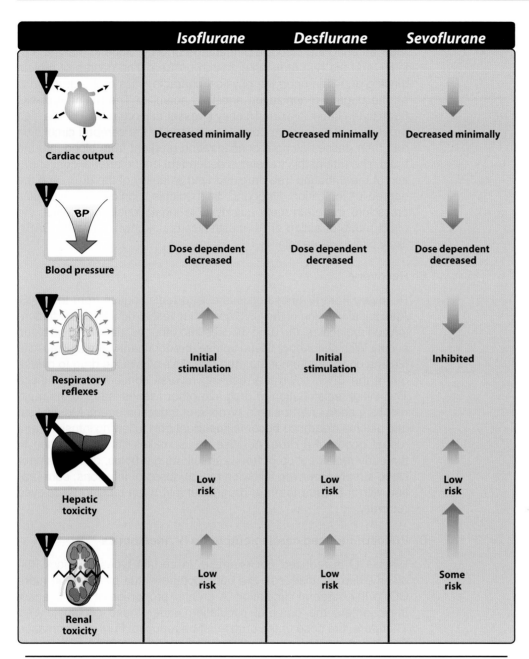

	Isoflurane	**Desflurane**	**Sevoflurane**
Cardiac output	↓ Decreased minimally	↓ Decreased minimally	↓ Decreased minimally
Blood pressure	↓ Dose dependent decreased	↓ Dose dependent decreased	↓ Dose dependent decreased
Respiratory reflexes	↑ Initial stimulation	↑ Initial stimulation	↓ Inhibited
Hepatic toxicity	↑ Low risk	↑ Low risk	↑ Low risk
Renal toxicity	↑ Low risk	↑ Low risk	↑ Some risk

Figure 13.9
Characteristics of some inhalation anesthetics.

V. INTRAVENOUS ANESTHETICS

IV anesthetics cause rapid induction of anesthesia often occurring in 1 minute or less. It is the most common way to induce anesthesia before maintenance of anesthesia with an inhalation agent. IV anesthetics may be used as single agents for short procedures or administered as infusions (TIVA) to help maintain anesthesia during longer surgeries. In lower doses, they may be used solely for sedation.

A. Induction

After entering the blood, a percentage of drug binds to plasma proteins, and the rest remains unbound or "free." The degree of protein binding depends upon the physical characteristics of the drug, such as the degree of ionization and lipid solubility. The majority of CO flows to the brain, liver, and kidney ("vessel-rich organs"). Thus, a high proportion of initial drug bolus is delivered to the cerebral circulation and then passes along a concentration gradient from blood into the brain. The rate of this transfer is dependent on the arterial concentration of the unbound free drug, the lipid solubility of the drug, and the degree of ionization. Unbound, lipid-soluble, nonionized molecules cross into the brain most quickly. Like inhalational anesthetics, the exact mode of action of IV anesthetics is unknown; however, GABA likely plays a large role.

B. Recovery

Recovery from IV anesthetics is due to redistribution from the CNS. After initial flooding of the CNS and other vessel-rich tissues with nonionized molecules, the drug diffuses into other tissues with less blood supply. With secondary tissue uptake, predominantly skeletal muscle, plasma concentration of the drug falls. This allows the drug to diffuse out of the CNS, down the resulting reverse concentration gradient. This initial redistribution of drug into other tissues leads to the rapid recovery seen after a single IV dose of induction agent. Metabolism and plasma clearance become important only following infusions and repeat doses of a drug. Adipose tissue makes little contribution to the early redistribution of free drug following a bolus, due to its poor blood supply. However, following repeat doses or infusions, equilibration with fat tissue forms a drug reservoir, often leading to delayed recovery.

C. Effect of reduced cardiac output on IV anesthetics

When CO is reduced (for example, in certain types of shock, the elderly, cardiac disease), the body compensates by diverting more CO to the cerebral circulation. A greater proportion of the IV anesthetic enters the cerebral circulation under these circumstances. Therefore, the dose of the drug must be reduced. Further, decreased CO causes prolonged circulation time. As global CO is reduced, it takes a longer time for an induction drug to reach the brain and exert its effects. **The slow titration of a reduced dose of an IV anesthetic is key to a safe induction in patients with reduced CO.**

D. Propofol

Propofol [PRO-puh-fol] is an IV sedative/hypnotic used for induction and/or maintenance of anesthesia. It is widely used and has replaced *thiopental* as the first choice for induction of general anesthesia and sedation. Because *propofol* is poorly water soluble, it is supplied as an emulsion containing soybean oil and egg phospholipid, giving it a milklike appearance.

1. **Onset:** Induction is smooth and occurs 30 to 40 seconds after administration. Plasma levels decline rapidly as a result of redistribution, followed by a more prolonged period of hepatic metabolism

and renal clearance. The initial redistribution half-life is 2 to 4 minutes. The pharmacokinetics of *propofol* are not altered by moderate hepatic or renal failure.

2. **Actions:** Although *propofol* depresses the CNS, it occasionally contributes to excitatory phenomena, such as muscle twitching, spontaneous movement, yawning, and hiccups. Transient pain at the injection site is common. *Propofol* decreases blood pressure without significantly depressing the myocardium. It also reduces intracranial pressure, mainly due to decreased cerebral blood flow and oxygen consumption. It has less of a depressant effect than volatile anesthetics on CNS-evoked potentials, making it useful for surgeries in which spinal cord function is monitored. It does not provide analgesia, so supplementation with narcotics is required. *Propofol* is commonly infused in lower doses to provide sedation. The incidence of postoperative nausea and vomiting (PONV) is very low secondary to its antiemetic properties.

E. Barbiturates

Thiopental [THYE-oh-PEN-tahl] is an ultra–short-acting barbiturate with high lipid solubility. It is a potent anesthetic but a weak analgesic. Barbiturates require supplementary analgesic administration during anesthesia. When given IV, agents such as *thiopental* and *methohexital* [meth-oh-HEX-uh-tall] quickly enter the CNS and depress function, often in less than 1 minute. However, diffusion out of the brain can also occur very rapidly because of redistribution to other tissues (Figure 13.10). These drugs may remain in the body for relatively long periods, because only about 15% of a dose entering the circulation is metabolized by the liver per hour. Thus, metabolism of *thiopental* is much slower than its redistribution. Barbiturates tend to decrease blood pressure, which may cause a reflex tachycardia. They decrease intracranial pressure through reductions in cerebral blood flow and oxygen consumption. *Thiopental* is no longer available in many countries, including the United States. *Methohexital* is still commonly used for electroconvulsive therapy.

F. Benzodiazepines

The benzodiazepines are used in conjunction with anesthetics for sedation and amnesia. The most commonly used is *midazolam* [meh-DAZ-o-lam]. *Diazepam* [dye-AZ-uh-pam] and *lorazepam* [lore-AZ-uh-pam] are alternatives. All three facilitate amnesia while causing sedation, enhancing the inhibitory effects of various neurotransmitters, particularly GABA. Minimal cardiovascular depressant effects are seen, but all are potential respiratory depressants (especially when administered IV). They are metabolized by the liver with variable elimination half-lives, and *erythromycin* may prolong effects of *midazolam*. Benzodiazepines can induce a temporary form of anterograde amnesia in which the patient retains memory of past events, but new information is not transferred into long-term memory. Therefore, important treatment information should be repeated to the patient after the effects of the drug have worn off.

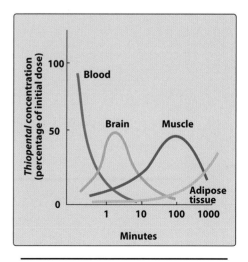

Figure 13.10
Redistribution of *thiopental* from the brain to muscle and adipose tissue.

G. Opioids

Because of their analgesic property, opioids are commonly combined with other anesthetics. The choice of opioid is based primarily on the duration of action needed. The most commonly used opioids are *fentanyl* [FEN-ta-nil] and its congeners, *sufentanil* [SOO-fen-ta-nil] and *remifentanil* [REMI-fen-ta-nil], because they induce analgesia more rapidly than *morphine*. They may be administered intravenously, epidurally, or intrathecally (into the cerebrospinal fluid). Opioids are not good amnestics, and they can all cause hypotension and respiratory depression, as well as nausea and vomiting. Opioid effects can be antagonized by *naloxone*.

H. Etomidate

Etomidate [ee-TOM-uh-date] is a hypnotic agent used to induce anesthesia, but it lacks analgesic activity. Its water solubility is poor, so it is formulated in a propylene glycol solution. Induction is rapid, and the drug is short-acting. Among its benefits are little to no effect on the heart and systemic vascular resistance. *Etomidate* is usually only used for patients with cardiovascular dysfunction or patients who are acutely critically ill. It inhibits 11-β hydroxylase involved in steroidogenesis, and adverse effects may include decreased plasma cortisol and aldosterone levels. *Etomidate* should not be infused for an extended time, because prolonged suppression of these hormones is dangerous. Injection site pain, involuntary skeletal muscle movements, and nausea and vomiting are common.

I. Ketamine

Ketamine [KET-uh-meen], a short-acting anti-NMDA receptor anesthetic and analgesic, induces a dissociated state in which the patient is unconscious (but may appear to be awake) with profound analgesia. *Ketamine* stimulates central sympathetic outflow, causing stimulation of the heart with increased blood pressure and CO. It is also a potent bronchodilator. Therefore, it is beneficial in patients with hypovolemic or cardiogenic shock as well as asthmatics. Conversely, it is contraindicated in hypertensive or stroke patients. The drug is lipophilic and enters the brain very quickly. Like the barbiturates, it redistributes to other organs and tissues. *Ketamine* has become popular as an adjunct to reduce opioid consumption during surgery. Of note, it may induce hallucinations, particularly in young adults, but pretreatment with benzodiazepines may help. *Ketamine* may be used illicitly, since it causes a dreamlike state and hallucinations similar to *phencyclidine* (PCP).

J. Dexmedetomidine

Dexmedetomidine [dex-med-eh-TOM-uh-deen] is a sedative used in intensive care settings and surgery. Like *clonidine*, it is an α_2 receptor agonist in certain parts of the brain. *Dexmedetomidine* has sedative, analgesic, sympatholytic, and anxiolytic effects that blunt many cardiovascular responses. It reduces volatile anesthetic, sedative, and analgesic requirements without causing significant respiratory depression. It has gained popularity for its ability to blunt emergence delirium in the pediatric population. Some therapeutic advantages and disadvantages of the anesthetic agents are summarized in Figure 13.11.

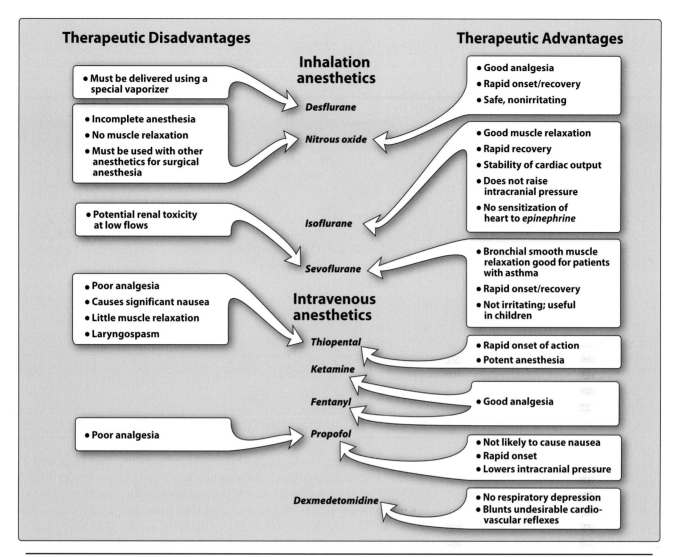

Figure 13.11
Therapeutic disadvantages and advantages of some anesthetic agents.

VI. NEUROMUSCULAR BLOCKERS

Neuromuscular blockers are crucial to the practice of anesthesia and used to facilitate endotracheal intubation and provide muscle relaxation when needed for surgery. Their mechanism of action is via blockade of nicotinic acetylcholine receptors on the skeletal muscle cell membrane. These agents include *cisatracurium*, *mivacurium*, *pancuronium*, *rocuronium*, *succinylcholine*, and *vecuronium* (see Chapter 5).

A. Sugammadex

Sugammadex [soo-GAM-ma-dex] is a selective relaxant-binding agent that terminates the action of both *rocuronium* and *vecuronium*. Its three-dimensional structure traps the neuromuscular blocker in a 1:1 ratio, terminating its action and making it water soluble. It is unique in that it produces rapid and effective reversal of both shallow and profound neuromuscular blockade. *Sugammadex* is eliminated via the kidneys.

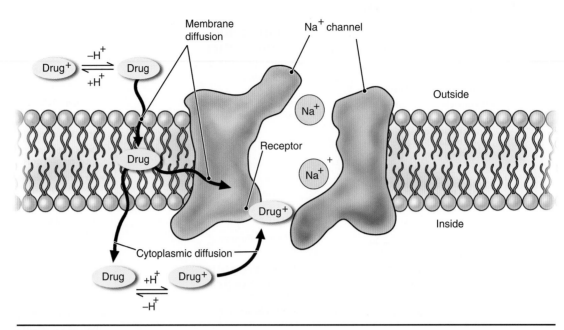

Figure 13.12
Mechanism of local anesthetic action.

VII. LOCAL ANESTHETICS

Local anesthetics block nerve conduction of sensory impulses and in higher concentrations block motor impulses from the periphery to the CNS. Sodium ion channels are blocked to prevent the transient increase in permeability of the nerve membrane to Na^+ that is required for an action potential (Figure 13.12). When propagation of action potentials is prevented, sensation cannot be transmitted from the source of stimulation to the brain. Delivery techniques include topical administration, infiltration, and perineural and neuraxial (spinal, epidural, or caudal) blocks. Small, unmyelinated nerve fibers for pain, temperature, and autonomic activity are most sensitive. Structurally, local anesthetics all include a lipophilic group joined by an amide or ester linkage to a carbon chain, which, in turn, is joined to a hydrophilic group (Figure 13.13). The most widely used local anesthetics are *bupivacaine* [byoo-PIV-uh-cane], *lidocaine* [LYE-doe-cane], *mepivacaine* [muh-PIV-uh-cane], *ropivacaine* [roe-PIV-uh-cane], and *tetracaine* [TET-truh-cane].

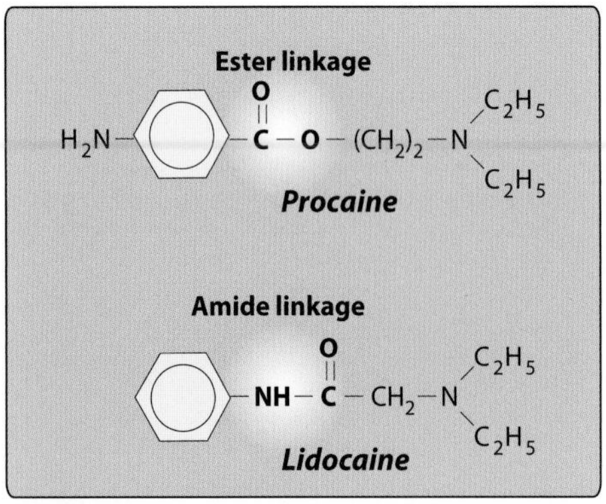

A. Actions

Local anesthetics cause vasodilation, which leads to a rapid diffusion away from the site of action and short duration when these drugs are administered alone. By adding the vasoconstrictor *epinephrine*, the rate of local anesthetic absorption and diffusion is decreased. This minimizes systemic toxicity and increases the duration of action. Hepatic function does not affect the duration of action of local anesthesia because that is determined by redistribution rather than biotransformation. Some local anesthetics have other therapeutic uses (for example, *lidocaine* is an IV antiarrhythmic).

Figure 13.13
Representative structures of ester and amide anesthetics.

B. Onset, potency, and duration of action

The onset of action of local anesthetics is influenced by several factors including tissue pH, nerve morphology, concentration, pKa, and lipid solubility of the drug. Of these, the pKa is most important. Local anesthetics with a lower pKa have a quicker onset, since more drug exists in the unionized form at physiologic pH, thereby allowing penetration of the nerve cell membrane. Once at the nerve membrane, the ionized form interacts with the protein receptor of the Na^+ channel to inhibit its function and achieve local anesthesia. The pH may drop in infected sites, causing onset to be delayed or even prevented. Potency and duration of these agents depend mainly on lipid solubility, with higher solubility correlating with increased potency and duration of action.

C. Metabolism

Biotransformation of amides occurs primarily in the liver. *Prilocaine* [PRY-low-cane], a dental anesthetic, is also metabolized in the plasma and kidney, and one of its metabolites may lead to methemoglobinemia. Esters are biotransformed by plasma cholinesterase (pseudocholinesterase). Patients with pseudocholinesterase deficiency may metabolize ester local anesthetics more slowly. At normal doses, this has little clinical effect. Reduced hepatic function predisposes patients to toxic effects, but should not significantly increase the duration of action of local anesthetics.

D. Allergic reactions

Patient reports of allergic reactions to local anesthetics are fairly common, but often times, reported "allergies" are actually side effects from the coadministered *epinephrine*. True allergy to an amide local anesthetic is exceedingly rare, while the ester *procaine* is more allergenic and has largely been removed from the market. Allergy to one ester rules out use of another ester, because the allergenic component is the metabolite para-aminobenzoic acid, produced by all esters. By contrast, allergy to one amide does not rule out the use of another amide. A patient may be allergic to other compounds in the local anesthetic, such as preservatives in multidose vials.

E. Local anesthetic systemic toxicity

Toxic blood levels of a local anesthetic may be due to repeated injections or could result from a single inadvertent IV injection. Each drug has a weight-based toxic threshold that should be calculated. This is especially important in children, the elderly, and women in labor (who are more susceptible to local anesthetics). Aspiration before every injection is imperative. The signs, symptoms, and timing of local anesthetic systemic toxicity (LAST) are unpredictable. One must consider the diagnosis in any patient with altered mental status, seizures, or cardiovascular instability following injection of local anesthetic. Treatment for LAST may include seizure suppression, airway management, and cardiopulmonary support. Administering a

CHARACTERISTIC	ESTERS	• Benzocaine • Procaine • Chloroprocaine • Tetracaine • Cocaine	AMIDES	• Bupivacaine • Prilocaine • Lidocaine • Ropivacaine • Mepivacaine
Metabolism		Rapid by plasma cholinesterase		Slow, hepatic
Systemic toxicity		Less likely		More likely
Allergic reaction		Possible—PABA derivatives form		Very rare
Stability in solution		Breaks down in ampules (heat, sun)		Very stable chemically
Onset of action		Slow as a general rule		Moderate to fast
pKa		Higher than physiologic pH (8.5–8.9)		Close to physiologic pH (7.6–8.1)

DRUG	POTENCY	ONSET	DURATION
Bupivacaine	High	Slow	Long
Chloroprocaine	Low	Rapid	Short
Lidocaine	Low	Rapid	Intermediate
Mepivacaine	Low	Moderate	Intermediate
Procaine	Low	Rapid	Short
Ropivacaine	High	Moderate	Long
Tetracaine	High	Slow	Long (spinal)

Figure 13.14
Summary of pharmacologic properties of some local anesthetics. PABA = para-aminobenzoic acid.

20% lipid emulsion infusion (lipid rescue therapy) is a valuable asset. Figure 13.14 summarizes pharmacologic properties of some local anesthetics.

VIII. ANESTHETIC ADJUNCTS

Adjuncts are a critical part of the practice of anesthesia and include drugs that affect gastrointestinal (GI) motility, PONV, anxiety, and analgesia. Adjuncts are used in collaboration to help make the anesthetic experience safe and pleasant.

A. Gastrointestinal medications

H_2-receptor antagonists (for example, *ranitidine*; see Chapter 40) and proton pump inhibitors (for example, *omeprazole*; see Chapter 40) help to reduce gastric acidity in the event of an aspiration. Nonparticulate antacids (*sodium citrate/citric acid*) are given occasionally to quickly increase the pH of stomach contents. These drugs are used in the obstetric population going to surgery, along with other patients with reflux. Finally, a dopamine receptor antagonist (*metoclopramide*) can be used as a prokinetic agent to speed gastric emptying and increase lower esophageal sphincter tone.

B. Medications for PONV

PONV can be a significant problem during and after surgery both for the clinician and the patient. Risk factors for PONV include female gender, nonsmoker, use of volatile and nitrous anesthetics, duration of surgery, and postoperative narcotic use. 5-HT$_3$ receptor antagonists (for example, *ondansetron*; see Chapter 40) are commonly used to prevent PONV and are usually administered toward the end of surgery. Caution is advised in patients with long QT intervals on electrocardiogram (ECG). An anticholinergic and antihistamine (*promethazine*) can also be used; however, sedation, delirium, and confusion can complicate the postoperative period, especially in the elderly. Glucocorticoids such as *dexamethasone* can be used to reduce PONV. The mechanism is unclear, but because of a longer onset, these agents are usually given at the start of surgery. The neurokinin-1 antagonist *aprepitant* has also been shown to reduce PONV. Lastly, transdermal *scopolamine* is given preoperatively to patients with multiple risk factors or a history of PONV. Caution is advised because it can produce central anticholinergic effects.

C. Anxiety medications

Anxiety is a common part of the surgical experience. Benzodiazepines (*midazolam, diazepam*), α$_2$ agonists (*clonidine, dexmedetomidine*), and H$_1$-receptor antagonists (*diphenhydramine*) can be used to alleviate anxiety. Benzodiazepines also elicit anterograde amnesia, which can help promote a more pleasant surgical experience.

D. Analgesia

While opioids are a mainstay in anesthesia for pain control, multimodal analgesia is becoming more common due to the long-term risks of opioid consumption in surgical patients. Nonsteroidal anti-inflammatory drugs (*ketorolac, celecoxib*; see Chapter 38) are common adjuncts to opioids. Caution should be used in patients with coagulopathies, and in those with a history of peptic ulcer or platelet aggregation abnormalities. *Acetaminophen* can be used both PO and IV, but caution is advised in impaired hepatic function. Analogs of GABA (*gabapentin, pregabalin*; see Chapter 12) are becoming more common as pretreatment to reduce opioid consumption both during and after surgery. They also have multiple uses in neuropathic pain and addiction medicine. The NMDA antagonist *ketamine* is used to reduce overall opioid consumption both intra- and postoperatively. Actions of anesthesia adjunct drugs are shown in Figure 13.15.

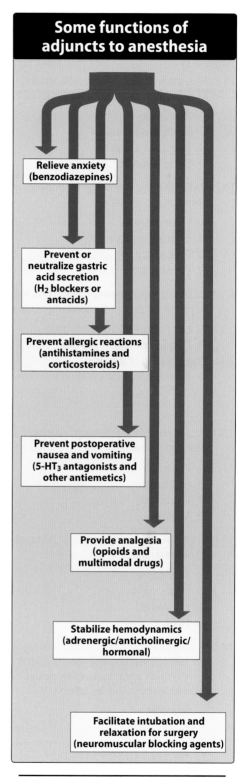

Figure 13.15
Actions of anesthesia adjunct drugs.

Study Questions

Choose the ONE best answer.

13.1 Regarding levels of sedation, which one applies to loss of perception and sensation to painful stimuli?

   A. Anxiolysis
   B. General anesthesia
   C. Moderate sedation
   D. Deep sedation

Correct answer = B. Anxiolysis is a state of relaxation, but consciousness remains. General anesthesia is a total loss of perception and sensation to stimuli. Moderate sedation maintains mentation with adequate airway and respiratory competency. Deep sedation has some response to stimuli, but respirations may be inadequate.

13.2 Which of the following decreases minimum alveolar concentration (MAC)?

   A. Hyperthermia
   B. Cocaine intoxication
   C. Pregnancy
   D. Chronic ethanol abuse

Correct answer = C. Pregnancy is the only choice that decreases minimum alveolar concentration. All the other options increase MAC.

13.3 Which of the following determines the speed of recovery from intravenous anesthetics used for induction?

   A. Liver metabolism of the drug
   B. Protein binding of the drug
   C. Ionization of the drug
   D. Redistribution of the drug from sites in the CNS

Correct answer = D. Following initial flooding of the CNS with nonionized molecules, the drug diffuses into other tissues. With secondary tissue uptake, the plasma concentration falls, allowing the drug to diffuse out of the CNS. This initial redistribution of drug into other tissues leads to the rapid recovery seen after a single dose of an IV induction drug. Protein binding, ionization, and lipid solubility affect the rate of transfer.

13.4 Which one of the following is a potent intravenous anesthetic and analgesic?

   A. Propofol
   B. Midazolam
   C. Ketamine
   D. Fentanyl

Correct answer = C. Ketamine is unique in its blockage of NMDA receptors, yielding both potent anesthetic and analgesic properties. Propofol is a potent anesthetic but a weak analgesic. Benzodiazepines such as midazolam have little analgesic effect, but can be a potent anesthetic at high doses. Fentanyl is a potent analgesic.

13.5 Which local anesthetic is metabolized by plasma cholinesterase?

   A. Tetracaine
   B. Bupivacaine
   C. Lidocaine
   D. Ropivacaine

Correct answer = A. Tetracaine is the only ester type local anesthetic of the choices. The other choices are amide-type local anesthetics, which are metabolized by biotransformation in the liver. Remember that esters usually have one "i" in the spelling, where amides typically have two "i"'s.

13.6 A 23-year-old patient with a history of severe postoperative nausea and vomiting is coming in for plastic surgery. Which anesthetic drug would be best to use for maintenance in this situation?

   A. Isoflurane
   B. Sevoflurane
   C. Nitrous oxide
   D. Propofol

Correct answer = D. A propofol infusion (TIVA) anesthetic would be best for this patient with a history of postoperative nausea and vomiting. Propofol is the only anesthetic listed with antiemetic properties. Both fluorinated hydrocarbons (isoflurane and sevoflurane) and nitrous oxide are linked to nausea and vomiting during surgery.

13.7 A 61-year-old patient with an acute myocardial infarction has severely reduced cardiac output. He has to undergo emergent coronary artery bypass surgery. Which of the following would you expect in this patient?

   A. Faster induction time with IV anesthetics
   B. Need for increased dosage of IV anesthetics
   C. Faster induction time with inhaled anesthetics
   D. Enhanced removal of inhaled anesthetics to peripheral tissues

Correct answer = C. For inhaled anesthetics during low CO, a longer period of time permits a larger concentration of gas to dissolve in the slowly moving bloodstream. Furthermore, this large bolus of drug has longer contact time to diffuse into neuronal tissue when it traverses the blood–brain barrier, yielding a faster induction time. The dose of an IV drug must be reduced (not increased). In addition, with reduced cardiac output, it takes a longer time for an IV induction drug to reach the brain, resulting in a slower induction time.

13.8 A 70-year-old patient in the intensive care unit needs sedation due to prolonged endotracheal intubation. Which of the following medications should be avoided for sedation in this patient?

A. Fentanyl
B. Etomidate
C. Propofol
D. Dexmedetomidine

Correct answer = B. Adverse effects of etomidate include decreased plasma cortisol and aldosterone levels by inhibiting the 11-β hydroxylase enzyme. Etomidate should not be infused for an extended time, because prolonged suppression of these hormones is dangerous. All of the other choices could be used for sedation in the ICU setting.

13.9 A 35-year-old man presents with appendicitis and requires a surgical intervention. He has a family history of malignant hyperthermia. Which anesthetic agent is most appropriate to use in this patient?

A. Isoflurane
B. Propofol
C. Succinylcholine
D. Sevoflurane

Correct answer = B. Propofol is the only medication listed that is safe in patients susceptible to malignant hyperthermia. All fluorinated hydrocarbons (isoflurane, sevoflurane, desflurane) as well as succinylcholine are contraindicated and considered triggering agents. Flushing of the anesthesia machine, removal of vaporizers, use of special filters, and availability of dantrolene are highly advised.

13.10 A 32-year-old woman presents for a right distal radius fracture. She requests regional anesthesia to help with her pain postoperatively. She reports that as a child, she had an allergic reaction to Novocain (procaine) at the dentist's office. Which local anesthetic is appropriate for use in this patient?

A. Chloroprocaine
B. Benzocaine
C. Ropivacaine
D. Tetracaine

Correct answer = C. Procaine is an ester local anesthetic. Since this patient has an allergy to procaine, other ester anesthetics (chloroprocaine, tetracaine, benzocaine) should not be used. Benzocaine is mostly used as a topical product for temporary relief of dental or oral pain. Ropivacaine is an amide local anesthetic commonly used in regional anesthesia to facilitate peripheral nerve blockade.

Opioids

Robin Moorman Li

14

I. OVERVIEW

Management of pain is one of clinical medicine's greatest challenges. Pain is defined as an unpleasant sensation that can be either acute or chronic and is a consequence of complex neurochemical processes in the peripheral and central nervous systems (CNS). It is subjective, and the clinician must rely on the patient's perception and description of pain. Alleviation of pain depends on the specific type of pain (nociceptive or neuropathic pain). For example, with mild to moderate arthritic pain (nociceptive pain), nonopioid analgesics such as nonsteroidal anti-inflammatory drugs (NSAIDs; see Chapter 38) are often effective. Neuropathic pain responds best to anticonvulsants, tricyclic antidepressants, or serotonin/norepinephrine reuptake inhibitors. However, for severe acute pain or chronic malignant or nonmalignant pain, opioids can be considered as part of the treatment plan in select patients (Figure 14.1). Opioids are natural, semisynthetic, or synthetic compounds that produce *morphine*-like effects (Figure 14.2). These agents are divided into chemical classes based on their chemical structure (Figure 14.3). All opioids act by binding to specific opioid receptors in the CNS to produce effects that mimic the action of endogenous peptide neurotransmitters (for example, endorphins, enkephalins, and dynorphins). Although the opioids have a broad range of effects, their primary use is to relieve intense pain that results from surgery, injury, or chronic disease. Unfortunately, widespread availability of opioids has led to abuse of agents with euphoric properties. Antagonists that reverse the actions of opioids are also clinically important for use in cases of overdose (Figure 14.1).

II. OPIOID RECEPTORS

The major effects of the opioids are mediated by three main receptor families, commonly designated as μ (mu, MOR), κ (kappa, KOR), and δ (delta, DOR). Each receptor family exhibits a different specificity for the drug(s) it binds. The analgesic properties of the opioids are primarily mediated by the mu receptors that modulate responses to thermal, mechanical, and chemical nociception. The κ receptors in the dorsal horn also contribute to analgesia by modulating the response to chemical and thermal nociception. The enkephalins interact more selectively with δ receptors in the periphery. All three opioid receptors are members of the G protein–coupled receptor family and inhibit adenylyl cyclase.

STRONG AGONISTS

Alfentanil ALFENTA
Fentanyl ABSTRAL, ACTIQ, DURAGESIC, FENTORA, IONSYS, LAZANDA, SUBSYS
Heroin GENERIC ONLY
Hydrocodone HYSINGLA, LORTAB*, NORCO*, VICODIN*, ZOHYDRO ER
Hydromorphone DILAUDID, EXALGO
Levorphanol GENERIC ONLY
Meperidine DEMEROL
Methadone DOLOPHINE, METHADOSE
Morphine ARYMO ER, KADIAN, MORPHABOND, MS CONTIN
Oxycodone OXAYDO, OXYCONTIN, PERCOCET*, ROXICODONE
Oxymorphone OPANA
Remifentanil ULTIVA
Sufentanil SUFENTA

MODERATE/LOW AGONISTS

Codeine GENERIC ONLY

MIXED AGONIST–ANTAGONIST AND PARTIAL AGONISTS

Buprenorphine BELBUCA, BUPRENEX, BUTRANS, PROBUPHINE
Butorphanol GENERIC ONLY
Nalbuphine GENERIC ONLY
Pentazocine TALWIN

ANTAGONISTS

Naloxone EVZIO, NARCAN
Naltrexone VIVITROL

OTHER ANALGESICS

Tapentadol NUCYNTA
Tramadol CONZIP, ULTRAM

Figure 14.1
Summary of opioid analgesics and antagonists with common trade names.
* = Contains *acetaminophen*.

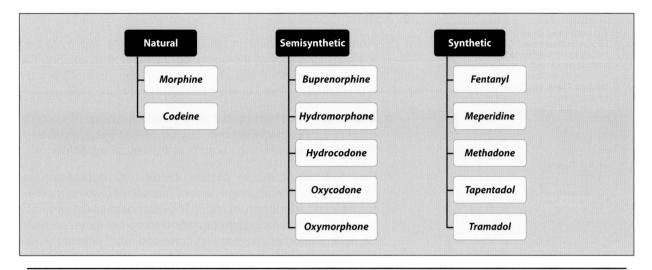

Figure 14.2
Origin of opioids: natural, semisynthetic, or synthetic.

They are also associated with ion channels, increasing postsynaptic K+ efflux (hyperpolarization) or reducing presynaptic Ca^{2+} influx, thus impeding neuronal firing and transmitter release in the spinal dorsal horn (Figure 14.4).

III. OPIOID AGONISTS

Morphine [MOR-feen] is the prototypical strong μ receptor agonist. *Codeine* [KOE-deen] is inherently less potent and the prototype of the weak μ opioid agonists. Currently available opioids have many differences, such as receptor affinity, pharmacokinetic profiles, available routes of administration, and adverse effect profiles. Some opioids are also available in abuse deterrent formulations. Comparing other available opioids to *morphine* is helpful in identifying the unique differences to guide the selection of a safe and effective pain management regimen (Figure 14.5).

A. Morphine

1. **Mechanism of action:** *Morphine* and other opioids exert analgesic effects by interacting stereospecifically with opioid receptors on the membranes of neuronal cells in the CNS and other anatomic structures, such as the smooth muscles of the gastrointestinal (GI) tract and the urinary bladder. *Morphine* is somewhat selective to the μ opioid receptor but has some affinity for the κ and δ receptors. *Morphine* also inhibits the release of many excitatory transmitters from nerve terminals carrying nociceptive (painful) stimuli. Some therapeutic uses of *morphine* and other opioids are listed in Figure 14.6.

Phenanthrenes	Action on Opioid Receptors
Morphine	Agonist
Codeine	Agonist
Oxycodone	Agonist
Oxymorphone	Agonist
Hydromorphone	Agonist
Hydrocodone	Agonist
Levorphanol	Agonist
Buprenorphine	Partial agonist/Antagonist
Nalbuphine	Mixed Agonist/Antagonist
Butorphanol	Mixed Agonist/Antagonist
Naloxone	Antagonist
Benzmorphan	
Pentazocine	Mixed Agonist/Antagonist
Phenylpiperidines	
Fentanyl	Agonist
Alfentanil	Agonist
Remifentanil	Agonist
Sufentanil	Agonist
Meperidine	Agonist
Diphenylheptane	
Methadone	Agonist
Phenylpropylamines	
Tramadol	Agonist
Tapentadol	Agonist

Figure 14.3
Pharmacological classes of opioids and actions on opioid receptors.

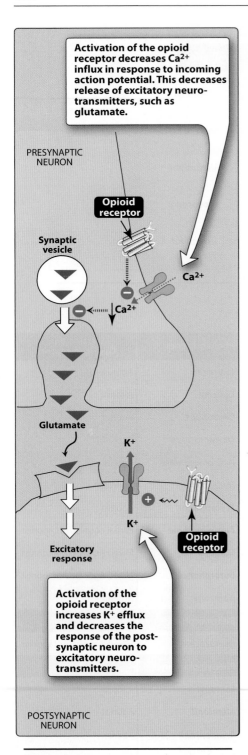

Figure 14.4
Mechanism of action of μ opioid receptor agonists in the spinal cord.

2. Actions

a. **Analgesia:** *Morphine* and other opioids relieve pain by raising the pain threshold at the spinal cord level and by altering the brain's perception of pain. The maximum analgesic efficacy for representative opioid agonists is shown in Figure 14.7.

b. **Euphoria:** *Morphine* produces a powerful sense of contentment and well-being. Euphoria may be caused by disinhibition of the dopamine-containing neurons of the ventral tegmental area.

c. **Respiration:** *Morphine* causes respiratory depression by reduction of the responsiveness of medullary respiratory center neurons to carbon dioxide. This can occur with ordinary doses of *morphine* in patients who are opioid naïve and can be accentuated as the dose is increased, until ultimately respiration ceases. Respiratory depression is the most common cause of death in acute opioid overdoses. Tolerance to this effect develops with repeated dosing, which allows for the safer use of *morphine* for the treatment of pain when the dose is correctly titrated.

d. **Depression of cough reflex:** Both *morphine* and *codeine* have antitussive properties. In general, cough suppression does not correlate closely with analgesic and respiratory depressant properties of opioid drugs. The receptors involved in the antitussive action appear to be different from those involved in analgesia.

e. **Miosis:** The pinpoint pupil (Figure 14.8) characteristic of *morphine* use results from stimulation of μ and κ receptors. There is little tolerance to this effect. [Note: This is important diagnostically, because many other causes of coma and respiratory depression produce dilation of the pupil.]

f. **Emesis:** *Morphine* directly stimulates the chemoreceptor trigger zone in the area postrema that causes vomiting.

g. **GI tract:** *Morphine* relieves diarrhea by decreasing the motility and increasing the tone of the intestinal circular smooth muscle. *Morphine* also increases the tone of the anal sphincter. *Morphine* and other opioids produce constipation, with little tolerance developing. *Morphine* can also increase biliary tract pressure due to contraction of the gallbladder and constriction of the biliary sphincter.

h. **Cardiovascular:** *Morphine* has no major effects on blood pressure or heart rate at lower dosages, but hypotension and bradycardia may occur at higher doses. Because of respiratory depression and carbon dioxide retention, cerebral vessels dilate and increase cerebrospinal fluid pressure. *Morphine* is usually contraindicated in individuals with head trauma or severe brain injury.

i. **Histamine release:** *Morphine* releases histamine from mast cells causing urticaria, sweating, and vasodilation. Because it can cause bronchoconstriction, *morphine* should be used with caution in patients with asthma.

Opioid	Routes of Administration	Comments
Morphine	PO (IR and ER), PR, IM, IV, SC, IA, SL, EA	• For all drugs listed: opioid class side effects. Metabolism through conjugation in liver and P-glycoprotein. • Active metabolites are renally eliminated and accumulate in renal impairment. • Metabolite M3G has no analgesic action, but can be neuroexcitatory. • Metabolite M6G is two to four times more potent than parent drug; accumulation can cause oversedation and respiratory depression. • Abuse deterrent formulations available.

Methadone	PO, IV, IM, SC	• No active metabolites.
		• Racemic mixture
		  • **Metabolized by many CYP450 isoenzymes:** high risk of drug interactions.
		  • **Substrate of P-glycoprotein**
		• Long and variable half-life increases risk of overdose.
		• Very lipophilic and redistributes to fat stores.
		• Duration of analgesia is much shorter than elimination half-life. Repeated dosing can lead to accumulation.
		• Can prolong QTc interval and cause torsades de pointes.
		• Warning: Conversion to and from *methadone* and other opioids should be done with great care, since equianalgesic dosing varies dramatically.

Fentanyl	IV, EA, IA, TD, OTFC, SL, Buccal, Nasal	• No active metabolites; option for patients with renal dysfunction but should be used with caution. • Metabolized by CYP3A4. • 100 times more potent than *morphine*. • Less histamine release, sedation, and constipation in comparison to *morphine*.
Oxycodone	PO (IR and CR)	• Metabolized by CYP2D6 and CYP3A4. • Black box warning: CYP3A4 drug interactions. • Less histamine release and nausea in comparison to *morphine*. • Abuse-deterrent formulation available.
Oxymorphone	PO (IR and ER), IV	• Immediate release has longer duration of action and elimination half-life (8 hours) compared to other immediate-release opioids. • Oral bioavailability increases with food. • Should be administered 1 to 2 hours after eating. • Bioavailability increased with coadministration of alcohol.
Hydromorphone	PO (IR and ER), PR, IV, SC, EA, IA	• Metabolized via glucuronidation to H6G and H3G which are renally eliminated and can cause CNS side effects in patients with renal insufficiency. • Abuse-deterrent formulation available.
Hydrocodone	PO (IR and ER)	• Active metabolite is *hydromorphone*. • Metabolized by CYP2D6 and CYP3A4. • Abuse-deterrent formulations available.
Tapentadol	PO (IR and ER)	• Centrally acting analgesic; μ agonist activity along with inhibition of norepinephrine reuptake. • Efficacy in treating nociceptive and neuropathic pain. • Metabolized predominately by glucuronidation; no CYP450 interactions. • Seizures and serotonin syndrome can occur in predisposed patients.

Tramadol	PO (IR and ER), Topical	• Metabolized by Phase 1 and 2. CYP2D6, CYP2B6, and CYP3A4 involved in metabolism; watch drug interactions.
		• Serotonin syndrome can occur due to drug interactions.
		• CI for treatment of pain in children <12 years old.
		• CI in children <18 y/o after removal of tonsils/adenoids.
		• Use is not recommended in 12–18 years old who are obese, have severe lung disease, or have sleep apnea
		• Use is not recommended in breastfeeding mothers due to adverse reactions in breastfed infants.
		• Warning:
		  • Renal impairment dosing required.
		  • Review dosing recommendations in severe hepatic impairment.

Codeine	PO, SC	• Prodrug: Metabolized by CYP2D6 to the active drug *morphine*. • Rapid metabolizers of CYP2D6 can experience toxicity. • Inhibitors of CYP2D6 will prevent conversion of *codeine* to *morphine*, thereby preventing pain control. • Do not use in patients with renal dysfunction. • Use only for mild or moderate pain. • CI in treatment of pain or cough in children <12 years old. • CI in children <18 years old after removal of tonsils/adenoids. • Use is not recommended in 12–18 years old who are obese, have severe lung disease, or have sleep apnea. • Use is not recommended in breastfeeding mothers due to adverse reactions in breastfed infants.
Meperidine	PO, IV, SC, EA, IA	• Not recommended as first-line opioid choice. • Active metabolite normeperidine accumulates with renal dysfunction, leading to toxicity. • *Naloxone* does not antagonize the effects of normeperidine; could worsen seizure activity. • Do not use in elderly, patients with renal dysfunction, or for chronic pain management.
Buprenorphine	SL, TD, IM, IV, Buccal (transmucosal), Implant	• Long duration of action; very lipophilic. • Incompletely reversible by *naloxone*. • Metabolized by CYP3A4; watch for drug interactions with strong CYP 3A4 inhibitors or inducers. • Can prolong QTc interval. • Transdermal patch is applied every 7 days. • Abuse-deterrent formulations available.

CI = contraindicated; CR = controlled-release; EA = epidural anesthesia; H3G = hydromorphone-3-glucuronide; H6G = hydromorphone-6-glucuronide; IA = intrathecal anesthesia; IM = intramuscular; IR = immediate release; IV = intravenous; M3G = morphine-3-glucuronide; M6G = morphine-6-glucuronide; OTFC = oral transmucosal fentanyl citrate; PO = orally; PR = rectally; SC = subcutaneous; SL = sublingual; TD = transdermal.
Note: Many different acronyms may be used to indicate a medication is extended-release. Examples include CR (controlled-release), LA (long-acting), ER (extended-release).

Figure 14.5
Summary of clinically relevant properties for selected opioids.

Therapeutic Use	Comments
Analgesia	*Morphine* is the prototype opioid agonist. Opioids are used for pain in trauma, cancer, and other types of severe pain.
Treatment of diarrhea	Opioids decrease the motility and increase the tone of intestinal circular smooth muscle. [Note: Agents commonly used include *diphenoxylate* and *loperamide* (see chapter 40).]
Relief of cough	*Morphine* does suppress the cough reflex, but *codeine* and *dextromethorphan* are more commonly used.
Treatment of acute pulmonary edema	Intravenous *morphine* dramatically relieves dyspnea caused by pulmonary edema associated with left ventricular failure, possibly via the vasodilatory effect. This, in effect, decreases cardiac preload and afterload, as well as anxiety experienced by the patient.
Anesthesia	Opioids are used as preanesthetic medications, for systemic and spinal anesthesia, and for postoperative analgesia.

Figure 14.6
Selected clinical uses of opioids.

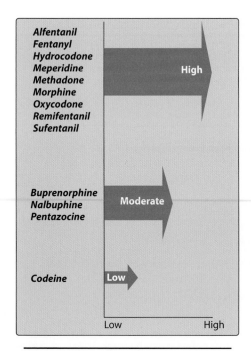

Figure 14.7
A comparison of opioid agonist efficacy.

j. Hormonal actions: Prolonged use of *morphine* may lead to opioid-induced androgen deficiency due to suppression of the hypothalamic–pituitary–gonadal axis (HPA). This results in decreased production of sex hormones, especially testosterone, resulting in many clinical symptoms (Figure 14.9).

k. Labor: *Morphine* may prolong the second stage of labor by transiently decreasing the strength, duration, and frequency of uterine contractions.

3. Pharmacokinetics

a. Administration: *Morphine* has a linear pharmacokinetic profile; however, absorption of morphine after oral administration is slow and erratic. Extended-release oral preparations provide more consistent plasma levels. Because significant first-pass metabolism of *morphine* occurs in the liver, subcutaneous and intravenous (IV) injections produce the most reliable response.

b. Distribution: *Morphine* rapidly enters all body tissues, including the fetuses of pregnant women. It should not be used for analgesia during labor. Infants born to addicted mothers show physical dependence on opioids and exhibit withdrawal symptoms if opioids are not administered. Only a small percentage of *morphine* crosses the blood–brain barrier, because *morphine* is the least lipophilic of the common opioids. By contrast, the more lipid-soluble opioids, such as *fentanyl* and *methadone*, readily penetrate the CNS.

c. Fate: *Morphine* is conjugated with glucuronic acid in the liver to two active metabolites (morphine-6-glucuronide [M6G] and morphine-3-glucuronide [M3G]), which are renally excreted. M6G is a very potent analgesic. M3G does not have analgesic activity but is believed to cause neuroexcitatory effects. The duration of action of *morphine* is 4 to 5 hours when administered systemically to opioid-naïve individuals but considerably longer when injected epidurally because the low lipophilicity prevents redistribution from the epidural space.

4. Adverse effects: Many adverse effects are common across the entire opioid class (Figure 14.10). With most mu agonists, severe respiratory depression can occur and may result in death from acute opioid overdose. Respiratory drive may be suppressed in patients with respiratory disorders such as obstructive sleep apnea, emphysema, or cor pulmonale, so close monitoring is necessary when using opioids. Opioid-induced constipation (OIC) is a common adverse effect. Initial management includes a nonprescription stimulant laxative such as *senna*. Peripherally acting μ-opioid receptor antagonists such as *methylnaltrexone*, *naloxegol*, and *naldemedine* are prescription drugs available for the treatment of OIC. [Note: *Lubiprostone* is a chloride channel activator that is indicated for OIC and irritable bowel syndrome; see Chapter 40.] *Morphine* should be used with caution in patients with liver disease and renal dysfunction.

5. **Tolerance and physical dependence:** Repeated use produces tolerance to the respiratory depressant, analgesic, euphoric, emetic, and sedative effects of *morphine*. Tolerance usually does not develop to miosis (constriction of the pupils) or constipation. Physical and psychological dependence can occur with *morphine* and other agonists. Withdrawal produces a series of autonomic, motor, and psychological responses that can be severe, although it is rare that withdrawal effects cause death.

6. **Drug interactions:** Drug interactions with *morphine* are possible. The depressant actions of *morphine* are enhanced by coadministration with CNS depressant medications such as phenothiazines, monoamine oxidase inhibitors (MAOIs), and benzodiazepines. Guidelines for opioid prescribing urge clinicians to avoid simultaneous prescribing of opioids and benzodiazepines. A black box warning also has been included on the labeling of both opioids and benzodiazepines to alert prescribers of this dangerous combination.

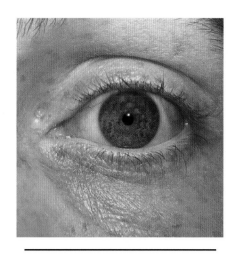

Figure 14.8
Characteristic pinpoint pupil associated with *morphine* use.

B. Codeine

Codeine [KOE-deen] is a naturally occurring opioid and a weak analgesic compared to *morphine*. It is used for mild to moderate pain. The analgesic actions of *codeine* are derived from its conversion to *morphine* by the CYP2D6 enzyme (see Chapter 1). CYP2D6 activity varies among patients, and ultrarapid metabolizers may experience higher levels of *morphine*, leading to possible overdose and toxicity. Life-threatening respiratory depression and death have been reported in children who received *codeine*, mostly following tonsillectomy and/or adenoidectomy. *Codeine* is commonly used in combination with *acetaminophen* for management of pain. The drug exhibits good antitussive activity at doses that do not cause analgesia. *Dextromethorphan* [dex-troe-meth-OR-fan] is a synthetic cough depressant that has relatively no analgesic action and much lower potential for abuse in usual antitussive doses. It is preferred over *codeine* in most situations where cough suppression is needed.

C. Oxycodone and oxymorphone

Oxymorphone [ox-ee-MOR-fone] and *oxycodone* [ok-see-KOE-done] are orally active, semisynthetic analogs of *morphine* and *codeine*, respectively. *Oxymorphone* given parenterally is approximately ten times more potent than *morphine*, but when administered orally, the potency drops to about three times that of *morphine*. *Oxymorphone* is available in both immediate-release and extended-release oral formulations. This agent has no clinically relevant drug interactions associated with the CYP450 enzyme system. *Oxycodone* is approximately two times more potent than *morphine* and is available in an immediate-release formulation, alone or in combination with *acetaminophen*, *aspirin*, *or ibuprofen*. An extended-release formulation is also available. *Oxycodone* is mainly metabolized via the CYP2D6 and CYP3A4 enzymes.

D. Hydromorphone and hydrocodone

Hydromorphone [hye-droe-MORE-fone] and *hydrocodone* [hye-droe-KOE-done] are orally active, semisynthetic analogs of *morphine* and *codeine*, respectively. Oral *hydromorphone* is approximately 4 to

7 times more potent than oral *morphine*. It is preferred over *morphine* in patients with renal dysfunction due to less accumulation of active metabolites. *Hydrocodone* is the methyl ether derivative of *hydromorphone*, but is a weaker analgesic than *hydromorphone*, with oral analgesic efficacy comparable to that of *morphine*. This agent is often combined with *acetaminophen* or *ibuprofen* to treat moderate to severe pain. It is also used as an antitussive. *Hydrocodone* is metabolized in the liver to several metabolites, one of which is *hydromorphone* via the actions of CYP2D6.

E. Fentanyl

Fentanyl [FEN-ta-nil] is a synthetic opioid chemically related to *meperidine*. *Fentanyl* has 100-fold the analgesic potency of *morphine* and is used for anesthesia and acute pain management. The drug is highly lipophilic and has a rapid onset and short duration of action (15 to 30 minutes). It is usually administered IV, epidurally, or intrathecally. *Fentanyl* is combined with local anesthetics to provide epidural analgesia for labor and postoperative pain. IV *fentanyl* is used in anesthesia for its analgesic and sedative effects. Many fast-acting transmucosal and nasal *fentanyl* products are available for cancer-related breakthrough pain in opioid-tolerant patients. The transdermal patch creates a reservoir of the drug in the skin and has a delayed onset of at least 12 hours and a prolonged offset. The patch is used for management of chronic severe pain. It is contraindicated in opioid-naïve patients and should not be used in management of acute or postoperative pain. *Fentanyl* is metabolized to inactive metabolites by CYP3A4, and drugs that inhibit this isoenzyme can potentiate the effect of *fentanyl*.

F. Sufentanil, alfentanil, remifentanil, and carfentanil

Sufentanil [soo-FEN-ta-nil], *alfentanil* [al-FEN-ta-nil], *remifentanil* [rem-ih-FEN-ta-nil], and *carfentanil* [car-FEN-ta-nil] are synthetic opioid agonists related to *fentanyl*. These agents differ in potency and metabolic disposition. *Sufentanil* and *carfentanil* are even more potent than *fentanyl*, whereas the other two are less potent and shorter acting. *Sufentanil*, *alfentanil*, and *remifentanil* are mainly used for their analgesic and sedative properties during surgical procedures requiring anesthesia. *Carfentanil* is about 100 times more potent than *fentanyl*. The drug is not used in clinical practice; however, it is of toxicological interest as it is used to lace *heroin* and has contributed to several opioid-related deaths.

G. Methadone

Methadone [METH-a-done] is a synthetic, orally effective opioid that has variable equianalgesic potency compared to that of *morphine*, and the conversion between the two products is not linear. *Methadone* is a μ agonist, an antagonist of the *N*-methyl-ᴅ-aspartate (NMDA) receptor, and a norepinephrine and serotonin reuptake inhibitor. Therefore, it is useful in the treatment of both nociceptive and neuropathic pain. *Methadone* may also be used for opioid withdrawal and maintenance therapy in the setting of prescription opioid and *heroin* abuse. The withdrawal syndrome with *methadone* is milder but more protracted (days to weeks) than that with other opioids. *Methadone* induces less euphoria and has a longer duration of

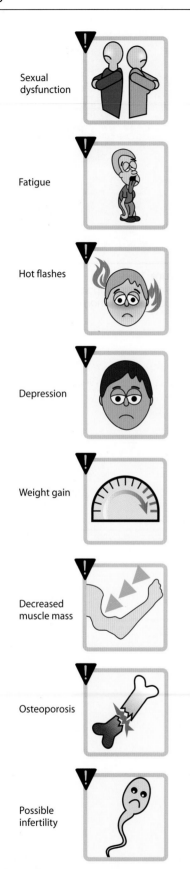

Figure 14.9
Clinical symptoms associated with opioid-induced androgen deficiency (OPIAD).

Sexual dysfunction

Fatigue

Hot flashes

Depression

Weight gain

Decreased muscle mass

Osteoporosis

Possible infertility

action than *morphine*. Unlike *morphine*, *methadone* is well absorbed after oral administration. *Methadone* is also constipating, but less so than *morphine*.

Understanding the pharmacokinetics of *methadone* is important to ensure proper use. After oral administration, *methadone* is biotransformed in the liver and excreted almost exclusively in the feces. *Methadone* is very lipophilic, rapidly distributed throughout the body, and released slowly during redistribution and elimination. This translates into a long half-life ranging from 12 to 40 hours, although it may extend up to 150 hours. Despite the extended half-life, the actual duration of analgesia ranges from 4 to 8 hours. Attainment of steady state can vary dramatically, ranging from 35 hours to 2 weeks, so dosage adjustments should occur only every 5 to 7 days. Upon repeated dosing, *methadone* can accumulate due to the long terminal half-life, leading to toxicity. Overdose is possible when prescribers are unaware of the long half-life, the incomplete cross-tolerance between *methadone* and other opioids, and the titration guidelines to avoid toxic accumulation. The metabolism is variable due to involvement of multiple CYP450 isoenzymes, some of which are affected by known genetic polymorphisms. As such, *methadone* is susceptible to many drug–drug interactions.

Methadone can produce physical dependence like that of *morphine*, but it has less neurotoxicity than *morphine* due to lack of active metabolites. *Methadone* can prolong the QT_c interval and cause torsades de pointes, possibly by interacting with cardiac potassium channels. Baseline and routine ECG monitoring is recommended.

H. Meperidine

Meperidine [me-PER-i-deen] is a lower-potency synthetic opioid structurally unrelated to *morphine*. It is used for acute pain and acts primarily as a κ agonist, with some μ agonist activity. *Meperidine* is very lipophilic and has anticholinergic effects, resulting in an increased incidence of delirium compared with other opioids. *Meperidine* has an active metabolite (normeperidine), which is potentially neurotoxic. Normeperidine is renally excreted, and in patients with renal insufficiency, accumulation of the metabolite may lead to delirium, hyperreflexia, myoclonus, and seizures. Due to the short duration of action and the potential for toxicity, *meperidine* should only be used for short-term (≤48 hours) management of pain. *Meperidine* should not be used in elderly patients or those with renal insufficiency, hepatic insufficiency, preexisting respiratory compromise, or concomitant or recent administration of MAOIs. Serotonin syndrome has been reported in patients receiving both *meperidine* and selective serotonin reuptake inhibitors (SSRIs).

IV. PARTIAL AGONISTS AND MIXED AGONIST–ANTAGONISTS

Partial agonists bind to the opioid receptor, but they have less intrinsic activity than full agonists (see Chapter 2). There is a ceiling to the pharmacologic effects of these agents. Drugs that stimulate one receptor but block another are termed mixed agonist–antagonists. The effects of these drugs depend on previous exposure to opioids. In individuals who

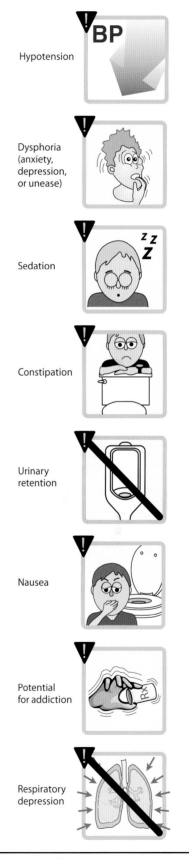

Figure 14.10
Adverse effects commonly observed in individuals treated with opioids.

are opioid-naïve, mixed agonist–antagonists show agonist activity and are used to relieve pain. In the presence of a full agonist, the agonist–antagonist drugs may precipitate opioid withdrawal symptoms.

A. Buprenorphine

Buprenorphine [byoo-pre-NOR-feen] acts as a potent partial agonist at the μ receptor and an antagonist at the κ receptors. *Buprenorphine* is very lipophilic and has a longer duration of action due to its high affinity for the opioid receptors when compared to *morphine*. Due to high affinity for the mu receptor, *buprenorphine* can displace full μ agonists, leading to withdrawal symptoms in an opioid-dependent patient. Because of the partial μ agonist activity, *buprenorphine* provides a "ceiling effect," causing less euphoric effects and a lower abuse potential than that of full agonists. Additionally, the risk of opioid-induced respiratory depression may be lower when compared with full agonists, except when combined with CNS depressants such as benzodiazepines. *Buprenorphine* is available in sublingual, transmucosal, buccal, parenteral, subdermal, and transdermal formulations. The drug is approved for moderate to severe pain. Certain formulations (for example, sublingual and subdermal) are approved for use in medication-assisted treatment of opioid addiction due to its ability to provide prolonged suppression of opioid withdrawal, the ability to block other μ agonists, and less frequent dosing requirements. In contrast to *methadone*, which is available only at specialized clinics when used for opioid detoxification or maintenance, *buprenorphine* is approved for office-based treatment of opioid dependence. It has been shown to have shorter and less severe withdrawal symptoms compared to *methadone* (Figure 14.11). Adverse effects include respiratory depression that cannot easily be reversed by *naloxone* and decreased (or, rarely, increased) blood pressure, nausea, and dizziness. Additionally, *buprenorphine* has been associated with prolongation of the QT_c interval. Although the clinical significance of this effect is controversial, current labeling for some *buprenorphine* products includes dosing restrictions due to the concern of QT_c prolongation. Risk factors to evaluate when considering *buprenorphine* include cardiovascular factors and concurrent drugs that may prolong.

B. Pentazocine

Pentazocine [pen-TAZ-oh-seen] acts as an agonist on κ receptors and is a weak antagonist or partial agonist at μ receptors. It can be administered either orally or parenterally. *Pentazocine* produces less euphoria compared to *morphine*, but in higher doses, respiratory depression, increased blood pressure, tachycardia, and hallucinations can occur. For these reasons, *pentazocine* is rarely used for management of pain. Despite its antagonist action, *pentazocine* does not antagonize the respiratory depression of *morphine*, but it can precipitate withdrawal effects in a *morphine* user. *Pentazocine* should be used with caution in patients with angina or coronary artery disease, since it can increase blood pressure.

C. Nalbuphine and butorphanol

Nalbuphine [NAL-byoo-feen] and *butorphanol* [byoo-TOR-fa-nole] are mixed opioid agonist–antagonists. Like *pentazocine*, they play a limited

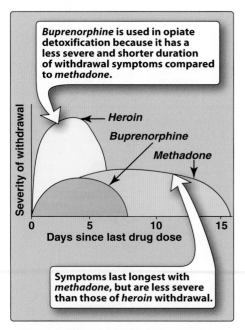

Figure 14.11
Severity of opioid withdrawal symptoms after abrupt withdrawal of equivalent doses of *heroin*, *buprenorphine*, and *methadone*.

role in the treatment of chronic pain. *Butorphanol* is available in a nasal spray that has been used for severe headaches, but it has been associated with abuse. Both products are available in an injectable formulation. Their propensity to cause psychotomimetic effects is less than that of *pentazocine*. In contrast to *pentazocine* and *butorphanol*, *nalbuphine* does not affect the heart or increase blood pressure. A benefit of all three medications is that they exhibit a ceiling effect for respiratory depression.

V. OTHER ANALGESICS

A. Tapentadol

Tapentadol [ta-PEN-ta-dol], a centrally acting analgesic, is an agonist at the μ opioid receptor and an inhibitor of norepinephrine reuptake. It is used to manage moderate to severe acute and chronic pain, including neuropathic pain associated with diabetic peripheral neuropathy. *Tapentadol* is mainly metabolized to inactive metabolites via glucuronidation, and it does not inhibit or induce the CYP450 enzyme system. Because *tapentadol* does not produce active metabolites, dosing adjustment is not necessary in mild to moderate renal impairment. *Tapentadol* should be avoided in patients who have received MAOIs within the past 14 days. It is available in an immediate-release and extended-release formulation.

B. Tramadol

Tramadol [TRA-ma-dole] is a centrally acting analgesic that binds to the μ opioid receptor. It undergoes extensive metabolism via CYP2D6, leading to an active metabolite, which has a much higher affinity for the mu receptor than the parent compound. In addition, it weakly inhibits reuptake of norepinephrine and serotonin. It is used to manage moderate to severe pain. Of note, *tramadol* has less respiratory-depressant activity compared to *morphine*. Administration of *naloxone* can only partially reverse *tramadol* toxicity and has been associated with an increased risk of seizures. Anaphylactoid reactions have been reported. Overdose or drug–drug interactions with SSRIs, MAOIs, and tricyclic antidepressants can lead to toxicity manifested by CNS excitation and seizures. *Tramadol* should be used with caution in patients with a history of seizures. As with other agents that bind the μ opioid receptor, *tramadol* has been associated with misuse and abuse.

VI. ANTAGONISTS

The opioid antagonists bind with high affinity to opioid receptors, but they fail to activate the receptor-mediated response. Administration of opioid antagonists produces no profound effects in individuals not taking opioids. In opioid-dependent patients, antagonists rapidly reverse the effect of agonists, such as *morphine* or any full μ agonist, and precipitate the symptoms of opioid withdrawal. Figure 14.12 summarizes some signs and symptoms of opioid withdrawal.

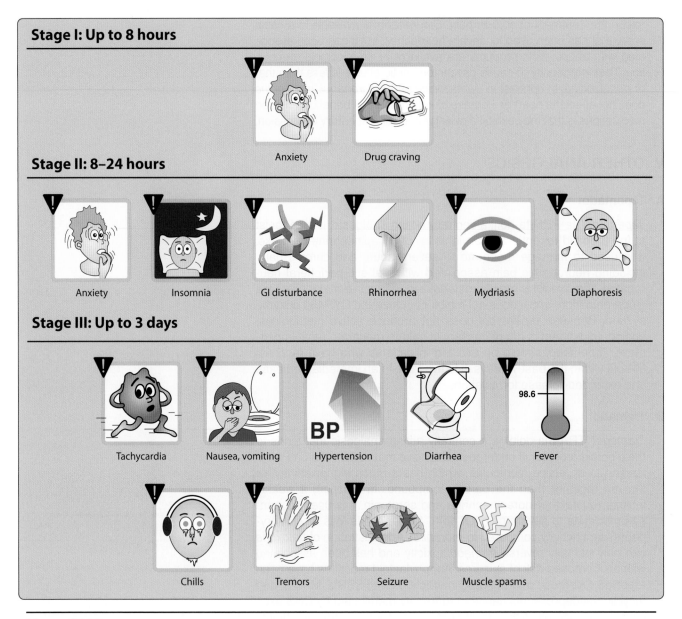

Figure 14.12
Opiate withdrawal syndrome. GI = gastrointestinal.

A. Naloxone

Naloxone [nal-OX-own] is a competitive antagonist at μ, κ, and δ receptors, with a 10-fold higher affinity for mu than for kappa receptors. It rapidly displaces all receptor-bound opioid molecules and, therefore, can reverse the effects of *morphine* overdose, such as respiratory depression and coma within 1 to 2 minutes of IV administration. *Naloxone* can also be administered intramuscularly, subcutaneously, and intranasally, with a slightly longer onset of 2 to 5 minutes; however, little to no clinical effect is seen with oral *naloxone* due to extensive first-pass metabolism. Since *naloxone* has a half-life of 30 to 81 minutes, a patient who has been treated for an overdose and recovered may lapse back into respiratory depression, depending on the opioid ingested and dosage form of that opioid. [Note: Much higher doses and continuous administration of *naloxone* are needed to reverse the effects of *buprenorphine* due to its high affinity for the mu receptor.]

Naloxone is available in an autoinjector and a nasal inhaler for community distribution for treatment of opioid overdose involving *heroin* or prescription opioids. It is imperative that prescribers counsel the patient and family members regarding the availability of these products, proper instructions for use, and the importance of calling emergency services in the case of overdose.

B. Naltrexone

Naltrexone [nal-TREX-own] has actions similar to those of *naloxone*, but it has a longer duration of action and can be given orally. For example, a single oral dose of *naltrexone* blocks the effect of injected *heroin* for up to 24 hours, and the intramuscular formulation blocks the effect for 30 days. *Naltrexone* in combination with *clonidine* (and, sometimes, with *buprenorphine*) is used for rapid opioid detoxification. *Naltrexone* has been reported to cause hepatotoxicity and monitoring of hepatic function is recommended.

Study Questions

Choose the ONE best answer.

14.1 Which of the agents listed is a phenanthrene opioid that exhibits a full and immediate response to treatment with naloxone in the case of overdose?

    A. Meperidine
    B. Morphine
    C. Buprenorphine
    D. Fentanyl

Correct answer = B. A morphine overdose can be effectively treated with naloxone, and morphine is a phenanthrene. Naloxone antagonizes the opioid by displacing it from the receptor, but there are cases in which naloxone is not effective. Meperidine is a phenylpiperidine, not a phenanthrene, and the active metabolite, normeperidine, is not reversible by naloxone. The effects of buprenorphine are only partially reversible by naloxone. In most cases of buprenorphine overdose, the dose of naloxone needs to be high and continuous due to the higher binding affinity to the mu receptor. Naloxone is effective for fentanyl overdoses; however, fentanyl is a phenylpiperidine, and not a phenanthrene.

14.2 A 76-year-old female with renal insufficiency has severe pain secondary to a compression fracture in the lumbar spine. She reports that the pain has been uncontrolled with tramadol, and it is decided to start treatment with an opioid. Which is the best opioid for this patient?

    A. Meperidine
    B. Fentanyl transdermal patch
    C. Hydrocodone/acetaminophen
    D. Morphine

Correct answer = C. Hydrocodone/acetaminophen is the best choice. It is very important to use a low dose and monitor closely for proper pain control and adverse effects. Meperidine should not be used for chronic pain, nor should it be used in a patient with renal insufficiency. The transdermal patch is not a good option, since her pain is considered acute and she is opioid naïve. Morphine is not the best choice due to the active metabolites that can accumulate in renal insufficiency.

14.3 Which statement about buprenorphine is correct?

    A. Buprenorphine has a much higher incidence of opioid-induced respiratory depression compared to other μ agonists.
    B. Buprenorphine has many dosage formulations, and all formulations can be prescribed for the treatment of pain or opioid dependence.
    C. Buprenorphine has a lower number of drug–drug interactions compared to methadone.
    D. Buprenorphine is a full μ agonist, an antagonist of the NMDA receptor, and a norepinephrine and serotonin reuptake inhibitor.

Correct answer = C. Buprenorphine is metabolized by the CYP3A4 system, so there are concerns about drug interactions; however, compared to methadone, which is metabolized by numerous CYP450 enzymes, the drug interaction concern for buprenorphine is much lower. Buprenorphine has a lower incidence of opioid-induced respiratory depression compared to the μ agonists due to the ceiling effect created by the partial μ agonist activity. Buprenorphine is available in many different dosage formulations, but these formulations are indicated for either pain management or medication-assisted treatment of opioid dependence, not both. Option D describes the mechanism of action of methadone. Buprenorphine is a potent partial μ agonist and a κ antagonist.

14.4 A 56-year-old patient has suffered with painful diabetic neuropathy and severe chronic back pain with radiculopathy secondary to spinal stenosis for many years. This patient has failed to receive relief from his neuropathic pain with first-line agents such as tricyclics, SNRIs, or anticonvulsants. Based on the mechanism of action, which opioid could be considered in this patient to treat both nociceptive and neuropathic pain?

    A. Meperidine

    B. Oxymorphone

    C. Morphine

    D. Tapentadol

> Correct answer = D. Tapentadol has a unique mechanism of action in comparison with the other choices given. Tapentadol has a dual mechanism of action (μ agonist and norepinephrine reuptake inhibition), which has been shown to effectively treat neuropathic pain associated with diabetic peripheral neuropathy. All other μ agonists could help manage neuropathic pain, but in some situations, higher doses of opioids are needed to achieve efficacy.

14.5 Which of the following statements regarding methadone is correct?

    A. Methadone is an excellent choice for analgesia in most patients because there are limited drug–drug interactions.

    B. The equianalgesic potency of methadone is similar to that of morphine.

    C. The duration of analgesia for methadone is much shorter than the elimination half-life.

    D. The active metabolites of methadone accumulate in patients with renal dysfunction.

> Correct Answer = C. The duration of analgesia is much shorter than the elimination half-life, leading to dangers of accumulation and increased potential for respiratory depression and death. The equianalgesic potency of methadone is extremely variable based on many factors, and only providers familiar with methadone should prescribe this agent. The drug interactions associated with methadone are numerous due to the multiple liver enzymes that metabolize the drug. Methadone does not have active metabolites, which makes it a treatment option in patients with renal dysfunction.

14.6 AN is a 57-year-old man who has been treated with oxycodone for chronic nonmalignant pain for over 2 years. He now reports increased pain in the afternoon while at work. Which of the following is a short-acting opioid and is the best choice for this patient's breakthrough pain?

    A. Methadone

    B. Fentanyl

    C. Hydrocodone

    D. Nalbuphine

> Correct answer = C. Hydrocodone is a commonly used short-acting agent that is commercially available in combination with either acetaminophen or ibuprofen. Methadone should not routinely be used for breakthrough pain due to the unique pharmacokinetics and should be reserved for practitioners who have experience with this agent and understand the variables associated with this drug. Fentanyl is available in formulations for treatment of breakthrough pain for cancer treatment. It is not appropriate to use fentanyl in this type of chronic pain setting. Nalbuphine is a mixed agonist/antagonist analgesic that could precipitate withdrawal in patients who are currently taking a full μ agonist such as oxycodone.

14.7 A 64-year-old man is preparing for a total knee replacement. He is taking many medications that are metabolized by the CYP450 enzyme system and is worried about drug interactions with the pain medication that will be used following surgery. Which of the following opioids would have the lowest chance of drug interactions in this patient?

    A. Methadone

    B. Tapentadol

    C. Tramadol

    D. Oxycodone

> Correct answer = B. Tapentadol is metabolized via glucuronidation and has not been shown to have any clinically relevant drug interactions associated with the CYP450 enzyme family. All other opioids listed are metabolized by one or more CYP450 enzymes and increase the risk of drug interactions.

14.8 Which of the following statements regarding adverse effects of opioid therapy is correct?

   A. The risk of respiratory depression is highest during an initial opioid initiation or following a dose increase.

   B. Opioid-induced constipation is only seen with the initiation of opioid therapy.

   C. The incidence of nausea and sedation increases with long-term use of opioid therapy.

   D. Decreased testosterone levels are commonly seen with short-term use of opioid therapy.

Correct answer = A. The risk of respiratory depression is highest when the opioid is first initiated or a dosage is raised (or sometimes a drug–drug interaction leads to higher opioid levels). Opioid-induced constipation can occur at any time during the therapy, and a patient does not develop a tolerance to this side effect. Side effects such as nausea and sedation commonly decrease after repeated dosing due to development of tolerance to these adverse effects. Chronic opioid exposure has been linked to decreased testosterone levels in males.

14.9 KM is a 64-year-old man who has been hospitalized following a car accident in which he sustained a broken leg and broken arm. He has been converted to oral morphine in anticipation of discharge from the hospital. Upon discharge, which medication should he receive along with the morphine?

   A. Diphenhydramine
   B. Methylphenidate
   C. Senna
   D. Docusate sodium

Correct answer = C. A bowel regimen should be prescribed with the initiation of the opioid since constipation is very common and can occur at any time, and tolerance to this adverse effect does not occur. Senna is a stimulant that is available over-the-counter. Docusate sodium is a stool softener that is ineffective in opioid-induced constipation when used as a single agent. Combination products that include both docusate and senna are commonly used and can be effective, mainly due to the actions of senna. Diphenhydramine can be used for urticaria that might occur with the initiation of an opioid, and methylphenidate has been used for opioid-induced sedation in certain situations, but these issues are not reported in this case.

14.10 AN is a 67-year-old man who has been treated with oxycodone for chronic nonmalignant pain with no changes in the dosing regimen for over 2 years. His pain has been fairly well controlled, and he remains active, reports satisfaction with his pain regimen, and denies any side effects. He has been recently diagnosed with COPD and obstructive sleep apnea (OSA). Which of the following options is the best treatment recommendation for him at this time?

   A. Taper off all opioids due to increased risk of opioid-induced respiratory depression.

   B. Prescribe naloxone nasal spray to have at home in case he experiences an opioid overdose.

   C. Prescribe oral naloxone tablets to have at home in case he experiences an opioid overdose.

   D. No action is needed at this time. His pain is well controlled, and he is reporting no side effects.

Correct answer = B. Because this patient has just been diagnosed with COPD and OSA, it is clear his risk for opioid-induced respiratory depression is greater. Since the pain is controlled and no side effects are reported, tapering off the opioids at this time is not the best answer. Because of the first-pass effect, naloxone is not clinically effective for management of an overdose when given orally. Therefore, the nasal spray is the best choice. Offering the at-home naloxone nasal spray, along with proper education, might be lifesaving if an overdose occurs. Providing proper education to the patient and caregivers on the importance of having the naloxone nasal spray at home and of calling emergency services is critical in case of an overdose situation.

CNS Stimulants

Jose A. Rey

15

I. OVERVIEW

Psychomotor stimulants and hallucinogens are two groups of drugs that act primarily to stimulate the central nervous system (CNS). The psychomotor stimulants cause excitement and euphoria, decrease feelings of fatigue, and increase motor activity. The hallucinogens produce profound changes in thought patterns and mood, with little effect on the brainstem and spinal cord. As a group, the CNS stimulants have diverse clinical uses and are also potential drugs of abuse, as are the CNS depressants (Chapter 9) and the opioids (Chapter 14). Figure 15.1 summarizes the CNS stimulants.

II. PSYCHOMOTOR STIMULANTS

A. Methylxanthines

The methylxanthines include *theophylline* [thee-OFF-i-lin], which is found in tea; *theobromine* [thee-oh-BROE-meen], which is found in cocoa; and *caffeine* [kaf-EEN]. *Caffeine*, the most widely consumed stimulant in the world, is found in highest concentration in certain coffee products (for example, espresso), but it is also present in tea, cola drinks, energy drinks, chocolate candy, and cocoa.

1. **Mechanism of action:** Several mechanisms have been proposed for the actions of methylxanthines, including translocation of extracellular calcium, increase in cyclic adenosine monophosphate and cyclic guanosine monophosphate caused by inhibition of phosphodiesterase, and blockade of adenosine receptors.

2. **Actions**

   a. **CNS:** The *caffeine* contained in one to two cups of coffee (100 to 200 mg) causes a decrease in fatigue and increased mental alertness as a result of stimulating the cortex and other areas of the brain. Consumption of 1.5 g of *caffeine* (12 to 15 cups of coffee) produces anxiety and tremors. The spinal cord is stimulated only by very high doses (2 to 5 g) of *caffeine*. Tolerance can rapidly develop to the stimulating properties of *caffeine*, and withdrawal consists of feelings of fatigue and sedation.

PSYCHOMOTOR STIMULANTS
Amphetamine ADDERALL, DYANAVEL, MYDAYIS
Armodafinil NUVIGIL
Atomoxetine STRATTERA
Caffeine CAFCIT, NO DOZ, VIVARIN
Cocaine GENERIC ONLY
Dexmethylphenidate FOCALIN
Dextroamphetamine DEXEDRINE, ZENZEDI
Lisdexamfetamine VYVANSE
Methamphetamine DESOXYN
Methylphenidate CONCERTA, COTEMPLA, DAYTRANA, RITALIN
Modafinil PROVIGIL
Nicotine NICODERM CQ, NICORETTE, NICOTROL
Theophylline ELIXOPHYLLIN, THEO-24, THEOCHRON
Varenicline CHANTIX

Figure 15.1
Summary of central nervous system (CNS) stimulants.

b. Cardiovascular system: A high dose of *caffeine* has positive inotropic and chronotropic effects on the heart. [Note: Increased contractility can be harmful to patients with angina pectoris. In others, an accelerated heart rate can trigger premature ventricular contractions.]

c. Diuretic action: *Caffeine* has a mild diuretic action that increases urinary output of sodium, chloride, and potassium.

d. Gastric mucosa: Because methylxanthines stimulate secretion of gastric acid, individuals with peptic ulcers should avoid foods and beverages containing methylxanthines.

3. **Therapeutic uses:** *Caffeine* and its derivatives relax the smooth muscles of the bronchioles. *Theophylline* has been largely replaced by other agents, such as β_2 agonists and corticosteroids, for the treatment of asthma (see Chapter 39). *Caffeine* is also used in combination with the analgesics *acetaminophen* and *aspirin* for the management of headaches in both prescription and over-the-counter products.

4. **Pharmacokinetics:** The methylxanthines are well absorbed orally. *Caffeine* distributes throughout the body, including the brain. These drugs cross the placenta to the fetus and are secreted into the breast milk. All methylxanthines are metabolized in the liver, generally by the CYP1A2 pathway, and the metabolites are excreted in the urine.

5. **Adverse effects:** Moderate doses of *caffeine* cause insomnia, anxiety, and agitation. A high dosage is required for toxicity, which is manifested by emesis and convulsions. The lethal dose is 10 g of *caffeine* (about 100 cups of coffee), which induces cardiac arrhythmias. Lethargy, irritability, and headache occur in users who routinely consume more than 600 mg of *caffeine* per day (roughly six cups of coffee per day) and then suddenly stop.

B. Nicotine

Nicotine [NIK-o-teen] is the active ingredient in tobacco. Although this drug is not currently used therapeutically (except in smoking cessation therapy), *nicotine* remains important because it is second only to *caffeine* as the most widely used CNS stimulant, and it is second only to alcohol as the most abused drug. In combination with the tars and carbon monoxide found in cigarette smoke, *nicotine* represents a serious risk factor for lung and cardiovascular disease, and other illnesses.

1. **Mechanism of action:** In low doses, *nicotine* causes ganglionic stimulation by depolarization. At high doses, *nicotine* causes ganglionic blockade. *Nicotine* receptors exist at a number of sites in the CNS, which participate in the stimulant attributes of the drug.

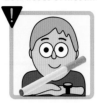

Low doses of *nicotine*

Arousal and relaxation

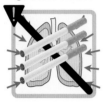

High doses of *nicotine*

Respiratory paralysis

Figure 15.2
Actions of *nicotine* on the CNS.

Potential for withdrawal

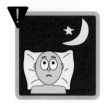

Insomnia

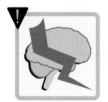

Headache

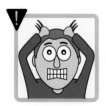

Irritability

Potential for addiction

Nicotine

Figure 15.3
Nicotine has potential for addiction and withdrawal.

2. Actions

a. CNS: *Nicotine* is highly lipid soluble and readily crosses the blood–brain barrier. Cigarette smoking or administration of low doses of *nicotine* produces some degree of euphoria and arousal, as well as relaxation. It improves attention, learning, problem solving, and reaction time. High doses of *nicotine* result in central respiratory paralysis and severe hypotension caused by medullary paralysis (Figure 15.2). *Nicotine* is also an appetite suppressant.

b. Peripheral effects: The peripheral effects of *nicotine* are complex. Stimulation of sympathetic ganglia as well as of the adrenal medulla increases blood pressure and heart rate. Thus, use of tobacco is particularly harmful in hypertensive patients. Many patients with peripheral vascular disease experience an exacerbation of symptoms with smoking. In addition, *nicotine*-induced vasoconstriction can decrease coronary blood flow, adversely affecting a patient with angina. Stimulation of parasympathetic ganglia also increases motor activity of the bowel. At higher doses, blood pressure falls and activity ceases in both the gastrointestinal (GI) tract and bladder musculature as a result of a *nicotine*-induced block of parasympathetic ganglia.

3. Pharmacokinetics: Because *nicotine* is highly lipid soluble, absorption readily occurs via the oral mucosa, lungs, GI mucosa, and skin. *Nicotine* crosses the placental membrane and is secreted in the breast milk. By inhaling tobacco smoke, the average smoker takes in 1 to 2 mg of *nicotine* per cigarette. The acute lethal dose is 60 mg. More than 90% of the *nicotine* inhaled in smoke is absorbed. Clearance of *nicotine* involves metabolism in the lung and the liver and urinary excretion. Tolerance to the toxic effects of *nicotine* develops rapidly, often within days.

4. Adverse effects: The CNS effects of *nicotine* include irritability and tremors. *Nicotine* may also cause intestinal cramps, diarrhea, and increased heart rate and blood pressure. In addition, cigarette smoking increases the rate of metabolism for a number of drugs.

5. Withdrawal syndrome: As with the other drugs in this class, *nicotine* is an addictive substance, and physical dependence develops rapidly and can be severe (Figure 15.3). Withdrawal is characterized by irritability, anxiety, restlessness, difficulty concentrating, headaches, and insomnia. Appetite is affected, and GI upset often occurs. The transdermal patch and chewing gum containing *nicotine* have been shown to reduce *nicotine* withdrawal symptoms and to help smokers stop smoking. For example, the blood concentration of *nicotine* obtained from *nicotine* chewing gum is typically about one-half the peak level observed with smoking (Figure 15.4). Other forms of *nicotine* replacement used for smoking cessation include the inhaler, nasal spray, and lozenges. *Bupropion*, an antidepressant (Chapter 10), can reduce the craving for cigarettes, assist in smoking cessation, and attenuate symptoms of withdrawal.

C. Varenicline

Varenicline [ver-EN-ih-kleen] is a partial agonist at neuronal nicotinic acetylcholine receptors in the CNS. Because *varenicline* is only a partial agonist at these receptors, it produces less euphoric effects than *nicotine* (*nicotine* is a full agonist). Thus, it is useful as an adjunct in the management of smoking cessation in patients with *nicotine* withdrawal symptoms. Patients taking *varenicline* should be monitored for suicidal thoughts, vivid nightmares, and mood changes.

D. Cocaine

Cocaine [koe-KANE] is a widely available and highly addictive drug. Because of its abuse potential, *cocaine* is classified as a Schedule II drug by the U.S. Drug Enforcement Agency. The primary mechanism of action underlying the effects of *cocaine* is blockade of reuptake of the monoamines (norepinephrine, serotonin, and dopamine) into the presynaptic terminals. This potentiates and prolongs the CNS and peripheral actions of these monoamines. In particular, the prolongation of dopaminergic effects in the brain's pleasure system (limbic system) produces the intense euphoria that *cocaine* initially causes. Chronic intake of *cocaine* depletes dopamine. This depletion triggers craving for *cocaine* (Figure 15.5). A full description of *cocaine* and its effects is provided in Chapter 45.

E. Amphetamine

Amphetamine [am-FET-a-meen] is a sympathetic amine that shows neurologic and clinical effects similar to those of *cocaine*. *Dextroamphetamine* [dex-troe-am-FET-a-meen] is the major member of this class of compounds. *Methamphetamine* [meth-am-FET-a-meen] (also known as "speed") is a derivative of *amphetamine* available for prescription use. *3,4-Methylenedioxymethamphetamine* (also known as MDMA, or ecstasy) is a synthetic derivative of *methamphetamine* with both stimulant and hallucinogenic properties (see Chapter 45).

1. **Mechanism of action:** As with *cocaine*, the effects of *amphetamine* on the CNS and peripheral nervous system are indirect. That is, both depend upon an elevation of the level of catecholamine neurotransmitters in synaptic spaces. *Amphetamine*, however, achieves this effect by releasing intracellular stores of catecholamines (Figure 15.6). Because *amphetamine* also inhibits monoamine oxidase (MAO) and is a weak reuptake transport inhibitor, high levels of catecholamines are present in synaptic spaces. Despite different mechanisms of action, the behavioral effects of *amphetamine* and its derivatives are similar to those of *cocaine*.

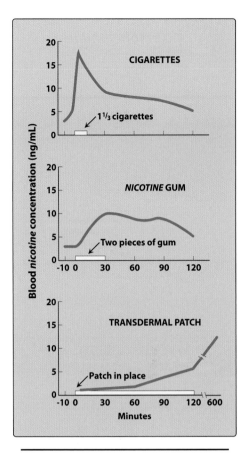

Figure 15.4
Blood concentrations of *nicotine* in individuals who smoked cigarettes, chewed *nicotine* gum, or received *nicotine* by transdermal patch.

Potential for addiction

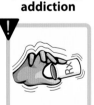

Cocaine amphetamine

Figure 15.5
Cocaine and *amphetamine* have potential for addiction.

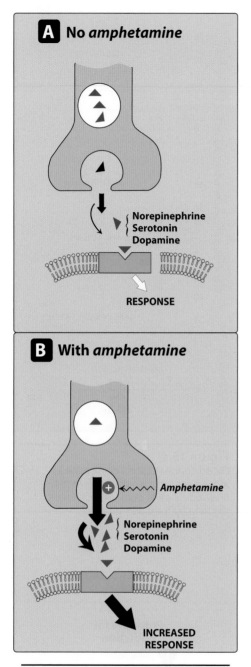

Figure 15.6
Mechanism of action of *amphetamine*.

2. Actions

a. CNS: The major behavioral effects of *amphetamine* result from a combination of its dopamine and norepinephrine release–enhancing properties. *Amphetamine* stimulates the entire cerebrospinal axis, cortex, brainstem, and medulla. This leads to increased alertness, decreased fatigue, depressed appetite, and insomnia. The CNS stimulant effects of *amphetamine* and its derivatives have led to their use in the treatment of hyperactivity in children, narcolepsy, and obesity. At high doses, psychosis and convulsions may occur.

b. Sympathetic nervous system: In addition to marked action on the CNS, *amphetamine* acts on the adrenergic system, indirectly stimulating the receptors through norepinephrine release.

3. Therapeutic uses: Factors that limit the therapeutic usefulness of *amphetamine* include psychological and physiologic dependence.

a. Attention deficit hyperactivity disorder (ADHD): Some children are hyperkinetic and lack the ability to be involved in any activity for longer than a few minutes. *Dextroamphetamine*, *methamphetamine*, the *mixed amphetamine salts*, and *methylphenidate* [meth-ill-FEN-ih-date] help improve attention span and alleviate many of the behavioral problems associated with this syndrome, in addition to reducing hyperkinesia. *Lisdexamfetamine* [lis-dex-am-FET-a-meen] is a prodrug that is converted to L-lysine and the active component *dextroamphetamine* through the hydrolytic actions of red blood cells. *Atomoxetine* [AT-oh-MOX-ih-teen] is a nonstimulant drug approved for ADHD in children and adults. Unlike *methylphenidate*, which blocks dopamine reuptake more than norepinephrine reuptake, *atomoxetine* is more selective for inhibition of norepinephrine reuptake. Therefore, it is not considered habit forming and is not a controlled substance.

b. Narcolepsy: Narcolepsy is a relatively rare sleep disorder that is characterized by uncontrollable bouts of sleepiness during the day. The sleepiness can be treated with drugs, such as the *mixed amphetamine salts* or *methylphenidate*. *Modafinil* [moe-DA-fi-nil] and its R-enantiomer derivative, *armodafinil* [ar-moe-DA-fi-nil], are considered first-line agents for the treatment of narcolepsy. *Modafinil* promotes wakefulness, but it produces less psychoactive and euphoric effects and fewer alterations in mood, perception, thinking, and feelings typical of other CNS stimulants. The mechanism of action remains unclear but may involve the adrenergic and dopaminergic systems. *Modafinil* is well distributed throughout the body and undergoes elimination via hepatic metabolism and excretion in the urine. Headaches, nausea, and nervousness are the primary adverse effects. *Modafinil* and *armodafinil* may have some potential for abuse and physical dependence, and both are classified as controlled substances.

c. **Appetite suppression:** *Phentermine* [FEN-ter-meen] and *diethylpropion* [dye-eth-ill-PROE-pee-on] are sympathomimetic amines that are related structurally to *amphetamine*. These agents are used for appetite suppressant effects in the management of obesity (see Chapter 37).

4. **Pharmacokinetics:** *Amphetamine* is completely absorbed from the GI tract, metabolized by the liver, and excreted in the urine. [Note: Administration of urinary alkalinizing agents such as *sodium bicarbonate* increase the nonionized species of the drug and enhance the reabsorption of *dextroamphetamine* from the renal tubules into the bloodstream.] *Amphetamine* abusers often administer the drug by IV injection and/or by smoking. The euphoria caused by *amphetamine* lasts 4 to 6 hours, or four- to eightfold longer than the effects of *cocaine*.

5. **Adverse effects:** The amphetamines may cause addiction, leading to dependence, tolerance, and drug-seeking behavior. In addition, they have the following undesirable effects:

a. **CNS effects:** Adverse effects of *amphetamine* usage include insomnia, irritability, weakness, dizziness, tremor, and hyperactive reflexes (Figure 15.7). *Amphetamine* can also cause confusion, delirium, panic states, and suicidal tendencies, especially in mentally ill patients. [Note: Benzodiazepines, such as *lorazepam*, are often used in the management of agitation and CNS stimulation secondary to *amphetamine* overdose.] Chronic *amphetamine* use produces a state of "*amphetamine* psychosis" that resembles the psychotic episodes associated with schizophrenia. Whereas long-term *amphetamine* use is associated with psychological and physical dependence, tolerance to its effects may occur within a few weeks. The anorectic effect of *amphetamine* is due to action in the lateral hypothalamic feeding center.

b. **Cardiovascular effects:** In addition to CNS effects, *amphetamine* may cause palpitations, cardiac arrhythmias, hypertension, anginal pain, and circulatory collapse. Headache, chills, and excessive sweating may also occur.

c. **Gastrointestinal effects:** *Amphetamine* acts on the GI system, causing anorexia, nausea, vomiting, abdominal cramps, and diarrhea.

d. **Contraindications:** Patients with hypertension, cardiovascular disease, hyperthyroidism, glaucoma, or a history of drug abuse or those taking MAO inhibitors should not be treated with *amphetamine*.

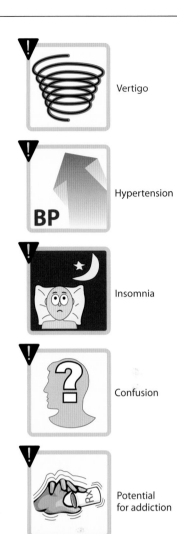

Vertigo

Hypertension

Insomnia

Confusion

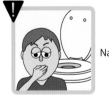

Potential for addiction

Nausea

Diarrhea

Figure 15.7
Adverse effects of amphetamines and *methylphenidate*.

F. Methylphenidate

Methylphenidate has CNS stimulant properties similar to those of *amphetamine* and is often used in the treatment of ADHD. *Methylphenidate* has abuse potential and is a Schedule II controlled substance. The pharmacologically active isomer, *dexmethylphenidate*, is also a Schedule II drug used for the treatment of ADHD.

1. **Mechanism of action:** Children with ADHD may produce weak dopamine signals, which suggest that once-interesting activities provide fewer rewards to these children. *Methylphenidate* is a dopamine and norepinephrine transport inhibitor and may act by increasing both dopamine and norepinephrine in the synaptic cleft.

2. **Therapeutic uses:** *Methylphenidate* is used in the treatment of ADHD. It is also effective in the treatment of narcolepsy. Unlike *methylphenidate*, *dexmethylphenidate* is not indicated in the treatment of narcolepsy.

3. **Pharmacokinetics:** Both *methylphenidate* and *dexmethylphenidate* are readily absorbed after oral administration. *Methylphenidate* is available in extended-release oral formulations and as a transdermal patch for once-daily application. The deesterified product, ritalinic acid, is excreted in urine.

4. **Adverse effects:** GI adverse effects are the most common and include abdominal pain and nausea. Other reactions include anorexia, insomnia, nervousness, and fever. In patients with epilepsy, *methylphenidate* may increase seizure frequency. The drug is contraindicated in patients with glaucoma. *Methylphenidate* can inhibit the metabolism of *warfarin*, *phenytoin*, *phenobarbital*, *primidone*, and the tricyclic antidepressants.

III. HALLUCINOGENS

A few drugs have, as their primary action, the ability to induce altered perceptual states reminiscent of dreams. Many of these altered states are accompanied by visions of bright, colorful changes in the environment and by a plasticity of constantly changing shapes and color. The individual under the influence of these drugs is incapable of normal decision-making because the drug interferes with rational thought. These compounds are known as hallucinogens, and *lysergic acid diethylamide (LSD)* and *tetrahydrocannabinol* (from marijuana) are examples of agents in this class. These agents are discussed in detail in Chapter 45.

Study Questions

Choose the ONE best answer.

15.1 A young male was brought to the emergency room by the police due to severe agitation. Psychiatric examination revealed that he had injected dextroamphetamine several times in the past few days. The last use was 10 hours prior. He was given an intramuscular drug that sedated him, and he fell asleep. Which drug was most likely used to counter this patient's symptoms of dextro-amphetamine withdrawal?

A. Trazodone
B. Lorazepam
C. Cocaine
D. Hydroxyzine

Correct answer = B. The anxiolytic properties of benzo-diazepines, such as lorazepam, make them the drugs of choice in treating the anxiety and agitation of amphetamine or cocaine abuse. Lorazepam also has hypnotic properties. Trazodone has hypnotic properties, but its anxiolytic properties are inferior to those of the benzodiazepines. Hydroxyzine, an antihistamine, is effective as a hypnotic, and it is sometimes used to deal with anxiety, especially if emesis is a problem but it is rarely used in the emergency situation when rapid anxiolytic and antiseizure treatment is warranted.

15.2 A 10-year-old boy is sent to a pediatric neurologist for an evaluation due to poor performance and inability to pay attention in school. He has also been fighting with other children. He is given a diagnosis of ADHD with impulsivity and irritability. Which is most appropriate for management of the ADHD?

A. Clonidine
B. Mirtazapine
C. Dextroamphetamine
D. Haloperidol

Correct answer = C. Dextroamphetamine is the only stimulant medication in the list that is approved for ADHD. Symptoms like fighting may improve with haloperidol, and hyperactivity may improve with clonidine, but these agents would not improve the patient's academic performance and the underlying problems.

15.3 A 10-year-old boy with ADHD has symptoms that are controlled with an oral psychostimulant. However, he and his family wish to avoid having to give a second dose of medication at school. They prefer an alternative treatment that can be administered in the morning and last the entire day. Which treatment option is best?

A. Mixed amphetamine salts in immediate-release oral tablet formulation
B. Methylphenidate in a transdermal delivery system
C. Nicotine in a chewing gum formulation for buccal absorption
D. Methylphenidate in immediate-release pills

Correct answer = B. Methylphenidate is also a psychostimulant, and the transdermal (patch) formulation is designed for once-daily use to avoid midday dosing. Immediate-release formulations require dosing at least twice daily.

15.4 Which of the following agents for ADHD is a controlled substance (Schedule II)?

A. Clonidine
B. Atomoxetine
C. Lisdexamfetamine
D. Desipramine

Correct answer = C. Lisdexamfetamine is the only controlled substance on the list and is schedule II. The other agents may assist in the management of ADHD but are not controlled substances.

15.5 Amphetamines may be used in patients with which of the following conditions?

A. Cardiovascular disease
B. Hypertension
C. Hyperthyroidism
D. Obesity

Correct answer = D. The use of amphetamines in the management of obesity should be closely monitored. Amphetamine analogs such as phentermine are approved for obesity. The other conditions are contraindications when considering the use of amphetamines.

15.6 Which of the following agents is considered a first-line treatment for narcolepsy?

A. Galantamine
B. Atomoxetine
C. Temazepam
D. Modafinil

Correct answer = D. Modafinil is the only drug listed that is approved for narcolepsy. Temazepam is indicated for insomnia, galantamine for Alzheimer's disease, and atomoxetine for ADHD.

15.7 Which of the following is a common adverse effect of amphetamines?

A. Bradycardia
B. Somnolence
C. Constipation
D. Hypertension

Correct answer = D. Hypertension is a possible adverse effect that warrants caution, especially in individuals with risk factors for increased blood pressure. Amphetamines cause tachycardia (not bradycardia), insomnia (not somnolence), and diarrhea (not constipation).

15.8 Which of the following CNS stimulants occurs naturally and can be found in certain candies?

A. Amphetamine
B. Modafinil
C. Caffeine
D. Atomoxetine

Correct answer = C. Caffeine is a naturally occurring substance found in cocoa, chocolate, and many forms of tea. Overuse of cola beverages and other caffeine-containing products may cause adverse effects, including anxiety and insomnia, and even increase the risk for seizures.

15.9 A 35-year-old man is interested in quitting smoking. In previous quit attempts, he has tried nicotine gum, the nicotine patch, and the "cold turkey" method. He has been unsuccessful in each of these attempts and resumed smoking within 4 to 6 weeks. Which may be useful to assist in his attempt to quit smoking?

A. Varenicline
B. Dextroamphetamine
C. Lorazepam
D. Methylphenidate

Correct answer = A. Varenicline is approved as an adjunctive treatment option for the management of nicotine dependence. It is believed to attenuate the withdrawal symptoms of smoking cessation, though monitoring is needed for changes in psychiatric status, including suicidal ideation. The use of dextroamphetamine, lorazepam, and methylphenidate bring the risk of addiction to another substance with abuse potential.

15.10 Which of the following agents carries the lowest risk for addiction?

A. Armodafinil
B. Lisdexamfetamine
C. Dexmethylphenidate
D. Varenicline

Correct answer = D. Varenicline is the only agent listed that is not a controlled substance. All of the other agents are considered to have a risk for addiction and/or dependence.

Antihypertensives

Benjamin Gross

16

I. OVERVIEW

Blood pressure is elevated when systolic blood pressure exceeds 120 mm Hg and diastolic blood pressure remains below 80 mm Hg. Hypertension occurs when systolic blood pressure exceeds 130 mm Hg or diastolic blood pressure exceeds 80 mm Hg on at least two occasions. Hypertension results from increased peripheral vascular arteriolar smooth muscle tone, which leads to increased arteriolar resistance and reduced capacitance of the venous system. In most cases, the cause of the increased vascular tone is unknown. Elevated blood pressure is a common disorder, affecting approximately 30% of adults in the United States. Although many patients have no symptoms, chronic hypertension can lead to heart disease and stroke, the top two causes of death in the world. Hypertension is also an important risk factor in the development of chronic kidney disease and heart failure. The incidence of morbidity and mortality significantly decreases when hypertension is diagnosed early and is properly treated. The drugs used in the treatment of hypertension are shown in Figure 16.1. In recognition of the progressive

DIURETICS
Amiloride MIDAMOR
Bumetanide BUMEX
Chlorthalidone GENERIC ONLY
Eplerenone INSPRA
Ethacrynic acid EDECRIN
Furosemide LASIX
Hydrochlorothiazide MICROZIDE
Indapamide GENERIC ONLY
Metolazone GENERIC ONLY
Spironolactone ALDACTONE
Triamterene DYRENIUM
Torsemide DEMADEX

β-BLOCKERS
Acebutolol GENERIC ONLY
Atenolol TENORMIN
Betaxolol GENERIC ONLY
Bisoprolol GENERIC ONLY
Carvedilol COREG, COREG CR
Esmolol BREVIBLOC
Labetalol TRANDATE
Metoprolol LOPRESSOR, TOPROL-XL
Nadolol CORGARD
Nebivolol BYSTOLIC
Pindolol GENERIC ONLY
Propranolol INDERAL LA, INNOPRAN XL

ANGIOTENSIN II RECEPTOR BLOCKERS
Azilsartan EDARBI
Candesartan ATACAND
Eprosartan GENERIC ONLY
Irbesartan AVAPRO
Losartan COZAAR
Olmesartan BENICAR
Telmisartan MICARDIS
Valsartan DIOVAN

RENIN INHIBITORS
Aliskiren TEKTURNA

ACE INHIBITORS
Benazepril LOTENSIN
Captopril GENERIC ONLY
Enalapril VASOTEC
Fosinopril GENERIC ONLY
Lisinopril PRINIVIL, ZESTRIL
Moexipril GENERIC ONLY
Quinapril ACCUPRIL
Perindopril GENERIC ONLY
Ramipril ALTACE
Trandolapril GENERIC ONLY

Figure 16.1
Summary of antihypertensive drugs. ACE = angiotensin converting enzyme.
(Figure continues on next page)

CALCIUM CHANNEL BLOCKERS

Amlodipine NORVASC
Clevidipine CLEVIPREX
Diltiazem CARDIZEM, CARTIA, TIAZAC
Felodipine GENERIC ONLY
Isradipine GENERIC ONLY
Nicardipine CARDENE
Nifedipine ADALAT, PROCARDIA
Nisoldipine SULAR
Verapamil CALAN, VERELAN

α-BLOCKERS

Doxazosin CARDURA
Prazosin MINIPRESS
Terazosin GENERIC ONLY

OTHERS

Clonidine CATAPRES, DURACLON
Fenoldopam CORLOPAM
Hydralazine GENERIC ONLY
Methyldopa GENERIC ONLY
Minoxidil GENERIC ONLY
Nitroprusside NIPRIDE, NITROPRESS

Figure 16.1 (continued)
Summary of antihypertensive drugs.

	Systolic mm Hg		Diastolic mm Hg
Normal	<120	and	<80
Elevated	120–129	or	<80
Stage 1 hypertension	130–139	or	80–89
Stage 2 hypertension	≥140	or	≥90

Figure 16.2
Classification of blood pressure.

nature of hypertension, hypertension is classified into four categories (Figure 16.2). The majority of current guidelines recommend treatment decisions based on goals of antihypertensive therapy, rather than the category of hypertension.

II. ETIOLOGY OF HYPERTENSION

Although hypertension may occur secondary to other disease processes, more than 90% of patients have essential hypertension (hypertension with no identifiable cause). A family history of hypertension increases the likelihood that an individual will develop hypertension. The prevalence of hypertension increases with age but decreases with education and income level. Non-Hispanic blacks have a higher incidence of hypertension than do both non-Hispanic whites and Hispanic whites. Persons with diabetes, obesity, or disability status are all more likely to have hypertension than those without these conditions. In addition, environmental factors, such as a stressful lifestyle, high dietary intake of sodium, and smoking, may further predispose an individual to hypertension.

III. MECHANISMS FOR CONTROLLING BLOOD PRESSURE

Arterial blood pressure is regulated within a narrow range to provide adequate perfusion of the tissues without causing damage to the vascular system, particularly the arterial intima (endothelium). Arterial blood pressure is directly proportional to cardiac output and peripheral vascular resistance (Figure 16.3). Cardiac output and peripheral resistance, in turn, are controlled mainly by two overlapping mechanisms: the baroreflexes and the renin–angiotensin–aldosterone system (Figure 16.4). Most antihypertensive drugs lower blood pressure by reducing cardiac output and/or decreasing peripheral resistance.

A. Baroreceptors and the sympathetic nervous system

Baroreflexes act by changing the activity of the sympathetic and parasympathetic nervous system. Therefore, they are responsible for the rapid, moment-to-moment regulation of blood pressure. A fall in blood pressure causes pressure-sensitive neurons (baroreceptors in the aortic arch and carotid sinuses) to send fewer impulses to cardiovascular centers in the spinal cord. This prompts a reflex response of increased sympathetic and decreased parasympathetic output to the heart and vasculature, resulting in vasoconstriction and increased cardiac output. These changes result in a compensatory rise in blood pressure (Figure 16.4).

B. Renin–angiotensin–aldosterone system

The kidney provides long-term control of blood pressure by altering the blood volume. Baroreceptors in the kidney respond to reduced arterial pressure (and to sympathetic stimulation of β_1-adrenoceptors) by releasing the enzyme renin (Figure 16.4). Low-sodium intake and greater sodium loss also increase renin release. Renin converts angiotensinogen to angiotensin I, which is converted in turn to angiotensin II, in the presence of angiotensin converting enzyme (ACE). Angiotensin II is a potent circulating vasoconstrictor, constricting both arterioles and veins, resulting in an increase in blood pressure. Angiotensin II exerts a preferential vasoconstrictor action on the efferent arterioles of the renal glomerulus, increasing glomerular filtration. Furthermore, angiotensin II stimulates aldosterone secretion, leading to increased renal sodium reabsorption and increased blood volume, which contribute to a further increase in blood pressure. These effects of angiotensin II are mediated by stimulation of angiotensin II type 1 (AT$_1$) receptors.

IV. TREATMENT STRATEGIES

The goal of antihypertensive therapy is to reduce cardiovascular and renal morbidity and mortality. For most patients, the blood pressure goal when treating hypertension is a systolic blood pressure of less than 130 mm Hg and a diastolic blood pressure of less than 80 mm Hg. Current recommendations are to initiate therapy with a thiazide diuretic, ACE inhibitor, angiotensin receptor blocker (ARB), or calcium channel blocker. However, initial drug therapy choice may vary depending on the guideline

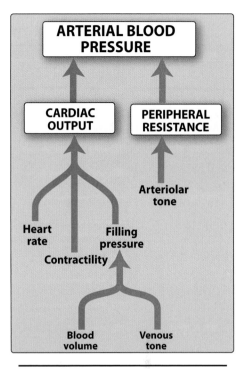

Figure 16.3
Major factors influencing blood pressure.

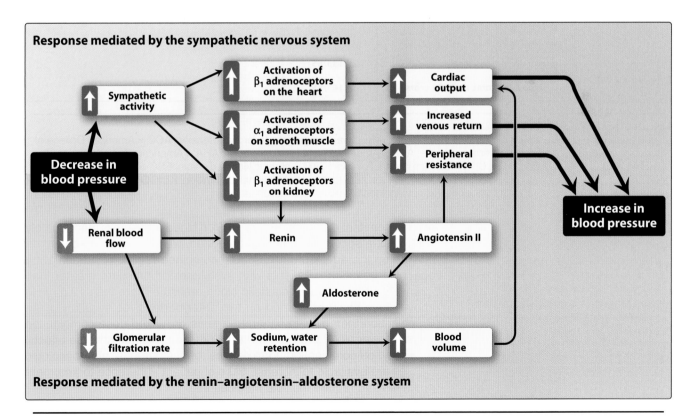

Figure 16.4
Response of the autonomic nervous system and the renin–angiotensin–aldosterone system to a decrease in blood pressure.

GUIDELINES	POPULATION DEMOGRAPHICS	GOAL BLOOD PRESSURE	INITIAL DRUG THERAPY OPTIONS
ACC/AHA 2017	General nonelderly	<130/80	Nonblack: thiazide diuretic, ACE inhibitor, ARB, CCB Black: thiazide diuretic or CCB
	Elderly >65 years old	<130/80	Use clinical judgment on blood pressure goal and drug choice if serious comorbidities
ADA 2017	Diabetes	<140/90	ACE inhibitor or ARB
KDIGO 2016	CKD with no proteinuria	<140/90	ACE inhibitor or ARB
	CKD and proteinuria	≤130/80	ACE inhibitor or ARB
ESH/ESC 2013	General nonelderly	<140/90	Thiazide diuretic, β-blocker, ACE inhibitor, or ARB
	General elderly <80 years old General elderly >80 years old	<150/90	Thiazide diuretic, β-blocker, ACE inhibitor, or ARB
	Diabetes	<140/85	ACE inhibitor or ARB
	CKD no proteinuria	<140/90	ACE inhibitor or ARB
	CKD plus proteinuria	<130/90	ACE inhibitor or ARB
JNC 8 2013	≥60 years old	<150/90	Nonblack: thiazide diuretic, ACE inhibitor, ARB, CCB Black: thiazide diuretic or CCB
	<60 years old	<140/90	
	Diabetes	<140/90	
	CKD	<140/90	ACE inhibitor or ARB
NICE 2011	>80 years old	<150/90	≥55 years old or black: CCB
	<80 years old	<140/90	<55 years old: ACE inhibitor or ARB
	White coat syndrome and <80 years old	<135/85	
	White coat syndrome and >80 years old	<145/85	

Figure 16.5
Comparison of blood pressure goals and initial drug therapy with various guidelines for hypertension. ACC = American College of Cardiology; ACE = angiotensin converting enzyme; ADA = American Diabetes Association; AHA = American Heart Association; ARB = angiotensin receptor blocker; CCB = calcium channel blocker; CKD = chronic kidney disease; ESC = European Society of Cardiology; ESH = European Society of Hypertension; JNC 8 = Eighth Joint National Committee; KDIGO = Kidney Disease: Improving Global Outcomes; NICE = National Institute for Health and Care Excellence.

and concomitant diseases (Figure 16.5). If blood pressure is inadequately controlled, a second drug should be added, with the selection based on minimizing the adverse effects of the combined regimen and achieving goal blood pressure. Patients with systolic blood pressure greater than 20 mm Hg above goal or diastolic blood pressure more than 10 mm Hg above goal should be started on two antihypertensives simultaneously. Combination therapy with separate agents or a fixed-dose combination pill may lower blood pressure more quickly with minimal adverse effects. A variety of combination formulations of the various pharmacologic classes are available to increase ease of patient adherence to treatment regimens that require multiple medications.

A. Individualized care

Hypertension may coexist with other conditions that can be aggravated by some of the antihypertensive drugs or that may benefit from

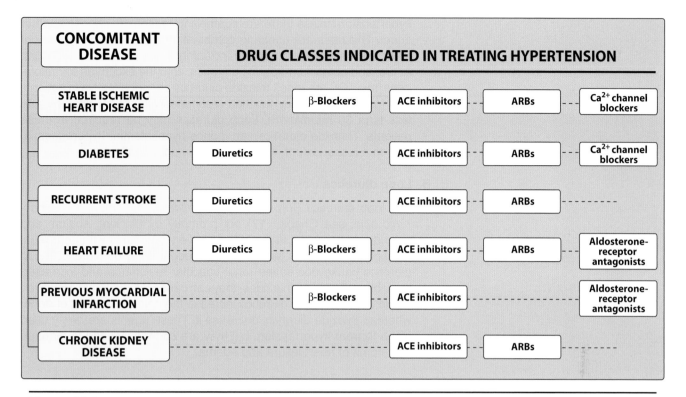

Figure 16.6
Treatment of hypertension in patients with concomitant diseases. [Note: Angiotensin receptor blockers (ARBs) are an alternative to angiotensin converting enzyme (ACE) inhibitors.]

the use of some antihypertensive drugs independent of blood pressure control. In such cases, it is important to match antihypertensive drugs to the particular patient. Figure 16.6 shows preferred therapies in hypertensive patients with concomitant diseases. In addition to the choice of therapy, blood pressure goals may also be individualized based on concurrent disease states and age (Figure 16.5).

V. DIURETICS

For all classes of diuretics, the initial mechanism of action is based upon decreasing blood volume, which ultimately leads to decreased blood pressure. Routine serum electrolyte monitoring should be done for all patients receiving diuretics. A complete discussion of the actions, therapeutic uses, pharmacokinetics, and adverse effects of diuretics can be found in Chapter 17.

A. Thiazide diuretics

Thiazide diuretics, such as *hydrochlorothiazide* [hye-droe-klor-oh-THYE-a-zide] and *chlorthalidone* [klor-THAL-ih-done], lower blood pressure initially by increasing sodium and water excretion. This causes a decrease in extracellular volume, resulting in a decrease in cardiac output and renal blood flow (Figure 16.7). With long-term treatment, plasma volume approaches a normal value, but a hypotensive effect persists that is related to a decrease in peripheral resistance. Thiazide diuretics can be used as initial drug therapy for

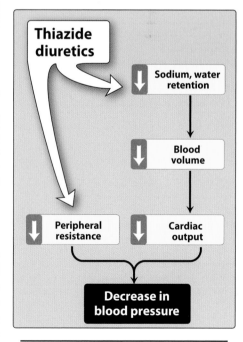

Figure 16.7
Actions of thiazide diuretics.

hypertension unless there are compelling reasons to choose another agent. Thiazides are useful in combination therapy with a variety of other antihypertensive agents, including β-blockers, ACE inhibitors, ARBs, and potassium-sparing diuretics. With the exception of *metolazone* [me-TOL-ah-zone], thiazide diuretics are not effective in patients with inadequate kidney function (estimated glomerular filtration rate less than 30 mL/min/m^2). Loop diuretics may be required in these patients. Thiazide diuretics can induce hypokalemia, hyperuricemia, and, to a lesser extent, hyperglycemia in some patients.

B. Loop diuretics

The loop diuretics (*furosemide*, *torsemide*, *bumetanide*, and *ethacrynic acid*; see Chapter 17) act promptly by blocking sodium and chloride reabsorption in the kidneys, even in patients with poor renal function or those who have not responded to thiazide diuretics. Loop diuretics cause decreased renal vascular resistance and increased renal blood flow. Like thiazides, they can cause hypokalemia. However, unlike thiazides, loop diuretics increase the calcium content of urine, whereas thiazide diuretics decrease it. These agents are rarely used alone to treat hypertension, but they are commonly used to manage symptoms of heart failure and edema.

C. Potassium-sparing diuretics

Amiloride [a-MIL-oh-ride] and *triamterene* [tri-AM-ter-een] are inhibitors of epithelial sodium transport at the late distal and collecting ducts, and *spironolactone* [speer-on-oh-LAK-tone] and *eplerenone* [eh-PLEH-reh-none] are aldosterone receptor antagonists. All of these agents reduce potassium loss in the urine. Aldosterone antagonists have the additional benefit of diminishing the cardiac remodeling that occurs in heart failure (see Chapter 18). Potassium-sparing diuretics are sometimes used in combination with loop diuretics and thiazides to reduce the amount of potassium loss induced by these diuretics.

VI. β-ADRENOCEPTOR–BLOCKING AGENTS

β-Blockers are a treatment option for hypertensive patients with concomitant heart disease or heart failure (Figure 16.6).

A. Actions

The β-blockers reduce blood pressure primarily by decreasing cardiac output (Figure 16.8). They may also decrease sympathetic outflow from the central nervous system (CNS) and inhibit the release of renin from the kidneys, thus decreasing the formation of angiotensin II and the secretion of aldosterone. The prototype β-blocker is *propranolol* [proe-PRAN-oh-lol], which acts at both β$_1$ and β$_2$ receptors. Selective blockers of β$_1$ receptors, such as *metoprolol* [met-OH-pro-lol] and *atenolol* [ah-TEN-oh-lol], are among the most commonly prescribed β-blockers. *Nebivolol* [ne-BIV-oh-lole] is a selective blocker of β$_1$ receptors, which also increases the production of nitric oxide, leading to vasodilation. The selective β-blockers may be administered cautiously to hypertensive patients who also have asthma. The nonselective β-blockers are contraindicated in patients with asthma due to their blockade of β$_2$-mediated bronchodilation. (See Chapter 7 for

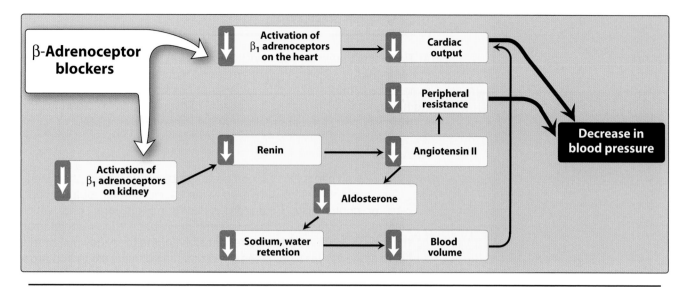

Figure 16.8
Actions of β-adrenoceptor–blocking agents.

an in-depth discussion of β-blockers.) β-Blockers should be used cautiously in the treatment of patients with acute heart failure or peripheral vascular disease.

B. Therapeutic uses

The primary therapeutic benefits of β-blockers are seen in hypertensive patients with concomitant heart disease, such as supraventricular tachyarrhythmia (for example, atrial fibrillation), previous myocardial infarction, stable ischemic heart disease, and chronic heart failure. Conditions that discourage the use of β-blockers include reversible bronchospastic disease such as asthma, second- and third-degree heart block, and severe peripheral vascular disease.

C. Pharmacokinetics

The β-blockers are orally active for the treatment of hypertension. *Propranolol* undergoes extensive and highly variable first-pass metabolism. Oral β-blockers may take several weeks to develop their full effects. *Esmolol, metoprolol,* and *propranolol* are available in intravenous formulations.

D. Adverse effects

1. **Common effects:** Figure 16.9 describes some of the adverse effects of β-blockers. The β-blockers may decrease libido and cause erectile dysfunction, which can severely reduce patient compliance.

2. **Alterations in serum lipid patterns:** Noncardioselective β-blockers may disturb lipid metabolism, decreasing high-density lipoprotein cholesterol and increasing triglycerides.

3. **Drug withdrawal:** Abrupt withdrawal may induce severe hypertension, angina, myocardial infarction, and even sudden death in patients with ischemic heart disease. Therefore, these drugs must be tapered over a few weeks in patients with hypertension and ischemic heart disease.

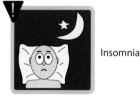

Hypotension

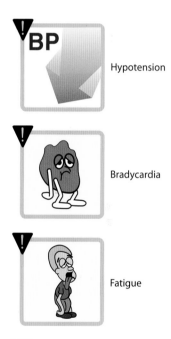

Bradycardia

Fatigue

Insomnia

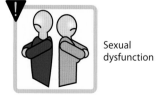

Sexual dysfunction

Figure 16.9
Some adverse effects of β-blockers.

VII. ACE INHIBITORS

ACE inhibitors such as *captopril* [KAP-toe-pril], *enalapril* [e-NAL-ah-pril], and *lisinopril* [lye-SIN-oh-pril] are recommended as first-line treatment of hypertension in patients with a variety of compelling indications, including high coronary disease risk or history of diabetes, stroke, heart failure, myocardial infarction, or chronic kidney disease (Figure 16.6).

A. Actions

The ACE inhibitors lower blood pressure by reducing peripheral vascular resistance without reflexively increasing cardiac output, heart rate, or contractility. These drugs block the enzyme ACE, which cleaves angiotensin I to form the potent vasoconstrictor angiotensin II (Figure 16.10). ACE is also responsible for the breakdown of bradykinin, a peptide that increases the production of nitric oxide and prostacyclin by the blood vessels. Both nitric oxide and prostacyclin are potent vasodilators. Vasodilation of both arterioles and veins occurs as a result of decreased vasoconstriction (from diminished levels of angiotensin II) and enhanced vasodilation (from increased bradykinin). By reducing circulating angiotensin II levels, ACE inhibitors also decrease the secretion of aldosterone, resulting in decreased sodium and water retention. ACE inhibitors reduce both cardiac preload and afterload, thereby decreasing workload on the heart.

B. Therapeutic uses

ACE inhibitors slow the progression of diabetic nephropathy and decrease albuminuria and, thus, have a compelling indication for use in patients with diabetic nephropathy. Beneficial effects on renal function may result from decreasing intraglomerular pressures, due to efferent arteriolar vasodilation. ACE inhibitors are a standard in the care of a patient following a myocardial infarction and first-line agents in the treatment of patients with systolic dysfunction. Chronic treatment with ACE inhibitors achieves sustained blood pressure reduction, regression of left ventricular hypertrophy, and prevention of ventricular remodeling after a myocardial infarction. ACE inhibitors are first-line drugs for treating heart failure, hypertensive patients with chronic kidney disease, and patients at increased risk of coronary

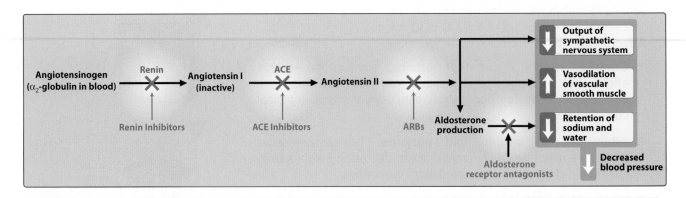

Figure 16.10
Effects of various drug classes on the renin–angiotensin–aldosterone system. *Blue* = drug target enzymes; *red* = drug class.

artery disease. All of the ACE inhibitors are equally effective in the treatment of hypertension at equivalent doses.

C. Pharmacokinetics

All of the ACE inhibitors are orally bioavailable as a drug or prodrug. All but *captopril* and *lisinopril* undergo hepatic conversion to active metabolites, so these agents may be preferred in patients with severe hepatic impairment. *Fosinopril* [foe-SIN-oh-pril] is the only ACE inhibitor that is not eliminated primarily by the kidneys. Therefore, it does not require dose adjustment in patients with renal impairment. *Enalaprilat* [en-AL-a-pril-AT] is the only drug in this class available intravenously.

D. Adverse effects

Figure 16.11 describes some of the common adverse effects of ACE inhibitors. The dry cough, which occurs in up to 10% of patients, is thought to be due to increased levels of bradykinin and substance P in the pulmonary tree, and it occurs more frequently in women. The cough resolves within a few days of discontinuation. Angioedema is a rare but potentially life-threatening reaction that may also be due to increased levels of bradykinin. Potassium levels must be monitored while on ACE inhibitors, and potassium supplements and potassium-sparing diuretics should be used with caution due to the risk of hyperkalemia. Serum creatinine levels should also be monitored, particularly in patients with underlying renal disease. However, an increase in serum creatinine of up to 30% above baseline is acceptable and by itself does not warrant discontinuation of treatment. ACE inhibitors can induce fetal malformations and should not be used by pregnant women.

VIII. ANGIOTENSIN II RECEPTOR BLOCKERS

The ARBs, such as *losartan* [LOW-sar-tan] and *irbesartan* [ir-be-SAR-tan], block the AT_1 receptors, decreasing the activation of AT_1 receptors by angiotensin II. Their pharmacologic effects are similar to those of ACE inhibitors in that they produce arteriolar and venous dilation and block aldosterone secretion, thus lowering blood pressure and decreasing salt and water retention (Figure 16.10). ARBs do not increase bradykinin levels. They may be used as first-line agents for the treatment of hypertension, especially in patients with a compelling indication of diabetes, heart failure, or chronic kidney disease (Figure 16.6). Adverse effects are similar to those of ACE inhibitors, although the risks of cough and angioedema are significantly decreased. ARBs should not be combined with an ACE inhibitor for the treatment of hypertension due to similar mechanisms and adverse effects. These agents are also teratogenic and should not be used by pregnant women. [Note: The ARBs are discussed more fully in Chapter 18.]

IX. RENIN INHIBITOR

A selective renin inhibitor, *aliskiren* [a-LIS-ke-rin], is available for the treatment of hypertension. *Aliskiren* directly inhibits renin and, thus, acts earlier in the renin–angiotensin–aldosterone system than ACE inhibitors

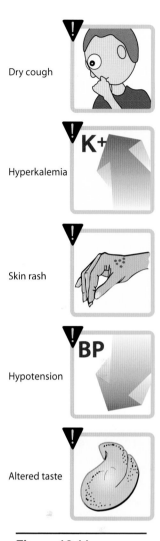

Dry cough

Hyperkalemia

Skin rash

Hypotension

Altered taste

Figure 16.11
Some common adverse effects of the ACE inhibitors.

or ARBs (Figure 16.10). *Aliskiren* should not be combined with an ACE inhibitor or ARB in the treatment of hypertension. *Aliskiren* can cause diarrhea, especially at higher doses. It also causes cough and angioedema but less often than ACE inhibitors. As with ACE inhibitors and ARBs, *aliskiren* is contraindicated during pregnancy. *Aliskiren* is metabolized by CYP3A4 and is subject to many drug interactions.

X. CALCIUM CHANNEL BLOCKERS

Calcium channel blockers are a recommended first-line treatment option in black patients. They may also be useful in hypertensive patients with diabetes or stable ischemic heart disease. High doses of short-acting calcium channel blockers should be avoided because of increased risk of myocardial infarction due to excessive vasodilation and marked reflex cardiac stimulation.

A. Classes of calcium channel blockers

The calcium channel blockers are divided into three chemical classes, each with different pharmacokinetic properties and clinical indications (Figure 16.12).

1. **Diphenylalkylamines:** *Verapamil* [ver-AP-a-mil] is the only member of this class that is available in the United States. *Verapamil* has significant effects on both cardiac and vascular smooth muscle cells. It is also used to treat angina and supraventricular tachyarrhythmias and to prevent migraine and cluster headaches.

2. **Benzothiazepines:** *Diltiazem* [dil-TYE-a-zem] is the only member of this class that is currently approved in the United States. Like *verapamil*, *diltiazem* affects both cardiac and vascular smooth muscle cells, but it has a less pronounced negative inotropic effect on the heart compared to that of *verapamil*. *Diltiazem* has a favorable side effect profile.

3. **Dihydropyridines:** This class of calcium channel blockers includes *nifedipine* [nye-FED-i-peen] (the prototype), *amlodipine* [am-LOE-di-peen], *felodipine* [fe-LOE-di-peen], *isradipine* [is-RAD-i-peen], *nicardipine* [nye-KAR-di-peen], and *nisoldipine* [nye-ZOL-di-peen]. These agents differ in pharmacokinetics, approved uses, and drug interactions. All dihydropyridines have a much greater affinity for vascular calcium channels than for calcium channels in the heart. They are, therefore, particularly beneficial in treating hypertension. The dihydropyridines have the advantage in that they show little interaction with other cardiovascular drugs, such as *digoxin* or *warfarin*, which are often used concomitantly with calcium channel blockers.

B. Actions

The intracellular concentration of calcium plays an important role in maintaining the tone of smooth muscle and in the contraction of the myocardium. Calcium channel antagonists block the inward movement of calcium by binding to L-type calcium channels in the heart and in smooth muscle of the coronary and peripheral arteriolar vasculature. This causes vascular smooth muscle to relax, dilating mainly arterioles. Calcium channel blockers do not dilate veins.

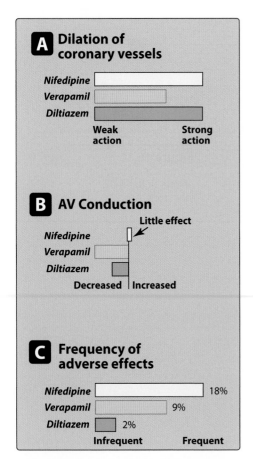

Figure 16.12
Actions of calcium channel blockers.
AV = atrioventricular.

C. Therapeutic uses

In the management of hypertension, CCBs may be used as an initial therapy or as add-on therapy. They are useful in the treatment of hypertensive patients who also have asthma, diabetes, and/or peripheral vascular disease, because unlike β-blockers, they do not have the potential to adversely affect these conditions. All CCBs are useful in the treatment of angina. In addition, *diltiazem* and *verapamil* are used in the treatment of atrial fibrillation.

D. Pharmacokinetics

Most of these agents have short half-lives (3 to 8 hours) following an oral dose. Sustained-release preparations are available and permit once-daily dosing. *Amlodipine* has a very long half-life and does not require a sustained-release formulation.

E. Adverse effects

First-degree atrioventricular block and constipation are common dose-dependent side effects of *verapamil*. *Verapamil* and *diltiazem* should be avoided in patients with heart failure or with atrioventricular block due to their negative inotropic (force of cardiac muscle contraction) and dromotropic (velocity of conduction) effects. Dizziness, headache, and a feeling of fatigue caused by a decrease in blood pressure are more frequent with dihydropyridines (Figure 16.13). Peripheral edema is another commonly reported side effect of this class. *Nifedipine* and other dihydropyridines may cause gingival hyperplasia.

XI. α-ADRENOCEPTOR–BLOCKING AGENTS

α-Adrenergic blockers used in the treatment of hypertension include *prazosin* [PRA-zoe-sin], *doxazosin* [dox-AH-zoe-sin], and *terazosin* [ter-AH-zoe-sin]. These agents produce a competitive block of α_1-adrenoceptors. They decrease peripheral vascular resistance and lower arterial blood pressure by causing relaxation of both arterial and venous smooth muscle. These drugs cause only minimal changes in cardiac output, renal blood flow, and glomerular filtration rate. Therefore, long-term tachycardia does not occur, but salt and water retention does. Reflex tachycardia and postural hypotension often occur at the onset of treatment and with dose increases, requiring slow titration of the drug in divided doses. Due to weaker outcome data and their side effect profile, α-blockers are no longer recommended as initial treatment for hypertension but may be used for refractory cases. Other α_1-blockers with greater selectivity for the prostate are used in the treatment of benign prostatic hyperplasia (see Chapter 41).

XII. α-/β-ADRENOCEPTOR–BLOCKING AGENTS

Labetalol [la-BAY-ta-lol] and *carvedilol* [kar-VE-di-lol] block α_1, β_1, and β_2 receptors. *Carvedilol* is indicated in the treatment of heart failure and hypertension. It has been shown to reduce morbidity and mortality

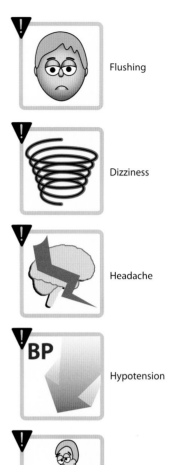

Flushing

Dizziness

Headache

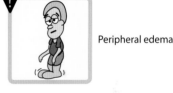

Hypotension

Peripheral edema

Figure 16.13
Some common adverse effects of the calcium channel blockers.

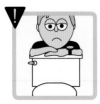

Constipation

Dry mouth

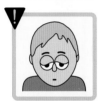

Drowsiness

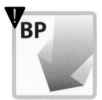

Hypotension

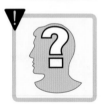

Confusion

Figure 16.14
Some adverse effects of *clonidine.*

associated with heart failure. *Labetalol* is used in the management of gestational hypertension and hypertensive emergencies.

XIII. CENTRALLY ACTING ADRENERGIC DRUGS

A. Clonidine

Clonidine [KLON-i-deen] acts centrally as an α_2 agonist to produce inhibition of sympathetic vasomotor centers, decreasing sympathetic outflow to the periphery. This leads to reduced total peripheral resistance and decreased blood pressure. *Clonidine* is used primarily for the treatment of hypertension that has not responded adequately to treatment with two or more drugs. *Clonidine* does not decrease renal blood flow or glomerular filtration and, therefore, is useful in the treatment of hypertension complicated by renal disease. *Clonidine* is well absorbed after oral administration and is excreted by the kidney. It is also available in a transdermal patch. Adverse effects include sedation, dry mouth, and constipation (Figure 16.14). Rebound hypertension occurs following abrupt withdrawal of *clonidine.* The drug should, therefore, be withdrawn slowly if discontinuation is required.

B. Methyldopa

Methyldopa [meth-ill-DOE-pa] is an α_2 agonist that is converted to methylnorepinephrine centrally to diminish adrenergic outflow from the CNS. The most common side effects of *methyldopa* are sedation and drowsiness. Its use is limited due to adverse effects and the need for multiple daily doses. It is mainly used for management of hypertension in pregnancy, where it has a record of safety.

XIV. VASODILATORS

The direct-acting smooth muscle relaxants, such as *hydralazine* [hye-DRAL-a-zeen] and *minoxidil* [min-OX-i-dill], are not used as primary drugs to treat hypertension. These vasodilators act by producing relaxation of vascular smooth muscle, primarily in arteries and arterioles. This results in decreased peripheral resistance and, therefore, blood pressure. Both agents produce reflex stimulation of the heart, resulting in the competing reflexes of increased myocardial contractility, heart rate, and oxygen consumption. These actions may prompt angina pectoris, myocardial infarction, or cardiac failure in predisposed individuals. Vasodilators also increase plasma renin concentration, resulting in sodium and water retention. These undesirable side effects can be blocked by concomitant use of a diuretic (to decrease sodium retention) and a β-blocker (to balance the reflex tachycardia). Together, the three drugs decrease cardiac output, plasma volume, and peripheral vascular resistance. *Hydralazine* is an accepted medication for controlling blood pressure in pregnancy-induced hypertension. Adverse effects of *hydralazine* include headache, tachycardia, nausea, sweating, arrhythmia, and precipitation of angina

(Figure 16.15). A lupus-like syndrome can occur with high dosages, but it is reversible upon discontinuation of the drug. *Minoxidil* treatment causes hypertrichosis (the growth of body hair). This drug is used topically to treat male pattern baldness.

XV. HYPERTENSIVE EMERGENCY

Hypertensive emergency is a rare but life-threatening situation characterized by severe elevations in blood pressure (systolic greater than 180 mm Hg or diastolic greater than 120 mm Hg) with evidence of impending or progressive target organ damage (for example, stroke, myocardial infarction). [Note: A severe elevation in blood pressure without evidence of target organ damage is considered a hypertensive urgency.] Hypertensive emergencies require timely blood pressure reduction with treatment administered intravenously to prevent or limit target organ damage. A variety of medications are used, including calcium channel blockers (*nicardipine* and *clevidipine*), nitric oxide vasodilators (*nitroprusside* and *nitroglycerin*), adrenergic receptor antagonists (*phentolamine*, *esmolol*, and *labetalol*), the vasodilator *hydralazine*, and the dopamine agonist *fenoldopam*. Treatment is directed by the type of target organ damage and/or comorbidities present.

XVI. RESISTANT HYPERTENSION

Resistant hypertension is defined as blood pressure that remains elevated (above goal) despite administration of an optimal three-drug regimen that includes a diuretic. The most common causes of resistant hypertension are poor compliance, excessive ethanol intake, concomitant conditions (diabetes, obesity, sleep apnea, hyperaldosteronism, high salt intake, and/or metabolic syndrome), concomitant medications (sympathomimetics, nonsteroidal anti-inflammatory drugs, or corticosteroids), insufficient dose and/or drugs, and use of drugs with similar mechanisms of action.

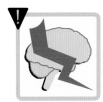
Headache

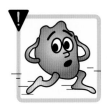
Tachycardia

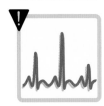
Palpitations

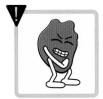
Angina

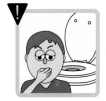
Nausea

Figure 16.15
Some adverse effects of *hydralazine*.

Study Questions

Choose the ONE best answer.

16.1 A 55-year-old non-Hispanic black male has hypertension. His past medical history also includes diabetes and hyperlipidemia. According to the ACC/AHA guidelines, which among the choices represents the most appropriate blood pressure goal for the patient?

A. Less than 140/85
B. Less than 135/85
C. Less than 130/80
D. Less than 140/80

Correct answer = C. Goals of therapy differ depending on which guidelines the clinician uses in practice. According to the ACC/AHA guidelines the goal blood pressure for a diabetic patient is less than 130/80.

16.2 A 59-year-old non-Hispanic white patient presents for treatment of hypertension. His past medical history also includes diabetes, hyperlipidemia, and hypertension. The patient's blood pressure is 150/93 (both today and at the last visit). Which is a recommended initial therapy to treat hypertension in this patient?

A. Enalapril
B. Hydralazine
C. Verapamil
D. Metoprolol

Correct answer = A. Enalapril is an ACE inhibitor and is recommended for first-line therapy in various patient populations, including those who have a compelling indication such as diabetes. The other therapies are not considered first-line therapy.

16.3 A 45-year-old male complains of constipation. He was recently started on two antihypertensives due to elevated systolic blood pressure (greater than 20 mm Hg above goal). His current medications include lisinopril, chlorthalidone, verapamil, rosuvastatin, and aspirin. Which is most likely contributing to his constipation?

A. Chlorthalidone
B. Verapamil
C. Aspirin
D. Lisinopril

Correct answer = B. Common side effects specific for verapamil include constipation and first-degree atrioventricular block, which typically are dose-dependent. Electrolyte disturbances are often associated with both diuretics (chlorthalidone) and ACE inhibitors (lisinopril).

16.4 Which antihypertensive medication can cause the rare side effect of angioedema?

A. Amlodipine
B. Fosinopril
C. Prazosin
D. Propranolol

Correct answer = B. ACE inhibitors (fosinopril), ARBs (for example, losartan), and renin inhibitors (aliskiren) can cause angioedema. The occurrence of angioedema is more common with ACE inhibitors. Amlodipine can cause dizziness, headache, and peripheral edema. Prazosin can cause reflex tachycardia and postural hypotension. Propranolol can cause insomnia, decreased libido, fatigue, and bradycardia.

16.5 A 52-year-old female has uncontrolled hypertension (blood pressure 154/82 mm Hg) on treatment with lisinopril. She recently had a myocardial infarction and her past medical history includes diabetes, hypertension, hyperlipidemia, and osteoarthritis. Considering her compelling indications, which agent may be appropriate to add to her antihypertensive therapy?

A. Clonidine
B. Olmesartan
C. Furosemide
D. Metoprolol

Correct answer = D. Individual patient care is warranted particularly in the case of a compelling indication for certain medication. Considering her recent myocardial infarction, the best choice is a β_1-blocker (metoprolol). It is not appropriate to combine an ACE inhibitor (lisinopril) and ARB (olmesartan). The other agents are not considered first-line therapy and do not have a compelling indication for addition to the regimen.

16.6 The blood pressure of a patient with essential hypertension is at goal on treatment with enalapril. Since initiation of enalapril, the serum creatinine has increased 25% above baseline. What is the appropriate next step for the enalapril therapy?

A. Discontinue enalapril.
B. Reduce dose of enalapril.
C. Continue current dose of enalapril.
D. Increase dose of enalapril.

Correct answer = C. The blood pressure is at goal. Electrolytes (such as potassium) and serum creatinine should be monitored in patients who initiate ACE inhibitors. Increases in serum creatinine up to 30% above baseline are acceptable and do not warrant discontinuation or reduction of treatment. Since the blood pressure is at goal, increasing the enalapril is not necessary.

16.7 Which of the following correctly outlines a major difference in electrolyte disturbances associated with thiazide and loop diuretics?

   A. Thiazide diuretics decrease potassium and loop diuretics increase potassium.

   B. Thiazide diuretics increase potassium and loop diuretics decrease potassium.

   C. Thiazide diuretics decrease calcium and loop diuretics increase calcium.

   D. Thiazide diuretics increase calcium and loop diuretics decrease calcium.

Correct answer = D. Thiazide and loop diuretics decrease potassium, sodium and magnesium. However, thiazide diuretics increase calcium (through reduced urinary excretion), while loop diuretics reduce calcium (through enhanced urinary excretion).

16.8 Which can precipitate a hypertensive crisis following abrupt cessation of therapy?

   A. Clonidine
   B. Diltiazem
   C. Valsartan
   D. Hydrochlorothiazide

Correct answer = A. Increased sympathetic nervous system activity occurs if clonidine therapy is abruptly stopped after prolonged administration. Uncontrolled elevation of blood pressure can occur. Patients should be slowly weaned from clonidine while other antihypertensive medications are initiated. The other drugs on the list do not produce this phenomenon.

16.9 Which of the following is a dihydropyridine calcium channel blocker?

   A. Amlodipine
   B. Metoprolol
   C. Verapamil
   D. Lisinopril

Correct answer = A. There are three classes of calcium channel blockers: nondihydropyridines (benzothiazepines, diphenylalkylamines) and dihydropyridines. Amlodipine is a member of the dihydropyridine class of calcium channel blockers, which also includes nifedipine and felodipine. Verapamil is a benzothiazepine calcium channel blocker, metoprolol is a β-blocker, and lisinopril is an ACE inhibitor.

16.10 A 45-year-old man was started on therapy for hypertension and developed a persistent, dry cough. Which is most likely responsible for this side effect?

   A. Lisinopril
   B. Losartan
   C. Nifedipine
   D. Atenolol

Correct answer = A. The cough is most likely an adverse effect of the ACE inhibitor lisinopril. Losartan is an ARB that has the same beneficial effects as an ACE inhibitor but is less likely to produce a cough. Nifedipine and atenolol do not cause this side effect.

Diuretics

Zachary L. Cox

17

I. OVERVIEW

Diuretics are drugs that increase the volume of urine excreted. Most diuretic agents are inhibitors of renal ion transporters that decrease the reabsorption of Na^+ at different sites in the nephron. As a result, Na^+ and other ions enter the urine in greater than normal amounts along with water, which is carried passively to maintain osmotic equilibrium. Diuretics, thus, increase the volume of urine and often change its pH, as well as the ionic composition of the urine and blood. The diuretic effect of the different classes of diuretics varies considerably with the site of action. In addition to the ion transport inhibitors, other types of diuretics include osmotic diuretics, aldosterone antagonists, and carbonic anhydrase inhibitors. While diuretics are most commonly used for management of excessive fluid retention (edema), many agents within this class are prescribed for non-diuretic indications or for systemic effects in addition to their actions on the kidney. Examples, which are discussed below, include use of thiazides in hypertension, use of carbonic anhydrase inhibitors in glaucoma, and use of aldosterone antagonists in heart failure. In this chapter, the diuretic drugs (Figure 17.1) are discussed according to the frequency of their use.

II. NORMAL REGULATION OF FLUID AND ELECTROLYTES BY THE KIDNEYS

Approximately 16% to 20% of the blood plasma entering the kidneys is filtered from the glomerular capillaries into Bowman's capsule. The filtrate, although normally free of proteins and blood cells, contains most of the low molecular weight plasma components in concentrations similar to that in the plasma. These include glucose, sodium bicarbonate, amino acids, and other organic solutes, as well as electrolytes, such as Na^+, K^+, and Cl^-. The kidney regulates the ionic composition and volume of urine by active reabsorption or secretion of ions and/or passive reabsorption of water at five functional zones along the nephron: 1) the proximal convoluted tubule, 2) the descending loop of Henle, 3) the ascending loop of Henle, 4) the distal convoluted tubule, and 5) the collecting tubule and duct (Figure 17.2).

A. Proximal convoluted tubule

In the proximal convoluted tubule located in the cortex of the kidney, almost all the glucose, bicarbonate, amino acids, and other metabolites

THIAZIDE DIURETICS
Chlorothiazide DIURIL
Chlorthalidone GENERIC ONLY
Hydrochlorothiazide (HCTZ) MICROZIDE
Indapamide GENERIC ONLY
Metolazone ZAROXOLYN

LOOP DIURETICS
Bumetanide BUMEX
Ethacrynic acid EDECRIN
Furosemide LASIX
Torsemide DEMADEX

POTASSIUM-SPARING DIURETICS
Amiloride MIDAMOR
Eplerenone INSPRA
Spironolactone ALDACTONE
Triamterene DYRENIUM

CARBONIC ANHYDRASE INHIBITORS
Acetazolamide DIAMOX

OSMOTIC DIURETICS
Mannitol OSMITROL

Figure 17.1
Summary of diuretic drugs.

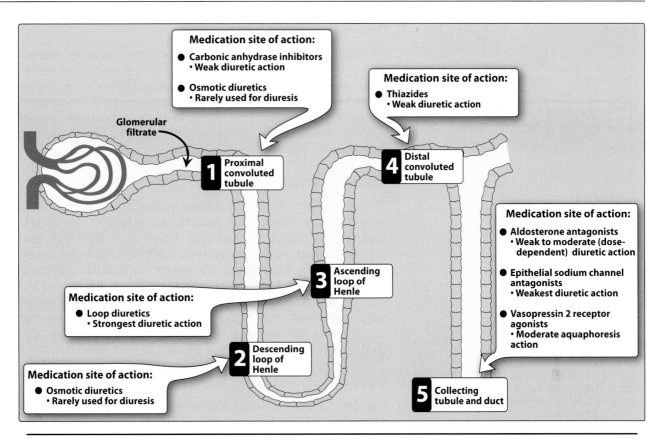

Figure 17.2
Major locations of ion and water exchange in the nephron, showing sites of action of the diuretic drugs.

are reabsorbed (Figure 17.3). Approximately 65% of the filtered Na^+ (and water) is reabsorbed. Given the high water permeability, about 60% of water is reabsorbed from the lumen to the blood to maintain osmolar equality. Chloride enters the lumen of the tubule in exchange for an anion, such as oxalate, as well as paracellularly through the lumen. The Na^+ that is reabsorbed is pumped into the interstitium by the Na^+/K^+-adenosine triphosphatase (ATPase) pump. Carbonic anhydrase in the luminal membrane and cytoplasm of the proximal tubular cells modulates the reabsorption of bicarbonate. Despite having the highest percentage of filtered Na^+ that is reabsorbed, diuretics working in the proximal convoluted tubule display weak diuretic properties. The presence of a high capacity Na^+ and water reabsorption area (loop of Henle) distal to the proximal convoluted tubule allows reabsorption of Na^+ and water kept in the lumen by diuretics acting in the proximal convoluted tubule, and limits effective diuresis.

The proximal tubule is the site of the organic acid and base secretory systems. The organic acid secretory system, located in the middle-third of the proximal tubule, secretes a variety of organic acids, such as uric acid, some antibiotics, and diuretics, from the bloodstream into the proximal tubular lumen. The organic acid secretory system is saturable, and diuretic drugs in the bloodstream compete for transfer with endogenous organic acids such as uric acid. A number of other interactions can also occur. For example, *probenecid* interferes with *penicillin* secretion. The organic base secretory system, located in the upper and middle segments of the proximal tubule, is responsible for the secretion of creatinine and choline.

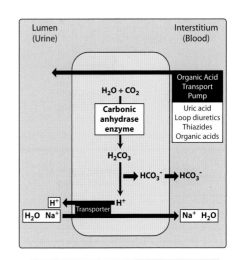

Figure 17.3
Proximal convoluted tubule cell.

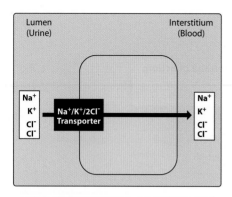

Figure 17.4
Ascending loop of Henle cell.

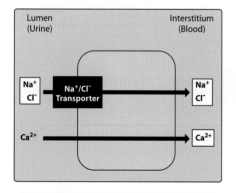

Figure 17.5
Distal convoluted tubule cell.

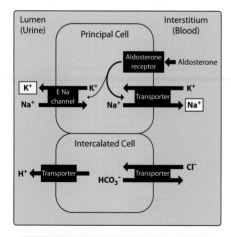

Figure 17.6
Collecting tubule and duct cells. E Na channel = Epithelial sodium channel.

B. Descending loop of Henle

The remaining filtrate, which is isotonic, next enters the descending limb of the loop of Henle and passes into the medulla of the kidney. The osmolarity increases along the descending portion of the loop of Henle because of the countercurrent mechanism that is responsible for water reabsorption. This results in a tubular fluid with a three-fold increase in Na^+ and Cl^- concentration. Osmotic diuretics exert part of their action in this region.

C. Ascending loop of Henle

The cells of the ascending tubular epithelium are unique in being impermeable to water. Active reabsorption of Na^+, K^+, and Cl^- is mediated by a $Na^+/K^+/2Cl^-$ cotransporter (Figure 17.4). Both Mg^{2+} and Ca^{2+} are reabsorbed via the paracellular pathway. Thus, the ascending loop dilutes the tubular fluid and raises the osmolarity of the medullary interstitium. Approximately 25% to 30% of the filtered sodium chloride is absorbed here. Because the ascending loop of Henle is a major site for salt reabsorption and no segments distally are capable of significant Na^+ and water reabsorption, drugs affecting this site, such as loop diuretics, have the greatest diuretic effect.

D. Distal convoluted tubule

The cells of the distal convoluted tubule are also impermeable to water. About 5% to 10% of the filtered sodium chloride is reabsorbed via a Na^+/Cl^- transporter, the target of thiazide diuretics. Calcium reabsorption, under the regulation of parathyroid hormone, is mediated by an apical channel and then transported by a Na^+/Ca^{2+}-exchanger into the interstitial fluid (Figure 17.5).

E. Collecting tubule and duct

The principal cells of the collecting tubule and duct are responsible for Na^+, K^+, and water transport, whereas the intercalated cells affect H^+ secretion (Figure 17.6). Approximately 1% to 2% of the filtered sodium enters the principal cells through epithelial sodium channels that are inhibited by *amiloride* and *triamterene*. Once inside the cell, Na^+ reabsorption relies on a Na^+/K^+-ATPase pump to be transported into the blood. Aldosterone receptors in the principal cells influence Na^+ reabsorption and K^+ secretion. Aldosterone increases the synthesis of epithelial sodium channels and of the Na^+/K^+-ATPase pump to increase Na^+ reabsorption and K+ excretion. Antidiuretic hormone (ADH; vasopressin) binds to V2 receptors to promote the reabsorption of water through aquaporin channels.

III. THIAZIDES

The thiazides are the most widely used diuretics because of their antihypertensive effects. However, the efficacy of thiazides for hypertension is not entirely dependent on their diuretic actions. These agents also reduce peripheral vascular resistance with long-term therapy. Despite being sulfonamide derivatives, thiazides do not generally cause hypersensitivity reactions in patients with allergies to sulfonamide antimicrobials such as *sulfamethoxazole.* All thiazides affect the distal convoluted tubule (Figure 17.2), and all have equal maximum diuretic effects, differing only in potency. Thiazides are sometimes called "low ceiling diuretics," because increasing the dose above normal therapeutic doses does not promote further diuretic response.

A. Thiazides

Chlorothiazide [klor-oh-THYE-ah-zide] was the first orally active thiazide, although *hydrochlorothiazide* [hye-dro-klor-oh-THYE-ah-zide] and *chlorthalidone* [klor-THAL-i-done] are now used more commonly due to better bioavailability. *Hydrochlorothiazide* is more potent, so the required dose is considerably lower than that of *chlorothiazide*, but the efficacy is comparable to that of the parent drug. In all other aspects, *hydrochlorothiazide* resembles *chlorothiazide*. *Chlorthalidone* is approximately twice as potent as *hydrochlorothiazide*. *Chlorthalidone*, *indapamide* [in-DAP-a-mide], and *metolazone* [me-TOL-ah-zone] are referred to as thiazide-like diuretics because they lack the characteristic benzothiadiazine chemical structure; however, their mechanism of action, indications, and adverse effects are similar to those of *hydrochlorothiazide*.

1. **Mechanism of action:** The thiazide and thiazide-like diuretics act mainly in the distal convoluted tubule to decrease the reabsorption of Na^+ by inhibition of a Na^+/Cl^- cotransporter (Figure 17.5). As a result, these drugs increase the concentration of Na^+ and Cl^- in the tubular fluid. Thiazides must be excreted into the tubular lumen at the proximal convoluted tubule to be effective (Figure 17.3). Therefore, decreasing renal function reduces the diuretic effects. The antihypertensive effects of thiazides may persist even when the glomerular filtration rate is below 30 mL/min/1.73 m^2. However, hypertension at this level of renal dysfunction is often exacerbated by hypervolemia, requiring a change to loop diuretics for volume status and, therefore, blood pressure control. The efficacy of thiazides may be diminished with concomitant use of nonsteroidal anti-inflammatory drugs (NSAIDs), such as *indomethacin*, which inhibit production of renal prostaglandins, thereby reducing renal blood flow.

2. **Actions**

   a. **Increased excretion of Na^+ and Cl^-:** Thiazide and thiazide-like diuretics cause diuresis with increased Na^+ and Cl^- excretion, which can result in the excretion of very hyperosmolar (concentrated) urine. This latter effect is unique, as the other diuretic classes are unlikely to produce a hyperosmolar urine. Figure 17.7 outlines relative changes in the ionic composition of the urine with thiazide and thiazide-like diuretics.

   b. **Decreased urinary calcium excretion:** Thiazide and thiazide-like diuretics decrease the Ca^{2+} content of urine by promoting the reabsorption of Ca^{2+} in the distal convoluted tubule where parathyroid hormone regulates reabsorption.

   c. **Reduced peripheral vascular resistance:** An initial reduction in blood pressure results from a decrease in blood volume and,

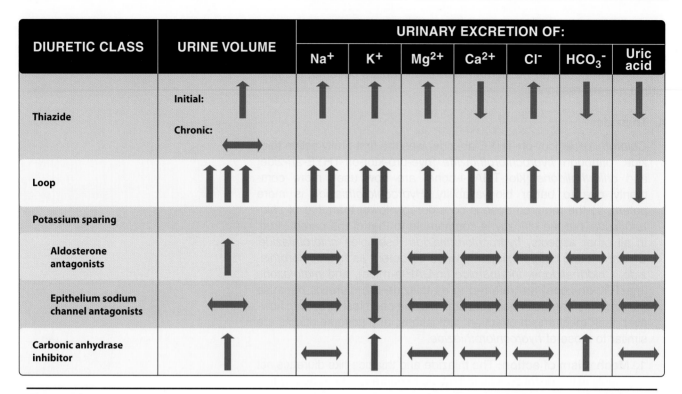

Figure 17.7
Urinary excretion from diuretic therapy.

therefore, a decrease in cardiac output. With continued therapy, blood volume returns to baseline. However, antihypertensive effects continue, resulting from reduced peripheral vascular resistance caused by relaxation of arteriolar smooth muscle.

3. Therapeutic uses

a. Hypertension: Clinically, thiazides are a mainstay of antihypertensive treatment, because they are inexpensive, convenient to administer, and well tolerated. Blood pressure can be lowered with a daily dose of thiazide. At doses equipotent to *hydrochlorothiazide*, *chlorthalidone* is considered a preferred option by some clinicians because of its longer half-life (50 to 60 hours) and improved control of blood pressure over the entire day. However, current treatment guidelines for hypertension do not recommend any thiazide preferentially.

b. Heart failure: Loop diuretics (not thiazides) are the diuretics of choice in reducing extracellular volume in heart failure. However, thiazide diuretics may be added in patients resistant to loop diuretics, with careful monitoring for hypokalemia. *Metolazone* is most frequently utilized as an addition to loop diuretics, although there is a lack of evidence that it is more effective than other thiazides for this indication when administered at equipotent doses. Historically, thiazides were prescribed to be administered 30 minutes prior to loop diuretics to allow the thiazide time to reach the site of action when combined to augment diuresis in diuretic resistance. This practice is unnecessary and not supported by current evidence.

c. **Hypercalciuria:** The thiazides can be useful in treating idiopathic hypercalciuria and calcium oxalate stones in the urinary tract, because they inhibit urinary Ca^{2+} excretion.

d. **Diabetes insipidus:** Thiazides have the unique ability to produce a hyperosmolar urine. Thiazides can be utilized as a treatment for nephrogenic diabetes insipidus. The urine volume of such individuals may drop from 11 to about 3 L/d when treated with thiazides.

4. **Pharmacokinetics:** As a class, thiazides are effective orally, with a bioavailability of 60% to 70%. *Chlorothiazide* has a much lower bioavailability (15% to 30%) and is the only thiazide with an intravenous dosage form. Most thiazides take 1 to 3 weeks to produce a stable reduction in blood pressure and exhibit a prolonged half-life (approximately 10 to 15 hours). *Indapamide* differs from the class because it undergoes hepatic metabolism and is excreted in both the urine and bile. Most thiazides are primarily excreted unchanged in the urine.

5. **Adverse effects:** These mainly involve problems in fluid and electrolyte balance (Figure 17.8).

a. **Hypokalemia:** Hypokalemia is the most frequent problem with the thiazide diuretics. Because thiazides increase Na^+ in the filtrate arriving at the distal tubule, more K^+ is also exchanged for Na^+, resulting in a continual loss of K^+ from the body with prolonged use of these drugs Thus, serum K^+ should be measured periodically (more frequently at the beginning of therapy) to monitor for the development of hypokalemia. Potassium supplementation or combination with a potassium-sparing diuretic may be required. Low-sodium diets blunt the potassium depletion caused by thiazide diuretics.

b. **Hypomagnesemia:** Urinary loss of magnesium can lead to hypomagnesemia.

c. **Hyponatremia:** Hyponatremia may develop due to elevation of ADH, as well as diminished diluting capacity of the kidney and increased thirst.

d. **Hyperuricemia:** Thiazides increase serum uric acid by decreasing the amount of acid excreted through competition in the organic acid secretory system. Being insoluble, uric acid deposits in the joints and may precipitate a gouty attack in predisposed individuals. Therefore, thiazides should be used with caution in patients with gout or high levels of uric acid.

e. **Hypovolemia:** This can cause orthostatic hypotension or light-headedness.

f. **Hypercalcemia:** Thiazides inhibit the secretion of Ca^{2+}, sometimes leading to hypercalcemia (elevated levels of Ca^{2+} in the blood).

g. **Hyperglycemia:** Therapy with thiazides can lead to mild elevations in serum glucose, possibly due to impaired release

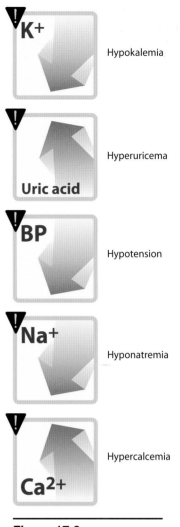

Figure 17.8
Summary of adverse effects commonly observed with thiazide and thiazide-like medications.

of insulin related to hypokalemia. Patients with diabetes still benefit from thiazide therapy, but should monitor glucose to assess the need for an adjustment in diabetes therapy if thiazides are initiated.

IV. LOOP DIURETICS

Bumetanide [byoo-MET-ah-nide], *furosemide* [fur-OH-se-mide], *torsemide* [TOR-se-mide], and *ethacrynic* [eth-a-KRIN-ik] *acid* have their major diuretic action on the ascending limb of the loop of Henle (Figure 17.2). Of all the diuretics, these drugs have the highest efficacy in mobilizing Na^+ and Cl^- from the body, producing copious amounts of urine. Similar to thiazides, loop diuretics do not generally cause hypersensitivity reactions in patients with allergies to sulfonamide antimicrobials such as *sulfamethoxazole* because of structural differences in their sulfonamide derivative. *Furosemide* is the most commonly used of these drugs. The use of *bumetanide* and *torsemide* is increasing, as these agents have better bioavailability and are more potent compared to *furosemide*. *Ethacrynic acid* is used infrequently due to its adverse effect profile.

A. Bumetanide, furosemide, torsemide, and ethacrynic acid

1. **Mechanism of action:** Loop diuretics inhibit the cotransport of $Na^+/K^+/2Cl^-$ in the luminal membrane in the ascending limb of the loop of Henle (Figure 17.4). Therefore, reabsorption of these ions into the renal medulla is decreased. By lowering the osmotic pressure in the medulla, less water is reabsorbed from water permeable segments, like the descending loop of Henle, causing diuresis. These agents have the greatest diuretic effect of all the diuretics because the ascending limb accounts for reabsorption of 25% to 30% of filtered NaCl and downstream sites are unable to compensate for the increased Na^+ load. Loop diuretics must be excreted into the tubular lumen at the proximal convoluted tubule to be effective (Figure 17.3). NSAIDs inhibit renal prostaglandin synthesis and can reduce the diuretic action of loop diuretics.

2. **Actions**

   a. **Diuresis:** Loop diuretics cause diuresis, even in patients with poor renal function or lack of response to other diuretics. Changes in the composition of the urine induced by loop diuretics are shown in Figure 17.7.

   Loop diuretics display a sigmoidal ("S"-shaped) dose-response curve with three parts: a threshold effect, a rapid increase in diuresis with small changes in drug concentration, and a ceiling effect (Figure 17.9). A dose must be selected to cross the response threshold, which is patient-specific. Reducing the effective dose with the intent of a reduction in diuresis can result in no diuresis, if the concentration of loop diuretic drops below the response threshold. Likewise, increasing the effective dose may not cause more diuresis because of the ceiling effect. Thus, after determination of an effective diuretic dose, the clinician should modify the frequency of administration to increase or decrease the daily diuresis.

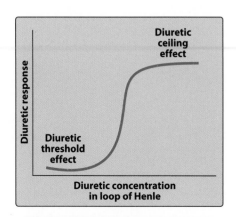

Figure 17.9
Loop diuretic dose-response curve.

b. Increased urinary calcium excretion: Unlike thiazides, loop diuretics increase the Ca^{2+} content of urine. In patients with normal serum Ca^{2+} concentrations, hypocalcemia does not result, because Ca^{2+} is reabsorbed in the distal convoluted tubule.

c. Venodilation: Prior to their diuretic actions, loop diuretics cause acute venodilation and reduce left ventricular filling pressures via enhanced prostaglandin synthesis.

3. Therapeutic uses

a. Edema: Loop diuretics are the drugs of choice for treatment of pulmonary edema and acute/chronic peripheral edema caused from heart failure or renal impairment. Because of their rapid onset of action, particularly when given intravenously, the drugs are useful in emergency situations such as acute pulmonary edema.

b. Hypercalcemia: Loop diuretics (along with hydration) are also useful in treating hypercalcemia, because they stimulate tubular Ca^{2+} excretion.

c. Hyperkalemia: Loop diuretics can be used with or without replacement intravenous fluid for the treatment of hyperkalemia.

4. Pharmacokinetics: Loop diuretics are administered orally or parenterally. *Furosemide* has unpredictable bioavailability of 10% to 90% after oral administration. *Bumetanide* and *torsemide* have reliable bioavailability of 80% to 100%, which makes these agents preferred for oral therapy. The duration of action is approximately 6 hours for *furosemide* and *bumetanide*, and moderately longer for *torsemide*, allowing patients to predict the window of diuresis.

5. Effects: Fluid and electrolyte issues are the predominant adverse effects (Figure 17.10).

a. Acute hypovolemia: Loop diuretics can cause a severe and rapid reduction in blood volume, with the possibility of hypotension, shock, and cardiac arrhythmias.

b. Hypokalemia: The heavy load of Na^+ presented to the collecting tubule results in increased exchange of tubular Na^+ for K^+, leading to hypokalemia, the most common adverse effect of the loop diuretics. The loss of K^+ from cells in exchange for H^+ leads to hypokalemic alkalosis. Use of potassium-sparing diuretics or supplementation with K^+ can prevent the development of hypokalemia.

c. Hypomagnesemia: Urinary loss of magnesium can lead to hypomagnesemia.

d. Ototoxicity: Reversible or permanent hearing loss may occur with loop diuretics, particularly when infused intravenously at fast rates, at high doses, or when used in conjunction with other ototoxic drugs (for example, aminoglycoside antibiotics). With current dosing and appropriate infusion rates,

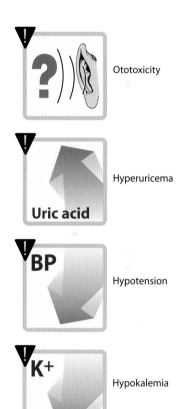

Ototoxicity

Hyperuricema

Hypotension

Hypokalemia

Hypomagnesemia

Figure 17.10
Summary of adverse effects commonly observed with loop diuretics.

ototoxicity is a rare occurrence. *Ethacrynic acid* is the most likely to cause ototoxicity. Although less common, vestibular function may also be affected, inducing vertigo.

e. Hyperuricemia: Loop diuretics compete with uric acid for the renal secretory systems, thus blocking its secretion and, in turn, may cause or exacerbate gouty attacks.

V. POTASSIUM-SPARING DIURETICS

Potassium-sparing diuretics act in the collecting tubule to inhibit Na^+ reabsorption and K^+ excretion (Figure 17.6). Potassium levels must be monitored in patients treated with potassium-sparing diuretics. These drugs should be used cautiously in moderate renal dysfunction and avoided in patients with severe renal dysfunction because of the increased risk of hyperkalemia. Within this class, there are drugs with two distinct mechanisms of action with different indications for use: aldosterone antagonists and epithelial sodium channel blockers. Changes in the composition of the urine induced by potassium-sparing diuretics are shown in Figure 17.7.

A. Aldosterone antagonists: spironolactone and eplerenone

1. **Mechanism of action:** *Spironolactone* [spear-oh-no-LAK-tone] and *eplerenone* [eh-PLEH-reh-none] are synthetic steroids that antagonize aldosterone receptors. This prevents translocation of the receptor complex into the nucleus of the target cell, ultimately resulting in a lack of intracellular proteins that stimulate the Na^+/K^+-exchange sites of the collecting tubule. Thus, aldosterone antagonists prevent Na^+ reabsorption and, therefore, K^+ and H^+ secretion. *Eplerenone* is more selective for aldosterone receptors and causes less endocrine effects (gynecomastia) than *spironolactone*, which also binds to progesterone and androgen receptors.

2. **Actions:** *Spironolactone* and *eplerenone* antagonize aldosterone receptors at renal sites, which causes diuresis, and nonrenal sites, which causes other effects. In most edematous states, blood levels of aldosterone are high, causing retention of Na^+. *Spironolactone* antagonizes the activity of aldosterone, resulting in retention of K^+ and excretion of Na^+.

3. **Therapeutic uses**

   a. Edema: Aldosterone antagonists are particularly effective diuretics when used in high doses for edema associated with secondary hyperaldosteronism, such as hepatic cirrhosis and nephrotic syndrome. *Spironolactone* is the diuretic of choice in patients with hepatic cirrhosis with fluid in the peritoneal cavity (ascites). By contrast, in patients who have no significant circulating levels of aldosterone, there is minimal diuretic effect with use of this drug.

   b. Hypokalemia: Although the aldosterone antagonists have a low efficacy in mobilizing Na^+ from the body in comparison with the other diuretics, they have the useful property of causing the retention of K^+. These agents are often given in conjunction with thiazide or loop diuretics to prevent K^+ excretion that occurs with those diuretics.

c. **Heart failure:** Aldosterone antagonists are employed at lower doses to prevent myocardial remodeling mediated by aldosterone. Use of these agents has been shown to decrease mortality associated with heart failure, particularly in those with reduced ejection fraction.

d. **Resistant hypertension:** Resistant hypertension, defined by the use of three or more medications without reaching the blood pressure goal, often responds well to aldosterone antagonists. This effect can be seen in those with or without elevated aldosterone levels.

e. **Polycystic ovary syndrome:** *Spironolactone* is often used off-label for the treatment of polycystic ovary syndrome. It blocks androgen receptors and inhibits steroid synthesis at high doses, thereby helping to offset increased androgen levels seen in this disorder.

4. **Pharmacokinetics:** Both *spironolactone* and *eplerenone* are well absorbed after oral administration. S*pironolactone* is extensively metabolized and converted to several active metabolites, which contribute to the therapeutic effects. *Eplerenone* is metabolized by cytochrome P450 3A4.

5. **Adverse effects**

a. **Hyperkalemia:** The most common side effect, hyperkalemia, is dose-dependent and increases with renal dysfunction or use of other potassium-sparing agents such as angiotensin-converting enzyme inhibitors and potassium supplements.

b. **Gynecomastia:** *Spironolactone*, but not *eplerenone*, may induce gynecomastia in approximately 10% of male patients and menstrual irregularities in female patients.

B. Triamterene and amiloride

Triamterene [trye-AM-ter-een] and *amiloride* [a-MIL-oh-ride] block epithelial sodium channels, resulting in a decrease in Na^+/K^+ exchange. Although they have a K^+-sparing diuretic action similar to that of the aldosterone antagonists, their ability to block the Na^+/K^+-exchange site in the collecting tubule does not depend on the presence of aldosterone. Like the aldosterone antagonists, these agents are not very efficacious diuretics. Both *triamterene* and *amiloride* are commonly used in combination with other diuretics, almost solely for their potassium-sparing properties.

VI. CARBONIC ANHYDRASE INHIBITOR

Acetazolamide [ah-set-a-ZOLE-a-mide] and other carbonic anhydrase inhibitors are more often used for their other pharmacologic actions than for their diuretic effect, because they are much less efficacious than the thiazide or loop diuretics.

A. Acetazolamide

1. **Mechanism of action:** *Acetazolamide* inhibits carbonic anhydrase located intracellularly (cytoplasm) and on the apical membrane of the proximal tubular epithelium (Figure 17.3). [Note: Carbonic anhydrase catalyzes the reaction of CO_2 and H_2O, leading to H_2CO_3, which spontaneously ionizes to H^+ and HCO_3^- (bicarbonate).] The decreased ability to exchange Na^+ for H^+ in the presence of *acetazolamide* results in a mild diuresis. Additionally, HCO_3^- is retained in the lumen, with marked elevation in urinary pH. The loss of HCO_3^- causes a hyperchloremic metabolic acidosis. Changes in the composition of urinary electrolytes induced by *acetazolamide* are summarized in Figure 17.7.

2. **Therapeutic uses**

    a. **Glaucoma:** Oral *acetazolamide* decreases the production of aqueous humor and reduces intraocular pressure in patients with chronic open-angle glaucoma, probably by blocking carbonic anhydrase in the ciliary body of the eye. Topical carbonic anhydrase inhibitors, such as *dorzolamide* and *brinzolamide*, have the advantage of not causing systemic effects.

    b. **Altitude sickness:** *Acetazolamide* can be used in the prophylaxis of symptoms of altitude sickness. *Acetazolamide* prevents weakness, breathlessness, dizziness, nausea, and cerebral as well as pulmonary edema characteristic of the syndrome.

3. **Pharmacokinetics:** *Acetazolamide* can be administered orally or intravenously. It is approximately 90% protein bound and eliminated renally by both active tubular secretion and passive reabsorption.

4. **Adverse effects:** Metabolic acidosis (mild), potassium depletion, renal stone formation, drowsiness, and paresthesia may occur. The drug should be avoided in patients with hepatic cirrhosis, because it could lead to a decreased excretion of NH_4^+.

VII. OSMOTIC DIURETICS

A number of simple, hydrophilic chemical substances that are filtered through the glomerulus, such as *mannitol* [MAN-i-tol], result in diuresis (Figure 17.2). Filtered substances that undergo little or no reabsorption result in a higher osmolarity of the tubular fluid. This prevents further water reabsorption at the descending loop of Henle and proximal convoluted tubule, resulting in osmotic diuresis with little additional Na^+ excretion (aquaresis). Therefore, these agents are not useful for treating conditions in which Na^+ retention occurs. They are used to maintain urine flow following acute toxic ingestion of substances capable of producing acute renal failure. Osmotic diuretics are a mainstay of treatment for patients with increased intracranial pressure. [Note: *Mannitol* is not absorbed when given orally and should be given intravenously.] Adverse effects include dehydration and extracellular water expansion from the osmotic effects in the systemic circulation. The expansion of extracellular water occurs because the presence of *mannitol* in the extracellular fluid extracts water from the cells and causes hyponatremia until diuresis occurs.

Study Questions

Choose the ONE best answer.

17.1 An elderly patient with a history of heart disease has difficulty breathing and is diagnosed with acute pulmonary edema. Which treatment is indicated?

A. Acetazolamide
B. Chlorthalidone
C. Furosemide
D. Spironolactone

Correct answer = C. This is a potentially fatal situation. It is important to administer a diuretic that reduces fluid accumulation in the lungs and improves oxygenation and heart function. The loop diuretics are most effective in removing large fluid volumes from the body and are the treatment of choice in this situation. In this situation, furosemide should be administered intravenously. The other choices are inappropriate.

17.2 A group of college students is planning a mountain climbing trip to the Andes. Which is most appropriate for them to take to prevent altitude sickness?

A. A thiazide diuretic such as hydrochlorothiazide
B. An anticholinergic such as atropine
C. A carbonic anhydrase inhibitor such as acetazolamide
D. A loop diuretic such as furosemide

Correct answer = C. Acetazolamide is used prophylactically for several days before an ascent above 10,000 feet. This treatment prevents the cerebral and pulmonary problems associated with altitude sickness as well as other difficulties, such as nausea.

17.3 An alcoholic male has developed hepatic cirrhosis. To control the ascites and edema, which should be prescribed?

A. Acetazolamide
B. Chlorthalidone
C. Furosemide
D. Spironolactone

Correct answer = D. Spironolactone is very effective in the treatment of hepatic edema. These patients are frequently resistant to the diuretic action of loop diuretics, although a combination with spironolactone may be beneficial. The other agents are not indicated.

17.4 A 55-year-old male with kidney stones needs a medication to decrease urinary calcium excretion. Which diuretic is best for this indication?

A. Torsemide
B. Hydrochlorothiazide
C. Spironolactone
D. Triamterene

Correct answer = B. Hydrochlorothiazide is effective in increasing calcium reabsorption, thus decreasing the amount of calcium excreted, and decreasing the formation of kidney stones that contain calcium phosphate or calcium oxalate. Furosemide increases the excretion of calcium, whereas the K^+-sparing diuretics, spironolactone, and triamterene do not have an effect.

17.5 A 75-year-old woman with hypertension and glaucoma is being treated with chlorthalidone, amlodipine, lisinopril, and acetazolamide. In clinic today, she complains of acute joint pain and redness in her great toe, which is diagnosed as gout. Which medication is most likely to have caused the gout attack?

A. Amlodipine
B. Acetazolamide
C. Chlorthalidone
D. Lisinopril

Correct answer = C. Thiazides such as chlorthalidone compete with uric acid for secretion into the lumen of the nephron at the proximal convoluted tubule. This competition decreases uric acid secretion, raising the serum concentration and increasing the risk of a gout attack. Loop diuretics have the same risk.

17.6 Which is contraindicated in a patient with hyperkalemia?

A. Acetazolamide
B. Chlorothiazide
C. Ethacrynic acid
D. Eplerenone

Correct answer = D. Eplerenone acts in the collecting tubule via aldosterone antagonism to inhibit Na^+ reabsorption and K^+ excretion. It is extremely important that patients who are treated with any potassium-sparing diuretic be closely monitored for potassium levels. Exogenous potassium supplementation is usually discontinued when potassium-sparing diuretic therapy is initiated. The other drugs promote the excretion of potassium.

17.7 A 59-year-old male patient in the intensive care unit has a metabolic alkalosis. Which therapy will treat this condition?

A. Amiloride

B. Hydrochlorothiazide

C. Mannitol

D. Acetazolamide

> Correct answer = D. Acetazolamide causes an increase in the urinary excretion of bicarbonate, lowering the pH of the blood.

17.8 A male patient is placed on a new medication and notes that his breasts have become enlarged and tender to the touch. Which medication is the most likely taking?

A. Furosemide

B. Hydrochlorothiazide

C. Spironolactone

D. Triamterene

> Correct answer = C. An adverse drug reaction to spironolactone is gynecomastia due to its effects on androgens and progesterone in the body. Eplerenone may be a suitable alternative if the patient is in need of an aldosterone antagonist but has a history of gynecomastia.

17.9 A patient with heart failure with reduced ejection fraction researched his medications on the Internet and found he was taking two "diuretics," bumetanide and spironolactone. He asks if this is a mistake with his therapy. What is the best response?

A. Spironolactone is used to prevent hyponatremia.

B. Spironolactone is used to reduce heart structure changes and decrease the risk of death.

C. Bumetanide is used to decrease the potassium lost from spironolactone therapy.

D. This is a duplication error and one diuretic should be stopped.

> Correct answer = B. Aldosterone antagonists are used at non-diuretic doses in heart failure to prevent myocardial remodeling and decrease mortality. Bumetanide is used as a diuretic to treat edema from heart failure. Both are appropriate to use together because of the unique indications. Spironolactone reduces the potassium lost from diuresis with bumetanide.

17.10 Which diuretic has been shown to improve blood pressure in resistant hypertension or those already treated with three blood pressure medications including a thiazide or thiazide-like medication?

A. Indapamide

B. Furosemide

C. Mannitol

D. Spironolactone

> Correct answer = D. Resistant hypertension, defined by the use of three or more medications without reaching the blood pressure goal, often responds well to aldosterone antagonists. This effect can be seen in those with or without elevated aldosterone levels.

Drugs for Heart Failure

18

Shawn Anderson and Katherine Vogel Anderson

I. OVERVIEW

Heart failure (HF) is a complex, progressive disorder in which the heart is unable to pump sufficient blood to meet the needs of the body. Its cardinal symptoms are dyspnea, fatigue, and fluid retention. HF is due to an impaired ability of the heart to adequately fill with and/or eject blood. It is often accompanied by abnormal increases in blood volume and interstitial fluid. Underlying causes of HF include, but are not limited to, atherosclerotic heart disease, hypertensive heart disease, valvular heart disease, and congenital heart disease.

A. Role of physiologic compensatory mechanisms in the progression of HF

Chronic activation of the sympathetic nervous system and the renin–angiotensin–aldosterone system (RAAS) is associated with remodeling of cardiac tissue, loss of myocytes, hypertrophy, and fibrosis. This prompts additional neurohormonal activation, creating a vicious cycle that, if left untreated, leads to death.

B. Goals of pharmacologic intervention in HF

Goals of treatment are to alleviate symptoms, slow disease progression, and improve survival. The following classes of drugs have been shown to be effective: 1) angiotensin-converting enzyme (ACE) inhibitors, 2) angiotensin receptor blockers, 3) aldosterone antagonists, 4) β-blockers, 5) diuretics, 6) direct vaso- and venodilators, 7) hyperpolarization-activated cyclic nucleotide-gated channel blockers, 8) inotropic agents, 9) the combination of a neprilysin inhibitor with an angiotensin receptor blocker, and 10) recombinant B-type natriuretic peptide (Figure 18.1). Depending on the severity of HF and individual patient factors, one or more of these classes of drugs are administered. Pharmacologic intervention provides the following benefits in HF: reduced myocardial work load, decreased extracellular fluid volume, improved cardiac contractility, and a reduced rate of cardiac remodeling. Knowledge of the physiology of cardiac muscle contraction is

ACE INHIBITORS
Captopril GENERIC ONLY
Enalapril VASOTEC
Fosinopril GENERIC ONLY
Lisinopril PRINIVIL, ZESTRIL
Quinapril ACCUPRIL
Ramipril ALTACE

ANGIOTENSIN RECEPTOR BLOCKERS
Candesartan ATACAND
Losartan COZAAR
Telmisartan MICARDIS
Valsartan DIOVAN

ARNI
Sacubitril/valsartan ENTRESTO

ALDOSTERONE ANTAGONISTS
Eplerenone INSPRA
Spironolactone ALDACTONE

β–ADRENORECEPTOR BLOCKERS
Bisoprolol GENERIC ONLY
Carvedilol COREG, COREG CR
Metoprolol succinate TOPROL XL
Metoprolol tartrate LOPRESSOR

DIURETICS
Bumetanide BUMEX
Furosemide LASIX
Metolazone ZAROXOLYN
Torsemide DEMADEX

DIRECT VASO - AND VENODILATORS
Hydralazine GENERIC ONLY
Isosorbide dinitrate DILATRATE-SR, ISORDIL
FDC Hydralazine/Isosorbide dinitrate BIDIL

HCN CHANNEL BLOCKER
Ivabradine CORLANOR

INOTROPIC AGENTS
Digoxin LANOXIN
Dobutamine DOBUTREX
Dopamine GENERIC ONLY
Milrinone GENERIC ONLY

B-TYPE NATRIURETIC PEPTIDE
Nesiritide NATRECOR

Figure 18.1
Summary of drugs used to treat HF. ACE = angiotensin-converting enzyme; ARB = angiotensin receptor blocker; ARNI = angiotensin receptor neprilysin inhibitor; FDC = fixed-dose combination; HCN = hyperpolarization-activated cyclic nucleotide-gated.

essential for understanding the compensatory responses evoked by the failing heart, as well as the actions of drugs used to treat HF.

II. PHYSIOLOGY OF MUSCLE CONTRACTION

The myocardium, like smooth and skeletal muscle, responds to stimulation by depolarization of the membrane, which is followed by shortening of the contractile proteins and ends with relaxation and return to the resting state (repolarization). Cardiac myocytes are interconnected in groups that respond to stimuli as a unit, contracting together whenever a single cell is stimulated.

A. Action potential

Cardiac myocytes are electrically excitable and have a spontaneous, intrinsic rhythm generated by specialized "pacemaker" cells located in the sinoatrial (SA) and atrioventricular (AV) nodes. Cardiac myocytes also have an unusually long action potential, which can be divided into five phases (0 to 4). Figure 18.2 illustrates the major ions contributing to depolarization and repolarization of cardiac myocytes.

B. Cardiac contraction

The force of contraction of the cardiac muscle is directly related to the concentration of free (unbound) cytosolic calcium. Therefore, agents that increase intracellular calcium levels (or that increase the sensitivity of the contractile machinery to calcium) increase the force of contraction (inotropic effect). The movement of calcium in cardiac myocytes is illustrated in Figure 18.3.

C. Compensatory physiological responses in HF

The failing heart evokes four major compensatory mechanisms to enhance cardiac output (Figure 18.4).

1. **Increased sympathetic activity:** Baroreceptors sense a decrease in blood pressure and activate the sympathetic nervous system. In an attempt to sustain tissue perfusion, this stimulation of β-adrenergic receptors results in an increased heart rate and a greater force of contraction of the heart muscle. In addition, vasoconstriction enhances venous return and increases cardiac preload. An increase in preload (stretch on the heart) increases stroke volume, which, in turn, increases cardiac output. These compensatory responses increase the workload of the heart, which, in the long term, contributes to further decline in cardiac function.

2. **Activation of the renin–angiotensin–aldosterone system (RAAS):** A fall in cardiac output decreases blood flow to the kidney, prompting the release of renin. Renin release is also stimulated by increased sympathetic activity resulting in increased formation of angiotensin II and release of aldosterone. This results in increased peripheral resistance (afterload) and retention of sodium and water. Blood volume increases, and more blood is returned to the heart. If the heart is unable to pump this extra volume, venous pressure increases and peripheral and pulmonary edema occur. In addition, high levels of angiotensin II and aldosterone have direct detrimental effects on cardiac muscle, favoring remodeling, fibrosis, and inflammatory changes. Again, these compensatory responses increase the workload of the heart, contributing to further decline in cardiac function.

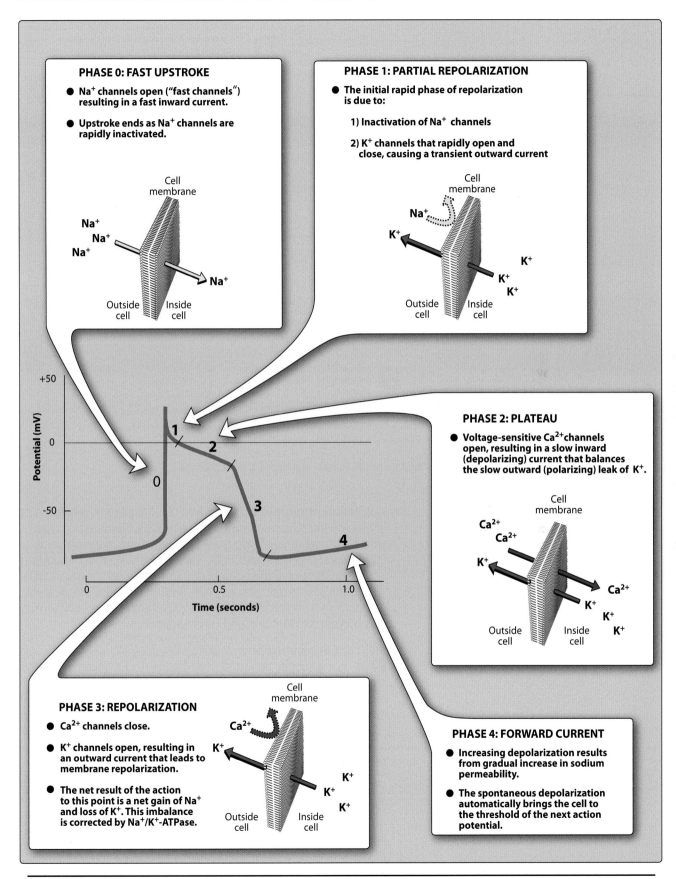

Figure 18.2
Action potential of a cardiac myocyte. ATPase = adenosine triphosphatase.

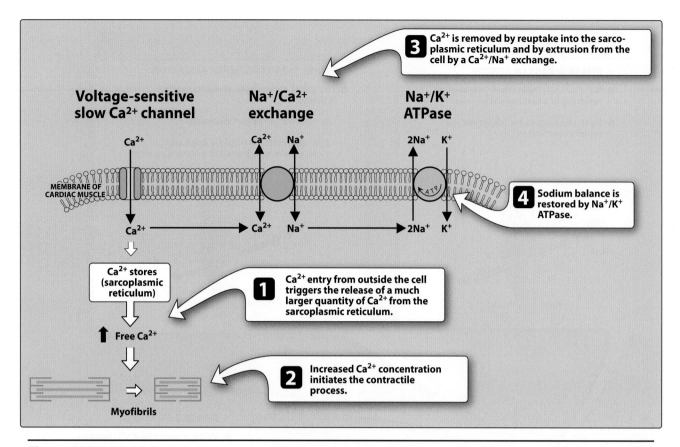

Figure 18.3
Ion movements during the contraction of cardiac muscle. ATPase = adenosine triphosphatase.

3. **Activation of natriuretic peptides:** An increase in preload also increases the release of natriuretic peptides. Natriuretic peptides, which include atrial, B-type, and C-type, have differing roles in HF; atrial and B-type natriuretic peptides are the most important. Activation of the natriuretic peptides ultimately results in vasodilation, natriuresis, inhibition of renin and aldosterone release, and a reduction in myocardial fibrosis. This beneficial response may improve cardiac function and HF symptoms.

4. **Myocardial hypertrophy:** Initially, stretching of the heart muscle leads to a stronger contraction of the heart. However, excessive elongation of the fibers results in weaker contractions and a diminished ability to eject blood. This type of failure is termed "systolic failure" or HF with reduced ejection fraction (HFrEF) and is the result of the ventricle being unable to pump effectively. Patients with HF may have "diastolic dysfunction," a term applied when the ability of the ventricles to relax and accept blood is impaired by structural changes such as hypertrophy. The thickening of the ventricular wall and subsequent decrease in ventricular volume decrease the ability of heart muscle to relax. In this case, the ventricle does not fill adequately, and the inadequacy of cardiac output is termed "diastolic HF" or HF with preserved ejection fraction (HFpEF). Diastolic dysfunction, in its pure form, is characterized by signs and symptoms of HF in the presence of a normal functioning left ventricle. However, both systolic and diastolic dysfunction commonly coexist in HF.

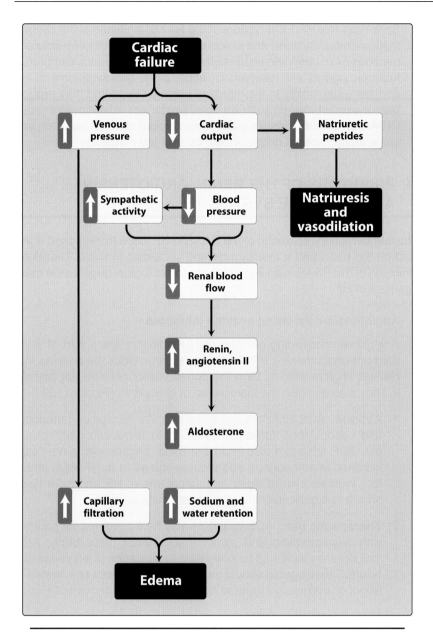

Figure 18.4
Cardiovascular consequences of HF.

D. Acute (decompensated) HF

If the compensatory mechanisms adequately restore cardiac output, HF is said to be compensated. If the compensatory mechanisms fail to maintain cardiac output, HF is decompensated and the patient develops worsening HF signs and symptoms. Typical HF signs and symptoms include dyspnea on exertion, orthopnea, paroxysmal nocturnal dyspnea, fatigue, and peripheral edema.

E. Therapeutic strategies in HF

Chronic HF is typically managed by fluid limitations (less than 1.5 to 2 L daily); low dietary intake of sodium (less than 2000 mg/d); treatment of comorbid conditions; and judicious use of diuretics.

Specifically for HFrEF, inhibitors of the RAAS, inhibitors of the sympathetic nervous system, and drugs that enhance activity of natriuretic peptides have been shown to improve survival and reduce symptoms. Inotropic agents are reserved for acute signs and symptoms of HF and are used mostly in the inpatient setting. Drugs that may precipitate or exacerbate HF, such as nonsteroidal anti-inflammatory drugs (NSAIDs), alcohol, nondihydropyridine calcium channel blockers, and some antiarrhythmic drugs, should be avoided if possible.

III. INHIBITORS OF THE RENIN–ANGIOTENSIN–ALDOSTERONE SYSTEM

The compensatory activation of the RAAS in HF leads to increased workload on the heart and a resultant decline in cardiac function. Therefore, inhibition of the RAAS is an important pharmacological target in the management of HF.

A. Angiotensin-converting enzyme inhibitors

Angiotensin-converting enzyme (ACE) inhibitors are a part of standard pharmacotherapy in HFrEF. These drugs block the enzyme that cleaves angiotensin I to form the potent vasoconstrictor angiotensin II. They also diminish the inactivation of bradykinin (Figure 18.5).

1. **Actions:** ACE inhibitors decrease vascular resistance (afterload) and venous tone (preload), resulting in increased cardiac output. ACE inhibitors also blunt the usual angiotensin II–mediated increase in epinephrine and aldosterone seen in HF. ACE inhibitors improve clinical signs and symptoms of HF and have been shown to significantly improve patient survival in HF.

2. **Therapeutic use:** ACE inhibitors may be considered for patients with asymptomatic and symptomatic HFrEF. Importantly, ACE inhibitors are indicated for patients with all stages of left ventricular failure. These agents should be started at low doses and titrated to target or maximally tolerated doses in the management of HFrEF.

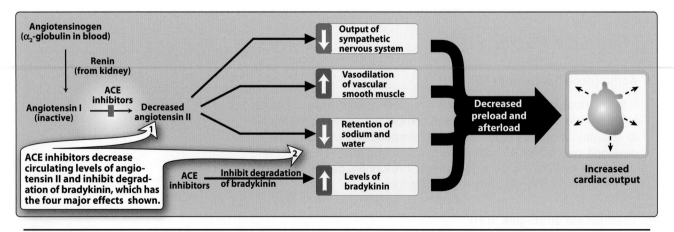

Figure 18.5
Effects of ACE inhibitors. [Note: The reduced retention of sodium and water results from two causes: decreased production of angiotensin II and aldosterone.]

ACE inhibitors are also used in the treatment of hypertension (see Chapter 16). Patients who have had a recent myocardial infarction or are at high risk for a cardiovascular event also benefit from long-term ACE inhibitor therapy.

3. **Pharmacokinetics:** ACE inhibitors are adequately absorbed following oral administration. Food may decrease the absorption of *captopril* [KAP-toe-pril], so it should be taken on an empty stomach. Except for *captopril* and injectable *enalaprilat* [en-AL-a-pril-at], ACE inhibitors are prodrugs that require activation by hydrolysis via hepatic enzymes. Renal elimination of the active moiety is important for most ACE inhibitors except *fosinopril* [foe-SIN-oh-pril], which also undergoes excretion in the feces. Plasma half-lives of active compounds vary from 2 to 12 hours, although the inhibition of ACE may be much longer.

4. **Adverse effects:** These include postural hypotension, renal insufficiency, hyperkalemia, a persistent dry cough, and angioedema (rare). Because of the risk of hyperkalemia, potassium levels must be monitored, particularly with concurrent use of potassium supplements, potassium-sparing diuretics, or aldosterone antagonists. Serum creatinine levels should also be monitored, particularly in patients with underlying renal disease. The potential for symptomatic hypotension with ACE inhibitors is much more common if used concomitantly with a diuretic. ACE inhibitors are teratogenic and should not be used in pregnant women. Please see Chapter 16 for a full discussion of ACE inhibitors.

B. Angiotensin receptor blockers

Angiotensin receptor blockers (ARBs) are orally active compounds that are competitive antagonists of the angiotensin II type 1 receptor. Because ACE inhibitors inhibit only one enzyme responsible for the production of angiotensin II, ARBs have the advantage of more complete blockade of the actions of angiotensin II. However, ARBs do not affect bradykinin levels. Although ARBs have actions similar to those of ACE inhibitors, they are not therapeutically identical. Even so, ARBs are a substitute for patients who cannot tolerate ACE inhibitors.

1. **Actions:** Although ARBs have a different mechanism of action than ACE inhibitors, their actions on preload and afterload are similar. Their use in HF is mainly as a substitute in patients who cannot tolerate ACE inhibitors due to cough or angioedema, which are thought to be mediated by elevated bradykinin levels. ARBs are also used in the treatment of hypertension (see Chapter 16).

2. **Pharmacokinetics:** ARBs are orally active and are dosed once daily, with the exception of *valsartan* [val-SAR-tan], which is dosed twice daily. They are highly plasma protein bound. *Losartan* [loe-SAR-tan] differs in that it undergoes extensive first-pass hepatic metabolism, including conversion to an active metabolite. The other drugs have inactive metabolites. Elimination of metabolites and parent compounds occurs in urine and feces.

3. **Adverse effects:** ARBs have an adverse effect and drug interaction profile similar to that of ACE inhibitors. However, the ARBs have a lower incidence of cough and angioedema. Like ACE inhibitors, ARBs are contraindicated in pregnancy.

C. Aldosterone receptor antagonists

Patients with HF have elevated levels of aldosterone due to angiotensin II stimulation and reduced hepatic clearance of the hormone. *Spironolactone* [spir-ON-oh-LAK-tone] and *eplerenone* [ep-LER-e-none] are antagonists of aldosterone at the mineralocorticoid receptor, thereby preventing salt retention, myocardial hypertrophy, and hypokalemia. *Spironolactone* also has affinity for androgen and progesterone receptors, and is associated with endocrine-related adverse effects such as gynecomastia and dysmenorrhea. Aldosterone antagonists are indicated in patients with symptomatic HFrEF or HFrEF and recent myocardial infarction. Please see Chapter 17 for a full discussion of aldosterone receptor antagonists.

IV. β-BLOCKERS

Although it may seem counterintuitive to administer drugs with negative inotropic activity in HF, evidence clearly demonstrates improved systolic function and reverse cardiac remodeling in patients receiving β-blockers. These benefits arise in spite of an occasional, initial exacerbation of symptoms. The benefit of β-blockers is attributed, in part, to their ability to prevent the changes that occur because of chronic activation of the sympathetic nervous system. These agents decrease heart rate and inhibit release of renin in the kidneys. In addition, β-blockers prevent the deleterious effects of norepinephrine on the cardiac muscle fibers, decreasing remodeling, hypertrophy, and cell death. Three β-blockers have shown benefit in HFrEF: *bisoprolol* [bis-oh-PROE-lol], *carvedilol* [KAR-ve-dil-ol], and long-acting *metoprolol succinate* [me-TOE-proe-lol SUK-si-nate]. *Carvedilol* is a nonselective β-adrenoreceptor antagonist that also blocks α-adrenoreceptors, whereas *bisoprolol* and *metoprolol succinate* are β_1-selective antagonists. [Note: The pharmacology of β-blockers is described in detail in Chapter 7.] β-Blockade is recommended for all patients with chronic, stable HFrEF. *Bisoprolol, carvedilol*, and *metoprolol succinate* reduce morbidity and mortality associated with HFrEF. Treatment should be started at low doses and gradually titrated to target doses based on patient tolerance and vital signs. Both *carvedilol* and *metoprolol* are metabolized by the cytochrome P450 2D6 isoenzyme, and inhibitors of this metabolic pathway may increase levels of these drugs and increase the risk of adverse effects. In addition, *carvedilol* is a substrate of P-glycoprotein (P-gp). Increased effects of *carvedilol* may occur if it is coadministered with P-gp inhibitors. β-Blockers should also be used with caution with other drugs that slow AV conduction, such as *amiodarone, verapamil*, and *diltiazem*.

V. DIURETICS

Diuretics reduce signs and symptoms of volume overload, such as dyspnea on exertion, orthopnea, and peripheral edema. Diuretics decrease plasma volume and, subsequently, decrease venous return to the heart (preload). This decreases cardiac workload and oxygen demand. Diuretics may also decrease afterload by reducing plasma volume, thereby decreasing blood pressure. Loop diuretics are the most commonly used diuretics in HF. These agents are used for patients who require extensive diuresis and those with renal insufficiency. Since diuretics have not been shown to improve survival in HF, they should only be used to treat signs and symptoms of volume excess. Please see Chapter 17 for a full discussion of diuretics.

VI. ANGIOTENSIN RECEPTOR–NEPRILYSIN INHIBITOR

Neprilysin is the enzyme responsible for breaking down vasoactive peptides, such as angiotensin I and II, bradykinin, and natriuretic peptides. Inhibition of neprilysin augments the activity of the vasoactive peptides. To maximize the effect of natriuretic peptides, stimulation of the RAAS must be offset without further increase in bradykinin. Therefore an ARB, instead of an ACE inhibitor, is combined with a neprilysin inhibitor to reduce the incidence of angioedema (Figure 18.6).

A. Sacubitril/valsartan

Sacubitril [sak-UE-bi-tril]/*valsartan* is the first available angiotensin receptor–neprilysin inhibitor (ARNI).

1. **Actions:** *Sacubitril/valsartan* combines the actions of an ARB with neprilysin inhibition. Inhibition of neprilysin results in increased concentration of vasoactive peptides, leading to natriuresis, diuresis, vasodilation, and inhibition of fibrosis. Together, the combination decreases afterload, preload, and myocardial fibrosis. An ARNI improves survival and clinical signs and symptoms of HF, as compared to therapy with an ACE inhibitor.

2. **Therapeutic use:** An ARNI should replace an ACE inhibitor or ARB in patients with HFrEF who remain symptomatic on optimal doses of a β-blocker and an ACE inhibitor or ARB.

3. **Pharmacokinetics:** *Sacubitril/valsartan* is orally active, administered with or without food, and quickly breaks down into the separate components. *Sacubitril* is transformed to active drug

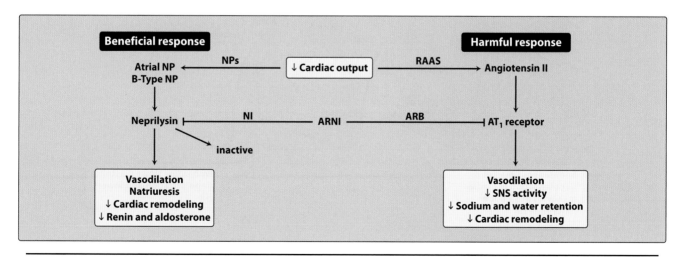

Figure 18.6
Effects of angiotensin receptor blocker–neprilysin inhibitors. ARB = angiotensin receptor blocker; ARNI = angiotensin receptor neprilysin inhibitor; AT1 = angiotensin type 1; NI, neprilysin inhibitor; NP = natriuretic peptide; RAAS = renin–angiotensin–aldosterone system; SNS = sympathetic nervous system.

by plasma esterases. Both drugs have a high volume of distribution and are highly bound to plasma proteins. *Sacubitril* is mainly excreted in the urine. The half-life of approximately 10 hours for both components allows for twice-daily dosing.

4. **Adverse effects:** The adverse effect profile is similar to that of an ACE inhibitor or ARB. Because of the added reduction of afterload, hypotension is more common with an ARNI. Due to inhibition of neprilysin with *sacubitril*, bradykinin levels may increase and angioedema may occur. Therefore, the combination is contraindicated in patients with a history of hereditary angioedema or angioedema associated with an ACE inhibitor or ARB. To minimize risk of angioedema, an ACE inhibitor must be stopped at least 36 hours prior to starting *sacubitril/valsartan*.

VII. HYPERPOLARIZATION-ACTIVATED CYCLIC NUCLEOTIDE–GATED CHANNEL BLOCKER

The hyperpolarization-activated cyclic nucleotide–gated (HCN) channel is responsible for the I_f current and setting the pace within the SA node. Inhibition of the HCN channel results in slowing of depolarization and a lower heart rate (Figure 18.7). Reduction in heart rate is use and dose dependent.

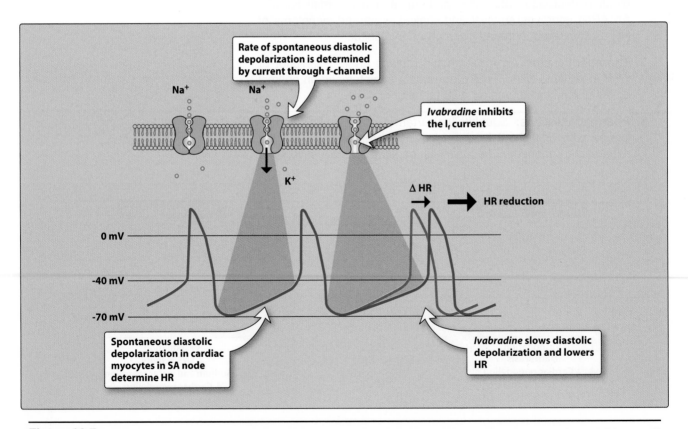

Figure 18.7
Effects of inhibition of I_f current with *ivabradine*. HR = heart rate; K^+ = potassium; Na^+ = sodium; SA = sinoatrial.

A. Ivabradine

Ivabradine [eye-VAB-ra-deen] is the only approved drug in the class of HCN channel blockers.

1. **Actions:** By selectively slowing the I_f current in the SA node, reduction of heart rate occurs without a reduction in contractility, AV conduction, ventricular repolarization, or blood pressure. In patients with HFrEF, a slower heart rate increases stroke volume and improves symptoms of HF.

2. **Therapeutic use:** *Ivabradine* is utilized in HFrEF to improve symptoms in patients who are in sinus rhythm with a heart rate above 70 beats per minute and are on optimized HF pharmacotherapy. Specifically, patients should be on an optimal dose of β-blocker or have a contraindication to β-blockers.

3. **Pharmacokinetics:** *Ivabradine* should be administered with meals to increase absorption. It undergoes extensive first-pass metabolism by cytochrome P450 3A4 to an active metabolite, which is also a 3A4 substrate. *Ivabradine* has a high volume of distribution and is 70% protein bound. The half-life is 6 hours, which allows for twice-daily dosing.

4. **Adverse effects:** Bradycardia may occur with *ivabradine*, which may improve with dose reduction. Because *ivabradine* is mostly selective for the SA node, it is not effective for rate control in atrial fibrillation and has been shown to increase the risk of atrial fibrillation. *Ivabradine* inhibits similar channels in the eye, and luminous phenomena may occur early in therapy. This enhanced brightness may be ameliorated by dose reduction. *Ivabradine* should not be used in pregnancy or breast-feeding, with more advanced heart block, or with potent 3A4 inhibitors.

VIII. VASO- AND VENODILATORS

Dilation of venous blood vessels leads to a decrease in cardiac preload by increasing venous capacitance. Nitrates are commonly used venous dilators to reduce preload for patients with chronic HF. Arterial dilators, such as *hydralazine* [hye-DRAL-a-zeen], reduce systemic arteriolar resistance and decrease afterload. If the patient is intolerant of ACE inhibitors or ARBs, or if additional vasodilator response is required, a combination of *hydralazine* and *isosorbide dinitrate* [eye-soe-SOR-bide dye-NYE-trate] may be used. A fixed-dose combination of these agents has been shown to improve symptoms and survival in black patients with HFrEF on standard HF treatment (β-blocker plus ACE inhibitor or ARB). Headache, dizziness, and hypotension are common adverse effects with this combination. Rarely, *hydralazine* has been associated with drug-induced lupus.

IX. INOTROPIC DRUGS

Positive inotropic agents enhance cardiac contractility and, thus, increase cardiac output. Although these drugs act by different mechanisms, the inotropic action is the result of an increased cytoplasmic calcium concentration that enhances the contractility of cardiac muscle. All positive inotropes in HFrEF that increase intracellular calcium concentration have been associated with reduced survival, especially in patients with HFrEF. For this reason, these agents, with the exception of *digoxin*, are only used for a short period mainly in the inpatient setting.

A. Digitalis glycosides

The cardiac glycosides are often called digitalis or digitalis glycosides, because most of the drugs come from the digitalis (foxglove) plant. They are a group of chemically similar compounds that can increase the contractility of the heart muscle and, therefore, are used in treating HF. The digitalis glycosides have a low therapeutic index, with only a small difference between a therapeutic dose and doses that are toxic or even fatal. The only available agent is *digoxin* [di-JOX-in].

1. Mechanism of action

a. Regulation of cytosolic calcium concentration: By inhibiting the Na^+/K^+-adenosine triphosphatase (ATPase) enzyme, *digoxin* reduces the ability of the myocyte to actively pump Na^+ from the cell (Figure 18.8). This ultimately results in a small but physiologically important increase in free Ca^{2+}, thereby leading to increased cardiac contractility.

b. Increased contractility of the cardiac muscle: *Digoxin* increases the force of cardiac contraction, causing cardiac output to more closely resemble that of the normal heart (Figure 18.9). Vagal tone is also enhanced, so both heart rate and myocardial oxygen demand decrease. *Digoxin* slows conduction velocity through the AV node, making it useful for atrial fibrillation.

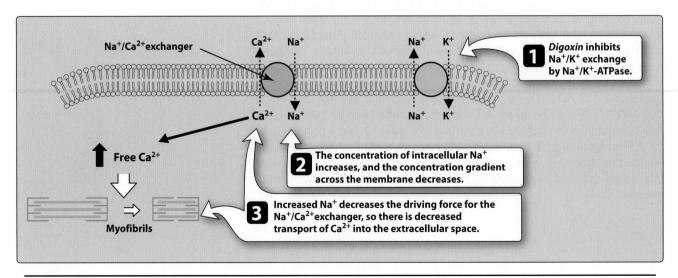

Figure 18.8
Mechanism of action of *digoxin*. ATPase = adenosine triphosphatase.

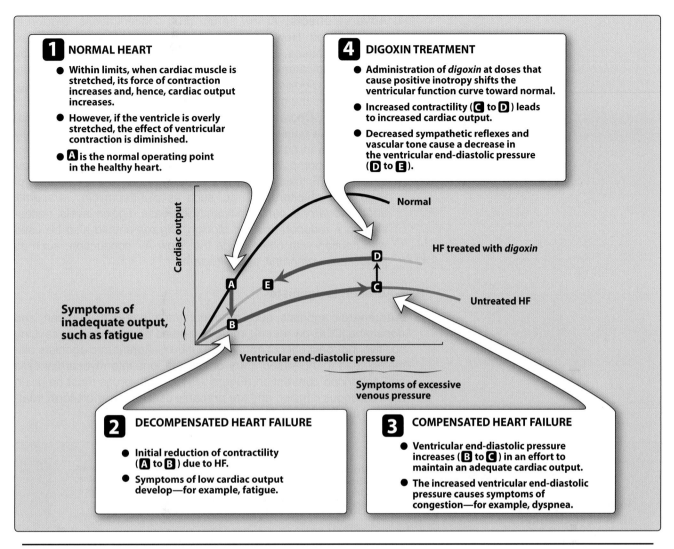

Figure 18.9
Ventricular function curves in the normal heart, in heart failure (HF), and in HF treated with *digoxin*.

    c. Neurohormonal inhibition: Although the exact mechanism of this effect has not been elucidated, low-dose *digoxin* inhibits sympathetic activation with minimal effects on contractility. This effect is the reason a lower serum drug concentration is targeted in HFrEF.

2. Therapeutic use: *Digoxin* therapy is indicated in patients with HFrEF who are symptomatic on optimal HF pharmacotherapy. A low serum drug concentration of *digoxin* (0.5 to 0.8 ng/mL) is beneficial in HFrEF.

3. Pharmacokinetics: *Digoxin* is available in oral and injectable formulations. It has a large volume of distribution, because it accumulates in muscle. The dosage is based on lean body weight. In acute situations, such as symptomatic atrial fibrillation, a loading dose regimen is used. *Digoxin* has a long half-life of 30 to 40 hours. It is mainly eliminated intact by the kidney, requiring dose adjustment in renal dysfunction.

4. **Adverse effects:** At low serum drug concentrations, *digoxin* is well tolerated. However, it has a very narrow therapeutic index. Anorexia, nausea, vomiting, blurred vision, or yellowish vision may be initial indicators of toxicity. When Na⁺/K⁺-ATPase is markedly inhibited by *digoxin*, the resting membrane potential may increase, which makes the membrane more excitable, increasing the risk of arrhythmias. Decreased levels of serum potassium (hypokalemia) predispose a patient to *digoxin* toxicity, because *digoxin* normally competes with potassium for the same binding site on the Na⁺/K⁺-ATPase pump. With the use of a lower serum drug concentration in HFrEF, toxic levels are infrequent. *Digoxin* is a substrate of P-gp, and inhibitors of P-gp, such as *clarithromycin*, *verapamil*, and *amiodarone*, can significantly increase *digoxin* levels, necessitating a reduced dose of *digoxin*. *Digoxin* should also be used with caution with other drugs that slow AV conduction, such as β-blockers, *verapamil*, and *diltiazem*.

B. β-Adrenergic agonists

β-Adrenergic agonists, such as *dobutamine* [doe-BUE-ta-meen] and *dopamine* [DOE-pa-meen], improve cardiac performance by causing positive inotropic effects and vasodilation. β-Adrenergic agonists ultimately lead to increased entry of calcium ions into myocardial cells and enhanced contraction (Figure 18.10). Both drugs must be given by intravenous infusion and are primarily used in the short-term treatment of acute HF in the hospital setting.

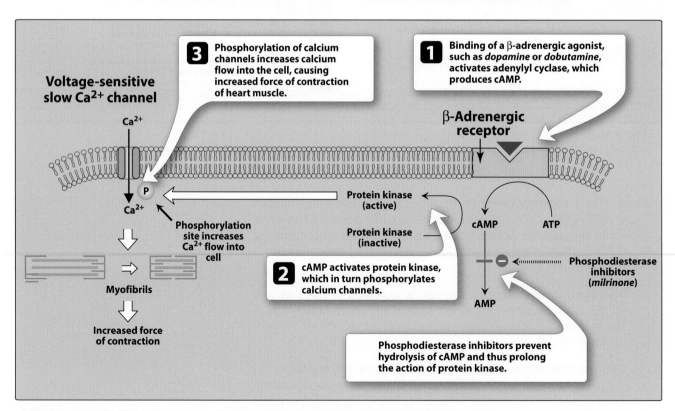

Figure 18.10
Sites of action by β-adrenergic agonists on heart muscle. AMP = adenosine monophosphate; ATP = adenosine triphosphate; cAMP = cyclic adenosine monophosphate; P = phosphate.

C. Phosphodiesterase inhibitors

Milrinone [MIL-ri-none] is a phosphodiesterase inhibitor that increases the intracellular concentration of cAMP (Figure 18.10). Like β-adrenergic agonists, this results in an increase of intracellular calcium and, therefore, cardiac contractility. *Milrinone* is usually given by intravenous infusion for short-term treatment of acute HF. However, *dobutamine* and *milrinone* may also be considered for intermediate-term treatment in the outpatient setting for palliative care.

X. RECOMBINANT B-TYPE NATRIURETIC PEPTIDE

In acute decompensated congestive HF, drugs that reduce preload result in improvement in HF symptoms such as dyspnea. Most often, IV diuretics are utilized in the acute setting to reduce preload. When IV diuretics are minimally effective, a recombinant B-type natriuretic peptide (BNP), or *nesiritide* [ness-EAR-a-tide], can be used as an alternative. Through binding to natriuretic peptide receptors, *nesiritide* stimulates natriuresis and diuresis and reduces preload and afterload. *Nesiritide* is administered intravenously as a bolus (most often) and continuous infusion. Like endogenous BNP, *nesiritide* has a short half-life of 20 minutes and is cleared by renal filtration, cleavage by endopeptidases and through internalization after binding to natriuretic peptide receptors. The most common adverse effects are hypotension and dizziness, and like diuretics, *nesiritide* can worsen renal function.

XI. ORDER OF THERAPY

Guidelines have classified HF into four stages, from least to most severe. Figure 18.11 shows a treatment strategy using this classification and the drugs described in this chapter. Note that as the disease progresses, polytherapy is initiated. In patients with overt HF, loop diuretics are often introduced first for relief of signs or symptoms of volume overload, such as dyspnea and peripheral edema. ACE inhibitors or ARBs (if ACE inhibitors are not tolerated) are added after the optimization of diuretic therapy. The dosage is gradually titrated to that which is maximally tolerated and/or produces optimal cardiac output. Historically, β-blockers were added after optimization of ACE inhibitor or ARB therapy; however, most patients newly diagnosed with HFrEF are initiated on both low doses of an ACE inhibitor and β-blocker after initial stabilization. These agents are slowly titrated to optimal levels to increase tolerability. Aldosterone antagonists and fixed-dose *hydralazine* and *isosorbide dinitrate* are initiated in patients who continue to have HF symptoms despite optimal doses of an ACE inhibitor and β-blocker. Once at an optimal ACE inhibitor or ARB dose and if the patient remains symptomatic, either can be replaced by *sacubitril/valsartan*. Lastly, *digoxin* and *ivabradine* are added for symptomatic benefit only in patients on optimal HF pharmacotherapy.

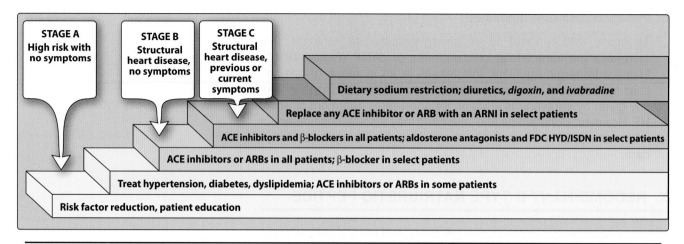

Figure 18.11
Treatment options for various stages of HF. ACE = angiotensin-converting enzyme; ARBs = angiotensin receptor blockers; FDC = fixed-dose combination; HYD = hydralazine; ISDN = isosorbide dinitrate. Stage D (refractory symptoms requiring special interventions) is not shown.

Study Questions

Choose the ONE best answer.

18.1 A patient is newly diagnosed with HFrEF and is asymptomatic. Which is the most appropriate drug to initiate for symptomatic and survival benefits?

   A. Dobutamine

   B. Furosemide

   C. Lisinopril

   D. Sacubitril/valsartan

> Correct answer = C. ACE inhibitors should be initiated in all patients, unless contraindicated, if they have HFrEF and are asymptomatic. This is known as stage B HF. Dobutamine and furosemide improve symptoms only. Sacubitril/valsartan will replace an ACE inhibitor if the patient remains symptomatic on optimal HF pharmacotherapy.

18.2 Which of the following statements best describes the action of ACE inhibitors on the failing heart?

   A. Increased vascular resistance.

   B. Decreased cardiac output.

   C. Reduced preload.

   D. Increased aldosterone.

> Correct answer = C. ACE inhibitors decrease vascular resistance, decrease preload, decrease afterload, and increase cardiac output. In addition, ACE inhibitors blunt aldosterone release.

18.3 A Hispanic man with HFrEF currently takes maximally tolerated doses of metoprolol succinate and enalapril, along with moderate-dose furosemide. He is euvolemic, but continues to have HF symptoms. The systolic blood pressure is low, but the patient does not have signs or symptoms of hypotension. Which is the best recommendation to improve HF symptoms and survival in this patient?

   A. Stop enalapril, wait 36 hours, and start sacubitril/valsartan.

   B. Start digoxin.

   C. Start fixed-dose hydralazine and isosorbide dinitrate.

   D. Start spironolactone.

> Correct answer = D. Because the patient is on optimal pharmacotherapy and continues to have symptoms, another agent is warranted. Adding low-dose spironolactone is unlikely to decrease the blood pressure and will confer a survival and symptomatic benefit. Changing to sacubitril/valsartan will likely worsen the low blood pressure. Digoxin will only improve symptoms and not improve survival. Fixed-dose hydralazine and isosorbide dinitrate would be appropriate if the patient were African American.

18.4 β-Blockers improve cardiac function in HF by

    A. decreasing cardiac remodeling

    B. increasing heart rate

    C. increasing renin release

    D. activating norepinephrine

> Correct answer = A. Although it seems counterintuitive to decrease heart rate in HF, β-blockers improve cardiac function by slowing heart rate, decreasing renin release, and preventing the direct effects of norepinephrine on cardiac muscle to decrease remodeling.

18.5 A 70-year-old woman has HFrEF and hypertension. She takes lisinopril and metoprolol tartrate. She feels well and has no cough, shortness of breath, or edema. Which of the following changes is most appropriate for her drug therapy?

    A. Initiate digoxin.

    B. Change lisinopril to losartan.

    C. Initiate ivabradine.

    D. Change metoprolol tartrate to metoprolol succinate.

> Correct answer = D. Metoprolol succinate should be used in HF, given that there is mortality benefit shown with metoprolol succinate in landmark HF trials. Digoxin and ivabradine are not indicated since symptoms are minimal and she is not yet on optimized guideline-directed medical therapy; there is no reason to change to an ARB since the patient has no cough or history of angioedema.

18.6 A 75-year-old white man has HFrEF and reports stable HF symptoms. His current drug therapy includes optimal-dose enalapril, carvedilol, and spironolactone. Which is the best recommendation to improve HF symptoms and survival?

    A. Start fixed-dose hydralazine/isosorbide dinitrate.

    B. Start ivabradine.

    C. Replace enalapril with sacubitril/valsartan.

    D. Start digoxin.

> Correct answer = C. Since patient is on optimal doses of HF medications and he continues to have symptoms, replacing enalapril with sacubitril/valsartan is the only option that improves both symptoms and survival in a white patient.

18.7 How is spironolactone beneficial in HF?

    A. Promotes potassium secretion

    B. Acts as aldosterone agonist

    C. Prevents cardiac hypertrophy

    D. Decreases blood glucose

> Correct answer = C. Spironolactone antagonizes aldosterone, which in turn prevents salt/water retention, cardiac hypertrophy, and hypokalemia. Spironolactone has endocrine effects on hormones, but not on glucose.

18.8 Which of the following is important to monitor in patients taking digoxin?

    A. Chloride

    B. Potassium

    C. Sodium

    D. Zinc

> Correct answer = B. Hypokalemia can lead to life-threatening arrhythmias and increases the potential of cardiac toxicity with digoxin.

18.9 Which of the following describes the mechanism of action of milrinone in HF?

    A. Decreases intracellular calcium

    B. Increases cardiac contractility

    C. Decreases cAMP

    D. Activates phosphodiesterase

> Correct answer = B. Milrinone is a phosphodiesterase inhibitor that leads to increased cAMP, increased intracellular calcium, and therefore increased contractility.

18.10 BH is a 52-year-old African American woman who has HFrEF. She is seen in clinic today reporting stable HF symptoms, but is having occasional peripheral brightness. Otherwise, vision is unchanged. Current medication regimen includes sacubitril/valsartan, carvedilol, fixed-dose hydralazine and isosorbide dinitrate, ivabradine, and bumetanide. Which is the best recommendation to minimize the adverse effect of peripheral brightness?

    A. Stop all HF medications immediately.

    B. Discontinue sacubitril/valsartan only.

    C. Do nothing; this adverse effect will slowly improve over time.

    D. Reduce the dose of ivabradine.

> Correct answer = D. Luminous phenomena can occur with ivabradine. This adverse effect can be minimized with dose reduction or discontinuation.

Antiarrhythmics

Shawn Anderson and Michelle Chung

19

I. OVERVIEW

In contrast to skeletal muscle, which contracts only when it receives a stimulus, the heart contains specialized cells that exhibit automaticity. That is, they intrinsically generate rhythmic action potentials in the absence of external stimuli. These "pacemaker" cells differ from other myocardial cells in showing a slow, spontaneous depolarization during diastole (phase 4), caused by an inward positive current carried by sodium and calcium ions. This depolarization is fastest in the sinoatrial (SA) node (the initiation site of the action potential), and it decreases throughout the normal conduction pathway through the atrioventricular (AV) node to the bundle of His and the Purkinje system. Dysfunction of impulse generation or conduction at any of a number of sites in the heart can cause an abnormality in cardiac rhythm. Figure 19.1 summarizes the drugs used to treat cardiac arrhythmias.

II. INTRODUCTION TO THE ARRHYTHMIAS

Arrhythmias are caused by abnormalities in impulse formation and conduction in the myocardium. Arrhythmias present as a complex family of disorders with a variety of symptoms. To make sense of this large group of disorders, it is useful to organize arrhythmias into groups according to anatomic site of the abnormality: the atria, the AV node, or the ventricles. Figure 19.2 summarizes several common arrhythmias.

A. Causes of arrhythmias

Most arrhythmias arise either from aberrations in impulse generation (abnormal automaticity) or from a defect in impulse conduction.

1. **Abnormal automaticity:** The SA node shows a faster rate of discharge than do other pacemaker cells, and thus, it normally sets the pace of contraction for the myocardium. If cardiac sites other than the SA node show enhanced automaticity, they may generate competing stimuli, and arrhythmias may arise. Most of the antiarrhythmic agents suppress automaticity by blocking either sodium (Na^+) or calcium (Ca^{2+}) channels to reduce the ratio of these ions to potassium (K^+). This decreases the slope of phase 4 (diastolic) depolarization and/or raises the threshold of discharge to a less

CLASS I (Na⁺-channel blockers)
Disopyramide (IA) NORPACE
Flecainide (IC) TAMBOCOR
Lidocaine (IB) XYLOCAINE
Mexiletine (IB) GENERIC ONLY
Procainamide (IA) GENERIC ONLY
Propafenone (IC) RYTHMOL
Quinidine (IA) GENERIC ONLY

CLASS II (β-adrenoreceptor blockers)
Atenolol TENORMIN
Esmolol BREVIBLOC
Metoprolol LOPRESSOR, TOPROL-XL

CLASS III (K⁺ channel blockers)
Amiodarone CORDARONE, PACERONE
Dofetilide TIKOSYN
Dronedarone MULTAQ
Ibutilide CORVERT
Sotalol BETAPACE, SORINE

CLASS IV (Ca²⁺ channel blockers)
Diltiazem CARDIZEM, CARTIA, TIAZAC
Verapamil CALAN, VERELAN

OTHER ANTIARRHYTHMIC DRUGS
Adenosine ADENOCARD
Digoxin LANOXIN
Magnesium sulfate GENERIC ONLY
Ranolazine RANEXA

Figure 19.1
Summary of antiarrhythmic drugs.

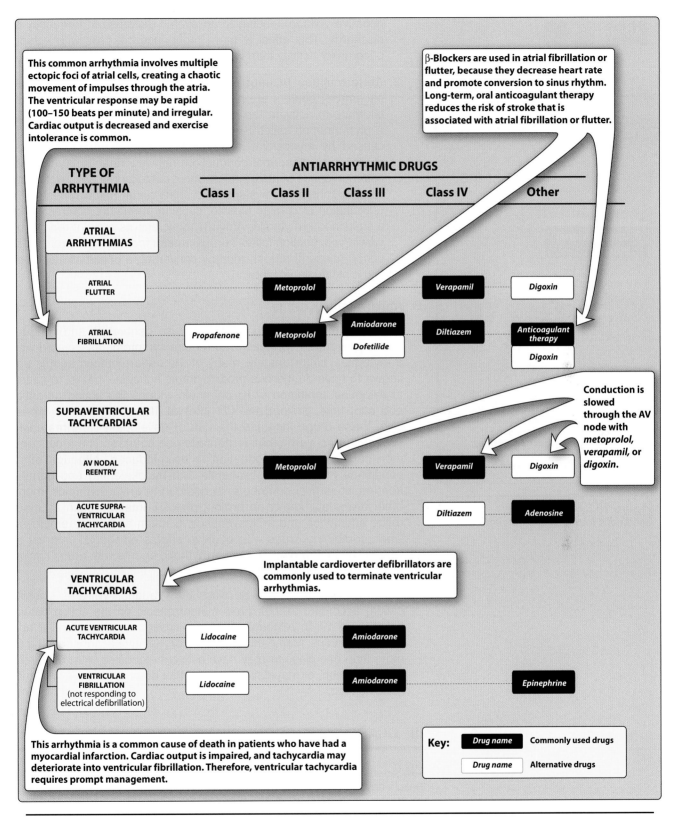

Figure 19.2
Therapeutic indications for some commonly encountered arrhythmias. AV = atrioventricular.

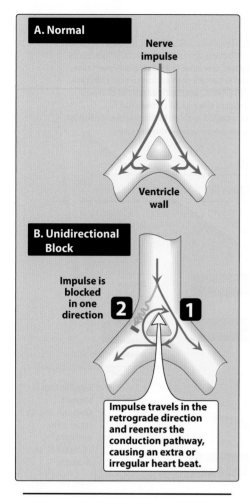

Figure 19.3
Schematic representation of reentry.

negative voltage, leading to an overall decrease in frequency of discharge. This effect is more pronounced in cells with ectopic pacemaker activity than in normal cells.

2. **Abnormalities in impulse conduction:** Impulses from higher pacemaker centers are normally conducted down pathways that bifurcate to activate the entire ventricular surface (Figure 19.3). A phenomenon called reentry can occur if a unidirectional block caused by myocardial injury or a prolonged refractory period results in an abnormal conduction pathway. Reentry is the most common cause of arrhythmias, and it can occur at any level of the cardiac conduction system. This short-circuit pathway results in reexcitation of cardiac muscle, causing premature contraction or a sustained arrhythmia. Antiarrhythmic agents prevent reentry by slowing conduction (class I drugs) and/or increasing the refractory period (class III drugs), thereby converting a unidirectional block into a bidirectional block.

B. Antiarrhythmic drugs

Antiarrhythmic drugs can modify impulse generation and conduction to prevent arrhythmias or to reduce symptoms associated with arrhythmias. Unfortunately, many of the antiarrhythmic agents are known to have dangerous proarrhythmic actions—that is, to cause arrhythmias. Inhibition of K^+ channels widens the action potential and can, thus, prolong the QT interval. If prolongation is excessive, these drugs increase the risk of developing life-threatening ventricular tachyarrhythmias (torsades de pointes). The most common cause of QT prolongation is drug-induced, although other conditions (for example, ischemia and hypokalemia) and genetic abnormalities may contribute. In addition to antiarrhythmics, many other drugs are known to prolong the QT interval, such as macrolide antibiotics and antipsychotics. Caution should be employed when combining drugs with additive effects on the QT interval or when giving QT-prolonging antiarrhythmic agents with drugs known to inhibit their metabolism.

Antiarrhythmic drugs can be classified (Vaughan-Williams classification) according to their predominant effects on the action potential (Figure 19.4). Although this classification is convenient, it has some limitations. Many antiarrhythmic drugs have actions relating to more than one class or may have active metabolites with a different class of action, or may have an action that does not meet any formal classification.

III. CLASS I ANTIARRHYTHMIC DRUGS

Class I antiarrhythmic drugs act by blocking voltage-sensitive Na^+ channels. They bind more rapidly to open or inactivated Na^+ channels than to channels that are fully repolarized. Therefore, these drugs show a greater degree of blockade in tissues that are frequently depolarizing. This property is called use dependence (or state dependence), and it enables these drugs to block cells that are discharging at an abnormally high frequency, without interfering with the normal beating of the heart.

CLASSIFICATION OF DRUG	MECHANISM OF ACTION	COMMENT
IA	Na⁺ channel blocker	Slows Phase 0 depolarization in ventricular muscle fibers
IB	Na⁺ channel blocker	Shortens Phase 3 repolarization in ventricular muscle fibers
IC	Na⁺ channel blocker	Markedly slows Phase 0 depolarization in ventricular muscle fibers
II	β-Adrenoreceptor blocker	Inhibits Phase 4 depolarization in SA and AV nodes
III	K⁺ channel blocker	Prolongs Phase 3 repolarization in ventricular muscle fibers
IV	Ca²⁺ channel blocker	Inhibits action potential in SA and AV nodes

Figure 19.4
Actions of antiarrhythmic drugs. SA = sinoatrial; AV = atrioventricular.

The use of Na⁺ channel blockers has declined due to their proarrhythmic effects, particularly in patients with reduced left ventricular function and atherosclerotic heart disease. Class I drugs are further subdivided into three groups according to their effect on the duration of the cardiac action potential (Figure 19.4).

A. Class IA antiarrhythmic drugs: Quinidine, procainamide, and disopyramide

Quinidine [KWIH-nih-deen] is the prototype class IA drug. Other agents in this class include *procainamide* [proe-KANE-a-mide] and *disopyramide* [dye-soe-PEER-a-mide]. Because of their concomitant class III activity, they can precipitate arrhythmias that can progress to ventricular fibrillation.

1. **Mechanism of action:** *Quinidine* binds to open and inactivated Na⁺ channels and prevents Na⁺ influx, thus slowing the rapid upstroke during phase 0 (Figure 19.5). It decreases the slope of phase 4 spontaneous depolarization, inhibits K⁺ channels, and blocks Ca²⁺ channels. Because of these actions, it slows conduction velocity and increases refractoriness. *Quinidine* also has mild α-adrenergic blocking and anticholinergic actions. Although *procainamide* and *disopyramide* have actions similar to those of *quinidine*, there is less anticholinergic activity with *procainamide* and more with *disopyramide*. Neither *procainamide* nor *disopyramide* has α-blocking activity. *Disopyramide* produces a greater negative inotropic effect, and unlike the other drugs, it causes peripheral vasoconstriction.

2. **Therapeutic uses:** *Quinidine* is used in the treatment of a wide variety of arrhythmias, including atrial, AV junctional, and ventricular tachyarrhythmias. *Procainamide* is only available in an intravenous formulation and may be used to treat acute atrial and ventricular arrhythmias. However, electrical cardioversion or defibrillation and *amiodarone* have mostly replaced *procainamide* in clinical practice. *Disopyramide* can be used as an alternative

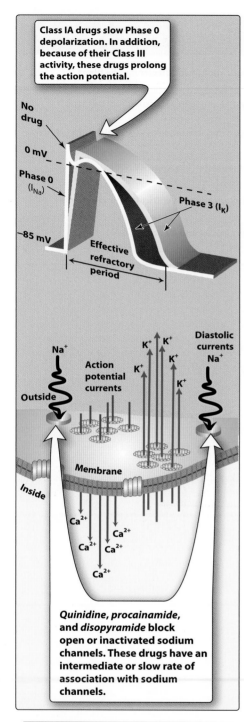

Class IA drugs slow Phase 0 depolarization. In addition, because of their Class III activity, these drugs prolong the action potential.

No drug

0 mV

Phase 0 (I_{Na})

Phase 3 (I_K)

–85 mV

Effective refractory period

Na^+

Action potential currents

K^+ K^+

K^+

K^+

K^+

Diastolic currents Na^+

Outside

Membrane

Inside

Ca^{2+}

Ca^{2+} Ca^{2+}

Ca^{2+} Ca^{2+}

Ca^{2+}

Quinidine, procainamide, and *disopyramide* block open or inactivated sodium channels. These drugs have an intermediate or slow rate of association with sodium channels.

Figure 19.5
Schematic diagram of the effects of class IA agents. I_{Na} and I_K are transmembrane currents due to the movement of Na^+ and K^+, respectively.

treatment of ventricular arrhythmias and may also be used for rhythm control in atrial fibrillation or flutter.

3. **Pharmacokinetics:** *Quinidine sulfate* or *gluconate* is rapidly and well absorbed after oral administration. It undergoes extensive metabolism primarily by the hepatic cytochrome P450 3A4 (CYP3A4) isoenzyme, forming active metabolites. A portion of *procainamide* is acetylated in the liver to *N*-acetylprocainamide (NAPA), which has the properties and adverse effects of a class III drug. NAPA is eliminated via the kidney; therefore, dosages of *procainamide* should be adjusted in patients with renal dysfunction. *Disopyramide* is well absorbed after oral administration and is metabolized in the liver by CYP3A4 to a less active metabolite and several inactive metabolites. About half of the drug is excreted unchanged by the kidneys.

4. **Adverse effects:** Due to enhanced proarrhythmic effects and ability to worsen heart failure symptoms, class IA drugs should not be used in patients with atherosclerotic heart disease or systolic heart failure. Large doses of *quinidine* may induce the symptoms of cinchonism (for example, blurred vision, tinnitus, headache, disorientation, and psychosis). Drug interactions are common with *quinidine* since it is an inhibitor of both CYP2D6 and P-glycoprotein. Intravenous administration of *procainamide* may cause hypotension. *Disopyramide* has the most anticholinergic adverse effects of the class IA drugs (for example, dry mouth, urinary retention, blurred vision, and constipation). Both *quinidine* and *disopyramide* should be used with caution with potent inhibitors of CYP3A4.

B. Class IB antiarrhythmic drugs: Lidocaine and mexiletine

The class IB agents rapidly associate and dissociate from Na^+ channels. Thus, the actions are greater when the cardiac cell is depolarized or firing rapidly. The class IB drugs *lidocaine* [LYE-doe-kane] and *mexiletine* [mex-IL-e-teen] are useful in treating ventricular arrhythmias.

1. **Mechanism of action:** In addition to Na^+ channel blockade, *lidocaine* and *mexiletine* shorten phase 3 repolarization and decrease the duration of the action potential (Figure 19.6). Neither drug contributes to negative inotropy.

2. **Therapeutic uses:** Although *amiodarone* is the drug of choice for ventricular fibrillation or ventricular tachycardia (VT), *lidocaine* may be used as an alternative. *Lidocaine* may also be used in combination with *amiodarone* for VT storm. The drug does not markedly slow conduction and, thus, has little effect on atrial or AV junction arrhythmias. *Mexiletine* is used for chronic treatment of ventricular arrhythmias, often in combination with *amiodarone*.

3. **Pharmacokinetics:** *Lidocaine* is given intravenously because of extensive first-pass transformation by the liver. The drug is dealkylated to two active metabolites, primarily by CYP1A2 with a minor role by CYP3A4. *Lidocaine* should be monitored closely when

given in combination with drugs affecting these CYP isoenzymes. *Mexiletine* is well absorbed after oral administration. It is metabolized in the liver primarily by CYP2D6 to inactive metabolites and excreted mainly via the biliary route.

4. **Adverse effects:** *Lidocaine* has a fairly wide therapeutic index. Central nervous system (CNS) effects include nystagmus (early indicator of toxicity), drowsiness, slurred speech, paresthesia, agitation, confusion, and convulsions, which often limit the duration of continuous infusions. *Mexiletine* has a narrow therapeutic index and caution should be used when administering the drug with inhibitors of CYP2D6. Nausea, vomiting, and dyspepsia are the most common adverse effects.

C. Class IC antiarrhythmic drugs: Flecainide and propafenone

These drugs slowly dissociate from resting Na+ channels and show prominent effects even at normal heart rates. Due to their negative inotropic and proarrhythmic effects, use of these agents is avoided in patients with structural heart disease (left ventricular hypertrophy, heart failure, atherosclerotic heart disease).

1. **Mechanism of action:** *Flecainide* [FLEK-a-nide] suppresses phase 0 upstroke in Purkinje and myocardial fibers (Figure 19.7). This causes marked slowing of conduction in all cardiac tissue, with a minor effect on the duration of the action potential and refractoriness. Automaticity is reduced by an increase in the threshold potential, rather than a decrease in slope of phase 4 depolarization. *Flecainide* also blocks K+ channels, leading to increased duration of the action potential. *Propafenone* [proe-PAF-e-none], like *flecainide*, slows conduction in all cardiac tissues but does not block K+ channels. It possesses weak β-blocking properties.

2. **Therapeutic uses:** *Flecainide* is useful in the maintenance of sinus rhythm in atrial flutter or fibrillation in patients without structural heart disease and in treating refractory ventricular arrhythmias. Use of *propafenone* is restricted mostly to atrial arrhythmias: rhythm control of atrial fibrillation or flutter and paroxysmal supraventricular tachycardia prophylaxis in patients with AV reentrant tachycardias.

3. **Pharmacokinetics:** *Flecainide* is well absorbed after oral administration and is metabolized by CYP2D6 to multiple metabolites. The parent drug and metabolites are mostly eliminated renally. *Propafenone* is metabolized to active metabolites primarily via CYP2D6, and also by CYP1A2 and CYP3A4. The metabolites are excreted in the urine and the feces.

4. **Adverse effects:** *Flecainide* is generally well tolerated, with blurred vision, dizziness, and nausea occurring most frequently. *Propafenone* has a similar side effect profile, but may cause bronchospasm and should be avoided in patients with asthma. *Propafenone* is also an inhibitor of P-glycoprotein. Both drugs should be used with caution with potent inhibitors of CYP2D6.

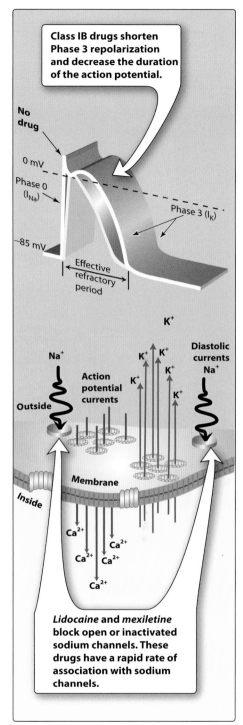

Figure 19.6
Schematic diagram of the effects of class IB agents. I_{Na} and I_K are transmembrane currents due to the movement of Na+ and K+, respectively.

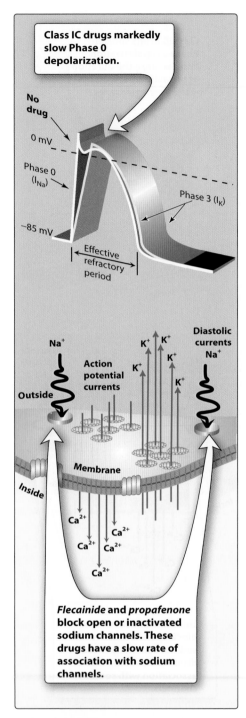

Class IC drugs markedly slow Phase 0 depolarization.

No drug

0 mV

Phase 0 (I_{Na})

Phase 3 (I_K)

−85 mV

Effective refractory period

Na$^+$

Action potential currents

K$^+$ K$^+$

K$^+$

K$^+$

K$^+$

Diastolic currents Na$^+$

Outside

Membrane

Inside

Ca^{2+}

Ca^{2+}

Ca^{2+} Ca^{2+}

Ca^{2+}

Flecainide and *propafenone* block open or inactivated sodium channels. These drugs have a slow rate of association with sodium channels.

Figure 19.7
Schematic diagram of the effects of class IC agents. I_{Na} and I_K are transmembrane currents due to the movement of Na$^+$ and K$^+$, respectively.

IV. CLASS II ANTIARRHYTHMIC DRUGS

Class II agents are β-adrenergic antagonists, or β-blockers. These drugs diminish phase 4 depolarization and, thus, depress automaticity, prolong AV conduction, and decrease heart rate and contractility. Class II agents are useful in treating tachyarrhythmias caused by increased sympathetic activity. They are also used for atrial flutter and fibrillation and for AV nodal reentrant tachycardia. In addition, β-blockers prevent life-threatening ventricular arrhythmias following a myocardial infarction.

Metoprolol [me-TOE-pro-lol] is the most widely used β-blocker for the treatment of cardiac arrhythmias. Compared to nonselective β-blockers, such as *propranolol* [pro-PRAN-oh-lol], it reduces the risk of bronchospasm. It is extensively metabolized by CYP2D6 and has CNS penetration (less than *propranolol*, but more than *atenolol* [a-TEN-oh-lol]). *Esmolol* [ES-moe-lol] is a very short and fast-acting β-blocker used for intravenous administration in acute arrhythmias that occur during surgery or emergency situations. *Esmolol* is rapidly metabolized by esterases in red blood cells. As such, there are no pharmacokinetic drug interactions. Common adverse effects with β-blockers include bradycardia, hypotension, and fatigue (see Chapter 7).

V. CLASS III ANTIARRHYTHMIC DRUGS

Class III agents block K$^+$ channels and, thus, diminish the outward K$^+$ current during repolarization of cardiac cells. These agents prolong the duration of the action potential without altering phase 0 of depolarization or the resting membrane potential (Figure 19.8). Instead, they prolong the effective refractory period, increasing refractoriness. All class III drugs have the potential to induce arrhythmias.

A. Amiodarone

1. **Mechanism of action:** *Amiodarone* [a-MEE-oh-da-rone] contains iodine and is related structurally to thyroxine. It has complex effects, showing class I, II, III, and IV actions, as well as α-blocking activity. Its dominant effect is prolongation of the action potential duration and the refractory period by blocking K$^+$ channels.

2. **Therapeutic uses:** *Amiodarone* is effective in the treatment of severe refractory supraventricular and ventricular tachyarrhythmias. *Amiodarone* has been a mainstay of therapy for the rhythm management of atrial fibrillation or flutter. Despite its adverse effect profile, *amiodarone* is thought to be the least proarrhythmic of the class I and III antiarrhythmic drugs.

3. **Pharmacokinetics:** *Amiodarone* is incompletely absorbed after oral administration. The drug is unusual in having a prolonged half-life of several weeks, and it distributes extensively in tissues. Full clinical effects may not be achieved until months after initiation of treatment, unless loading doses are employed.

4. **Adverse effects:** *Amiodarone* shows a variety of toxic effects, including pulmonary fibrosis, neuropathy, hepatotoxicity, corneal

deposits, optic neuritis, blue-gray skin discoloration, and hypo- or hyperthyroidism. However, use of low doses and close monitoring reduce toxicity, while retaining clinical efficacy. *Amiodarone* is subject to numerous drug interactions, since it is metabolized by CYP3A4 and serves as an inhibitor of CYP1A2, CYP2C9, CYP2D6, and P-glycoprotein.

B. Dronedarone

Dronedarone [droe-NE-da-rone] is a benzofuran *amiodarone* derivative, which is less lipophilic and has a shorter half-life than *amiodarone*. It does not have the iodine moieties that are responsible for thyroid dysfunction associated with *amiodarone*. Like *amiodarone*, it has class I, II, III, and IV actions. *Dronedarone* has a better adverse effect profile than does *amiodarone* but may still cause liver failure. The drug is contraindicated in those with symptomatic heart failure or permanent atrial fibrillation due to an increased risk of death. Currently, *dronedarone* is used to maintain sinus rhythm in atrial fibrillation or flutter, but it is less effective than *amiodarone*.

C. Sotalol

Sotalol [SOE-ta-lol], although a class III antiarrhythmic agent, also has nonselective β-blocker activity. The levorotatory isomer (*L-sotalol*) has β-blocking activity and *D-sotalol* has class III antiarrhythmic action. *Sotalol* blocks a rapid outward K⁺ current, known as the delayed rectifier current. This blockade prolongs both repolarization and duration of the action potential, thus lengthening the effective refractory period. *Sotalol* is used for maintenance of sinus rhythm in patients with atrial fibrillation, atrial flutter, or refractory paroxysmal supraventricular tachycardia and in the treatment of ventricular arrhythmias. Since *sotalol* has β-blocking properties, it is commonly used for these indications in patients with left ventricular hypertrophy or atherosclerotic heart disease. This drug can cause the typical adverse effects associated with β-blockers but has a low rate of adverse effects when compared to other antiarrhythmic agents. The dosing interval should be extended in patients with renal disease, since the drug is renally eliminated. To reduce the risk of proarrhythmic effects, *sotalol* should be initiated in the hospital to monitor QT interval.

D. Dofetilide

Dofetilide [doe-FET-i-lide] is a pure K⁺ channel blocker. It can be used as a first-line antiarrhythmic agent in patients with persistent atrial fibrillation and heart failure or in those with coronary artery disease. Because of the risk of proarrhythmia, *dofetilide* initiation is limited to the inpatient setting. The half-life of this oral drug is 10 hours. The drug is mainly excreted unchanged in the urine. Drugs that inhibit active tubular secretion are contraindicated with *dofetilide*.

E. Ibutilide

Ibutilide [eye-BUE-til-ide] is a K⁺ channel blocker that also activates the inward Na⁺ current (mixed class III and IA actions). *Ibutilide* is the drug of choice for chemical conversion of atrial flutter, but electri-

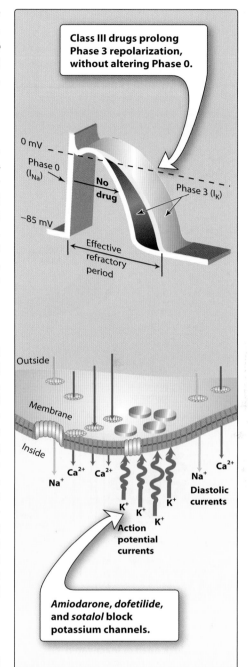

Figure 19.8
Schematic diagram of the effects of class III agents. I_{Na} and I_K are transmembrane currents due to the movement of Na⁺ and K⁺, respectively.

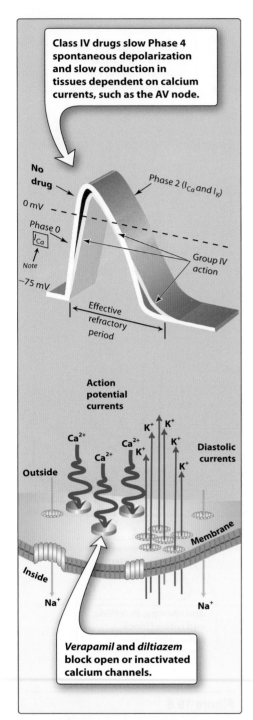

Class IV drugs slow Phase 4 spontaneous depolarization and slow conduction in tissues dependent on calcium currents, such as the AV node.

No drug

Phase 2 (I_{Ca} and I_K)

0 mV

Phase 0
I_{Ca}

Note

Group IV action

−75 mV

Effective refractory period

Action potential currents

Ca^{2+}

Ca^{2+}

Ca^{2+}

K^+ K^+

K^+

K^+

K^+

Diastolic currents

Outside

Membrane

Inside

Na^+

Na^+

Verapamil and diltiazem block open or inactivated calcium channels.

Figure 19.9
Schematic diagram of the effects of class IV agents. I_{Ca} and I_K are transmembrane currents due to the movement of Ca^{2+} and K^+, respectively. AV = atrioventricular.

cal cardioversion has supplanted its use. It undergoes extensive first-pass metabolism and is not used orally. Initiation is also limited to the inpatient setting due to the risk of arrhythmia.

VI. CLASS IV ANTIARRHYTHMIC DRUGS

Class IV drugs are the nondihydropyridine Ca^{2+} channel blockers *verapamil* [ver-AP-a-mil] and *diltiazem* [dil-TYE-a-zem]. Although voltage-sensitive Ca^{2+} channels occur in many different tissues, the major effect of Ca^{2+} channel blockers is on vascular smooth muscle and the heart. Both drugs show greater action on the heart than on vascular smooth muscle, but more so with *verapamil*. In the heart, *verapamil* and *diltiazem* bind only to open depolarized voltage-sensitive channels, thus decreasing the inward current carried by Ca^{2+}. These drugs are use dependent in that they prevent repolarization until the drug dissociates from the channel, resulting in a decreased rate of phase 4 spontaneous depolarization. They also slow conduction in tissues that are dependent on Ca^{2+} currents, such as the AV and SA nodes (Figure 19.9). These agents are more effective against atrial than against ventricular arrhythmias. They are useful in treating reentrant supraventricular tachycardia and in reducing the ventricular rate in atrial flutter and fibrillation. Common adverse effects include bradycardia, hypotension, and peripheral edema. Both drugs are metabolized in the liver by CYP3A4. Dosage adjustments may be needed in patients with hepatic dysfunction. Both agents are subject to many drug interactions as they are CYP3A4 inhibitors, as well as substrates and inhibitors of P-glycoprotein.

VII. OTHER ANTIARRHYTHMIC DRUGS

A. Digoxin

Digoxin [di-JOX-in] inhibits the Na^+/K^+-ATPase pump, ultimately shortening the refractory period in atrial and ventricular myocardial cells while prolonging the effective refractory period and diminishing conduction velocity in the AV node. *Digoxin* is used to control ventricular response rate in atrial fibrillation and flutter; however, sympathetic stimulation easily overcomes the inhibitory effects of *digoxin*. At toxic concentrations, *digoxin* causes ectopic ventricular beats that may result in VT and fibrillation. [Note: Serum trough concentrations of 1.0 to 2.0 ng/mL are desirable for atrial fibrillation or flutter, whereas lower concentrations of 0.5 to 0.8 ng/mL are targeted for systolic heart failure.]

B. Adenosine

Adenosine [ah-DEN-oh-seen] is a naturally occurring nucleoside, but at high doses, the drug decreases conduction velocity, prolongs the refractory period, and decreases automaticity in the AV node. Intravenous *adenosine* is the drug of choice for converting acute supraventricular tachycardias. It has low toxicity but causes flushing, chest pain, and hypotension. *Adenosine* has an extremely short duration of action (approximately 10 to 15 seconds) due to rapid uptake by erythrocytes and endothelial cells.

C. Magnesium sulfate

Magnesium is necessary for the transport of Na$^+$, Ca^{2+}, and K$^+$ across cell membranes. It slows the rate of SA node impulse formation and prolongs conduction time along the myocardial tissue. Intravenous *magnesium sulfate* is the salt used to treat arrhythmias, as oral *magnesium* is not effective in the setting of arrhythmia. Most notably, *magnesium* is the drug of choice for treating the potentially fatal arrhythmia torsades de pointes and *digoxin*-induced arrhythmias.

D. Ranolazine

Ranolazine [ra-NOE-la-zeen] is an antianginal drug with antiarrhythmic properties similar to *amiodarone*. However, its main effect is to shorten repolarization and decrease the action potential duration similar to *mexiletine*. It is used to treat refractory atrial and ventricular arrhythmias, often in combination with other antiarrhythmic drugs. It is well tolerated with dizziness and constipation as the most common adverse effects. *Ranolazine* is extensively metabolized in the liver by CYP3A and CYP2D6 isoenzymes and is mainly excreted by the kidney. Concomitant use with strong CYP3A inducers or inhibitors is contraindicated.

Study Questions

Choose the ONE best answer.

19.1 A 60-year-old woman had a myocardial infarction. Which agent should be used to prevent life-threatening arrhythmias that can occur post myocardial infarction in this patient?

A. Digoxin
B. Flecainide
C. Metoprolol
D. Procainamide

> Correct answer = C. β-Blockers such as metoprolol prevent arrhythmias that occur subsequent to a myocardial infarction. None of the other drugs has been shown to be effective in preventing postinfarct arrhythmias. Flecainide should be avoided in patients with structural heart disease.

19.2 Suppression of arrhythmias resulting from a reentry focus is most likely to occur if the drug:

A. has vagomimetic effects on the AV node
B. is a β-blocker
C. converts a unidirectional block to a bidirectional block
D. slows conduction through the atria

> Correct answer = C. Current theory holds that a reentrant arrhythmia is caused by damaged heart muscle, so that conduction is slowed through the damaged area in only one direction. A drug that prevents conduction in either direction through the damaged area interrupts the reentrant arrhythmia. Class I antiarrhythmics, such as lidocaine, are capable of producing bidirectional block. The other choices do not have any direct effects on the direction of blockade of conduction through damaged cardiac muscle.

19.3 A 57-year-old man is being treated for an atrial arrhythmia. He complains of dry mouth, blurred vision, and urinary hesitancy. Which antiarrhythmic drug is he mostly like taking?

A. Metoprolol
B. Disopyramide
C. Dronedarone
D. Sotalol

> Correct answer = B. The clustered symptoms of dry mouth, blurred vision, and urinary hesitancy are characteristic of anticholinergic adverse effects, which are caused by class IA agents (in this case, disopyramide). The other drugs do not cause anticholinergic effects.

19.4 A 58-year-old woman is being treated for chronic suppression of a ventricular arrhythmia. After 1 week of therapy, she complains of severe upset stomach and heartburn. Which antiarrhythmic drug is the likely cause of these symptoms?

A. Amiodarone
B. Digoxin
C. Mexiletine
D. Propranolol

Correct answer = C. The patient is exhibiting a classic adverse effect of mexiletine. None of the other agents listed are likely to cause dyspepsia.

19.5 A 78-year-old woman has been newly diagnosed with atrial fibrillation. She is not currently having symptoms of palpitations or fatigue. Which is appropriate to initiate for rate control as an outpatient?

A. Dronedarone
B. Esmolol
C. Flecainide
D. Metoprolol

Correct answer = D. Only B and D are options to control rate. The other options are used for rhythm control in patients with atrial fibrillation. Since esmolol is IV only, the only option to start as an outpatient is metoprolol.

19.6 Which of the following is correct regarding digoxin when used for atrial fibrillation?

A. Digoxin works by blocking voltage-sensitive calcium channels.
B. Digoxin is used for rhythm control in patients with atrial fibrillation.
C. Digoxin increases conduction velocity through the AV node.
D. Digoxin levels of 1 to 2 ng/mL are desirable in the treatment of atrial fibrillation.

Correct answer = D. Digoxin works by inhibiting the Na^+/K^+-ATPase pump. It decreases conduction velocity through the AV node and is used for rate control in atrial fibrillation (not rhythm control). Digoxin levels between 1 and 2 ng/mL are more likely to exhibit negative chronotropic effects desired in atrial fibrillation or flutter. A serum drug concentration between 0.5 and 0.8 ng/mL is for symptomatic management of heart failure.

19.7 All of the following are adverse effects of amiodarone except:

A. Cinchonism
B. Hypothyroidism
C. Pulmonary fibrosis
D. Blue skin discoloration

Correct answer = A. Cinchonism is a constellation of symptoms (blurred vision, tinnitus, headache, psychosis) that is known to occur with quinidine. All other options are adverse effects with amiodarone that require close monitoring.

19.8 Which arrhythmia can be treated with lidocaine?

A. Paroxysmal supraventricular ventricular tachycardia
B. Atrial fibrillation
C. Atrial flutter
D. Ventricular tachycardia

Correct answer = D. Lidocaine has little effect on atrial or AV nodal tissue; thus, it used for ventricular arrhythmias such as ventricular tachycardia.

19.9 A clinician would like to initiate a drug for rhythm control of atrial fibrillation. Which of the following coexisting conditions would allow for initiation of flecainide?

A. Hypertension
B. Left ventricular hypertrophy
C. Coronary artery disease
D. Heart failure

Correct answer = A. Since flecainide can increase the risk of sudden cardiac death in those with a history of structural heart disease, only coexisting hypertension will allow for flecainide initiation. Structural heart disease includes left ventricular hypertrophy, heart failure, and atherosclerotic heart disease.

19.10 Which statement regarding dronedarone is correct?

A. Dronedarone is more effective than is amiodarone.
B. QT interval prolongation is not a risk with dronedarone.
C. Dronedarone increases the risk of death in patients with permanent atrial fibrillation or symptomatic heart failure.
D. There is no need to monitor liver function with dronedarone.

Correct answer = C. Dronedarone is not as effective as amiodarone, QT prolongation is a risk with this drug, and liver function should be monitored when taking dronedarone since it increases the risk of liver failure. The drug is contraindicated in those with symptomatic heart failure or permanent atrial fibrillation due to an increased risk of death.

Antianginal Drugs

20

Kristyn Pardo

I. OVERVIEW

Atherosclerotic disease of the coronary arteries, also known as coronary artery disease (CAD) or ischemic heart disease (IHD), is the most common cause of mortality worldwide. Atherosclerotic lesions in coronary arteries can obstruct blood flow, leading to an imbalance in myocardial oxygen supply and demand that presents as stable angina or an acute coronary syndrome (myocardial infarction [MI] or unstable angina). Spasms of vascular smooth muscle may also impede cardiac blood flow, reducing perfusion and causing ischemia and angina pain. Typical angina pectoris is a characteristic sudden, severe, crushing chest pain that may radiate to the neck, jaw, back, and arms. All patients with IHD and angina should receive guideline-directed medical therapy with emphasis on lifestyle modifications (smoking cessation, physical activity, weight management) and management of modifiable risk factors (hypertension, diabetes, dyslipidemia) to reduce cardiovascular morbidity and mortality. Medications used for the management of stable angina are summarized in Figure 20.1.

II. TYPES OF ANGINA

Angina pectoris has three patterns: 1) stable, effort-induced, classic, or typical angina; 2) unstable angina; and 3) Prinzmetal, variant, vasospastic, or rest angina. They are caused by varying combinations of increased myocardial oxygen demand and decreased myocardial perfusion.

A. Stable angina, effort-induced angina, classic or typical angina

Classic or typical angina pectoris is the most common form of angina. It is usually characterized by a short-lasting burning, heavy, or squeezing feeling in the chest. Some ischemic episodes may present "atypically"—with extreme fatigue, nausea, or diaphoresis—while others may not be associated with any symptoms (silent angina). Atypical presentations are more common in women, diabetic patients, and the elderly.

Classic angina is caused by the reduction of coronary perfusion due to a fixed obstruction of a coronary artery produced by atherosclerosis. Increased myocardial oxygen demand, such as that produced by

β-BLOCKERS
Atenolol TENORMIN
Bisoprolol GENERIC ONLY
Metoprolol LOPRESSOR, TOPROL XL
Propranolol INDERAL, INNOPRAN XL
CALCIUM CHANNEL BLOCKERS (DIHYDROPYRIDINES)
Amlodipine NORVASC
Felodipine PLENDIL
Nifedipine ADALAT, PROCARDIA
CALCIUM CHANNEL BLOCKERS (NONDIHYDROPYRIDINE)
Diltiazem CARDIZEM, CARTIA, TIAZAC
Verapamil CALAN, VERELAN
NITRATES
Nitroglycerin MINITRAN, NITRO-DUR, NITROSTAT
Isosorbide dinitrate DILATRATE-SR, ISORDIL
Isosorbide mononitrate GENERIC ONLY
SODIUM CHANNEL BLOCKER
Ranolazine RANEXA

Figure 20.1
Summary of antianginal drugs.

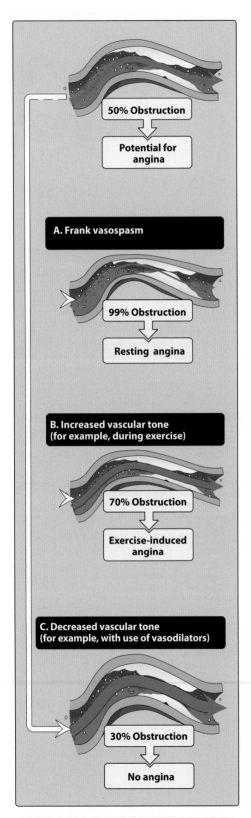

Figure 20.2
Blood flow in a coronary artery partially blocked with atherosclerotic plaques.

physical activity, emotional stress or excitement, or any other cause of increased cardiac workload (Figure 20.2), may induce ischemia. Typical angina pectoris is promptly relieved by rest or *nitroglycerin* [nye-troe-GLIS-er-in]. When the pattern of chest pain and the amount of effort needed to trigger the chest pain does not vary over time, the angina is named "stable angina."

B. Unstable angina

Unstable angina is chest pain that occurs with increased frequency, duration, and intensity and can be precipitated by progressively less effort. Any episode of rest angina longer than 20 minutes, any new-onset angina, any increasing (crescendo) angina, or even sudden development of shortness of breath is suggestive of unstable angina. The symptoms are not relieved by rest or *nitroglycerin*. Unstable angina is a form of acute coronary syndrome and requires hospital admission and more aggressive therapy to prevent progression to MI and death.

C. Prinzmetal, variant, vasospastic, or rest angina

Prinzmetal angina is an uncommon pattern of episodic angina that occurs at rest and is due to decreased blood flow to the heart muscle caused by spasm of the coronary arteries. Although individuals with this form of angina may have significant coronary atherosclerosis, the angina attacks are unrelated to physical activity, heart rate, or blood pressure. Prinzmetal angina generally responds promptly to coronary vasodilators, such as *nitroglycerin* and calcium channel blockers.

D. Acute coronary syndrome

Acute coronary syndrome is an emergency that commonly results from rupture of an atherosclerotic plaque and partial or complete thrombosis of a coronary artery. If the thrombus occludes most of the blood vessel, and, if the occlusion is untreated, necrosis of the cardiac muscle may ensue. MI (necrosis) is typified by increases in the serum levels of biomarkers such as troponins and creatine kinase. The acute coronary syndrome may present as ST-segment elevation myocardial infarction, non–ST-segment elevation myocardial infarction, or as unstable angina. [Note: In unstable angina, increases in biomarkers of myocardial necrosis are not present.]

III. TREATMENT STRATEGIES

Four types of drugs, used either alone or in combination, are commonly used to manage patients with stable angina: β-blockers, calcium channel blockers, organic nitrates, and the sodium channel–blocking drug, *ranolazine* (Figure 20.1). These agents help to balance the cardiac oxygen supply and demand equation by affecting blood pressure, venous return, heart rate, and contractility. Figure 20.3 summarizes the treatment of angina in patients with concomitant diseases, and Figure 20.4 provides a treatment algorithm for patients with stable angina.

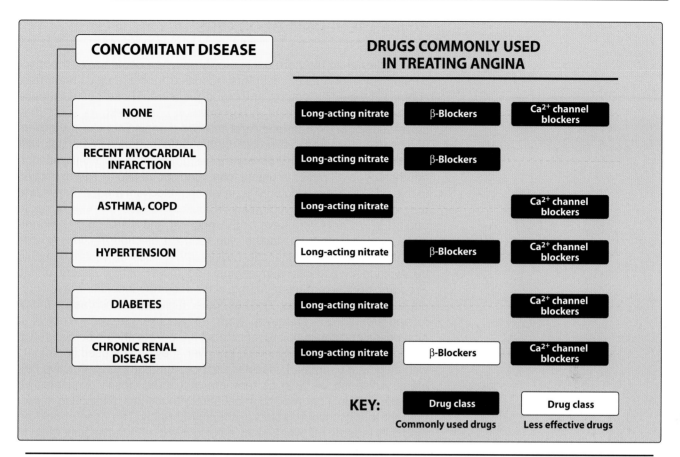

Figure 20.3
Treatment of angina in patients with concomitant diseases. COPD = chronic obstructive pulmonary disease.

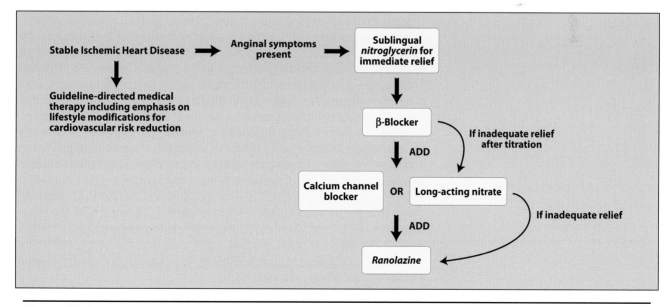

Figure 20.4
Treatment algorithm for improving symptoms in patients with stable angina.

IV. β-ADRENERGIC BLOCKERS

The β-adrenergic blockers decrease the oxygen demands of the myocardium by blocking β₁ receptors, resulting in decreased heart rate, contractility, cardiac output, and blood pressure. These agents reduce myocardial oxygen demand during exertion and at rest. As such, they can reduce both the frequency and severity of angina attacks. β-Blockers can be used to increase exercise duration and tolerance in patients with effort-induced angina. β-Blockers are recommended as initial antianginal therapy in all patients unless contraindicated. [Note: The exception to this rule is vasospastic angina, in which β-blockers are ineffective and may actually worsen symptoms.] β-Blockers reduce the risk of death and MI in patients who have had a prior MI and also improve mortality in patients with heart failure with reduced ejection fraction. Agents with intrinsic sympathomimetic activity (ISA) such as *pindolol* should be avoided in patients with angina and those with a history of MI. *Propranolol* is the prototype for this class of compounds, but it is not cardioselective (see Chapter 7). Thus, other β-blockers, such as *metoprolol* and *atenolol*, are preferred. [Note: All β-blockers are nonselective at high doses and can inhibit β₂ receptors.] β-Blockers should be avoided in patients with severe bradycardia; however, they can be used in patients with diabetes, peripheral vascular disease, and chronic obstructive pulmonary disease, as long as they are monitored closely. Nonselective β-blockers should be avoided in patients with asthma. [Note: It is important not to discontinue β-blocker therapy abruptly. The dose should be gradually tapered off over 2 to 3 weeks to avoid rebound angina, MI, and hypertension.]

V. CALCIUM CHANNEL BLOCKERS

Calcium is essential for muscular contraction. Calcium influx is increased in ischemia because of the membrane depolarization that hypoxia produces. In turn, this promotes the activity of several ATP-consuming enzymes, thereby depleting energy stores and worsening the ischemia. The calcium channel blockers protect the tissue by inhibiting the entrance of calcium into cardiac and smooth muscle cells of the coronary and systemic arterial beds. All calcium channel blockers are, therefore, arteriolar vasodilators that cause a decrease in smooth muscle tone and vascular resistance. These agents primarily affect the resistance of peripheral and coronary arteriolar smooth muscle. In the treatment of effort-induced angina, calcium channel blockers reduce myocardial oxygen consumption by decreasing vascular resistance, thereby decreasing afterload. Their efficacy in vasospastic angina is due to relaxation of the coronary arteries. [Note: *Verapamil* mainly affects the myocardium, whereas *amlodipine* exerts a greater effect on smooth muscle in the peripheral vasculature. *Diltiazem* is intermediate in its actions.] All calcium channel blockers lower blood pressure.

A. Dihydropyridine calcium channel blockers

Amlodipine [am-LOE-di-peen], an oral dihydropyridine, has minimal effect on cardiac conduction and functions mainly as an arteriolar vasodilator. The vasodilatory effect of *amlodipine* is useful in the treatment of variant angina caused by spontaneous coronary spasm. *Nifedipine* [ni-FED-i-pine] is another agent in this class; it is usually administered as an extended-release oral formulation. [Note: Short-acting dihydropyridines should be avoided in CAD because of evidence of increased mortality after an MI and an increase in acute MI in hypertensive patients.]

B. Nondihydropyridine calcium channel blockers

Verapamil [ver-AP-a-mil] slows atrioventricular (AV) conduction directly and decreases heart rate, contractility, blood pressure, and oxygen demand. *Verapamil* has greater negative inotropic effects than *amlodipine*, but it is a weaker vasodilator. *Verapamil* is contraindicated in patients with preexisting depressed cardiac function or AV conduction abnormalities. *Diltiazem* [dil-TYE-a-zem] also slows AV conduction, decreases the rate of firing of the sinus node pacemaker, and is also a coronary artery vasodilator. *Diltiazem* can relieve coronary artery spasm and is particularly useful in patients with variant angina. Nondihydropyridine calcium channel blockers can worsen heart failure due to their negative inotropic effect, and their use should be avoided in this population.

VI. ORGANIC NITRATES

These compounds cause a reduction in myocardial oxygen demand, followed by relief of symptoms. They are effective in stable, unstable, and variant angina.

A. Mechanism of action

Organic nitrates relax vascular smooth muscle by their intracellular conversion to nitrite ions and then to nitric oxide, which in turn activates guanylate cyclase and increases synthesis of cyclic guanosine monophosphate (cGMP). Elevated cGMP ultimately leads to dephosphorylation of the myosin light chain, resulting in vascular smooth muscle relaxation (Figure 20.5). Nitrates such as *nitroglycerin* cause dilation of the large veins, which reduces preload (venous return to the heart) and, therefore, reduces the work of the heart. Nitrates also dilate the coronary vasculature, providing an increased blood supply to the heart muscle.

B. Pharmacokinetics

Nitrates differ in their onset of action and rate of elimination. The onset of action varies from 1 minute for *nitroglycerin* to 30 minutes for

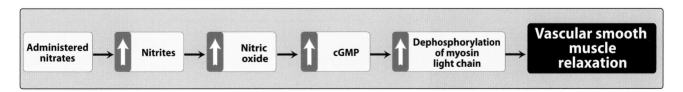

Figure 20.5
Effects of nitrates and nitrites on smooth muscle. cGMP = cyclic guanosine 3′,5′-monophosphate.

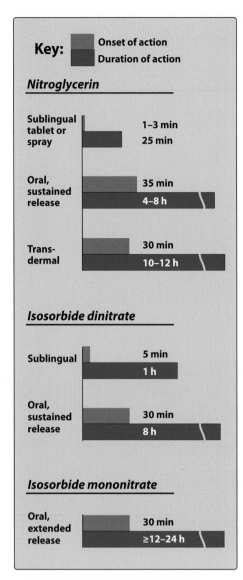

Figure 20.6
Time to peak effect and duration of action for some common organic nitrate preparations.

isosorbide [eye-soe-SOR-bide] *mononitrate* (Figure 20.6). Sublingual *nitroglycerin*, available in tablet or spray formulation, is the drug of choice for prompt relief of an angina attack precipitated by exercise or emotional stress. All patients should have *nitroglycerin* on hand to treat acute angina attacks. Significant first-pass metabolism of *nitroglycerin* occurs in the liver. Therefore, it is commonly administered via the sublingual or transdermal route (patch or ointment), thereby avoiding the hepatic first-pass effect. *Isosorbide mononitrate* owes its improved bioavailability and long duration of action to its stability against hepatic breakdown. Oral *isosorbide dinitrate* undergoes denitration to two mononitrates, both of which possess antianginal activity.

C. Adverse effects

Headache is the most common adverse effect of nitrates. High doses of nitrates can also cause postural hypotension, facial flushing, and tachycardia. Phosphodiesterase type 5 inhibitors such as *sildenafil* potentiate the action of the nitrates. To preclude the dangerous hypotension that may occur, this combination is contraindicated.

Tolerance to the actions of nitrates develops rapidly as the blood vessels become desensitized to vasodilation. Tolerance can be overcome by providing a daily "nitrate-free interval" to restore sensitivity to the drug. The nitrate-free interval of 10 to 12 hours is usually taken at night when myocardial oxygen demand is decreased. However, variant angina worsens early in the morning, perhaps due to circadian catecholamine surges. Therefore, the nitrate-free interval in patients with variant angina should occur in the late afternoon. *Nitroglycerin* patches are worn for 12 hours and then removed for 12 hours to provide the nitrate-free interval.

VII. SODIUM CHANNEL BLOCKER

Ranolazine [ra-NOE-la-zeen] inhibits the late phase of the sodium current (late I_{Na}), improving the oxygen supply and demand equation. Inhibition of late I_{Na} reduces intracellular sodium and calcium overload, thereby improving diastolic function. *Ranolazine* has antianginal as well as antiarrhythmic properties. It is most often used in patients who have failed other antianginal therapies. The antianginal effects of *ranolazine* are considerably less in women than in men. The reason for this difference in effect is unknown. *Ranolazine* is extensively metabolized in the liver, mainly by the CYP3A family and also by CYP2D6. It is also a substrate of P-glycoprotein. As such, *ranolazine* is subject to numerous drug interactions. In addition, *ranolazine* can prolong the QT interval and should be avoided with other drugs that cause QT prolongation.

Figure 20.7 provides a summary of characteristics of the antianginal drugs.

DRUG CLASS	COMMON ADVERSE EFFECTS	DRUG INTERACTIONS	NOTES
β-Blockers *atenolol* *metoprolol* *propranolol*	Bradycardia, worsening peripheral vascular disease, fatigue, sleep disturbance, depression, blunt hypoglycemia awareness, inhibit β$_2$-mediated bronchodilation in asthmatics	β$_2$ Agonists (blunted effect); non-dihydropyridine calcium channel blockers (additive effects)	β$_1$-Selective agents preferred (*atenolol, metoprolol*). Avoid agents with ISA for angina therapy (*pindolol*).
Dihydropyridine calcium channel blockers *amlodipine* *felodipine* *nifedipine*	Peripheral edema, headache, flushing, rebound tachycardia (immediate-release formulations), hypotension	CYP 3A4 substrates (will increase drug concentrations)	Avoid short-acting agents as they can worsen angina (may use extended-release formulations)
Nondihydropyridine calcium channel blockers *diltiazem* *verapamil*	Bradycardia, constipation, heart failure exacerbations, gingival hyperplasia (*verapamil*), edema (*diltiazem*)	CYP 3A4 substrates (will increase drug concentrations); increase *digoxin* levels; β-blockers and other drugs affecting AV node conduction (additive effects)	Avoid in patients with heart failure Adjust dose of both agents in patients with hepatic dysfunction
Organic nitrates *isosorbide dinitrate* *isosorbide mononitrate* *nitroglycerin*	Headache, hypotension, flushing, tachycardia	Contraindicated with PDE5 inhibitors (*sildenafil* and others)	Ensure nitrate-free interval to prevent tolerance
Sodium-channel inhibitor *ranolazine*	Constipation, headache, edema, dizziness, QT interval prolongation	Avoid use with CYP 3A4 inducers (*phenytoin, carbamazepine, St. John's wort*) and strong inhibitors (*clarithromycin*, azole antifungals) and agents that prolong QT interval (*citalopram, quetiapine*, others)	No effect on hemodynamic parameters

Figure 20.7
Summary of characteristics of antianginal drugs. CYP = cytochrome P450; ISA = intrinsic sympathomimetic activity; PDE5 = phosphodiesterase type 5.

Study Questions

Choose the ONE best answer.

20.1 Which of the following best describes stable angina?

A. Angina that occurs more frequently or with progressively less exercise or stress than before

B. Angina due to spasm of coronary arteries

C. Angina due to increased myocardial demand which is reproducible and relieved by rest or nitroglycerin

D. Angina pain accompanied by increases in serum biomarkers of myocardial necrosis

Correct answer = C. When the pattern of the chest pain and the amount of effort needed to trigger the chest pain does not vary over time, the angina is named "stable angina."

20.2 Which medication should be prescribed to all angina patients to treat an acute attack?

A. Isosorbide dinitrate

B. Nitroglycerin patch

C. Nitroglycerin sublingual tablet or spray

D. Ranolazine

Correct answer = C. The other options will not provide prompt relief of angina and should not be used to treat an acute attack.

20.3 Which of the following instructions is important to communicate to a patient receiving a prescription for the nitroglycerin patch?

    A. Apply the patch at onset of angina symptoms for quick relief.

    B. Remove the old patch after 24 hours of use, then immediately apply the next patch to prevent any breakthrough angina pain.

    C. Do not use sublingual nitroglycerin in combination with the patch.

    D. Have a nitrate-free interval of 10 to 12 hours every day to prevent development of nitrate tolerance.

> Correct answer = D. Nitrate-free intervals help prevent the development of nitrate tolerance. Sublingual nitroglycerin should be used to treat breakthrough angina due to its quick onset of action; transdermal nitroglycerin has a delayed onset of action.

20.4 A 64-year-old man was prescribed atenolol and sublingual nitroglycerin after his recent hospitalization for unstable angina. Which of his current medications should be discontinued?

    A. Sildenafil

    B. Amlodipine

    C. Metformin

    D. Lisinopril

> Correct answer = A. Sildenafil and other PDE-5 inhibitors can potentiate the vasodilator effects of nitrates and cause an unsafe drop in blood pressure. Concomitant use of nitrates and PDE-5 inhibitors should be avoided.

20.5 Which of the following correctly ranks the calcium channel blockers from most active on the myocardium to most peripherally active?

    A. Diltiazem, amlodipine, verapamil

    B. Verapamil, diltiazem, nifedipine

    C. Nifedipine, verapamil, diltiazem

    D. Amlodipine, diltiazem, verapamil

> Correct answer = B. Verapamil has the most negative inotropic effects, nifedipine is a peripheral vasodilator, and diltiazem is intermediate with actions on both myocardial and peripheral calcium channels.

20.6 A 76-year-old man with uncontrolled hypertension is experiencing typical angina pain that is relieved with rest and sublingual nitroglycerin. He has a high blood pressure (178/92 mm Hg) and a low heart rate (54 bpm). Which is the most appropriate therapy for his angina at this time?

    A. Ranolazine

    B. Verapamil

    C. Metoprolol

    D. Amlodipine

> Correct answer = D. Amlodipine is the best choice because it will improve angina as well as help control blood pressure, without further reducing the heart rate. Adding verapamil or metoprolol may worsen the bradycardia. Ranolazine may help the angina, but it will not improve the hypertension.

20.7 A 65-year-old male experiences uncontrolled angina attacks that limit his ability to do household chores. He is adherent to a maximized dose of β-blocker with a low heart rate and low blood pressure. He is unable to tolerate an increase in isosorbide mononitrate due to headache. Which is the most appropriate addition to his antianginal therapy?

    A. Nifedipine

    B. Aspirin

    C. Ranolazine

    D. Verapamil

> Correct answer = C. Ranolazine is the best answer. The patient's blood pressure is low, and verapamil and nifedipine may drop blood pressure further. Verapamil may also decrease heart rate. Ranolazine can be used when other agents are maximized, especially when blood pressure is well controlled. The patient will need a baseline ECG and lab work to ensure safe use of this medication.

20.8 A 62-year-old man with ischemic heart disease complains of angina pain that has been getting progressively worse over the past 30 minutes despite use of nitroglycerin. Which of the following is the best course of action?

A. Change nitroglycerin to a long-acting nitrate.

B. Initiate metoprolol.

C. Initiate ranolazine.

D. Refer him to the nearest emergency department for immediate evaluation.

Correct answer = C. Crescendo angina is indicative of unstable angina that requires immediate evaluation.

20.9 Which is correct regarding antianginal therapy in patients with heart failure with reduced ejection fraction?

A. β-Blockers have been associated with reduced mortality.

B. Dihydropyridine calcium channel blockers should be avoided.

C. β-Blockers with ISA are preferred over those without ISA.

D. Nondihydropyridine calcium channel blockers should be used in patients with heart failure with reduced ejection fraction who cannot tolerate β-blockers.

Correct answer = A. β-Blockers have been shown to reduce mortality in heart failure with reduced ejection fraction, but β-blockers with ISA should be avoided in these patients. Dihydropyridine calcium channel blockers can be used in patients with heart failure with reduced ejection fraction, but nondihydropyridine calcium channel blockers should be avoided due to negative inotropic effects.

20.10 A 45-year-old woman with type 1 diabetes has been diagnosed with Prinzmetal angina. Which of the following is correct regarding management of angina in this patient?

A. β-Blockers are the treatment of choice but should be avoided because of her diabetes.

B. Nitroglycerin is not beneficial for this type of angina.

C. She should be counseled to take nitroglycerin before physical activity to prevent symptoms.

D. Felodipine will be more effective than verapamil.

Correct answer = D. Prinzmetal or vasospastic angina responds well to vasodilators, including the dihydropyridine calcium channel blocker felodipine. Verapamil is a weak vasodilator. Beta-blockers may be used with caution in patients with diabetes, but these drugs are less effective options for Prinzmetal angina. Nitrates are also effective, but Prinzmetal angina is provoked by coronary artery vasospasm rather than physical activity.

Anticoagulants and Antiplatelet Agents

21

Katherine Vogel Anderson and Kaylie Smith

I. OVERVIEW

This chapter describes drugs that are useful in the treatment of disorders of hemostasis. Thrombosis, the formation of an unwanted clot within a blood vessel, is the most common abnormality of hemostasis. Thrombotic disorders include acute myocardial infarction (MI), deep vein thrombosis (DVT), pulmonary embolism (PE), and acute ischemic stroke. These conditions are treated with drugs such as anticoagulants and fibrinolytics. Bleeding disorders related to the failure of hemostasis are less common than thromboembolic disorders. Bleeding disorders include hemophilia, which is treated with transfusion of recombinant factor VIII, and vitamin K deficiency, which is treated with vitamin K supplementation. Figure 21.1 summarizes agents used for the treatment of dysfunctions of hemostasis.

II. THROMBUS VERSUS EMBOLUS

A clot that adheres to a vessel wall is called a "thrombus," whereas an intravascular clot that floats in the blood is termed an "embolus." Thus, a detached thrombus becomes an embolus. Both thrombi and emboli are dangerous, because they may occlude blood vessels and deprive tissues of oxygen and nutrients. Arterial thrombosis most often occurs in medium-sized vessels rendered thrombogenic by atherosclerosis. Arterial thrombosis usually consists of a platelet-rich clot. In contrast, venous thrombosis is triggered by blood stasis or inappropriate activation of the coagulation cascade. Venous thrombosis typically involves a clot that is rich in fibrin, with fewer platelets than are observed with arterial clots.

III. PLATELET RESPONSE TO VASCULAR INJURY

Physical trauma to the vascular system, such as a puncture or a cut, initiates a complex series of interactions between platelets, endothelial cells, and the coagulation cascade. These interactions lead to hemostasis or the cessation of blood loss from a damaged blood vessel. Platelets are central in this process. Initially, there is vasospasm of the damaged blood

PLATELET INHIBITORS
Abciximab REOPRO
Aspirin VARIOUS
Cangrelor KENGREAL
Cilostazol GENERIC ONLY
Clopidogrel PLAVIX
Dipyridamole PERSANTINE
Eptifibatide INTEGRILIN
Prasugrel EFFIENT
Ticagrelor BRILINTA
Ticlopidine GENERIC ONLY
Tirofiban AGGRASTAT
ANTICOAGULANTS
Apixaban ELIQUIS
Argatroban GENERIC ONLY
Betrixaban BEVYXXA
Bivalirudin ANGIOMAX
Dabigatran PRADAXA
Dalteparin FRAGMIN
Desirudin IPRIVASK
Edoxaban SAVAYSA
Enoxaparin LOVENOX
Fondaparinux ARIXTRA
Heparin VARIOUS
Rivaroxaban XARELTO
Warfarin COUMADIN, JANTOVEN
THROMBOLYTIC AGENTS
Alteplase (tPA) ACTIVASE
Tenecteplase TNKASE
TREATMENT OF BLEEDING
Aminocaproic acid AMICAR
Idarucizumab PRAXBIND
Protamine sulfate GENERIC ONLY
Tranexamic acid CYKLOKAPRON, LYSTEDA
Vitamin K$_1$ (phytonadione) MEPHYTON

Figure 21.1
Summary of drugs used in treating dysfunctions of hemostasis.

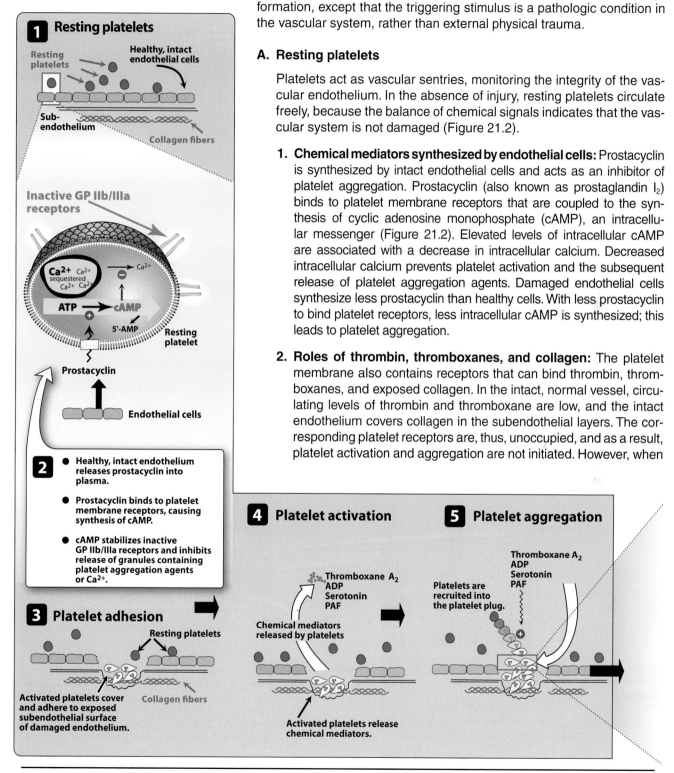

vessel to prevent further blood loss. The next step involves the formation of a platelet–fibrin plug at the site of the puncture. The creation of an unwanted thrombus involves many of the same steps as normal clot formation, except that the triggering stimulus is a pathologic condition in the vascular system, rather than external physical trauma.

A. Resting platelets

Platelets act as vascular sentries, monitoring the integrity of the vascular endothelium. In the absence of injury, resting platelets circulate freely, because the balance of chemical signals indicates that the vascular system is not damaged (Figure 21.2).

1. **Chemical mediators synthesized by endothelial cells:** Prostacyclin is synthesized by intact endothelial cells and acts as an inhibitor of platelet aggregation. Prostacyclin (also known as prostaglandin I_2) binds to platelet membrane receptors that are coupled to the synthesis of cyclic adenosine monophosphate (cAMP), an intracellular messenger (Figure 21.2). Elevated levels of intracellular cAMP are associated with a decrease in intracellular calcium. Decreased intracellular calcium prevents platelet activation and the subsequent release of platelet aggregation agents. Damaged endothelial cells synthesize less prostacyclin than healthy cells. With less prostacyclin to bind platelet receptors, less intracellular cAMP is synthesized; this leads to platelet aggregation.

2. **Roles of thrombin, thromboxanes, and collagen:** The platelet membrane also contains receptors that can bind thrombin, thromboxanes, and exposed collagen. In the intact, normal vessel, circulating levels of thrombin and thromboxane are low, and the intact endothelium covers collagen in the subendothelial layers. The corresponding platelet receptors are, thus, unoccupied, and as a result, platelet activation and aggregation are not initiated. However, when

Figure 21.2
Formation of a hemostatic plug. GP = glycoprotein; ATP = adenosine triphosphate; cAMP = cyclic adenosine monophosphate;
(Figure continues on next page)

occupied, each of these receptor types triggers a series of reactions leading to the release into the circulation of intracellular granules by the platelets. This ultimately stimulates platelet aggregation.

B. Platelet adhesion

When the endothelium is injured, platelets adhere to and virtually cover the exposed collagen of the subendothelium (Figure 21.2). This triggers a complex series of chemical reactions, resulting in platelet activation.

C. Platelet activation

Receptors on the surface of the adhering platelets are activated by the collagen of the underlying connective tissue. This causes morphologic changes in platelets (Figure 21.3) and the release of platelet granules containing chemical mediators, such as adenosine diphosphate (ADP), thromboxane A_2, serotonin, platelet activation factor, and thrombin (Figure 21.2). These signaling molecules bind to receptors in the outer membrane of resting platelets circulating nearby. These receptors function as sensors that are activated by the signals sent from the adhering platelets. The previously dormant platelets become activated and start to aggregate. These actions are mediated by several messenger systems that ultimately result in elevated levels of calcium and a decreased concentration of cAMP within the platelet.

D. Platelet aggregation

The increase in cytosolic calcium accompanying activation is due to a release of sequestered stores within the platelet (Figure 21.2). This leads to 1) the release of platelet granules containing mediators, such as ADP and serotonin that activate other platelets; 2) activation of thromboxane A_2 synthesis; and 3) activation of glycoprotein (GP) IIb/IIIa receptors that bind fibrinogen and, ultimately, regulate platelet–platelet interaction and thrombus formation. Fibrinogen, a soluble

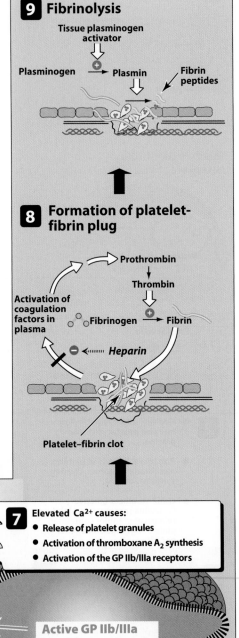

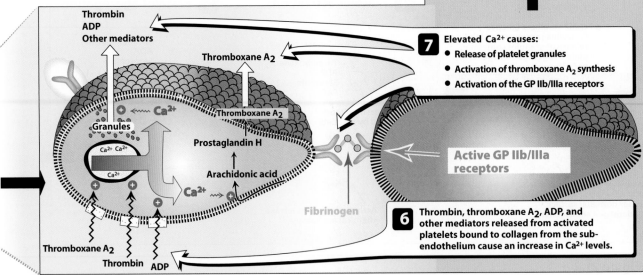

Figure 21.2 (continued)
ADP = adenosine diphosphate; PAF = platelet activation factor.

plasma GP, simultaneously binds to GP IIb/IIIa receptors on two separate platelets, resulting in platelet cross-linking and platelet aggregation. This leads to an avalanche of platelet aggregation, because each activated platelet can recruit other platelets (Figure 21.4).

E. Formation of a clot

Local stimulation of the coagulation cascade by tissue factors released from the injured tissue and by mediators on the surface of platelets results in the formation of thrombin (factor IIa). In turn, thrombin, a serine protease, catalyzes the hydrolysis of fibrinogen to fibrin, which is incorporated into the clot. Subsequent cross-linking of the fibrin strands stabilizes the clot and forms a hemostatic platelet–fibrin plug (Figure 21.2).

F. Fibrinolysis

During clot formation, the fibrinolytic pathway is locally activated. Plasminogen is enzymatically processed to plasmin (fibrinolysin) by plasminogen activators in the tissue (Figure 21.2). Plasmin limits the growth of the clot and dissolves the fibrin network as wounds heal.

IV. PLATELET AGGREGATION INHIBITORS

Platelet aggregation inhibitors decrease the formation of a platelet-rich clot or decrease the action of chemical signals that promote platelet aggregation (Figure 21.5). The platelet aggregation inhibitors described below inhibit cyclooxygenase-1 (COX-1), block GP IIb/IIIa, or block ADP receptors, thereby interfering with the signals that promote platelet aggregation. These agents are beneficial in the prevention and treatment of occlusive cardiovascular diseases, in the maintenance of vascular grafts and arterial patency, and as adjuncts to thrombin inhibitors or thrombolytic therapy in MI.

A. Aspirin

1. **Mechanism of action:** Stimulation of platelets by thrombin, collagen, and ADP results in activation of platelet membrane phospholipases that liberate arachidonic acid from membrane phospholipids. Arachidonic acid is first converted to prostaglandin H_2 by COX-1 (Figure 21.6). Prostaglandin H_2 is further metabolized to thromboxane A_2, which is released into plasma. Thromboxane A_2 promotes the aggregation process that is essential for the rapid formation of a hemostatic plug. *Aspirin* [AS-pir-in] inhibits thromboxane A_2 synthesis by acetylation of a serine residue on the active site of COX-1, thereby irreversibly inactivating the enzyme (Figure 21.7). This shifts the balance of chemical mediators to favor the antiaggregatory effects of prostacyclin, thereby preventing platelet aggregation. The inhibitory effect is rapid, and *aspirin*-induced suppression of thromboxane A_2 and the resulting suppression of platelet aggregation last for the life of the platelet, which is approximately 7 to 10 days. Repeated administration of *aspirin* has a cumulative effect on the function of platelets. *Aspirin* is the only antiplatelet agent that irreversibly inhibits platelet function.

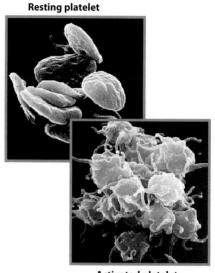

Resting platelet

Activated platelet

Figure 21.3
Scanning electron micrograph of platelets.

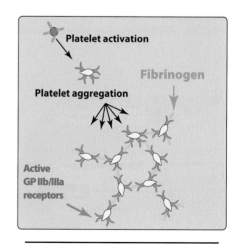

Figure 21.4
Activation and aggregation of platelets. GP = glycoprotein.

Medication	Adverse Effects	Drug Interactions	Monitoring Parameters
Oral Agents:			
Aspirin	Angioedema Bleeding Bronchospasm GI disturbances Reye syndrome SJS	Anticoagulants, P2Y12 inhibitors, NSAIDs —increased bleeding *cidofovir*—nephrotoxicity *probenecid*—decreased uricosuric effects	CBC LFT
Cilostazol	Bleeding GI disturbances Headache Peripheral edema SJS	Food (administer on empty stomach)	CBC
Clopidogrel	Bleeding SJS	Strong CYP2C19 inhibitors reduce antiplatelet effect (e.g., *omeprazole*)	CBC LFT
Dipyridamole	Bleeding Dizziness GI discomfort Rash	Salicylates—increased bleeding Thrombolytic agents—increased bleeding	None for oral administration
Prasugrel	Angioedema Bleeding Headache Hyperlipidemia Hypertension	Anticoagulants—increased bleeding Other antiplatelets—increased bleeding	CBC
Ticagrelor	Bleeding Dyspnea Headache Raised SCr	Strong CYP3A4 inhibitors (e.g., *ketoconazole*)—increased bleeding Strong CYP3A4 inducers (e.g., *rifampin*)—decreased efficacy	CBC LFT
Injectable Agents:			
Abciximab	**For all agents:** Hypotension Nausea Vomiting Thrombocytopenia	**For all agents:** Increased bleeding: *Ginkgo biloba* Antiplatelets Salicylates SSRIs and SNRIs	**For all agents:** APTT clotting time H/H platelet count thrombin time
Eptifibatide			
Tirofiban			

Figure 21.5
Summary of characteristics of platelet aggregation inhibitors. APTT = activated partial thromboplastin time, CBC = complete blood count, GI = gastrointestinal, H/H = hemoglobin and hematocrit, LFT = liver function test, NSAID = nonsteroidal anti-inflammatory drug, SCr = serum creatinine, SJS = Stevens-Johnson Syndrome, SNRI = serotonin-norepinephrine reuptake inhibitor, SSRI = selective serotonin reuptake inhibitor.

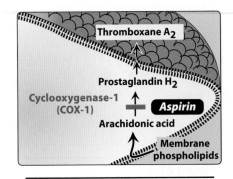

Figure 21.6
Aspirin irreversibly inhibits platelet cyclooxygenase-1.

2. **Therapeutic use:** *Aspirin* is used in the prophylactic treatment of transient cerebral ischemia, to reduce the incidence of recurrent MI, and to decrease mortality in the setting of primary and secondary prevention of MI. Complete inactivation of platelets occurs with 75 mg of *aspirin* given daily. The recommended antiplatelet dose of *aspirin* ranges from 50 to 325 mg daily.

3. **Pharmacokinetics:** When given orally, *aspirin* is absorbed by passive diffusion and quickly hydrolyzed to salicylic acid in the liver. Salicylic acid is further metabolized in the liver and some is excreted unchanged in the urine. The half-life of *aspirin* ranges from 15 to 20 minutes and for salicylic acid is 3 to 12 hours.

4. **Adverse effects:** Higher doses of *aspirin* increase drug-related toxicities as well as the probability that *aspirin* may also inhibit prostacyclin production. Bleeding time is prolonged by *aspirin* treatment, causing complications that include an increased incidence

of hemorrhagic stroke and gastrointestinal (GI) bleeding, especially at higher doses of the drug. Nonsteroidal anti-inflammatory drugs, such as *ibuprofen*, inhibit COX-1 by transiently competing at the catalytic site. *Ibuprofen*, if taken within the 2 hours prior to *aspirin*, can obstruct the access of *aspirin* to the serine residue and, thereby, antagonize platelet inhibition by *aspirin*. Therefore, immediate-release *aspirin* should be taken at least 60 minutes before or at least 8 hours after *ibuprofen*.

B. P2Y$_{12}$ receptor antagonists

Ticlopidine [ti-KLOE-pi-deen], *clopidogrel* [kloh-PID-oh-grel], *prasugrel* [PRA-soo-grel], *ticagrelor* [tye-KA-grel-or], and *cangrelor* [KAN-grel-or] are P2Y$_{12}$ ADP receptor inhibitors that also block platelet aggregation but by a mechanism different from that of *aspirin*. All of these agents are administered orally, with the exception of *cangrelor*, which is an injectable formulation.

1. **Mechanism of action:** These drugs inhibit the binding of ADP to the P2Y$_{12}$ receptor on platelets and, thereby, inhibit the activation of the GP IIb/IIIa receptors required for platelets to bind to fibrinogen and to each other (Figure 21.8). *Ticagrelor* and *cangrelor* bind to the P2Y$_{12}$ ADP receptor in a reversible manner. The other agents bind irreversibly. The maximum inhibition of platelet aggregation is achieved in 2 minutes with intravenous (IV) *cangrelor*, 1 to 3 hours with *ticagrelor*, 2 to 4 hours with *prasugrel*, 3 to 4 days with *ticlopidine*, and 3 to 5 days with *clopidogrel*. When treatment is suspended, the platelet system requires time to recover.

2. **Therapeutic use:** *Clopidogrel* is approved for prevention of atherosclerotic events in patients with a recent MI or stroke and in those with established peripheral arterial disease. It is also approved for prophylaxis of thrombotic events in acute coronary syndromes (unstable angina or non–ST-elevation MI). Additionally, *clopidogrel* is used to prevent thrombotic events associated with percutaneous coronary intervention (PCI) with or without coronary stenting. *Ticlopidine* is similar in structure to *clopidogrel*. It is indicated for the prevention of transient ischemic attacks (TIA) and strokes in patients with a prior cerebral thrombotic event. However, due to life-threatening hematologic adverse reactions, *ticlopidine* is generally reserved for patients who are intolerant to other therapies. *Prasugrel* is approved to decrease thrombotic cardiovascular events in patients with acute coronary syndromes (unstable angina, non–ST-elevation MI, and ST-elevation MI managed with PCI). *Ticagrelor* is approved for the prevention of arterial thromboembolism in patients with unstable angina and acute MI, including those undergoing PCI. *Cangrelor* is approved as an adjunct during PCI to reduce thrombotic events in select patients.

3. **Pharmacokinetics:** These agents require oral loading doses for quicker antiplatelet effect, except *cangrelor* that has a fast onset of action with intravenous administration. Food interferes with the absorption of *ticlopidine* but not with the other agents. After oral ingestion, the drugs are extensively bound to plasma proteins. They undergo hepatic metabolism by the cytochrome P-450 (CYP) system to active metabolites. Elimination of the drugs and metabolites occurs by both the renal and fecal routes. *Clopidogrel* is a prodrug,

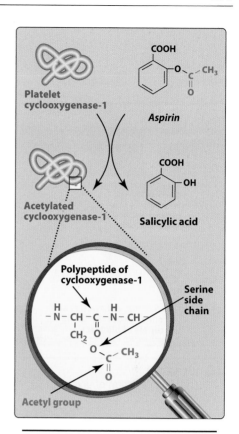

Figure 21.7
Acetylation of cyclooxygenase-1 by *aspirin*.

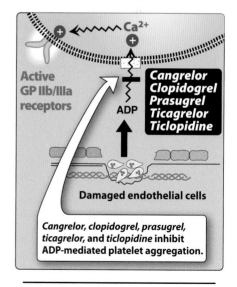

Cangrelor, clopidogrel, prasugrel, ticagrelor, and ticlopidine inhibit ADP-mediated platelet aggregation.

Figure 21.8
Mechanism of action of P2Y$_{12}$ receptor antagonists. ADP = adenine diphosphate; GP = glycoprotein.

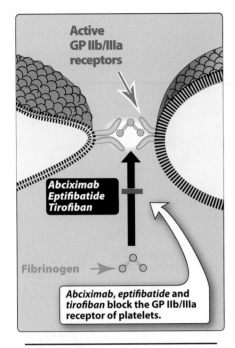

Figure 21.9
Mechanism of action of glycoprotein
(GP) IIb/IIIa receptor blockers.

and its therapeutic efficacy relies on its active metabolite, which is produced via metabolism by CYP 2C19. Genetic polymorphism of CYP 2C19 leads to a reduced clinical response in patients who are "poor metabolizers" of *clopidogrel*. Tests are currently available to identify poor metabolizers, and it is recommended that other antiplatelet agents (*prasugrel* or *ticagrelor*) be prescribed for these patients. In addition, other drugs that inhibit CYP 2C19, such as *omeprazole* and *esomeprazole*, should be avoided while on *clopidogrel*.

4. **Adverse effects:** These agents can cause prolonged bleeding for which there is no antidote. *Ticlopidine* is associated with severe hematologic reactions that limit its use, such as agranulocytosis, thrombotic thrombocytopenic purpura (TTP), and aplastic anemia. *Clopidogrel* causes fewer adverse reactions, and the incidence of neutropenia is lower. However, TTP has been reported as an adverse effect for both *clopidogrel* and *prasugrel* (but not for *ticagrelor*). *Prasugrel* is contraindicated in patients with history of TIA or stroke. *Prasugrel, ticagrelor*, and *cangrelor* carry black box warnings for bleeding. Additionally, *ticagrelor* carries a black box warning for diminished effectiveness with concomitant use of *aspirin* doses above 100 mg.

C. Glycoprotein IIb/IIIa inhibitors

1. **Mechanism of action:** The GP IIb/IIIa receptor plays a key role in stimulating platelet aggregation. A chimeric monoclonal antibody fragment, *abciximab* [ab-SIKS-eh-mab], inhibits the GP IIb/IIIa receptor complex. By binding to GP IIb/IIIa, *abciximab* blocks the binding of fibrinogen and von Willebrand factor and, consequently, aggregation does not occur (Figure 21.9). *Eptifibatide* [ep-ti-FIB-ih-tide] and *tirofiban* [tye-roe-FYE-ban] act similarly to *abciximab*, by blocking the GP IIb/IIIa receptor. *Eptifibatide* is a cyclic peptide that binds to GP IIb/IIIa at the site that interacts with the arginine–glycine–aspartic acid sequence of fibrinogen. *Tirofiban* is not a peptide, but it blocks the same site as *eptifibatide*.

2. **Therapeutic use:** These agents are given intravenously, along with *heparin* and *aspirin*, as an adjunct to PCI for the prevention of cardiac ischemic complications. *Abciximab* is also approved for patients with unstable angina not responding to conventional medical therapy when PCI is planned within 24 hours.

3. **Pharmacokinetics:** *Abciximab* is given by IV bolus, followed by IV infusion, achieving peak platelet inhibition within 30 minutes. The metabolism of *abciximab* is unknown. After cessation of *abciximab* infusion, platelet function gradually returns to normal, with the antiplatelet effect persisting for 24 to 48 hours. When IV infusion of *eptifibatide* or *tirofiban* is stopped, both agents are rapidly cleared from the plasma. *Eptifibatide* and its metabolites are excreted by the kidney. *Tirofiban* is excreted largely unchanged by the kidney and to a lesser extent in the feces.

4. **Adverse effects:** The major adverse effect of these agents is bleeding, especially if used with anticoagulants.

D. Dipyridamole

Dipyridamole [dye-peer-ID-a-mole], a coronary vasodilator, increases intracellular levels of cAMP by inhibiting phosphodiesterase, thereby resulting in decreased thromboxane A_2 synthesis. The drug may potentiate the effect of prostacyclin and, therefore, decrease platelet adhesion to thrombogenic surfaces (Figure 21.2). *Dipyridamole* is used for stroke prevention and is usually given in combination with *aspirin*. *Dipyridamole* has variable bioavailability following oral administration. It is highly protein bound. The drug undergoes hepatic metabolism, mainly glucuronidation, and is excreted primarily in the feces. Patients with unstable angina should not use *dipyridamole* because of its vasodilating properties, which may worsen ischemia (coronary steal phenomenon). *Dipyridamole* commonly causes headache and dizziness and can lead to orthostatic hypotension (especially if administered IV).

E. Cilostazol

Cilostazol [sill-AH-sta-zole] is an oral antiplatelet agent that also has vasodilating activity. *Cilostazol* and its active metabolites inhibit phosphodiesterase type III, which prevents the degradation of cAMP, thereby increasing levels of cAMP in platelets and vascular tissues. The increase in cAMP prevents platelet aggregation and promotes vasodilation of blood vessels, respectively. *Cilostazol* is approved to reduce the symptoms of intermittent claudication. *Cilostazol* is extensively metabolized in the liver by the CYP 3A4 and 2C19 isoenzymes. As such, this agent has many drug interactions that require dose modification. The primary route of elimination is via the kidney. Headache and GI side effects (diarrhea, abnormal stools, dyspepsia, and abdominal pain) are the most common adverse effects observed with *cilostazol*. Rarely, thrombocytopenia or leukopenia has been reported. Phosphodiesterase type III inhibitors have been shown to increase mortality in patients with advanced heart failure. As such, *cilostazol* is contraindicated in patients with heart failure.

V. BLOOD COAGULATION

The coagulation process that generates thrombin consists of two interrelated pathways, the extrinsic and the intrinsic systems. The extrinsic system is initiated by the activation of clotting factor VII by tissue factor (also known as thromboplastin). Tissue factor is a membrane protein that is normally separated from the blood by the endothelial cells that line the vasculature. However, in response to vascular injury, tissue factor becomes exposed to blood. There, it can bind and activate factor VII, initiating the extrinsic pathway. The intrinsic system is triggered by the activation of clotting factor XII. This occurs when blood comes into contact with the collagen in the damaged wall of a blood vessel.

A. Formation of fibrin

Both the extrinsic and the intrinsic systems involve a cascade of enzyme reactions that sequentially transform various plasma factors (proenzymes) to their active (enzymatic) forms. [Note: The active form of a clotting factor is denoted by the letter "a."] Ultimately, factor Xa is produced, which converts prothrombin (factor II) to thrombin (factor IIa; Figure 21.10). Thrombin plays a key role in coagulation, because it is responsible for generation of fibrin, which forms the mesh-like matrix of the blood clot. If thrombin is not formed or if its function is impeded (for example, by antithrombin III), coagulation is inhibited.

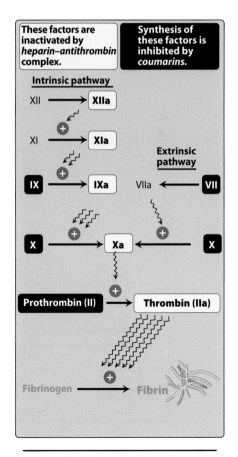

Figure 21.10
Formation of a fibrin clot.

B. Inhibitors of coagulation

It is important that coagulation is restricted to the local site of vascular injury. Endogenously, protein C, protein S, antithrombin III, and tissue factor pathway inhibitor all inhibit coagulation factors. The mechanism of action of several anticoagulant agents, including *heparin* and *heparin*-related products, involves activation of these endogenous inhibitors (primarily antithrombin III).

VI. PARENTERAL ANTICOAGULANTS

The anticoagulant drugs inhibit either the action of the coagulation factors (for example, *heparin*) or interfere with the synthesis of the coagulation factors (*warfarin*).

A. Heparin and low molecular weight heparins

Heparin [HEP-a-rin] is an injectable, rapidly acting anticoagulant that is often used acutely to interfere with the formation of thrombi. *Heparin* occurs naturally as a macromolecule complexed with histamine in mast cells, where its physiologic role is unknown. It is extracted for commercial use from porcine intestinal mucosa. Unfractionated *heparin* is a mixture of straight-chain, anionic glycosaminoglycans with a wide range of molecular weights. It is strongly acidic because of the presence of sulfate and carboxylic acid groups. The realization that low molecular weight forms of *heparin* (LMWHs) can also act as anticoagulants led to the isolation of *enoxaparin* [e-NOX-a-par-in] and *dalteparin* [DAL-te-PAR-in], produced by depolymerization of unfractionated *heparin*. The LMWHs are heterogeneous compounds about one-third the size of unfractionated *heparin*.

1. **Mechanism of action:** *Heparin* acts at a number of molecular targets, but its anticoagulant effect is a consequence of binding to antithrombin III, with the subsequent rapid inactivation of coagulation factors (Figure 21.11). Antithrombin III is an α globulin that inhibits serine proteases of thrombin (factor IIa) and factor Xa. In the absence of *heparin*, antithrombin III interacts very

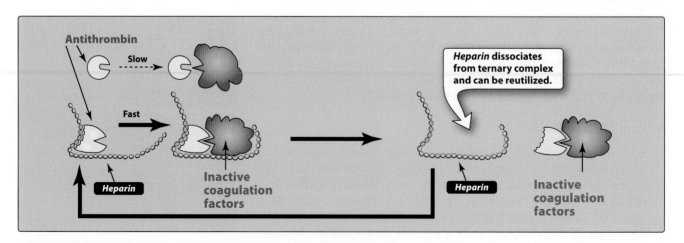

Figure 21.11
Heparin accelerates inactivation of coagulation factors by antithrombin.

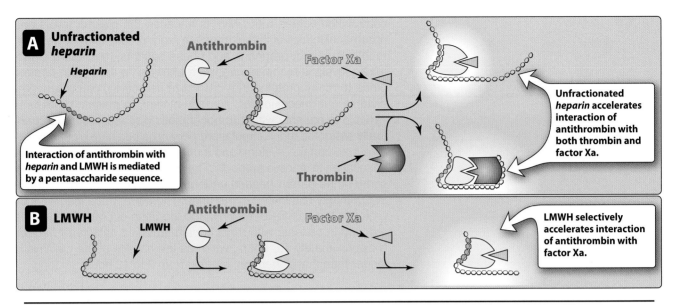

Figure 21.12
Heparin-mediated and low molecular weight heparin (LMWH)-mediated inactivation of thrombin or factor Xa.

slowly with thrombin and factor Xa. When *heparin* molecules bind to antithrombin III, a conformational change occurs that catalyzes the inhibition of thrombin about 1000-fold. LMWHs complex with antithrombin III and inactivate factor Xa (including that located on platelet surfaces) but do not bind as avidly to thrombin. A unique pentasaccharide sequence contained in *heparin* and LMWHs permits their binding to antithrombin III (Figure 21.12).

2. **Therapeutic use:** *Heparin* and the LMWHs limit the expansion of thrombi by preventing fibrin formation. These agents are used for the treatment of acute venous thromboembolism (DVT or PE). *Heparin* and LMWHs are also used for prophylaxis of postoperative venous thrombosis in patients undergoing surgery (for example, hip replacement) and those with acute MI. These drugs are the anticoagulants of choice for treating pregnant women, because they do not cross the placenta, due to their large size and negative charge. LMWHs do not require the same intense monitoring as *heparin*, thereby saving laboratory costs and nursing time. These advantages make LMWHs useful for both inpatient and outpatient therapy.

3. **Pharmacokinetics:** *Heparin* must be administered subcutaneously or intravenously, because the drug does not readily cross membranes (Figure 21.13). The LMWHs are usually administered subcutaneously. [Note: *Enoxaparin* can be administered intravenously in the treatment of MI.] *Heparin* is often initiated as an intravenous bolus to achieve immediate anticoagulation. This is followed by lower doses or continuous infusion of *heparin*, titrated to the desired level of anticoagulation according to the activated partial thromboplastin time (aPTT) or anti-Xa level. Whereas the anticoagulant effect with *heparin* occurs within minutes of IV administration (or 1 to 2 hours after subcutaneous injection), the maximum anti–factor Xa activity of the LMWHs occurs about 4 hours after subcutaneous injection. It is usually not necessary to monitor

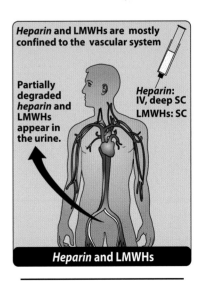

Figure 21.13
Administration and fate of *heparin* and low molecular weight heparins (LMWHs).

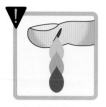

Bleeding

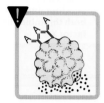

Hypersensitivity

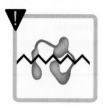

Thrombo-
cytopenia

Figure 21.14
Adverse effects of *heparin*.

coagulation values with LMWHs because the plasma levels and pharmacokinetics of these drugs are more predictable. However, in renally impaired, pregnant, and obese patients, monitoring of factor Xa levels is recommended with LMWHs. In the blood, *heparin* binds to many proteins that neutralize its activity, causing unpredictable pharmacokinetics. *Heparin* binding to plasma proteins is variable in patients with thromboembolic diseases. Although generally restricted to the circulation, *heparin* is taken up by the monocyte/macrophage system, and it undergoes depolymerization and desulfation to inactive products. The inactive metabolites, as well as some of the parent *heparin* undergo renal excretion. The LMWHs are primarily eliminated in the urine. Therefore, renal insufficiency prolongs the half-life of LMWH, and the dose of LMWH should be reduced in patients with renal impairment. The half-life of *heparin* is approximately 1.5 hours, whereas the half-life of the LMWHs is longer than that of *heparin*, ranging from 3 to 12 hours.

4. **Adverse effects:** The chief complication of *heparin* and LMWH therapy is bleeding (Figure 21.14). Careful monitoring of the patient and laboratory parameters is required to minimize bleeding. Excessive bleeding may be managed by discontinuing the drug or by treating with *protamine sulfate*. When infused slowly, the latter combines ionically with *heparin* to form a stable, 1:1 inactive complex. It is important that the dosage of *protamine sulfate* is carefully titrated (1 mg for every 100 units of *heparin* administered), because *protamine sulfate* is a weak anticoagulant, and excess amounts may trigger bleeding episodes or worsen bleeding potential. *Heparin* preparations are obtained from porcine sources and, therefore, may be antigenic. Possible adverse reactions include chills, fever, urticaria, and anaphylactic shock. *Heparin*-induced thrombocytopenia (HIT) is a serious condition, in which circulating blood contains an abnormally low number of platelets. This reaction is immune mediated and carries a risk of venous and arterial embolism. *Heparin* therapy should be discontinued when patients develop HIT or show severe thrombocytopenia. In cases of HIT, *heparin* can be replaced by another anticoagulant, such as *argatroban*. [Note: LMWHs can have cross-sensitivity and are not recommended in patients with HIT.] In addition, osteoporosis has been observed in patients on long-term *heparin* therapy. *Heparin* and LMWHs are contraindicated in patients who have hypersensitivity to *heparin*, bleeding disorders, alcoholism, or who have had recent surgery of the brain, eye, or spinal cord.

B. Argatroban

Argatroban [ar-GA-troh-ban] is a synthetic parenteral anticoagulant that is derived from L-arginine. It is a direct thrombin inhibitor. *Argatroban* is used for the prophylaxis or treatment of venous thromboembolism in patients with HIT, and it is also approved for use during PCI in patients who have or are at risk for developing HIT. Anticoagulant effects are immediate. *Argatroban* is metabolized in the liver and has a half-life of about 39 to 51 minutes. Dose reduction is recommended for patients with hepatic impairment. Monitoring includes aPTT, hemoglobin, and hematocrit. As with other anticoagulants, the major side effect is bleeding.

C. Bivalirudin and desirudin

Bivalirudin [bye-VAL-ih-ruh-din] and *desirudin* [deh-SIHR-uh-din] are parenteral anticoagulants that are analogs of hirudin, a thrombin inhibitor derived from saliva of the medicinal leech. These drugs are selective direct thrombin inhibitors that reversibly inhibit the catalytic site of both free and clot-bound thrombin. *Bivalirudin* is an alternative to *heparin* in patients undergoing PCI who have or are at risk for developing HIT and also in patients with unstable angina undergoing angioplasty. In patients with normal renal function, the half-life of *bivalirudin* is 25 minutes. Dosage adjustments are required in patients with renal impairment. *Desirudin* is indicated for the prevention of DVT in patients undergoing hip replacement surgery. Like the others, bleeding is the major side effect of these agents.

D. Fondaparinux

Fondaparinux [fawn-da-PARE-eh-nux] is a synthetically derived pentasaccharide anticoagulant that selectively inhibits factor Xa. By selectively binding to antithrombin III, *fondaparinux* potentiates (300- to 1000-fold) the innate neutralization of factor Xa by antithrombin III. *Fondaparinux* is approved for use in the treatment of DVT and PE and for the prophylaxis of venous thromboembolism in the setting of orthopedic and abdominal surgery. The drug is well absorbed from the subcutaneous route with a predictable pharmacokinetic profile and, therefore, requires less monitoring than *heparin*. *Fondaparinux* is eliminated in the urine mainly as unchanged drug with an elimination half-life of 17 to 21 hours. It is contraindicated in patients with severe renal impairment. Bleeding is the major side effect of *fondaparinux*. There is no available agent for the reversal of bleeding associated with *fondaparinux*. HIT is less likely with *fondaparinux* than with *heparin* but is still a possibility.

VII. VITAMIN K ANTAGONISTS

Coumarin anticoagulants owe their action to the ability to antagonize the cofactor functions of vitamin K. The only coumarin anticoagulant available in the United States is *warfarin* [WAR-far-in]. The international normalized ratio (INR) is the standard by which the anticoagulant activity of *warfarin* therapy is monitored. *Warfarin* has a narrow therapeutic index. Therefore, it is important that the INR is maintained within the optimal range as much as possible, and frequent monitoring may be required.

A. Warfarin

1. **Mechanism of action:** Factors II, VII, IX, and X (Figure 21.10) require vitamin K as a cofactor for their synthesis by the liver. These factors undergo vitamin K–dependent posttranslational modification, whereby a number of their glutamic acid residues are carboxylated to form γ-carboxyglutamic acid residues (Figure 21.15). The γ-carboxyglutamyl residues bind calcium ions, which are essential for interaction between the coagulation factors and platelet membranes. In the carboxylation reactions, the vitamin K–dependent

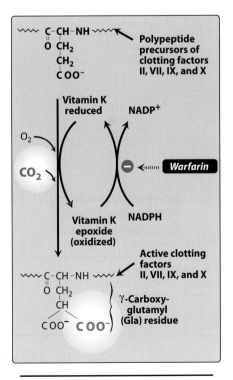

Figure 21.15
Mechanism of action of *warfarin*. NADP+ = oxidized form of nicotinamide adenine dinucleotide phosphate; NADPH = reduced form of nicotinamide adenine dinucleotide phosphate.

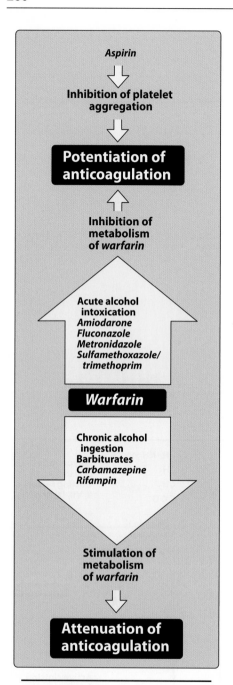

Figure 21.16
Drugs affecting the anticoagulant
effect of *warfarin*.

carboxylase fixes CO_2 to form the new COOH group on glutamic acid. The reduced vitamin K cofactor is converted to vitamin K epoxide during the reaction. Vitamin K is regenerated from the epoxide by vitamin K epoxide reductase, the enzyme that is inhibited by *warfarin*. *Warfarin* treatment results in the production of clotting factors with diminished activity (10% to 40% of normal), due to the lack of sufficient γ-carboxyglutamyl side chains. Unlike *heparin*, the anticoagulant effects of *warfarin* are not observed immediately after drug administration. Instead, peak effects may be delayed for 72 to 96 hours, which is the time required to deplete the pool of circulating clotting factors. The anticoagulant effects of *warfarin* can be overcome by the administration of *vitamin K*. However, reversal following administration of *vitamin K* takes approximately 24 hours (the time necessary for degradation of already synthesized clotting factors).

2. **Therapeutic use:** *Warfarin* is used in the prevention and treatment of DVT and PE, stroke prevention, stroke prevention in the setting of atrial fibrillation and/or prosthetic heart valves, protein C and S deficiency, and antiphospholipid syndrome. It is also used for prevention of venous thromboembolism following orthopedic surgery.

3. **Pharmacokinetics:** *Warfarin* is rapidly absorbed after oral administration (100% bioavailability with little individual patient variation). *Warfarin* is highly bound to plasma albumin, which prevents its diffusion into the cerebrospinal fluid, urine, and breast milk. However, drugs that have a greater affinity for the albumin-binding site, such as sulfonamides, can displace the anticoagulant and lead to a transient, elevated activity. Drugs that affect *warfarin* binding to plasma proteins can lead to variability in the therapeutic response to *warfarin*. *Warfarin* readily crosses the placental barrier. The mean half-life of *warfarin* is approximately 40 hours, but this value is highly variable among individuals. *Warfarin* is metabolized by the CYP450 system (mainly CYP2C9) to inactive components. After conjugation to glucuronic acid, the inactive metabolites are excreted in urine and feces. Agents that affect the metabolism of *warfarin* may alter its therapeutic effects. *Warfarin* has numerous drug interactions that may potentiate or attenuate its anticoagulant effect. The list of interacting drugs is extensive. A summary of some of the important interactions is shown in Figure 21.16.

4. **Adverse effects:** The principal adverse effect of *warfarin* is bleeding. Minor bleeding may be treated by withdrawal of the drug or administration of oral *vitamin K*, but severe bleeding may require greater doses of *vitamin K* given intravenously. Whole blood, frozen plasma, and plasma concentrates of blood factors may also be used for rapid reversal of *warfarin*. Skin lesions and necrosis are rare complications of *warfarin* therapy. Purple toe syndrome, a rare, painful, blue-tinged discoloration of the toe caused by cholesterol emboli from plaques, has also been observed with *warfarin* therapy. *Warfarin* is teratogenic and is contraindicated in pregnancy.

VIII. DIRECT ORAL ANTICOAGULANTS

A. Dabigatran

1. **Mechanism of action:** *Dabigatran etexilate* [da-bi-GAT-ran e-TEX-i-late] is the prodrug of the active moiety *dabigatran*, which is an oral direct thrombin inhibitor. Both clot-bound thrombin and free thrombin are inhibited by *dabigatran*.

2. **Therapeutic use:** *Dabigatran* is approved for the prevention of stroke and systemic embolism in patients with nonvalvular atrial fibrillation. It may also be used in the treatment of DVT and PE in patients who have already received parenteral anticoagulants and as prophylaxis to prevent or reduce the risk of recurrence of DVT and PE. The drug is contraindicated in patients with mechanical prosthetic heart valves and is not recommended in patients with bioprosthetic heart valves.

3. **Pharmacokinetics:** *Dabigatran etexilate* is administered orally. It is hydrolyzed to the active drug, *dabigatran*, by various plasma esterases. *Dabigatran* is metabolized by esterases. It is a substrate for P-glycoprotein (P-gp) and is eliminated renally.

4. **Adverse effects:** The major adverse effect, like other anticoagulants, is bleeding. *Dabigatran* should be used with caution in renal impairment or in patients over the age of 75, as the risk of bleeding is higher in these groups. *Idarucizumab* may be used to reverse bleeding in severe cases. GI adverse effects are common with *dabigatran* and may include dyspepsia, abdominal pain, esophagitis, and GI bleeding. Abrupt discontinuation should be avoided, as patients may be at increased risk for thrombotic events.

B. Direct oral factor Xa inhibitors

1. **Mechanism of action:** *Apixaban* [a-PIX-a-ban], *betrixaban* [be-TRIX-a-ban], *edoxaban* [e-DOX-a-ban], and *rivaroxaban* [RIV-a-ROX-a-ban] are oral inhibitors of factor Xa. Inhibition of factor Xa reduces the production of thrombin (IIa) from prothrombin (Figure 21.10).

2. **Therapeutic use:** With the exception of *betrixaban*, these agents are approved for prevention of stroke in nonvalvular atrial fibrillation, as well as the treatment of DVT and PE. *Rivaroxaban* and *apixaban* are also used as prophylaxis to prevent or reduce the risk of recurrence of DVT and PE. *Betrixaban* is indicated for the prophylaxis of DVT and PE in at-risk hospitalized medical patients.

3. **Pharmacokinetics:** These drugs are adequately absorbed after oral administration. *Rivaroxaban* is metabolized by the CYP 3A4/5 and CYP 2J2 isoenzymes to inactive metabolites. About one-third of the drug is excreted unchanged in the urine, and the inactive metabolites are excreted in the urine and feces. *Apixaban* is primarily metabolized by CYP 3A4, with CYP enzymes 1A2, 2C8, 2C9, 2C19, and 2J2 all sharing minor metabolic roles; approximately 27% is excreted renally. *Edoxaban* and *betrixaban* are minimally metabolized and are eliminated primarily unchanged in the urine and feces, respectively. All of these drugs are substrates of P-gp,

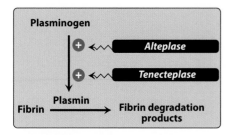

Figure 21.17
Activation of plasminogen by thrombolytic drugs.

and dosages should be reduced (in some cases concomitant use should be avoided) with P-gp inhibitors such as *clarithromycin*, *verapamil*, and *amiodarone*. Concomitant administration of *apixaban* and *rivaroxaban* with drugs that are strong P-gp and CYP 3A4 inducers (for example, *phenytoin*, *carbamazepine*, *rifampin*, *St. John's wort*) should be avoided due to the potential for reduced efficacy of the factor Xa inhibitors.

4. **Adverse effects:** Bleeding is the most serious adverse effect. Currently there is no antidote, but recombinant factor Xa products are in development. Declining kidney function can prolong the effect of these drugs and, therefore, increase the risk of bleeding. Renal dosage adjustments are recommended for these agents. Abrupt discontinuation of the factor Xa inhibitors should be avoided.

IX. THROMBOLYTIC DRUGS

Acute thromboembolic disease in selected patients may be treated by the administration of drugs that activate the conversion of plasminogen to plasmin, a serine protease that hydrolyzes fibrin and, thus, dissolves clots.

A. Common characteristics of thrombolytic agents

1. **Mechanism of action:** The thrombolytic agents act either directly or indirectly to convert plasminogen to plasmin, which, in turn, cleaves fibrin, thus lysing thrombi (Figure 21.17). Clot dissolution and reperfusion occur with a higher frequency when therapy is initiated early after clot formation because clots become more resistant to lysis as they age. Unfortunately, increased local thrombi may occur as the clot dissolves, leading to enhanced platelet aggregation and thrombosis. Strategies to prevent this include administration of antiplatelet drugs, such as *aspirin*, or antithrombotics such as *heparin*.

2. **Therapeutic use:** Originally used for the treatment of DVT and serious PE, thrombolytic drugs are currently used less frequently because of tendency to cause serious bleeding. For MI, intracoronary delivery of the drugs is the most reliable in terms of achieving recanalization. However, cardiac catheterization may not be possible in the 2- to 6-hour "therapeutic window," beyond which significant myocardial salvage becomes less likely. Thus, thrombolytic agents are usually administered intravenously. Thrombolytic agents are helpful in restoring catheter and shunt function, by lysing clots causing occlusions. They are also used to dissolve clots that result in strokes.

3. **Adverse effects:** Thrombolytic agents do not distinguish between the fibrin of an unwanted thrombus and the fibrin of a beneficial hemostatic plug. Thus, hemorrhage is a major adverse effect. For example, a previously unsuspected lesion, such as a gastric ulcer, may hemorrhage following injection of a thrombolytic agent (Figure 21.18). These drugs are contraindicated in pregnancy and in patients with healing wounds, a history of cerebrovascular accident, brain tumor, head trauma, intracranial bleeding, and metastatic cancer.

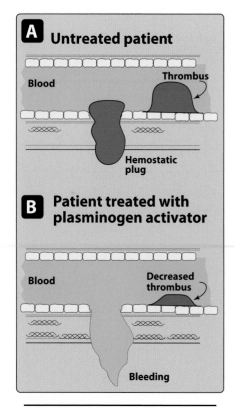

Figure 21.18
Degradation of an unwanted thrombus and a beneficial hemostatic plug by plasminogen activators.

B. Alteplase and tenecteplase

Alteplase [AL-teh-place] (formerly known as *tissue plasminogen activator* or *tPA*) is a serine protease originally derived from cultured human melanoma cells. It is now obtained as a product of recombinant DNA technology. *Tenecteplase* [ten-EK-te-place] is recombinant tPA with a longer half-life and greater binding affinity for fibrin than *alteplase*. *Alteplase* has a low affinity for free plasminogen in the plasma, but it rapidly activates plasminogen that is bound to fibrin in a thrombus or a hemostatic plug. Thus, *alteplase* is said to be "fibrin selective" at low doses. *Alteplase* is approved for the treatment of MI, massive PE, and acute ischemic stroke. *Tenecteplase* is approved only for use in acute MI.

Alteplase has a very short half-life (5 to 30 minutes), and therefore, a portion of the total dose is injected intravenously as a bolus, and the remaining drug is administered over 1 to 3 hours, depending on the indication. *Tenecteplase* has a longer half-life and, therefore, may be administered as an intravenous bolus. *Alteplase* may cause angioedema, and there may be an increased risk of this effect when combined with angiotensin-converting enzyme (ACE) inhibitors.

X. DRUGS USED TO TREAT BLEEDING

Bleeding problems may have their origin in naturally occurring pathologic conditions, such as hemophilia, or as a result of fibrinolytic states that may arise after surgery. The use of anticoagulants may also give rise to hemorrhage. Certain natural proteins and *vitamin K*, as well as synthetic antagonists, are effective in controlling this bleeding (Figure 21.19). Concentrated preparations of coagulation factors are available from human donors. However, these preparations carry the risk of transferring viral infections. Blood transfusion is also an option for treating severe hemorrhage.

Medication	Antidote for Bleeding Caused by	Adverse Effects	Monitoring Parameters
Aminocaproic acid *Tranexamic acid*	**Fibrinolytic state**	**Muscle necrosis** **Thrombosis** **CVA** **Seizure**	**CBC** **Muscle enzymes** **Blood pressure**
Idarucizumab	*Dabigatran*	**Hypokalemia** **Thrombosis**	**aPTT** **Clotting time** **Thrombin time**
Protamine sulfate	*Heparin*	**Flushing** **Nausea/vomiting** **Dyspnea** **Bradyarrhythmia** **Hypotension** **Anaphylaxis**	**Coagulation monitoring** **Blood pressure** **Heart rate**
Vitamin K1	*Warfarin*	**Skin reaction** **Anaphylaxis**	**PT/INR**

Figure 21.19
Summary of drugs used to treat bleeding. aPTT = activated partial thromboplastin time, CBC = complete blood count, CVA = cerebrovascular accident, INR = international normalized ratio, PT = prothrombin time.

A. Aminocaproic acid and tranexamic acid

Fibrinolytic states can be controlled by the administration of *aminocaproic* [a-mee-noe-ka-PROE-ic] *acid* or *tranexamic* [tran-ex-AM-ic] *acid*. Both agents are synthetic, orally active, excreted in the urine, and inhibit plasminogen activation. *Tranexamic acid* is 10 times more potent than *aminocaproic acid*. A potential side effect is intravascular thrombosis.

B. Protamine sulfate

Protamine [PROE-ta-meen] *sulfate* antagonizes the anticoagulant effects of *heparin*. This protein is derived from fish sperm or testes and is high in arginine content, which explains its basicity. The positively charged *protamine* interacts with the negatively charged *heparin*, forming a stable complex without anticoagulant activity. Adverse effects of drug administration include hypersensitivity as well as dyspnea, flushing, bradycardia, and hypotension when rapidly injected.

C. Vitamin K

Vitamin K_1 (*phytonadione*) administration can stop bleeding problems due to *warfarin* by increasing the supply of active *vitamin K_1*, thereby inhibiting the effect of *warfarin*. *Vitamin K_1* may be administered via the oral, subcutaneous, or intravenous route. [Note: Intravenous *vitamin K* should be administered by slow IV infusion to minimize the risk of hypersensitivity or anaphylactoid reactions.] For the treatment of bleeding, the subcutaneous route of *vitamin K_1* is less preferred, as it is not as effective as oral or IV administration. The response to *vitamin K_1* is slow, requiring about 24 hours to reduce INR (time to synthesize new coagulation factors). Thus, if immediate hemostasis is required, fresh frozen plasma should be infused.

D. Idarucizumab

Idarucizumab [EYE-da-roo-KIZ-ue-mab] is a monoclonal antibody fragment used to reverse bleeding caused by *dabigatran*. By binding to *dabigatran* and its metabolites, *idarucizumab* neutralizes anticoagulation. *Idarucizumab* is administered intravenously and is rapidly eliminated. *Idarucizumab* is used in emergency situations, in the inpatient setting. Because it reverses the effect of *dabigatran*, thrombosis is the most serious adverse effect of *idarucizumab*.

Study Questions

Choose the ONE best answer.

21.1 Which of the P2Y$_{12}$ ADP receptor antagonists reversibly binds the receptor?

A. Clopidogrel
B. Prasugrel
C. Ticagrelor
D. Ticlopidine

Correct answer = C. Of the P2Y$_{12}$ ADP receptor antagonists listed, ticagrelor is the only one that reversibly binds the receptor. This is important when it comes to compliance. If a patient is not compliant, then the antiplatelet activity of ticagrelor stops when the drug is missed (since the platelets are not irreversibly inhibited as they would be with aspirin, clopidogrel, or prasugrel).

21.2 A 70-year-old woman is diagnosed with nonvalvular atrial fibrillation. Her past medical history is significant for chronic kidney disease, and her renal function is moderately diminished. Which anticoagulant for atrial fibrillation avoids the need for renal dose adjustment in this patient?

A. Apixaban
B. Dabigatran
C. Rivaroxaban
D. Warfarin

Correct answer = D. Warfarin does not require dosage adjustment in renal dysfunction. The INR is monitored and dosage adjustments are made on the basis of this information. All of the other agents are renally cleared to some extent and require dosage adjustments in renal dysfunction.

21.3 An 80-year-old man is taking warfarin indefinitely for the prevention of deep venous thrombosis. He is compliant, has a stable INR, and denies bleeding or bruising. He is diagnosed with a urinary tract infection and is prescribed sulfamethoxazole/trimethoprim. What are the expected effects on his warfarin therapy?

A. Decreased anticoagulant effect of warfarin
B. Increased anticoagulant effect of warfarin
C. Activation of platelet activity
D. No change in anticoagulation status

Correct answer = B. Sulfamethoxazole/trimethoprim has a significant drug interaction with warfarin, such that it inhibits warfarin metabolism. Therefore, sulfamethoxazole/trimethoprim will cause increased anticoagulant effects, and the patient will need to have his warfarin dose decreased and INR checked frequently while he is on this antibiotic.

21.4 A 47-year-old woman presents to the emergency room with severe bleeding. Upon evaluation of the medical record, you discover that she takes dabigatran for a history of multiple DVTs. What is the appropriate reversal agent to administer to the patient at this time?

A. Protamine
B. Vitamin K
C. Idarucizumab
D. A reversal agent does not exist for this medication

Correct answer = C. Idarucizumab is used to reverse bleeding caused by dabigatran. By binding to dabigatran and its metabolites, idarucizumab neutralizes anticoagulation. It would be important to monitor this patient for any signs of thrombosis due to reversal of her anticoagulation. Vitamin K is the antidote for warfarin, and protamine is the antidote for heparin.

21.5 Which must heparin bind to in order to exert its anticoagulant effect?

A. GP IIb/IIIa receptor
B. Thrombin
C. Antithrombin III
D. von Willebrand factor

Correct answer = C. Heparin binds to antithrombin III, causing a conformational change. This heparin/antithrombin III complex then inactivates thrombin and factor Xa.

21.6 Which is considered "fibrin selective" because it rapidly activates plasminogen that is bound to fibrin?

A. Alteplase
B. Fondaparinux
C. Argatroban
D. Bivalirudin

Correct answer = A. Alteplase has a low affinity for free plasminogen in the plasma, but it rapidly activates plasminogen that is bound to fibrin in a thrombus or a hemostatic plug. It has the advantage of lysing only fibrin, without unwanted degradation of other proteins (notably fibrinogen).

21.7 A 56-year-old man presents to the emergency room with complaints of swelling, redness, and pain in his right leg. The patient is diagnosed with acute DVT, and the provider wants to start an oral agent. Which drug is most appropriate for treatment of DVT in this patient?

A. Rivaroxaban
B. Betrixaban
C. Enoxaparin
D. Clopidogrel

Correct answer = A. Betrixaban is only approved for the prophylaxis of DVT and PE; it is not approved for the treatment of acute DVT. Enoxaparin is used for the treatment of DVT, but it is an injectable medication. Clopidogrel is an antiplatelet medication that is not appropriate for acute treatment of DVT.

21.8 Which is most appropriate for reversing the anticoagulant effects of heparin?

  A. Aminocaproic acid
  B. Protamine sulfate
  C. Vitamin K_1
  D. Tranexamic acid

Correct answer = B. Excessive bleeding may be managed by ceasing administration of heparin or by treating with protamine sulfate. Infused slowly, protamine sulfate combines ionically with heparin to form a stable, inactive complex. Aminocaproic acid and tranexamic acid are approved for the treatment of hemorrhage but do not specifically reverse the effects of heparin to stop bleeding. Vitamin K_1 is used to help reverse the effects of warfarin-induced bleeding.

21.9 A 62-year-old man taking warfarin for stroke prevention in atrial fibrillation presents to his primary care physician with an elevated INR of 10.5 without bleeding. He is instructed to hold his warfarin dose and given oral vitamin K_1. When would the effects of vitamin K on the INR most likely be noted in this patient?

  A. 1 hour
  B. 6 hours
  C. 24 hours
  D. 72 hours

Correct answer = C. Vitamin K_1 takes about 24 hours to see a reduction in the INR. This is due to the time required for the body to synthesize new coagulation factors.

21.10 A 58-year-old man receives intravenous alteplase treatment for acute stroke. Five minutes following completion of alteplase infusion, he develops angioedema. Which of the following drugs may have increased the risk of developing angioedema in this patient?

  A. ACE inhibitor
  B. GP IIb/IIIa receptor antagonist
  C. Phosphodiesterase inhibitor
  D. Thiazide diuretic

Correct answer = A. ACE inhibitors, aspirin, and prasugrel all have possible adverse effects including angioedema. In the setting of alteplase administration, ACE inhibitors have been associated with an increased risk of developing angioedema with concomitant use.

Drugs for Hyperlipidemia

22

Karen Sando and Kevin Cowart

I. OVERVIEW

Coronary heart disease (CHD) is the leading cause of death worldwide. CHD is correlated with elevated levels of low-density lipoprotein cholesterol (LDL-C) and triglycerides, and low levels of high-density lipoprotein cholesterol (HDL-C). Other risk factors for CHD include cigarette smoking, hypertension, obesity, diabetes, chronic kidney disease, and advanced age. Elevated cholesterol levels (hyperlipidemia) may be due to lifestyle factors (for example, lack of exercise or diet containing excess saturated fats). Hyperlipidemia can also result from an inherited defect in lipoprotein metabolism or, more commonly, from a combination of genetic and lifestyle factors. Appropriate lifestyle changes, along with drug therapy, can lead to a 30% to 40% reduction in CHD mortality. Antihyperlipidemic drugs (Figure 22.1) are often taken indefinitely to reduce the risk of atherosclerotic cardiovascular disease (ASCVD) in select patients and to control plasma lipid levels. [Note: ASCVD includes CHD, stroke, and peripheral arterial disease.] Figure 22.2 illustrates the normal metabolism of serum lipoproteins and the characteristics of the major genetic hyperlipidemias.

II. TREATMENT GOALS

Plasma lipids consist mostly of lipoproteins, which are spherical complexes of lipids and specific proteins. The clinically important lipoproteins, listed in decreasing order of atherogenicity, are LDL, very–low-density lipoprotein (VLDL) and chylomicrons, and HDL. The occurrence of CHD is positively associated with high total cholesterol and has an even stronger correlation with elevated LDL-C. In contrast to LDL-C, high levels of HDL-C have been associated with a decreased risk for CHD (Figure 22.3). According to cholesterol guidelines, the need for antihyperlipidemic drug therapy should be determined based on an assessment of risk for ASCVD, in conjunction with evaluation of lipoprotein levels (for example, LDL-C; Figure 22.4). [Note: Therapeutic lifestyle changes, such as diet, exercise, and weight loss, may help reduce cholesterol levels; however, lifestyle modifications do not replace the need for drug therapy in patients who fall into one of the four statin benefit groups (see Figure 22.4).]

HMG CoA REDUCTASE INHIBITORS (STATINS)
Atorvastatin LIPITOR
Fluvastatin LESCOL
Lovastatin ALTOPREV
Pitavastatin LIVALO
Pravastatin PRAVACHOL
Rosuvastatin CRESTOR
Simvastatin ZOCOR

NIACIN
Niacin NIASPAN, SLO-NIACIN

FIBRATES
Gemfibrozil LOPID
Fenofibrate TRICOR, TRIGLIDE

BILE ACID SEQUESTRANTS
Colesevelam WELCHOL
Colestipol COLESTID
Cholestyramine PREVALITE, QUESTRAN

CHOLESTEROL ABSORPTION INHIBITOR
Ezetimibe ZETIA

OMEGA-3 FATTY ACIDS
Docosahexaenoic and *eicosapentaenoic acids* LOVAZA, VARIOUS OTC PREPARATIONS
Icosapent ethyl VASCEPA

PCSK9 INHIBITORS
Alirocumab PRALUENT
Evolocumab REPATHA

Figure 22.1
Summary of antihyperlipidemic drugs. HMG CoA = 3-hydroxy-3-methylglutaryl coenzyme A; OTC = over-the-counter; PCSK9 = proprotein convertase subtilisin kexin type 9.

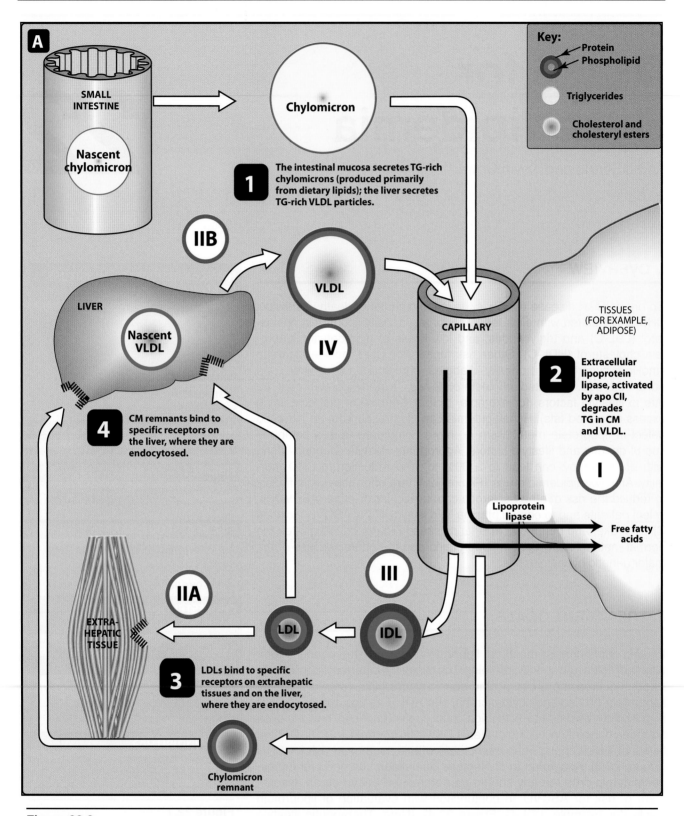

Figure 22.2
Metabolism of plasma lipoproteins and related genetic diseases. Roman numerals in the *white circles* refer to specific genetic types of hyperlipidemias summarized on the facing page. apo CII = apolipoprotein CII found in chylomicrons and VLDL; CM = chylomicron; IDL = intermediate-density lipoprotein; LDL = low-density lipoprotein; PCSK9 = proprotein convertase subtilisin kexin type 9; TG = triglyceride; VLDL = very–low-density lipoprotein.

(Figure continues on next page)

B **Type I (FAMILIAL HYPERCHYLOMICRONEMIA)**

- Massive fasting hyperchylomicronemia, even following normal dietary fat intake, resulting in greatly elevated serum TG levels.
- Deficiency of lipoprotein lipase or deficiency of normal apolipoprotein CII (rare).
- Type I is not associated with an increase in coronary heart disease.
- Treatment: Low-fat diet. No drug therapy is effective for Type I hyperlipidemia.

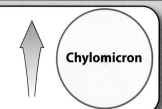

Type IIA (FAMILIAL HYPERCHOLESTEROLEMIA)

- Elevated LDL with normal VLDL levels due to a block in LDL degradation. This results in increased serum cholesterol but normal TG levels.
- Caused by defects in the synthesis or processing of LDL receptors.
- Ischemic heart disease is greatly accelerated.
- Treatment: Diet. Heterozygotes: *Cholestyramine* and *niacin*, a statin, or a statin and a PCSK9 inhibitor.

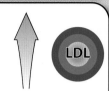

Type IIB (FAMILIAL COMBINED [MIXED] HYPERLIPIDEMIA)

- Similar to Type IIA except that VLDL is also increased, resulting in elevated serum TG as well as cholesterol levels.
- Caused by overproduction of VLDL by the liver.
- Relatively common.
- Treatment: Diet. Drug therapy is similar to that for Type IIA.

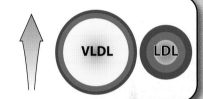

Type III (FAMILIAL DYSBETALIPOPROTEINEMIA)

- Serum concentrations of IDL are increased, resulting in increased TG and cholesterol levels.
- Cause is either overproduction or underutilization of IDL due to mutant apolipoprotein E.
- Xanthomas and accelerated vascular disease develop in patients by middle age.
- Treatment: Diet. Drug therapy includes *niacin* and *fenofibrate*, or a statin.

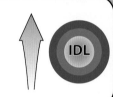

Type IV (FAMILIAL HYPERTRIGLYCERIDEMIA)

- VLDL levels are increased, whereas LDL levels are normal or decreased, resulting in normal to elevated cholesterol and greatly elevated circulating TG levels.
- Cause is overproduction and/or decreased removal of VLDL and TG in serum.
- This is a relatively common disease. It has few clinical manifestations other than accelerated ischemic heart disease. Patients with this disorder are frequently obese, diabetic, and hyperuricemic.
- Treatment: Diet. If necessary, drug therapy includes *niacin* and/or *fenofibrate*.

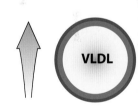

Type V (FAMILIAL MIXED HYPERTRIGLYCERIDEMIA)

- Serum VLDL and chylomicrons are elevated. LDL is normal or decreased. This results in elevated cholesterol and greatly elevated TG levels.
- Cause is either increased production or decreased clearance of VLDL and chylomicrons. Usually, it is a genetic defect.
- Occurs most commonly in adults who are obese and/or diabetic.
- Treatment: Diet. If necessary, drug therapy includes *niacin*, and/or *fenofibrate*, or a statin.

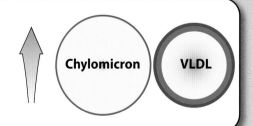

Figure 22.2 (continued)

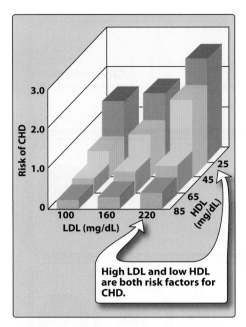

Figure 22.3
Effect of circulating low-density lipoprotein (LDL) and high-density lipoprotein (HDL) on the risk of coronary heart disease (CHD).

III. DRUGS FOR HYPERLIPIDEMIA

Antihyperlipidemic drugs include the statins, *niacin*, fibrates, bile acid sequestrants, a cholesterol absorption inhibitor, proprotein convertase subtilisin kexin type 9 (PCSK9) inhibitors, and omega-3 fatty acids. These agents may be used alone or in combination. However, drug therapy should always be accompanied by lifestyle modifications, such as exercise and a diet low in saturated fats.

A. HMG CoA reductase inhibitors

3-Hydroxy-3-methylglutaryl coenzyme A (HMG CoA) reductase inhibitors (commonly known as statins) lower LDL-C, resulting in a substantial reduction in coronary events and death from CHD. Therapeutic benefits include atherosclerotic plaque stabilization, improvement of coronary endothelial function, inhibition of platelet thrombus formation, and vascular anti-inflammatory activity. They are first-line treatment for patients with elevated risk of ASCVD to reduce the occurrence of ASCVD events (see Figure 22.4). [Note: The intensity of statin therapy should be guided by the patient's absolute risk for an ASCVD event.]

1. **Mechanism of action:** *Lovastatin* [LOE-vah-stat-in], *simvastatin* [sim-vah-STAT-in], *pravastatin* [PRAH-vah-stat-in], *atorvastatin* [a-TOR-vah-stat-in], *fluvastatin* [FLOO-vah-stat-in], *pitavastatin* [pit-AV-a-STAT-in], and *rosuvastatin* [roe-SOO-va-stat-in] are competitive inhibitors of HMG CoA reductase, the rate-limiting step in cholesterol synthesis. By inhibiting de novo cholesterol synthesis, they deplete the intracellular supply of cholesterol (Figure 22.5). Depletion of intracellular cholesterol causes the cell to increase the number of cell surface LDL receptors that can bind and internalize circulating LDL-C. Thus, plasma cholesterol is reduced, by both decreased cholesterol synthesis and increased LDL-C catabolism. *Rosuvastatin* and *atorvastatin* are the most potent LDL-C lowering statins, followed by *pitavastatin*, *simvastatin*, *lovastatin*, *pravastatin*, and *fluvastatin*. [Note: Because these agents undergo a marked first-pass extraction by the liver, their dominant effect is on that organ.] The HMG CoA reductase inhibitors also decrease triglyceride levels and may increase HDL-C in some patients.

2. **Therapeutic uses:** These drugs are used to lower the risk of ASCVD events for patients in the four statin benefit groups. Statins are effective in lowering plasma cholesterol levels in all types of hyperlipidemias. However, patients who are homozygous for familial hypercholesterolemia lack LDL receptors and, therefore, benefit much less from treatment with these drugs.

3. **Pharmacokinetics:** *Lovastatin* and *simvastatin* are lactones that are hydrolyzed to the active drug. The remaining statins are all administered in their active form. Absorption of the statins is variable (30% to 85%) following oral administration. All statins are metabolized by cytochrome P450 (CYP450) isoenzymes in the liver, except *pravastatin*. Excretion takes place principally through bile and feces, but some urinary elimination also occurs. Some characteristics of the statins are summarized in Figure 22.6.

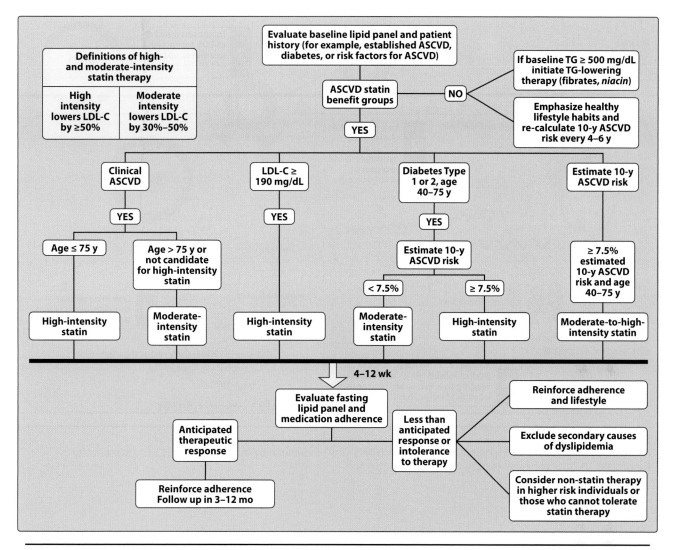

Figure 22.4
Treatment guidelines for hyperlipidemia. ASCVD = atherosclerotic cardiovascular disease; LDL-C = low-density lipoprotein cholesterol; TG = triglycerides.

4. **Adverse effects:** Elevated liver enzymes may occur with statin therapy. Therefore, liver function should be evaluated prior to starting therapy or if a patient has symptoms consistent with liver dysfunction. [Note: Hepatic insufficiency can cause drug accumulation.] Myopathy and rhabdomyolysis (disintegration of skeletal muscle; rare) have been reported (Figure 22.7). Risk factors for rhabdomyolysis, include renal insufficiency, vitamin D deficiency, hypothyroidism, advanced age, female sex, and use of drugs that increase the risk of muscle adverse effects, such as azole antifungals, protease inhibitors, *cyclosporine*, *erythromycin*, *gemfibrozil*, or *niacin*. *Simvastatin* is metabolized by CYP450 3A4, and inhibitors of this enzyme may increase the risk of rhabdomyolysis. Plasma creatine kinase levels should be determined in patients with muscle complaints. The HMG CoA reductase inhibitors may also increase the effect of *warfarin*. Thus, it is important to evaluate the international normalized ratio (INR) when initiating a statin or changing the dosage. These drugs are contraindicated during pregnancy, lactation, and active liver disease.

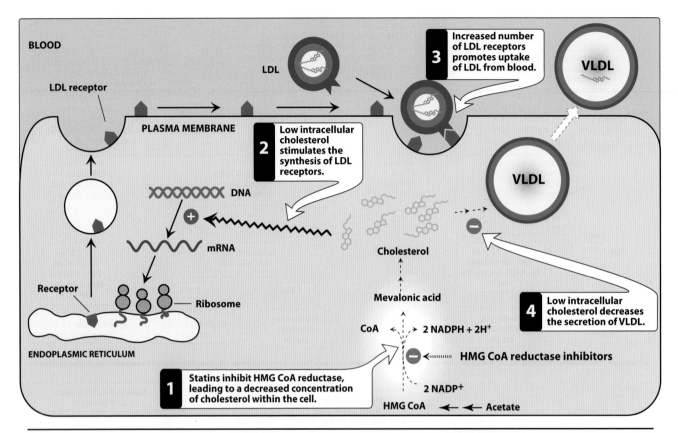

Figure 22.5
Inhibition of 3-hydroxy-3-methylglutaryl coenzyme A (HMG CoA) reductase by the statin drugs. LDL = low-density lipoprotein; VLDL = very–low-density lipoprotein.

Characteristic	Atorvastatin	Fluvastatin	Lovastatin	Pitavastatin	Pravastatin	Rosuvastatin	Simvastatin
Serum LDL cholesterol reduction produced (%)	55	24	34	43	34	60	41
Serum triglyceride reduction produced (%)	29	10	16	18	24	18	18
Serum HDL cholesterol increase produced (%)	6	8	9	8	12	8	12
Plasma half-life (h)	14	2–3	2	12	1–2	19	1–2
Penetration of central nervous system	No	No	Yes	Yes	No	No	Yes
Renal excretion of absorbed dose (%)	2	< 6	10	15	20	10	13

Figure 22.6
Summary of 3-hydroxy-3-methylglutaryl coenzyme A (HMG CoA) reductase inhibitors. LDL = low-density lipoprotein; HDL = high-density lipoprotein.

B. Niacin (nicotinic acid)

Niacin [NYE-uh-sin] reduces LDL-C by 10% to 20% and is the most effective agent for increasing HDL-C. It also lowers triglycerides by 20% to 35% at typical doses of 1.5 to 3 g/day. *Niacin* can be used in combination with statins, and fixed-dose combinations of long-acting *niacin* with *lovastatin* and *simvastatin* are available. [Note: the addition of *niacin* to statin therapy has not been shown to reduce the risk of ASCVD events.]

1. **Mechanism of action:** At gram doses, *niacin* strongly inhibits lipolysis in adipose tissue, thereby reducing production of free fatty acids (Figure 22.8). The liver normally uses circulating free fatty acids as a major precursor for triglyceride synthesis. Reduced liver triglyceride levels decrease hepatic VLDL production, which in turn reduces LDL-C plasma concentrations.

2. **Therapeutic uses:** Because *niacin* lowers plasma levels of both cholesterol and triglycerides, it is useful in the treatment of familial hyperlipidemias. It is also used to treat other severe hypercholesterolemias, often in combination with other agents.

3. **Pharmacokinetics:** *Niacin* is administered orally. It is converted in the body to nicotinamide, which is incorporated into the cofactor nicotinamide adenine dinucleotide (NAD⁺). *Niacin*, its nicotinamide derivative, and other metabolites are excreted in the urine. [Note: Administration of nicotinamide alone does not decrease plasma lipid levels.]

4. **Adverse effects:** The most common adverse effects of *niacin* are an intense cutaneous flush accompanied by an uncomfortable feeling of warmth and pruritus. Administration of *aspirin* prior to taking *niacin* decreases the flush, which is prostaglandin-mediated. Some patients also experience nausea and abdominal pain. Slow titration of the dosage or use of the sustained-release formulation of *niacin* reduces bothersome initial adverse effects. *Niacin* inhibits tubular secretion of uric acid and, thus, predisposes patients to hyperuricemia and gout. Impaired glucose tolerance and hepatotoxicity have also been reported. The drug should be avoided in active hepatic disease or in patients with an active peptic ulcer.

C. Fibrates

Fenofibrate [fen-oh-FIH-brate] and *gemfibrozil* [jem-FI-broh-zill] are derivatives of fibric acid that lower serum triglycerides and increase HDL-C.

1. **Mechanism of action:** The peroxisome proliferator–activated receptors (PPARs) are members of the nuclear receptor family that regulate lipid metabolism. PPARs function as ligand-activated transcription factors. Upon binding to their natural ligands (fatty acids or eicosanoids) or antihyperlipidemic drugs, PPARs are activated. They then bind to peroxisome proliferator response elements, which ultimately leads to decreased triglyceride concentrations through increased expression

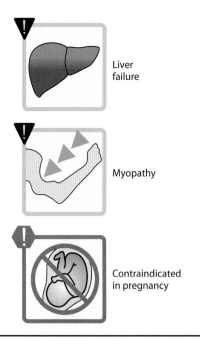

Figure 22.7
Some adverse effects and precautions associated with 3-hydroxy-3-methylglutaryl coenzyme A (HMG CoA) reductase inhibitors.

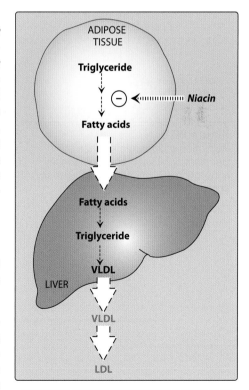

Figure 22.8
Niacin inhibits lipolysis in adipose tissue, resulting in decreased hepatic very–low-density lipoprotein (VLDL) synthesis and production of low-density lipoprotein (LDL) in the plasma.

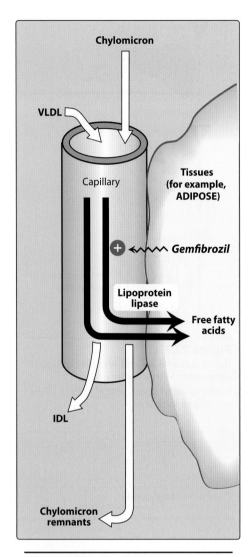

Figure 22.9
Activation of lipoprotein lipase by *gemfibrozil*. VLDL = very-low-density lipoprotein; IDL = intermediate-density lipoprotein.

of lipoprotein lipase (Figure 22.9) and decreased apolipoprotein (apo) CII concentration. *Fenofibrate* is more effective than *gemfibrozil* in lowering triglyceride levels. Fibrates also increase HDL-C by increasing the expression of apo AI and apo AII.

2. **Therapeutic uses:** The fibrates are used in the treatment of hypertriglyceridemias. They are particularly useful in treating type III hyperlipidemia (dysbetalipoproteinemia), in which intermediate-density lipoprotein particles accumulate.

3. **Pharmacokinetics:** *Gemfibrozil* and *fenofibrate* are completely absorbed after oral administration and distribute widely, bound to albumin. *Fenofibrate* is a prodrug, which is converted to the active moiety fenofibric acid. Both drugs undergo extensive biotransformation and are excreted in the urine as glucuronide conjugates.

4. **Adverse effects:** The most common adverse effects are mild gastrointestinal (GI) disturbances. These lessen as the therapy progresses. Because these drugs increase biliary cholesterol excretion, there is a predisposition to form gallstones. Myositis (inflammation of a voluntary muscle) can occur, and muscle weakness or tenderness should be evaluated. Patients with renal insufficiency may be at risk. Myopathy and rhabdomyolysis have been reported in patients taking *gemfibrozil* and statins together. The use of *gemfibrozil* is contraindicated with *simvastatin*, and, in general, the use of *gemfibrozil* with any statin should be avoided. Both fibrates may increase the effects of *warfarin*. Therefore, INR should be monitored more frequently when a fibrate is initiated. Fibrates should not be used in patients with severe hepatic or renal dysfunction, in patients with preexisting gallbladder disease or biliary cirrhosis.

D. Bile acid sequestrants

Bile acid sequestrants (resins) have significant LDL-C lowering effects, although the benefits are less than those observed with statins.

1. **Mechanism of action:** *Cholestyramine* [koe-LES-tir-a-meen], *colestipol* [koe-LES-tih-pole], and *colesevelam* [koh-le-SEV-e-lam] are anion-exchange resins that bind negatively charged bile acids and bile salts in the small intestine (Figure 22.10). The resin/bile acid complex is excreted in the feces, thus lowering the bile acid concentration. This causes hepatocytes to increase conversion of cholesterol to bile acids, which are essential components of the bile. Consequently, intracellular cholesterol concentrations decrease, which activates an increased hepatic uptake of cholesterol-containing LDL-C particles, leading to a decrease in plasma LDL-C. [Note: This increased uptake is mediated by an up-regulation of cell surface LDL receptors.]

2. **Therapeutic uses:** The bile acid sequestrants are useful (often in combination with diet or *niacin*) for treating type IIA and type IIB hyperlipidemias. [Note: In those rare individuals who are homozygous for type IIA and functional LDL receptors are totally lacking, these drugs have little effect on plasma LDL levels.] *Cholestyramine* can also relieve pruritus caused by accumulation of bile acids in patients with biliary stasis. *Colesevelam* is also indicated for type 2 diabetes due to its glucose-lowering effects.

3. **Pharmacokinetics:** Bile acid sequestrants are insoluble in water and have large molecular weights. After oral administration, they are neither absorbed nor metabolically altered by the intestine. Instead, they are totally excreted in feces.

4. **Adverse effects:** The most common adverse effects are GI disturbances, such as constipation, nausea, and flatulence. *Colesevelam* has fewer GI side effects than other bile acid sequestrants. These agents may impair the absorption of the fat-soluble vitamins (A, D, E, and K), and they interfere with the absorption of many drugs (for example, *digoxin*, *warfarin*, and thyroid hormone). Therefore, other drugs should be taken at least 1 to 2 hours before, or 4 to 6 hours after, the bile acid sequestrants. These agents may raise triglyceride levels and are contraindicated in patients with significant hypertriglyceridemia (greater than 400 mg/dL).

E. Cholesterol absorption inhibitor

Ezetimibe [eh-ZEH-teh-mibe] selectively inhibits absorption of dietary and biliary cholesterol in the small intestine, leading to a decrease in the delivery of intestinal cholesterol to the liver. This causes a reduction of hepatic cholesterol stores and an increase in clearance of cholesterol from the blood. *Ezetimibe* lowers LDL-C by approximately 18% to 23%. Due its modest LDL-C lowering, *ezetimibe* is often used as an adjunct to maximally tolerated statin therapy in patients with high ASCVD risk, or in statin-intolerant patients. *Ezetimibe* is primarily metabolized in the small intestine and liver via glucuronide conjugation, with subsequent biliary and renal excretion. Patients with moderate to severe hepatic insufficiency should not be treated with *ezetimibe*. Adverse effects are uncommon with the use of *ezetimibe*.

F. Proprotein convertase subtilisin kexin type 9 inhibitors

Proprotein convertase subtilisin kexin type 9 (PCSK9) is an enzyme predominately produced in the liver. PCSK9 binds to the LDL receptor on the surface of hepatocytes, leading to the degradation of LDL receptors (Figure 22.11). By inhibiting the PCSK9 enzyme, more LDL receptors are available to clear LDL-C from the serum. *Alirocumab* [al-i-ROK-ue-mab] and *evolocumab* [e-voe-LOK-ue-mab] are PCSK9 inhibitors, which are fully humanized monoclonal antibodies. These agents are used in addition to maximally tolerated statin therapy in patients with heterozygous or homozygous familial hypercholesterolemia, or in patients with clinical ASCVD who require additional LDL-C lowering. When combined with statin therapy, PCSK9 inhibitors provide potent LDL-C lowering (50% to 70%). They may also be considered for patients with high ASCVD risk and statin intolerance. PCSK9 inhibitors are only available as subcutaneous injections and are administered every two to four weeks. Monoclonal antibodies are not eliminated by the kidneys and have been used in dialysis patients or those with severe renal impairment. PCSK9 inhibitors are generally well tolerated. The most common adverse drug reactions are injection site reactions, immunologic or allergic reactions, nasopharyngitis, and upper respiratory tract infections.

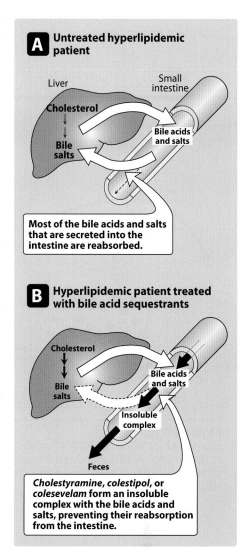

A Untreated hyperlipidemic patient

Liver
Small intestine
Cholesterol
Bile salts
Bile acids and salts

Most of the bile acids and salts that are secreted into the intestine are reabsorbed.

B Hyperlipidemic patient treated with bile acid sequestrants

Cholesterol
Bile salts
Bile acids and salts
Insoluble complex
Feces

Cholestyramine, colestipol, or *colesevelam* form an insoluble complex with the bile acids and salts, preventing their reabsorption from the intestine.

Figure 22.10
Mechanism of bile acid sequestrants.

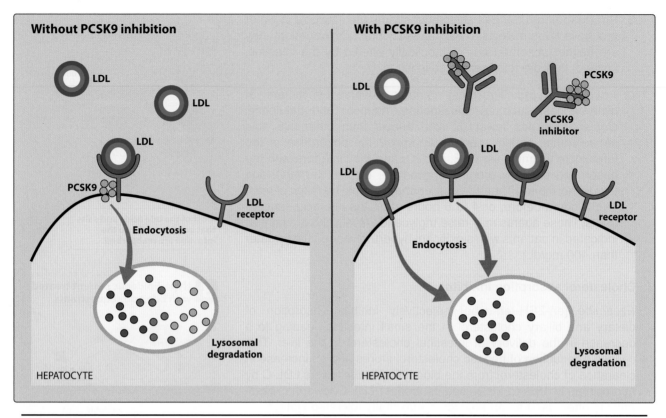

Figure 22.11
Mechanism of action of PCSK9 inhibitors. PCSK9 binds to the LDL receptor on the surface of hepatocytes, leading
to degradation of LDL receptors. Inhibition of PCSK9 prevents degradation of LDL receptors and promotes greater
clearance of LDL-C from the serum. LDL = low-density lipoprotein cholesterol; PCSK9 = proprotein convertase subtilisin
kexin type 9.

G. Omega-3 fatty acids

Omega-3 polyunsaturated fatty acids (PUFAs) are essential fatty
acids that are predominately used for triglyceride lowering. Essential
fatty acids inhibit VLDL and triglyceride synthesis in the liver. The
omega-3 PUFAs eicosapentaenoic acid (EPA) and docosahexaenoic
acid (DHA) are found in marine sources such as tuna, halibut, and
salmon. Approximately 4 g of marine-derived omega-3 PUFAs daily
decreases serum triglyceride concentrations by 25% to 30%, with
small increases in LDL-C and HDL-C. Over-the-counter or prescription fish oil capsules (EPA/DHA) can be used for supplementation,
as it is difficult to consume enough omega-3 PUFAs from dietary
sources alone. *Icosapent* [eye-KOE-sa-pent] *ethyl* is a prescription
product that contains only EPA and, unlike other fish oil supplements,
does not significantly raise LDL-C. Omega-3 PUFAs can be considered as an adjunct to other lipid-lowering therapies for individuals
with elevated triglycerides ($\geq$500 mg/dL). Although effective for triglyceride lowering, omega-3 PUFA supplementation has not been
shown to reduce cardiovascular morbidity and mortality. The most
common side effects of omega-3 PUFAs include GI effects (abdominal pain, nausea, diarrhea) and a fishy aftertaste. Bleeding risk can
be increased in those who are concomitantly taking anticoagulants or
antiplatelet agents.

TYPE OF DRUG	EFFECT ON LDL	EFFECT ON HDL	EFFECT ON TRIGLYCERIDES
HMG CoA reductase inhibitors (statins)	↓↓↓↓	↑↑	↓↓
Fibrates	↓	↑↑↑	↓↓↓↓
Niacin	↓↓	↑↑↑↑	↓↓↓
Bile acid sequestrants	↓↓↓	↑	↑
Cholesterol absorption inhibitor	↓	↑	↓
PCSK9 inhibitors	↓↓↓↓↓	↑↑	↓

Figure 22.12
Characteristics of antihyperlipidemic drug families. HDL = high-density lipoprotein; HMG CoA = 3-hydroxy-3-methylglutaryl coenzyme A; LDL = low-density lipoprotein.

H. Combination drug therapy

It is sometimes necessary to use two antihyperlipidemic drugs to achieve treatment goals. Patients with established ASCVD, an elevated 10-year risk of ASCVD, or those that do not achieve intended LDL-C reductions on maximally tolerated statin therapy may be considered for combination therapy. *Ezetimibe* and PCSK9 inhibitors can be considered for add-on therapy, since there is evidence that these combinations further reduce ASCVD events in patients already taking statin therapy. Combination drug therapy is not without risks. Liver and muscle toxicity occur more frequently with lipid-lowering drug combinations. Figure 22.12 summarizes some actions of the antihyperlipidemic drugs.

Study Questions

Choose the ONE best answer.

22.1 Which of the following is the most common adverse effect of antihyperlipidemic drug therapy?

A. Elevated blood pressure
B. Gastrointestinal disturbance
C. Neurologic problems
D. Heart palpitations

Correct answer = B. Gastrointestinal disturbances frequently occur as an adverse effect of antihyperlipidemic drug therapy. The other choices are not seen as often.

22.2 Which of the following hyperlipidemias is characterized by elevated plasma levels of chylomicrons and has no drug therapy available to lower the plasma lipoprotein levels?

A. Type I
B. Type II
C. Type III
D. Type IV

Correct answer = A. Type I hyperlipidemia (hyperchylomicronemia) is treated with a low-fat diet. No drug therapy is effective for this disorder.

22.3 Which of the following drugs decreases cholesterol synthesis by inhibiting the enzyme 3-hydroxy-3-methyl-glutaryl coenzyme A reductase?

A. Fenofibrate

B. Cholestyramine

C. Lovastatin

D. Gemfibrozil

Correct answer = C. Lovastatin decreases cholesterol synthesis by inhibiting HMG CoA reductase. Fenofibrate and gemfibrozil increase the activity of lipoprotein lipase, thereby increasing the removal of VLDL from plasma. Cholestyramine lowers the amount of bile acids returning to the liver via the enterohepatic circulation.

22.4 Which of the following nonstatin drugs lowers LDL-C most effectively?

A. Niacin

B. Alirocumab

C. Cholestyramine

D. Ezetimibe

Correct answer = B. Alirocumab is a PCSK9 inhibitor that can lower LDL-C by up to 70% in patients on statin therapy. Niacin primarily raises HDL-C and decreases triglycerides, with less potent effects on LDL-C lowering. Cholestyramine and ezetimibe both lower LDL-C, although not as potently as PCSK9 inhibitors.

22.5 Which of the following drugs binds bile acids in the intestine, thus preventing their return to the liver via the enterohepatic circulation?

A. Niacin

B. Fenofibrate

C. Cholestyramine

D. Fluvastatin

Correct answer = C. Cholestyramine is an anion-exchange resin that binds negatively charged bile acids and bile salts in the small intestine. The resin/bile acid complex is excreted in the feces, thus preventing the bile acids from returning to the liver by the enterohepatic circulation. The other choices do not bind intestinal bile acids.

22.6 A 65-year-old man has type 2 diabetes mellitus and an LDL-C of 165 mg/dL. Which is the best option to lower LDL-C and decrease the risk of ASCVD events in this patient?

A. Fenofibrate

B. Colesevelam

C. Rosuvastatin

D. Ezetimibe

Correct answer = C. Rosuvastatin, an HMG CoA reductase inhibitor (statin), is the most effective option for lowering LDL-C, achieving reductions of up to 60% from baseline levels. Statins are the primary modality for reducing ASCVD risk when drug therapy is indicated. Fenofibrate is more effective at lowering triglyceride levels or raising HDL-C. Colesevelam can reduce LDL-C, but not as effectively as statins. Ezetimibe lowers LDL-C modestly compared to the LDL-C reduction achieved by statins.

22.7 A 62-year-old female with hyperlipidemia and hypothyroidism is prescribed cholestyramine and levothyroxine (thyroid hormone). What advice would you give this patient to avoid a drug interaction between her cholestyramine and levothyroxine?

A. Stop taking the levothyroxine as it can interact with cholestyramine.

B. Take levothyroxine 1 hour before cholestyramine on an empty stomach.

C. Switch cholestyramine to colesevelam as this eliminates the interaction.

D. Switch cholestyramine to colestipol as this eliminates the interaction.

Correct answer = B. Cholestyramine and the bile acid sequestrants can bind several medications, causing decreased absorption of medications such as levothyroxine. Administration of levothyroxine 1 hour before or 4 to 6 hours after cholestyramine can help to avoid this interaction. Choices C and D are incorrect, as all bile acid sequestrants cause this interaction. Choice A is incorrect, as this patient should not stop her thyroid medication.

22.8 A 42-year-old man was started on sustained-release niacin 2 weeks ago. He reports uncomfortable flushing and itchiness that he thinks is related to the niacin. Which of the following can help manage this adverse effect of niacin therapy?

A. Administer aspirin 30 minutes prior to taking niacin.

B. Administer aspirin 30 minutes after taking niacin.

C. Increase the dose of niacin.

D. Change the sustained-release niacin to immediate-release niacin.

Correct answer = A. Flushing associated with niacin is prostaglandin mediated; therefore, use of aspirin (a prostaglandin inhibitor) can help to minimize this adverse effect. It must be administered 30 minutes before the dose of the niacin; therefore, choice B is incorrect. Increasing the dose of niacin is likely to increase these complaints; therefore, choice C is incorrect. The sustained-release formulation of niacin has less incidence of flushing versus that of the immediate release; therefore, choice D is incorrect.

22.9 A 72-year-old man with hyperlipidemia and renal insufficiency has been treated with high-intensity atorvastatin for 6 months. His LDL-C is 131 mg/dL; triglycerides, 710 mg/dL; and HDL-C, 32 mg/dL. His physician wishes to add another agent for hyperlipidemia. Which is the best option to address the hyperlipidemia in this patient?

A. Fenofibrate
B. Niacin
C. Colestipol
D. Gemfibrozil

Correct answer = B. This patient has significantly elevated triglycerides and low HDL-C. Niacin can lower triglycerides by 35% to 50% and also raise HDL-C. The fibrates (fenofibrate and gemfibrozil) should not be used due to the history of renal insufficiency. In addition, the use of gemfibrozil with statins should be avoided. Colestipol should not be used because triglycerides are greater than 400 mg/dL.

22.10 Which patient population is most likely to experience myalgia (muscle pain) or myopathy with use of HMG CoA reductase inhibitors?

A. Patients with renal insufficiency
B. Patients with gout
C. Patients with hypertriglyceridemia
D. Patients taking warfarin (blood thinner)

Correct answer = A. Patients with a history of renal insufficiency have a higher incidence of developing myalgias, myopathy, and rhabdomyolysis with use of HMG CoA reductase inhibitors (statins), especially with those that are renally eliminated as drug accumulation can occur. The other populations have not been reported to have a higher incidence of this adverse effect with HMG CoA reductase inhibitors.

Pituitary and Thyroid

23

Shannon Miller and Karen Whalen

I. OVERVIEW

The endocrine system releases hormones into the bloodstream, which carries chemical messengers to target cells throughout the body. Hormones have a much broader range of response time than do nerve impulses, requiring from seconds to days, or longer, to cause a response that may last for weeks or months. [Note: Nerve impulses generally act within milliseconds.] An important function of the hypothalamus is to connect the nervous system with the endocrine system via the pituitary gland. This chapter presents the central role of hypothalamic and pituitary hormones in regulating body functions. In addition, drugs affecting thyroid hormone synthesis and/or secretion are discussed (Figure 23.1). Chapters 24 to 26 focus on drugs that affect the synthesis and/or secretion of specific hormones and their actions.

II. HYPOTHALAMIC AND ANTERIOR PITUITARY HORMONES

The hormones secreted by the hypothalamus and the pituitary are peptides or glycoproteins that act by binding to specific receptor sites on target tissues. The hormones of the anterior pituitary are regulated by neuropeptides that are called either "releasing" or "inhibiting" factors or hormones. These are produced in the hypothalamus, and they reach the pituitary by the hypophyseal portal system (Figure 23.2). The interaction of the releasing hormones with receptors results in the activation of genes that promote the synthesis of protein precursors. The protein precursors then undergo posttranslational modification to produce hormones, which are released into the circulation. Each hypothalamic regulatory hormone controls the release of a specific hormone from the

HYPOTHALAMIC AND ANTERIOR PITUITARY HORMONES
Corticotropin H.P. ACTHAR
Cosyntropin CORTROSYN
Follitropin alfa GONAL-F
Follitropin beta FOLLISTIM AQ
Goserelin ZOLADEX
Histrelin SUPPRELIN LA, VANTAS
Lanreotide SOMATULINE DEPOT
Leuprolide LUPRON
Menotropins MENOPUR
Nafarelin SYNAREL
Octreotide SANDOSTATIN
Somatropin HUMATROPE, GENOTROPIN
Urofollitropin BRAVELLE
POSTERIOR PITUITARY HORMONES
Desmopressin DDAVP
Oxytocin PITOCIN
Vasopressin **(ADH)** VASOSTRICT
DRUGS AFFECTING THE THYROID
Iodine and potassium iodide LUGOL'S SOLUTION
Levothyroxine SYNTHROID
Liothyronine CYTOMEL
Liotrix THYROLAR
Methimazole TAPAZOLE
Propylthiouracil **(PTU)** GENERIC ONLY

Figure 23.1
Hormones and drugs affecting the hypothalamus, pituitary, and thyroid.

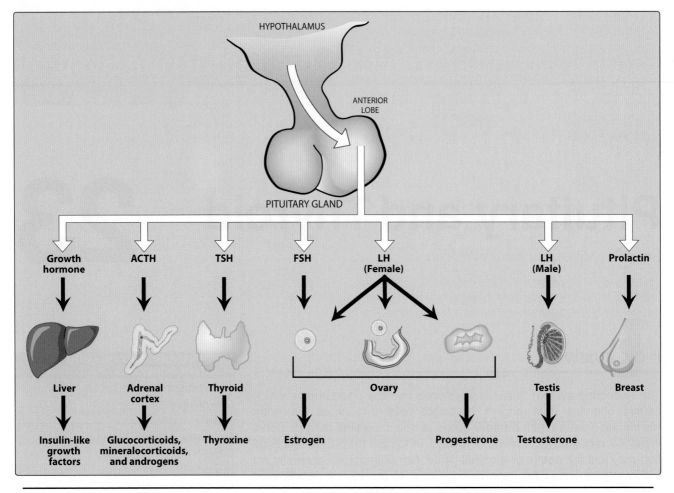

Figure 23.2
Anterior pituitary hormones. ACTH = adrenocorticotropic hormone; TSH = thyroid-stimulating hormone; FSH = follicle-stimulating hormone; LH = luteinizing hormone.

anterior pituitary. Pituitary hormone preparations are currently used for specific hormonal deficiencies, although most of the agents have limited therapeutic applications. Hormones of the anterior pituitary are administered intramuscularly (IM), subcutaneously, or intranasally because their peptidyl nature makes them susceptible to destruction by proteolytic enzymes of the digestive tract.

A. Adrenocorticotropic hormone (corticotropin)

Corticotropin-releasing hormone (CRH) is responsible for the synthesis and release of the peptide proopiomelanocortin by the pituitary (Figure 23.3). *Adrenocorticotropic hormone* (ACTH) or *corticotropin* [kor-ti-koe-TROE-pin] is a product of the posttranslational processing of this precursor polypeptide. [Note: CRH is used diagnostically to differentiate between Cushing syndrome and ectopic ACTH-producing cells.] Normally, ACTH is released from the pituitary in pulses with an overriding diurnal rhythm, with the highest concentration occurring in early morning and the lowest in late evening. Stress stimulates its secretion, whereas cortisol acting via negative feedback suppresses its release.

1. **Mechanism of action:** ACTH binds to receptors on the surface of the adrenal cortex, thereby activating G protein–coupled processes that ultimately stimulate the rate-limiting step in the adrenocorticosteroid synthetic pathway (cholesterol to pregnenolone; Figure 23.3). This pathway ends with the synthesis and release of adrenocorticosteroids and the adrenal androgens.

2. **Therapeutic uses:** The availability of synthetic adrenocorticosteroids with specific properties has limited the use of *corticotropin* mainly to serving as a diagnostic tool for differentiating between primary adrenal insufficiency (Addison disease, associated with adrenal atrophy) and secondary adrenal insufficiency (caused by inadequate secretion of ACTH by the pituitary). Therapeutic *corticotropin* preparations are extracts from the anterior pituitaries of domestic animals or synthetic human ACTH. The latter, *cosyntropin* [ko-sin-TROE-pin], is preferred for the diagnosis of adrenal insufficiency. ACTH is also used in the treatment of infantile spasms and multiple sclerosis.

3. **Adverse effects:** Short-term use of ACTH for diagnostic purposes is usually well tolerated. With longer use, toxicities are similar to glucocorticoids and include hypertension, peripheral edema, hypokalemia, emotional disturbances, and increased risk of infection.

B. Growth hormone (somatotropin)

Somatotropin is released by the anterior pituitary in response to growth hormone (GH)-releasing hormone (Figure 23.4). Conversely, secretion of GH is inhibited by the hormone somatostatin (see below). GH is released in a pulsatile manner, with the highest levels occurring during sleep. With increasing age, GH secretion decreases, accompanied by a decrease in lean muscle mass. Somatotropin influences a wide variety of biochemical processes (for example, cell proliferation and bone growth). Synthetic human GH (*somatropin* [soe-mah-TROE-pin]) is produced using recombinant DNA technology.

1. **Mechanism of action:** Although many physiologic effects of GH are exerted directly at its targets, others are mediated through the somatomedins—insulin-like growth factors 1 and 2 (IGF-1 and IGF-2). [Note: In acromegaly (a syndrome of excess GH due to hormone-secreting tumors), IGF-1 levels are consistently high, reflecting elevated GH.]

2. **Therapeutic uses:** *Somatropin* is used in the treatment of GH deficiency, growth failure in children, treatment of HIV patients with cachexia, and GH replacement in adults with confirmed deficiency. [Note: GH administered to adults increases lean body mass, bone density, and skin thickness, and decreases adipose tissue. Many consider GH an "antiaging" hormone. This has led to off-label use of GH by older individuals and by athletes seeking to enhance performance.] *Somatropin* is administered

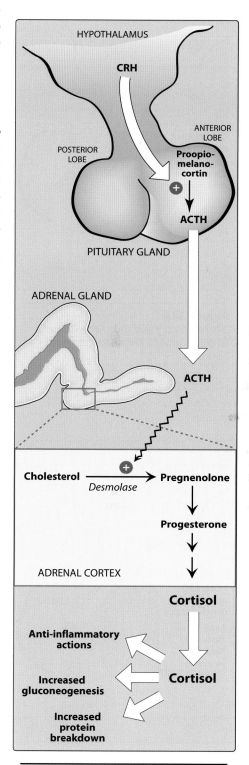

Figure 23.3
Secretion and actions of adrenocorticotropic hormone (ACTH). CRH = corticotropin-releasing hormone.

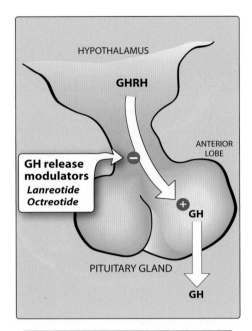

Figure 23.4
Secretion of growth hormone (GH).
GHRH = growth hormone–releasing
hormone.

by subcutaneous or IM injection. Although the half-life of GH is short (approximately 25 minutes), it induces release of IGF-1 from the liver, which is responsible for subsequent GH-like actions.

3. **Adverse effects:** Adverse effects of *somatropin* include pain at the injection site, edema, arthralgias, myalgias, nausea, and an increased risk of diabetes. *Somatropin* should not be used in pediatric patients with closed epiphyses, patients with diabetic retinopathy, or obese patients with Prader-Willi syndrome.

C. Somatostatin (growth hormone–inhibiting hormone)

In the pituitary, somatostatin binds to receptors that suppress GH and thyroid-stimulating hormone (TSH) release. Originally isolated from the hypothalamus, somatostatin is a small polypeptide found in neurons throughout the body as well as in the intestine, stomach, and pancreas. Somatostatin not only inhibits release of GH but also insulin, glucagon, and gastrin. *Octreotide* [ok-TREE-oh-tide] and *lanreotide* [lan-REE-oh-tide] are synthetic analogs of somatostatin with longer half-lives. Depot formulations of these agents allow for administration every 4 weeks. They have found use in the treatment of acromegaly and in severe diarrhea/flushing episodes associated with carcinoid tumors. An intravenous infusion of *octreotide* is also used for the treatment of bleeding esophageal varices. Adverse effects of *octreotide* include bradycardia, diarrhea, abdominal pain, flatulence, nausea, and steatorrhea. Gallbladder emptying is delayed, and asymptomatic cholesterol gallstones can occur with long-term treatment.

D. Gonadotropin-releasing hormone

Pulsatile secretion of gonadotropin-releasing hormone (GnRH) from the hypothalamus is essential for release of the gonadotropins follicle-stimulating hormone (FSH) and luteinizing hormone (LH) from the anterior pituitary. However, continuous administration of GnRH inhibits gonadotropin release through down-regulation of GnRH receptors on the pituitary. Continuous administration of synthetic GnRH analogs, such as *leuprolide* [loo-PROE-lide], is effective in suppressing production of FSH and LH (Figure 23.5). Suppression of gonadotropins, in turn, leads to reduced production of gonadal steroid hormones (androgens and estrogens). Thus, these agents are effective in the treatment of prostate cancer, endometriosis, and precocious puberty. *Leuprolide* is also used to suppress the LH surge and prevent premature ovulation in women undergoing controlled ovarian stimulation protocols for the treatment of infertility. [Note: GnRH antagonists such as *cetrorelix* (set-roe-REL-iks) and *ganirelix* (ga-ni-REL-iks) can also be used to inhibit LH secretion in infertility protocols.] In women, the GnRH analogs may cause hot flushes and sweating, as well as diminished libido, depression, and ovarian cysts. They are contraindicated in pregnancy and breast-feeding. In men, they initially cause a rise in testosterone that can result in bone pain. Hot flushes, edema, gynecomastia, and diminished libido may also occur.

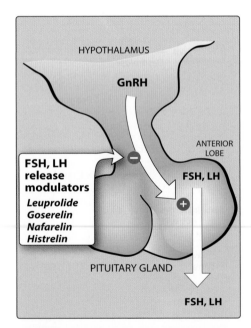

Figure 23.5
Secretion of follicle-stimulating hormone
(FSH) and luteinizing hormone (LH).
GnRH = gonadotropin-releasing
hormone.

E. Gonadotropins

The gonadotropins (FSH and LH) are produced in the anterior pituitary. The regulation of gonadal steroid hormones depends on these agents. They find use in the treatment of infertility. *Menotropins* [men-oh-TROE-pinz] (also known as *human menopausal gonadotropins* or *hMG*) are obtained from urine of postmenopausal women and contain both FSH and LH. *Urofollitropin* [yoor-oh-fol-li-TROE-pin] is FSH obtained from postmenopausal women and is devoid of LH. *Follitropin* [fol-ih-TROE-pin] *alfa* and *follitropin beta* are human FSH products manufactured using recombinant DNA technology. *Human chorionic gonadotropin* (*hCG*) is a placental hormone that is excreted in urine of pregnant women. The effects of *hCG* and *choriogonadotropin* [kore-ee-oh-goe-NAD-oh-troe-pin] *alfa* (made using recombinant DNA technology) are essentially identical to those of LH. All of these hormones are injected via the IM or subcutaneous route. Injection of *hMG* or FSH products over a period of 5 to 12 days causes ovarian follicular growth and maturation, and with subsequent injection of *hCG*, ovulation occurs. Adverse effects include ovarian enlargement and possible ovarian hyperstimulation syndrome, which may be life threatening. Multiple births can occur.

F. Prolactin

Prolactin is a peptide hormone secreted by the anterior pituitary. Its primary function is to stimulate and maintain lactation. In addition, it decreases sexual drive and reproductive function. Thyrotropin-releasing hormone stimulates the release of prolactin, and secretion is inhibited by dopamine acting at D_2 receptors (Figure 23.6). [Note: Drugs that act as dopamine antagonists (for example, *metoclopramide* and some antipsychotics) can increase the secretion of prolactin.] Hyperprolactinemia, which is associated with galactorrhea and hypogonadism, is treated with D_2 receptor agonists, such as *bromocriptine* and *cabergoline*. Both of these agents also find use in the treatment of pituitary microadenomas. *Bromocriptine* is also indicated for treatment of type 2 diabetes. Among their adverse effects are nausea, headache and, less frequently, psychosis.

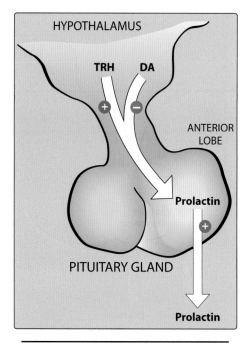

Figure 23.6
Secretion and action of prolactin. DA = dopamine; TRH = thyrotropin-releasing hormone.

III. HORMONES OF THE POSTERIOR PITUITARY

In contrast to the hormones of the anterior lobe of the pituitary, those of the posterior lobe, *vasopressin* and *oxytocin*, are not regulated by releasing hormones. Instead, they are synthesized in the hypothalamus, transported to the posterior pituitary, and released in response to specific physiologic signals, such as high plasma osmolarity or parturition. Both hormones are administered intravenously and have very short half-lives. Their actions are summarized in Figure 23.7.

A. Oxytocin

Oxytocin [ok-se-TOE-sin] is used in obstetrics to stimulate uterine contraction and induce labor. *Oxytocin* also causes milk ejection by contracting the myoepithelial cells around the mammary alveoli. Although toxicities are uncommon with proper drug use,

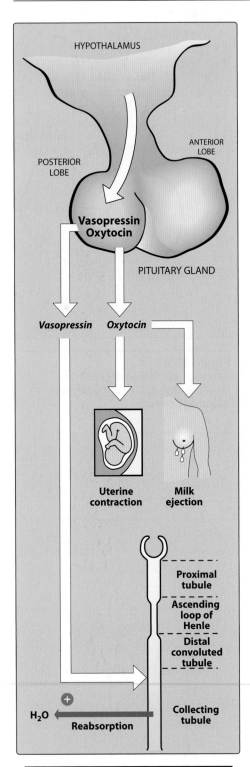

Figure 23.7
Actions of *oxytocin* and *vasopressin*.

hypertension, uterine rupture, water retention, and fetal death may occur. Its antidiuretic and pressor activities are much less than those of *vasopressin*.

B. Vasopressin

Vasopressin [vas-oh-PRESS-in] (antidiuretic hormone) is structurally related to *oxytocin*. *Vasopressin* has both antidiuretic and vasopressor effects (Figure 23.7). In the kidney, it binds to the V_2 receptor to increase water permeability and reabsorption in the collecting tubules. Thus, the major use of *vasopressin* is to treat diabetes insipidus. It also finds use in septic shock and in controlling bleeding due to esophageal varices. Other effects of *vasopressin* are mediated by the V_1 receptor, which is found in the liver, vascular smooth muscle (where it causes constriction), and other tissues. The major toxicities of *vasopressin* are water intoxication and hyponatremia. Abdominal pain, tremor, and vertigo can also occur. *Desmopressin* [des-moe-PRESS-in], an analog of *vasopressin*, has minimal activity at the V_1 receptor, making it largely free of pressor effects. This analog is longer acting than *vasopressin* and is preferred for the treatment of diabetes insipidus and nocturnal enuresis. For these indications, *desmopressin* is administered intranasally or orally. [Note: The nasal spray should not be used for enuresis due to reports of seizures in children using this formulation.] Local irritation may occur with the nasal spray.

IV. THYROID HORMONES

The thyroid gland facilitates normal growth and maturation by maintaining a level of metabolism in the tissues that is optimal for normal function. The two major thyroid hormones are triiodothyronine (T_3; the most active form) and thyroxine (T_4). Inadequate secretion of thyroid hormone (hypothyroidism) results in bradycardia, cold intolerance, and mental and physical slowing. In children, this can cause mental retardation and dwarfism. By contrast, excess secretion of thyroid hormones (hyperthyroidism) can cause tachycardia and cardiac arrhythmias, body wasting, nervousness, tremor, and heat intolerance.

A. Thyroid hormone synthesis and secretion

The thyroid gland is made up of multiple follicles that consist of a single layer of epithelial cells surrounding a lumen filled with thyroglobulin (the storage form of thyroid hormone). Thyroid function is controlled by TSH (thyrotropin), which is synthesized by the anterior pituitary (Figure 23.8). [Note: The hypothalamic thyrotropin-releasing hormone (TRH) governs the generation of TSH.] TSH action is mediated by cAMP and leads to stimulation of iodide (I^-) uptake by the thyroid gland. Oxidation to iodine (I_2) by a peroxidase is followed by iodination of tyrosines on thyroglobulin. [Note: Antibodies to thyroid peroxidase are diagnostic for Hashimoto thyroiditis, a common cause of hypothyroidism.] Condensation of two diiodotyrosine residues gives rise to T_4, whereas condensation of a monoiodotyrosine residue with a diiodotyrosine residue generates T_3. The hormones are released following proteolytic cleavage of the thyroglobulin. A summary of the steps in thyroid hormone synthesis and secretion is shown in Figure 23.9.

B. Mechanism of action

Most circulating T_3 and T_4 is bound to thyroxine-binding globulin in the plasma. The hormones must dissociate from thyroxine-binding globulin prior to entry into cells. In the cell, T_4 is enzymatically deiodinated to T_3, which enters the nucleus and attaches to specific receptors. The activation of these receptors promotes the formation of RNA and subsequent protein synthesis, which is responsible for the effects of T_4.

C. Pharmacokinetics

Both T_4 and T_3 are absorbed after oral administration. Food, calcium preparations, iron salts, and aluminum-containing antacids can decrease the absorption of T_4. Deiodination is the major route of metabolism of T_4. T_3 also undergoes sequential deiodination. The hormones are also metabolized via conjugation with glucuronides and sulfates and excreted into bile.

D. Treatment of hypothyroidism

Hypothyroidism usually results from autoimmune destruction of the gland and is diagnosed by elevated TSH. *Levothyroxine* (T_4) [leh-vo-thye-ROK-sin] is preferred over T_3 (*liothyronine* [lye-oh-THYE-roe-neen]) or T_3/T_4 combination products (*liotrix* [LYE-oh-trix]) for the treatment of hypothyroidism. *Levothyroxine* is better tolerated than T_3 preparations and has a longer half-life. It is dosed once daily, and

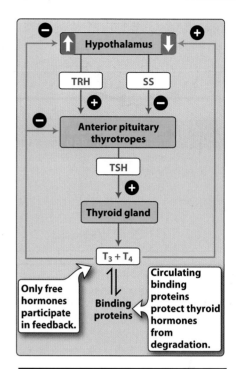

Figure 23.8
Feedback regulation of thyroid hormone release. SS = somatostatin; T_3 = triiodothyronine; T_4 = thyroxine; TRH = thyrotropin-releasing hormone; TSH = thyroid-stimulating hormone.

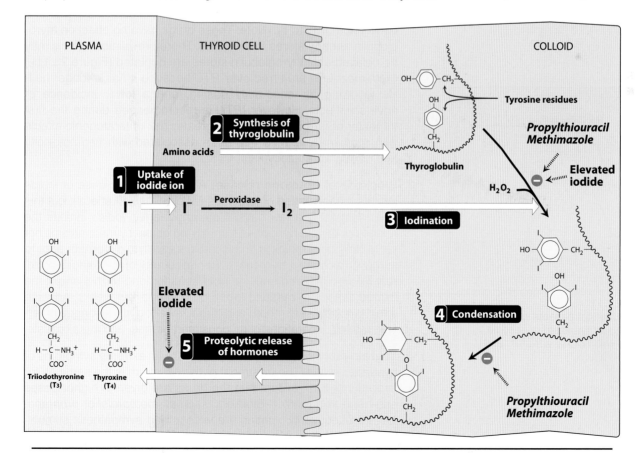

Figure 23.9
Biosynthesis of thyroid hormones.

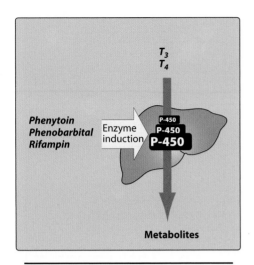

Figure 23.10
Enzyme induction can increase the metabolism of the thyroid hormones. T_3 = triiodothyronine; T_4 = thyroxine.

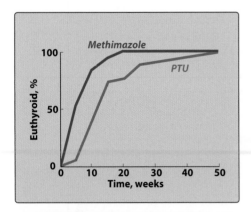

Figure 23.11
Time required for patients with Graves hyperthyroidism to become euthyroid with normal serum T_4 and T_3 concentrations.

steady state is achieved in 6 to 8 weeks. Toxicity is directly related to T_4 levels and manifests as nervousness, palpitations and tachycardia, heat intolerance, and unexplained weight loss. Drugs that induce the cytochrome P-450 enzymes, such as *phenytoin*, *rifampin*, and *phenobarbital*, accelerate metabolism of thyroid hormones and may decrease the effectiveness (Figure 23.10).

E. Treatment of hyperthyroidism (thyrotoxicosis)

Graves disease, an autoimmune disease that affects the thyroid, is the most common cause of hyperthyroidism. In these situations, TSH levels are low due to negative feedback. [Note: Feedback inhibition of TRH occurs with high levels of circulating thyroid hormone, which, in turn, decreases secretion of TSH.] The goal of therapy is to decrease synthesis and/or release of additional hormone. This can be accomplished by removing part or all of the thyroid gland, by inhibiting synthesis of the hormones, or by blocking release of hormones from the follicle.

1. **Removal of the thyroid:** This can be accomplished surgically or by destruction of the gland with radioactive iodine (^{131}I), which is selectively taken up by the thyroid follicular cells. Most patients become hypothyroid after radioactive iodine and require treatment with *levothyroxine*.

2. **Inhibition of thyroid hormone synthesis:** The thioamides, *propylthiouracil* [proe-pil-thye-oh-YOOR-ah-sil] (*PTU*) and *methimazole* [me-THIM-ah-zole], are concentrated in the thyroid, where they inhibit both the oxidative processes required for iodination of tyrosyl groups and the condensation (coupling) of iodotyrosines to form T_3 and T_4 (Figure 23.9). *PTU* also blocks the peripheral conversion of T_4 to T_3. [Note: These drugs have no effect on thyroglobulin already stored in the gland. Therefore, clinical effects may be delayed until thyroglobulin stores are depleted (Figure 23.11).] *Methimazole* is preferred over *PTU* because it has a longer half-life, allowing for once-daily dosing, and a lower incidence of adverse effects. However, *PTU* is recommended during the first trimester of pregnancy due to a greater risk of teratogenic effects with *methimazole*. *PTU* has been associated with hepatotoxicity and, rarely, agranulocytosis.

3. **Blockade of hormone release:** A pharmacologic dose of *iodide* inhibits the iodination of tyrosines ("Wolff-Chaikoff effect"), but this effect lasts only a few days. More importantly, *iodide* inhibits the release of thyroid hormones from thyroglobulin by mechanisms not yet understood. *Iodide* is employed to treat thyroid storm or prior to surgery, because it decreases the vascularity of the thyroid gland. *Iodide*, administered orally, is not useful for long-term therapy; the thyroid ceases to respond to the drug after a few weeks. Adverse effects include sore mouth and throat, swelling of the tongue or larynx, rashes, ulcerations of mucous membranes, and metallic taste.

4. **Thyroid storm:** Thyroid storm presents with extreme symptoms of hyperthyroidism. The treatment of thyroid storm is the same as for hyperthyroidism, except that the drugs are given in higher doses and more frequently. β-Blockers, such as *metoprolol* or *propranolol*, are effective in blunting the widespread sympathetic stimulation that occurs in hyperthyroidism.

Study Questions

Choose the ONE best answer.

23.1 Which option is most appropriate for a patient with newly diagnosed hyperthyroidism in the first trimester of pregnancy?

A. Methimazole

B. Propylthiouracil (PTU)

C. Radioactive iodine

D. Surgical removal of the thyroid

Correct answer = B. Methimazole is generally preferred over PTU because it has a longer half-life and lower incidence of adverse effects. However, PTU is recommended in the first trimester of pregnancy due to a greater risk of teratogenic effects with methimazole. Surgery is not ideal in a pregnant patient. Radioactive iodine is contraindicated due to potential effects on the fetus.

23.2 Which drug is beneficial in the treatment of patients with acromegaly?

A. Cosyntropin

B. Lanreotide

C. Oxytocin

D. Somatropin

Correct answer = B. Lanreotide is a synthetic analog of somatostatin, which inhibits GH. Acromegaly is characterized by an excess of GH. Cosyntropin is used as a diagnostic tool in adrenal insufficiency. Oxytocin is used for induction of labor. Somatropin is synthetic human GH, so it would not be beneficial.

23.3 A 40-year-old female is undergoing infertility treatments. Which drug might be included in her treatment regimen?

A. Cabergoline

B. Follitropin

C. Methimazole

D. Vasopressin

Correct answer = B. Follitropin is a recombinant version of FSH that causes ovarian follicular growth and maturation. Cabergoline is a dopamine agonist that is used for hyperprolactinemia. Methimazole is the treatment of choice for hyperthyroidism. Vasopressin is an antidiuretic hormone.

23.4 A 29-year-old female has a TSH of 13.5 mIU/L (normal 0.5 to 4.7 mIU/L). Which agent is most appropriate to treat the TSH abnormality?

A. Levothyroxine

B. Liothyronine

C. Liotrix

D. Propylthiouracil

Correct answer = A. This patient presents with hypothyroidism as evidenced by high TSH. Levothyroxine is preferred due to its long half-life and better tolerability. Liothyronine (T_3) and liotrix (T_3/T_4) are not as well tolerated. Propylthiouracil is used in the treatment of hyperthyroidism.

23.5 Which agent is correctly paired with an appropriate clinical use of the drug?

A. Desmopressin—treatment of diabetes insipidus

B. Goserelin—growth hormone deficiency

C. hCG—treatment of bleeding esophageal varices

D. Octreotide—treatment of infertility

Correct answer = A. Goserelin is a GnRH analog that is used for the treatment of prostate cancer or endometriosis. HCG is used in the treatment of infertility. Octreotide is used in the treatment of bleeding esophageal varices.

23.6 Which agent is used in infertility treatment to mimic the action of luteinizing hormone and stimulate ovulation?

A. Cetrorelix

B. Choriogonadotropin alfa

C. Ganirelix

D. Leuprolide

Correct answer = B. Effects of choriogonadotropin alfa (recombinant hCG) are similar to LH and trigger ovulation. The other agents (leuprolide, a GnRH analog; cetrorelix and ganirelix, GnRH antagonists) are all used to inhibit LH secretion.

23.7 A patient was recently placed on levothyroxine. Which of her medications may affect the levothyroxine dosage requirements?

A. Bromocriptine

B. Calcium carbonate

C. Metoprolol

D. Vitamin D

Correct answer = B. Calcium carbonate may reduce the absorption of levothyroxine. The other medications should not interact with the levothyroxine.

23.8 Which is a common side effect that should be communicated to a patient prescribed octreotide?

A. Weight gain
B. Low blood sugar
C. Myalgia
D. Abdominal pain

Correct answer = D. Common side effects of octreotide are gastrointestinal in nature and include diarrhea, abdominal pain, nausea, and steatorrhea.

23.9 Which symptom indicates that a patient may need a lower dosage of levothyroxine?

A. Bradycardia
B. Cold intolerance
C. Palpitations
D. Weight gain

Correct answer = C. Palpitations are an adverse effect of too much thyroid supplementation. The other symptoms are indicative of untreated or undertreated hypothyroidism and may require an increase in thyroid supplementation.

23.10 The adrenocorticosteroid synthetic pathway is responsible for the synthesis and release of cortisol. Which of the following effects is expected after cortisol is released?

A. Insulin release
B. Production of inflammation
C. Increased gluconeogenesis
D. Decreased protein breakdown

Correct answer = C. See Figure 23.3. Cortisol has anti-inflammatory actions, increases gluconeogenesis, and increases protein breakdown.

Drugs for Diabetes

24

Karen Whalen and Cynthia Moreau

I. OVERVIEW

The pancreas produces the peptide hormones insulin, glucagon, and somatostatin. The peptide hormones are secreted from cells in the islets of Langerhans (β-cells produce insulin, α cells produce glucagon, and δ cells produce somatostatin). These hormones play an important role in regulating metabolic activities of the body, particularly glucose homeostasis. A relative or absolute lack of insulin, as seen in diabetes mellitus, can cause serious hyperglycemia. Left untreated, retinopathy, nephropathy, neuropathy, and cardiovascular complications may result. Administration of insulin preparations or other glucose-lowering agents (Figure 24.1) can reduce morbidity and mortality associated with diabetes.

II. DIABETES MELLITUS

The incidence of diabetes is growing rapidly in the United States and worldwide. An estimated 30.3 million people in the United States and 422 million people worldwide are afflicted with diabetes. Diabetes is not a single disease. Rather, it is a heterogeneous group of syndromes characterized by elevated blood glucose attributed to a relative or absolute deficiency of insulin. The American Diabetes Association (ADA) recognizes four clinical classifications of diabetes: type 1 diabetes, type 2 diabetes, gestational diabetes, and diabetes due to other causes such as genetic defects or medications. Figure 24.2 summarizes the characteristics of type 1 and type 2 diabetes. Gestational diabetes is defined as carbohydrate intolerance with onset or first recognition during pregnancy.

A. Type 1 diabetes

Type 1 diabetes most commonly afflicts children, adolescents, or young adults, but some latent forms occur later in life. The disease is characterized by an absolute deficiency of insulin due to destruction of β cells. Without functional β cells, the pancreas fails to respond to glucose, and a person with type 1 diabetes shows classic symptoms of insulin deficiency (polydipsia, polyphagia, polyuria, and weight loss).

Figure 24.1
Summary of drugs used in the treatment of diabetes. GLP-1 = glucagon-like peptide-1.

INSULIN
Inhaled insulin AFREZZA
Insulin aspart NOVOLOG
Insulin degludec TRESIBA
Insulin detemir LEVEMIR
Insulin glargine BASAGLAR, LANTUS, TOUJEO
Insulin glulisine APIDRA
Insulin lispro HUMALOG
NPH insulin suspension HUMULIN N, NOVOLIN N
Regular insulin HUMULIN R, NOVOLIN R

AMYLIN ANALOG
Pramlintide SYMLIN

ORAL AGENTS
Acarbose PRECOSE
Alogliptin NESINA
Bromocriptine CYCLOSET
Canagliflozin INVOKANA
Colesevelam WELCHOL
Dapagliflozin FARXIGA
Empagliflozin JARDIANCE
Ertugliflozin STEGLATRO
Glimepiride AMARYL
Glipizide GLUCOTROL
Glyburide DIABETA, GLYNASE PRESTAB
Linagliptin TRADJENTA
Metformin FORTAMET, GLUCOPHAGE
Miglitol GLYSET
Nateglinide STARLIX
Pioglitazone ACTOS
Repaglinide PRANDIN
Rosiglitazone AVANDIA
Saxagliptin ONGLYZA
Sitagliptin JANUVIA
Tolbutamide GENERIC ONLY

GLP-1 RECEPTOR AGONISTS
Albiglutide TANZEUM
Dulaglutide TRULICITY
Exenatide BYETTA, BYDUREON
Liraglutide VICTOZA
Lixisenatide ADLYXIN
Semaglutide OZEMPIC

	Type 1	Type 2
Age at onset	Usually during childhood or puberty	Commonly over age 35
Nutritional status at time of onset	Commonly undernourished	Obesity usually present
Prevalence among diagnosed diabetics	5%–10%	90%–95%
Genetic predisposition	Moderate	Very strong
Defect or deficiency	β Cells are destroyed, eliminating the production of insulin	Inability of β cells to produce appropriate quantities of insulin; insulin resistance; other defects

Figure 24.2
Comparison of type 1 and type 2 diabetes.

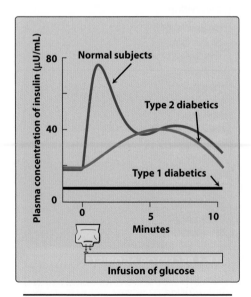

Figure 24.3
Release of insulin that occurs in response to an IV glucose load in normal subjects and diabetic patients.

1. **Cause:** Loss of β-cell function in type 1 diabetes results from autoimmune-mediated processes that may be triggered by viruses or other environmental toxins. In patients without diabetes, constant β-cell secretion maintains low basal levels of circulating insulin. This suppresses lipolysis, proteolysis, and glycogenolysis. A burst of insulin secretion occurs within 2 minutes after ingesting a meal, in response to transient increases in circulating glucose and amino acids. This lasts for up to 15 minutes, followed by the postprandial secretion of insulin. However, without functional β cells, those with type 1 diabetes can neither maintain basal secretion of insulin nor respond to variations in circulating glucose (Figure 24.3).

2. **Treatment:** A person with type 1 diabetes must rely on exogenous insulin to control hyperglycemia, avoid ketoacidosis, and maintain acceptable levels of glycosylated hemoglobin (HbA_{1c}). [Note: HbA_{1c} is a marker of overall glucose control and is used to monitor diabetes in clinical practice. The rate of formation of HbA_{1c} is proportional to the average blood glucose concentration over the previous 3 months. A higher average glucose results in a higher HbA_{1c}.] The goal of insulin therapy in type 1 diabetes is to maintain blood glucose as close to normal as possible and to avoid wide fluctuations in glucose. The use of home blood glucose monitors facilitates frequent self-monitoring and treatment with insulin.

B. Type 2 diabetes

Type 2 diabetes accounts for greater than 90% of cases. Type 2 diabetes is influenced by genetic factors, aging, obesity, and peripheral insulin resistance, rather than autoimmune processes. The metabolic alterations are generally milder than those observed with type 1 diabetes (for example, patients with type 2 diabetes typically are not ketotic), but the long-term clinical consequences are similar.

1. **Cause:** Type 2 diabetes is characterized by a lack of sensitivity of target organs to insulin (Figure 24.4). In type 2 diabetes, the pancreas retains some β-cell function, but insulin secretion is insufficient to maintain glucose homeostasis (Figure 24.3) in the face of increasing peripheral insulin resistance. The β-cell mass may gradually decline over time in type 2 diabetes. In contrast to patients with type 1 diabetes, those with type 2 diabetes are often obese. Obesity contributes to insulin resistance, which is considered the major underlying defect of type 2 diabetes.

2. **Treatment:** The goal in treating type 2 diabetes is to maintain blood glucose within normal limits and to prevent the development of long-term complications. Weight reduction, exercise, and dietary modification decrease insulin resistance and correct hyperglycemia in some patients with type 2 diabetes. However, most patients require pharmacologic intervention with oral glucose-lowering agents. As the disease progresses, β-cell function declines, and insulin therapy is often needed to achieve satisfactory glucose levels (Figure 24.5).

III. INSULIN AND INSULIN ANALOGS

Insulin [IN-su-lin] is a polypeptide hormone consisting of two peptide chains that are connected by disulfide bonds. It is synthesized as a precursor (proinsulin) that undergoes proteolytic cleavage to form insulin and C-peptide, both of which are secreted by the β cells of the pancreas. [Note: Because insulin undergoes significant hepatic and renal extraction, plasma insulin levels may not accurately reflect insulin production. Thus, measurement of C-peptide provides a better index of insulin levels.] Insulin secretion is regulated by blood glucose levels, certain amino acids, other hormones, and autonomic mediators. Secretion is most often triggered by increased blood glucose, which is taken up by the glucose transporter into the β cells of the pancreas. There, it is phosphorylated by glucokinase, which acts as a glucose sensor. The products of glucose metabolism enter the mitochondrial respiratory chain and generate adenosine triphosphate (ATP). The rise in ATP levels causes a blockade of K^+ channels, leading to membrane depolarization and an influx of Ca^{2+}. The increase in intracellular Ca^{2+} causes pulsatile insulin exocytosis.

A. Mechanism of action

Exogenous insulin is administered to replace absent insulin secretion in type 1 diabetes or to supplement insufficient insulin secretion in type 2 diabetes.

B. Pharmacokinetics

Human insulin is produced by recombinant DNA technology using strains of Escherichia coli or yeast that are genetically altered to contain the gene for human insulin. Modification of the amino acid sequence of human insulin produces insulins with different pharmacokinetic properties. Insulin preparations vary primarily in their onset and duration of activity. Dose, injection site, blood supply, temperature, and physical activity can also affect the onset and duration of various insulin preparations. Because insulin is a polypeptide, it is degraded in the gastrointestinal tract if taken orally. Therefore, it is generally administered by subcutaneous injection, although an inhaled insulin formulation is also available. [Note: In a hyperglycemic emergency, *regular insulin* is administered intravenously (IV).] Continuous subcutaneous insulin infusion (also called the insulin pump) is another method of insulin delivery. This method of administration may be more convenient for some patients, eliminating multiple daily injections of insulin. The pump is programmed to deliver a basal rate of insulin. In addition, it allows the patient to deliver a bolus of insulin to cover mealtime carbohydrate intake and compensate for high blood glucose.

C. Adverse effects

Hypoglycemia is the most serious and common adverse reaction to insulin (Figure 24.6). Other adverse effects include weight gain, local injection site reactions, and lipodystrophy. Lipodystrophy can be minimized by rotation of injection sites. Diabetics with renal insufficiency may require a decrease in insulin dose. Due to the potential for bronchospasm with inhaled insulin, patients with asthma, chronic obstructive pulmonary disease, and smokers should not use this formulation.

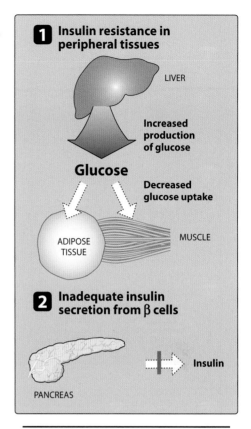

Figure 24.4
Major factors contributing to hyperglycemia observed in type 2 diabetes.

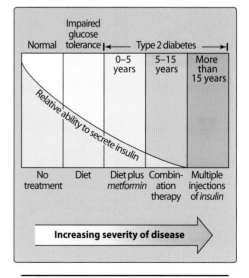

Figure 24.5
Duration of type 2 diabetes mellitus, sufficiency of endogenous insulin, and recommended sequence of therapy.

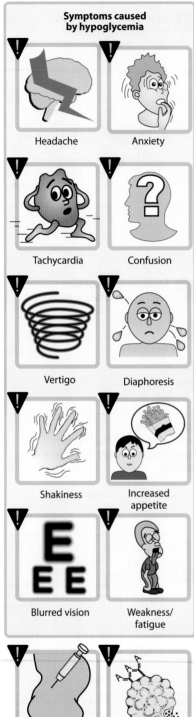

Symptoms caused by hypoglycemia

Headache   Anxiety

Tachycardia   Confusion

Vertigo   Diaphoresis

Shakiness   Increased appetite

Blurred vision   Weakness/fatigue

Lipodystrophy   Hypersensitivity

Figure 24.6
Adverse effects observed with *insulin*. [Note: Lipodystrophy is a local atrophy or hypertrophy of subcutaneous fatty tissue at the site of injections.]

IV. INSULIN PREPARATIONS AND TREATMENT

Insulin preparations are classified as rapid-, short-, intermediate-, or long-acting. Figure 24.7 summarizes onset of action, timing of peak level, and duration of action for the various types of insulin. It is important that clinicians exercise caution when adjusting insulin treatment, paying strict attention to the dose and type of insulin.

A. Rapid-acting and short-acting insulin preparations

Five preparations fall into this category: *regular insulin, insulin lispro* [LIS-proe], *insulin aspart* [AS-part], *insulin glulisine* [gloo-LYSE-een], and *inhaled insulin*. *Regular insulin* is a short-acting, soluble, crystalline zinc insulin. *Insulin lispro, aspart,* and *glulisine* are classified as rapid-acting insulins. Modification of the amino acid sequence of *regular insulin* produces analogs that are rapid-acting insulins. This modification results in more rapid absorption, a quicker onset, and a shorter duration of action after subcutaneous injection. Peak levels of *insulin lispro* are seen at 30 to 90 minutes, as compared with 50 to 120 minutes for *regular insulin*. *Insulin aspart* and *insulin glulisine* have pharmacokinetic and pharmacodynamic properties similar to those of *insulin lispro*. *Inhaled insulin* is also considered rapid-acting. This dry powder formulation is inhaled and absorbed through pulmonary tissue, with peak levels achieved within 45 to 60 minutes. Rapid- or short-acting insulins are administered to mimic the prandial (mealtime) release of insulins and to control postprandial glucose. They may also be used in cases where swift correction of elevated glucose is needed. Rapid- and short-acting insulins are usually used in conjunction with a longer-acting basal insulin that provides control of fasting glucose. *Regular insulin* should be injected subcutaneously 30 minutes before a meal, whereas rapid-acting insulins are administered in the 15 minutes preceding a meal or within 15 to 20 minutes after starting a meal. Rapid-acting insulin suspensions are commonly used in external insulin pumps, and they are suitable for IV administration, although *regular insulin* is most commonly used when the IV route is needed.

B. Intermediate-acting insulin

Neutral protamine Hagedorn (NPH) insulin is an intermediate-acting insulin formed by the addition of zinc and protamine to *regular insulin*. [Note: Another name for this preparation is *insulin isophane*.] The combination with protamine forms a complex that is less soluble, resulting in delayed absorption and a longer duration of action. *NPH insulin* is used for basal (fasting) control in type 1 or 2 diabetes and is usually given along with rapid- or short-acting insulin for mealtime control. *NPH insulin* should be given only subcutaneously (*never IV*), and it should not be used when rapid glucose lowering is needed (for example, diabetic ketoacidosis). Figure 24.8 shows common regimens that use combinations of insulins.

C. Long-acting insulin preparations

The isoelectric point of *insulin glargine* [GLAR-geen] is lower than that of human insulin, leading to formation of a precipitate at the injection site that releases insulin over an extended period. It has a slower

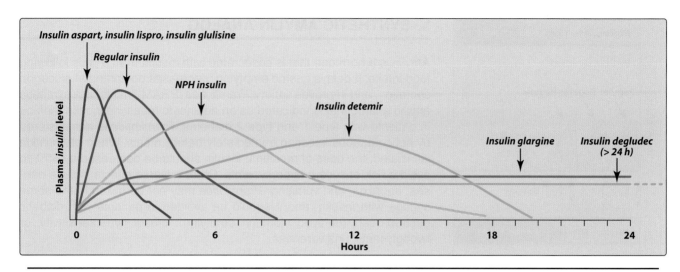

Figure 24.7
Onset and duration of action of human insulin and insulin analogs. NPH = neutral protamine Hagedorn.

onset than *NPH insulin* and a flat, prolonged hypoglycemic effect with no peak (Figure 24.7). *Insulin detemir* [deh-TEE-meer] has a fatty acid side chain that enhances association to albumin. Slow dissociation from albumin results in long-acting properties similar to those of *insulin glargine. Insulin degludec* [de-GLOO-dek] remains in solution at physiologic pH, with a slow release over an extended period. It has the longest half-life of the long-acting insulins. As with *NPH insulin, insulin glargine, insulin detemir,* and *insulin degludec* are used for basal control and should only be administered subcutaneously. Long-acting insulins should not be mixed in the same syringe with other insulins, because doing so may alter the pharmacodynamic profile.

D. Insulin combinations

Various premixed combinations of human insulins, such as 70% *NPH insulin* plus 30% *regular insulin* (Figure 24.8) or 50% of each of these, are also available. Use of premixed combinations decreases the number of daily injections but makes it more difficult to adjust individual components of the insulin regimen.

E. Standard treatment versus intensive treatment

Standard insulin therapy involves twice daily injections. In contrast, intensive treatment utilizes three or more injections daily with frequent monitoring of blood glucose levels. The ADA recommends a target mean blood glucose level of 154 mg/dL or less (HbA$_{1c}$ ≤ 7%) for most patients, and intensive treatment is more likely to achieve this goal. The frequency of hypoglycemic episodes, coma, and seizures is higher with intensive insulin regimens (Figure 24.9A). However, patients on intensive therapy show a significant reduction in microvascular complications of diabetes such as retinopathy, nephropathy, and neuropathy compared to patients receiving standard care (Figure 24.9B). Intensive therapy should not be recommended for patients with long-standing diabetes, significant microvascular complications, advanced age, and those with hypoglycemic unawareness.

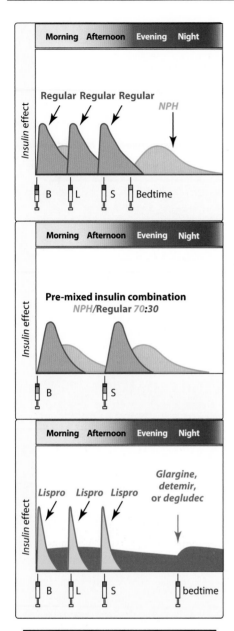

Figure 24.8
Examples of three regimens that provide both prandial and basal *insulin* replacement. B = breakfast; L = lunch; S = supper; NPH = neutral protamine Hagedorn.

V. SYNTHETIC AMYLIN ANALOG

Amylin is a hormone that is cosecreted with insulin from β cells following food intake. It delays gastric emptying, decreases postprandial glucagon secretion, and improves satiety. *Pramlintide* [PRAM-lin-tide] is a synthetic amylin analog that is indicated as an adjunct to mealtime insulin therapy in patients with type 1 and type 2 diabetes. *Pramlintide* is administered by subcutaneous injection immediately before meals. When *pramlintide* is initiated, the dose of mealtime insulin should be decreased by 50% to avoid a risk of severe hypoglycemia. Other adverse effects include nausea, anorexia, and vomiting. *Pramlintide* may not be mixed in the same syringe with insulin, and it should be avoided in patients with diabetic gastroparesis (delayed stomach emptying), cresol hypersensitivity, or hypoglycemic unawareness.

VI. GLUCAGON-LIKE PEPTIDE RECEPTOR AGONISTS

Oral intake of glucose results in a higher secretion of insulin than occurs when an equal load of glucose is given IV. This effect is referred to as the "incretin effect" and is markedly reduced in type 2 diabetes. The incretin effect occurs because the gut releases incretin hormones, notably glucagon-like peptide-1 (GLP-1) and glucose-dependent insulinotropic polypeptide (GIP), in response to a meal. Incretin hormones are responsible for 60% to 70% of postprandial insulin secretion. *Albiglutide* [al-bi-GLOO-tide], *dulaglutide* [doo-la-GLOO-tide], *exenatide* [EX-e-nah-tide], *liraglutide* [LIR-a-GLOO-tide], *lixisenatide* [lix-i-SEN-a-tide], and *semaglutide* [sem-a-GLOO-tide] are injectable GLP-1 receptor agonists used for the treatment of type 2 diabetes. *Liraglutide* is also approved to reduce the risk of cardiovascular events and cardiovascular mortality in patients with type 2 diabetes and cardiovascular disease. Two premixed preparations of long-acting insulins and GLP-1 receptor agonists are available: *insulin glargine* plus *lixisenatide* and *insulin degludec* plus *liraglutide*. Use of these combinations may decrease daily insulin requirements and the number of daily injections.

A. Mechanism of action

These agents are analogs of GLP-1 that exert their activity by improving glucose-dependent insulin secretion, slowing gastric emptying time, reducing food intake by enhancing satiety (a feeling of fullness), decreasing postprandial glucagon secretion, and promoting β-cell proliferation. Consequently, postprandial hyperglycemia is reduced, HbA_{1c} levels decline, and weight loss may occur.

B. Pharmacokinetics

GLP-1 receptor agonists are administered subcutaneously, since they are polypeptides. *Albiglutide*, *dulaglutide*, *liraglutide*, and *semaglutide* are considered long-acting GLP-1 receptor agonists. *Albiglutide*, *dulaglutide*, and *semaglutide* are dosed once weekly, while *liraglutide* is available as a once-daily injection. *Lixisenatide* is a short-acting GLP-1 receptor agonist that is dosed once daily. *Exenatide* is available as both a short-acting (dosed twice daily) and extended-release preparation (dosed once weekly). *Exenatide* should be avoided in patients with severe renal impairment.

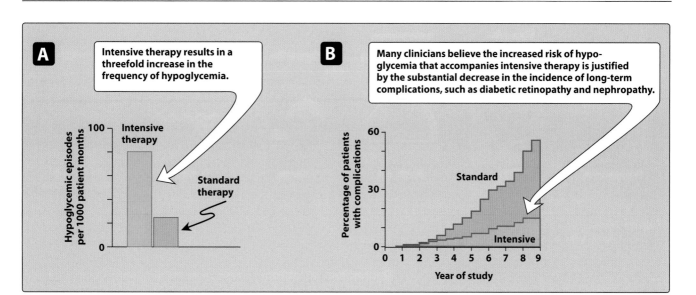

Figure 24.9
A. Effect of tight glucose control on hypoglycemic episodes in a population of patients with type 1 diabetes receiving intensive or standard therapy. **B.** Effect of standard and intensive care on the long-term complications of diabetes.

C. Adverse effects

The main adverse effects of the incretin mimetics consist of nausea, vomiting, diarrhea, and constipation. GLP-1 receptor agonists have been associated with pancreatitis and should be avoided in patients with chronic pancreatitis. Longer-acting agents have been associated with thyroid C-cell tumors in rodents. It is unknown if GLP-1 receptor agonists cause these tumors or thyroid carcinoma in humans, although they are contraindicated in patients with a history of medullary thyroid carcinoma or multiple endocrine neoplasia type 2.

VII. ORAL AGENTS

Oral agents are useful in the treatment of patients who have type 2 diabetes that is not controlled with diet. Patients who developed diabetes after age 40 and have had diabetes less than 5 years are most likely to respond well to oral glucose-lowering agents. Patients with long-standing disease may require a combination of oral agents with or without insulin to control hyperglycemia. Figure 24.10 summarizes the duration of action of some of the oral glucose-lowering drugs, and Figure 24.11 illustrates some of the common adverse effects.

A. Sulfonylureas

These agents are classified as insulin secretagogues, because they promote insulin release from the β cells of the pancreas. The sulfonylureas most used in clinical practice are the second-generation drugs *glyburide* [GLYE-byoor-ide], *glipizide* [GLIP-ih-zide], and *glimepiride* [GLYE-me-pih-ride].

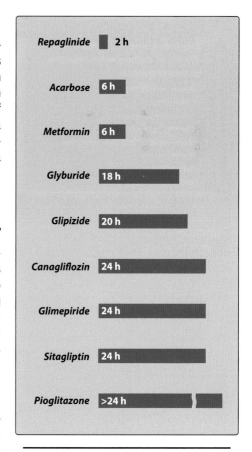

Figure 24.10
Duration of action of some oral hypoglycemic agents.

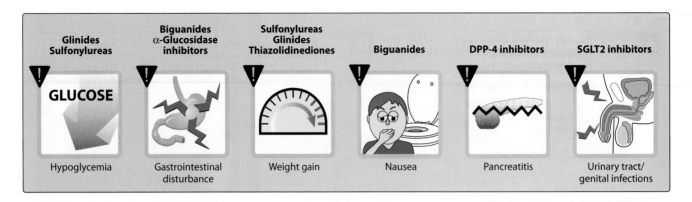

Figure 24.11
Some adverse effects observed with oral hypoglycemic agents.

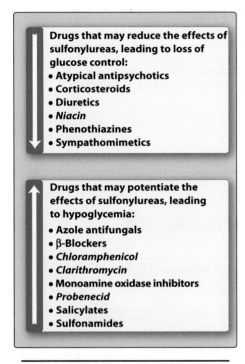

Figure 24.12
Drugs interacting with sulfonylureas.

1. **Mechanism of action:** These agents stimulate insulin release from the β cells of the pancreas. Sulfonylureas block ATP-sensitive K$^+$ channels, resulting in depolarization, Ca^{2+} influx, and insulin exocytosis. In addition, sulfonylureas may reduce hepatic glucose production and increase peripheral insulin sensitivity.

2. **Pharmacokinetics:** Given orally, these drugs bind to serum proteins, are metabolized by the liver, and are excreted in the urine and feces. The duration of action ranges from 12 to 24 hours.

3. **Adverse effects:** Adverse effects of the sulfonylureas include hypoglycemia, hyperinsulinemia, and weight gain. They should be used with caution in hepatic or renal insufficiency, since accumulation of sulfonylureas may cause hypoglycemia. Renal impairment is a particular problem for *glyburide*, as it may increase the duration of action and increase the risk of hypoglycemia significantly. *Glipizide* or *glimepiride* are safer options in renal dysfunction and in elderly patients. Figure 24.12 summarizes some drug interactions with sulfonylureas.

B. Glinides

This class of agents includes *repaglinide* [re-PAG-lin-ide] and *nateglinide* [nuh-TAY-gli-nide]. Glinides are also considered insulin secretagogues.

1. **Mechanism of action:** Like the sulfonylureas, the glinides stimulate insulin secretion. In contrast to the sulfonylureas, the glinides have a rapid onset and a short duration of action. They are particularly effective in the early release of insulin that occurs after a meal and are categorized as postprandial glucose regulators. Glinides should not be used in combination with sulfonylureas due to overlapping mechanisms of action and increased risk of serious hypoglycemia.

2. **Pharmacokinetics:** Glinides should be taken prior to a meal and are well absorbed after oral administration. Both glinides are metabolized to inactive products by cytochrome P450 3A4 (CYP3A4; see Chapter 1) in the liver and are excreted through the bile.

3. **Adverse effects:** Although glinides cause hypoglycemia and weight gain, the incidence is lower than that with sulfonylureas. By inhibiting hepatic metabolism, the lipid-lowering drug *gemfibrozil* may significantly increase the effects of *repaglinide*, and concurrent use is contraindicated. These agents should be used with caution in patients with hepatic impairment.

C. Biguanides

Metformin [met-FOR-min], the only biguanide, is classified as an insulin sensitizer. It increases glucose uptake and use by target tissues, thereby decreasing insulin resistance. Unlike sulfonylureas, *metformin* does not promote insulin secretion. Therefore, the risk of hypoglycemia is far less than that with sulfonylureas. *Metformin* is also useful in the treatment of polycystic ovary syndrome, as it reduces insulin resistance seen in this disorder.

1. **Mechanism of action:** The main mechanism of action of *metformin* is reduction of hepatic gluconeogenesis. [Note: Excess glucose produced by the liver is a major source of high blood glucose in type 2 diabetes, accounting for high fasting blood glucose.] *Metformin* also slows intestinal absorption of sugars and improves peripheral glucose uptake and utilization. Weight loss may occur because *metformin* causes loss of appetite. The ADA recommends *metformin* as the initial drug of choice for type 2 diabetes. *Metformin* may be used alone or in combination with other oral agents or insulin. Hypoglycemia may occur when *metformin* is taken in combination with insulin or insulin secretagogues, so adjustment in dosage may be required.

2. **Pharmacokinetics:** *Metformin* is well absorbed after oral administration, is not bound to serum proteins, and is not metabolized. Excretion is via the urine.

3. **Adverse effects:** These are largely gastrointestinal, including diarrhea, nausea, and vomiting. These effects can be alleviated by titrating the dose of *metformin* slowly and administering doses with meals. *Metformin* is contraindicated in renal dysfunction due to the risk of lactic acidosis. It should be discontinued in cases of acute myocardial infarction, exacerbation of heart failure, sepsis, or other disorders that can cause acute renal failure. *Metformin* should be used with caution in patients older than 80 years and in those with heart failure or alcohol abuse. It should be temporarily discontinued in patients undergoing procedures requiring IV radiographic contrast. Rarely, potentially fatal lactic acidosis has occurred. Long-term use may be associated with vitamin B_{12} deficiency, and periodic measurement of vitamin B_{12} levels is recommended, especially in patients with anemia or peripheral neuropathy.

D. Thiazolidinediones

The thiazolidinediones (TZDs) are also insulin sensitizers. The two agents in this class are *pioglitazone* [pye-oh-GLI-ta-zone] and *rosiglitazone* [roe-si-GLIH-ta-zone]. Although insulin is required for their action, the TZDs do not promote its release from the β cells, so hyperinsulinemia is not a risk.

1. **Mechanism of action:** The TZDs lower insulin resistance by acting as agonists for the peroxisome proliferator–activated receptor-γ (PPARγ), a nuclear hormone receptor. Activation of PPARγ regulates the transcription of several insulin responsive genes, resulting in increased insulin sensitivity in adipose tissue, liver, and skeletal muscle. The TZDs can be used as monotherapy or in combination with other glucose-lowering agents or insulin. The dose of insulin may have to be lowered when used in combination with these agents. The ADA recommends *pioglitazone* as a second- or third-line agent for type 2 diabetes. *Rosiglitazone* is less utilized due to concerns regarding cardiovascular adverse effects.

2. Pharmacokinetics: *Pioglitazone* and *rosiglitazone* are well absorbed after oral administration and are extensively bound to serum albumin. Both undergo extensive metabolism by different CYP450 isozymes (see Chapter 1). Some metabolites of *pioglitazone* have activity. Renal elimination of *pioglitazone* is negligible, with the majority of active drug and metabolites excreted in the bile and eliminated in the feces. Metabolites of *rosiglitazone* are primarily excreted in the urine. No dosage adjustment is required in renal impairment.

3. Adverse effects: Liver toxicity has occasionally been reported with these drugs, and baseline and periodic monitoring of liver function is recommended. Weight gain can occur because TZDs may increase subcutaneous fat and cause fluid retention. [Note: Fluid retention can worsen heart failure. These drugs should be avoided in patients with severe heart failure.] TZDs have been associated with osteopenia and increased fracture risk in women. *Pioglitazone* may also increase the risk of bladder cancer. Additionally, *rosiglitazone* carries a boxed warning about the potential increased risk of myocardial infarction and angina with the use of this agent.

E. α-Glucosidase inhibitors

Acarbose [AY-car-bose] and *miglitol* [MIG-li-tol] are oral agents used for the treatment of type 2 diabetes.

1. Mechanism of action: Located in the intestinal brush border, α-glucosidase enzymes break down carbohydrates into glucose and other simple sugars that can be absorbed. *Acarbose* and *miglitol* reversibly inhibit α-glucosidase enzymes. When taken at the start of a meal, these drugs delay the digestion of carbohydrates, resulting in lower postprandial glucose levels. Since they do not stimulate insulin release or increase insulin sensitivity, these agents do not cause hypoglycemia when used as monotherapy. However, when used with insulin secretagogues or insulin, hypoglycemia may develop. [Note: It is important that hypoglycemia in this context be treated with glucose rather than sucrose, because sucrase is also inhibited by these drugs.]

2. Pharmacokinetics: *Acarbose* is poorly absorbed. It is metabolized primarily by intestinal bacteria, and some of the metabolites are absorbed and excreted into the urine. *Miglitol* is very well absorbed but has no systemic effects. It is excreted unchanged by the kidney.

3. Adverse effects: The most common adverse effects are flatulence, diarrhea, and abdominal cramping. Adverse effects limit the use of these agents in clinical practice. Patients with inflammatory bowel disease, colonic ulceration, or intestinal obstruction should not use these drugs.

F. Dipeptidyl peptidase-4 inhibitors

Alogliptin [al-oh-GLIP-tin], *linagliptin* [lin-a-GLIP-tin], *saxagliptin* [sax-a-GLIP-tin], and *sitagliptin* [si-ta-GLIP-tin] are oral dipeptidyl peptidase-4 (DPP-4) inhibitors used for the treatment of type 2 diabetes.

1. Mechanism of action: These drugs inhibit the enzyme DPP-4, which is responsible for the inactivation of incretin hormones such as GLP-1 (Figure 24.13). Prolonging the activity of incretin hormones increases release of insulin in response to meals and

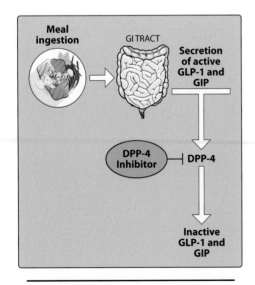

Figure 24.13
Mechanism of action of DPP-4 inhibitors. DPP-4 = dipeptidyl peptidase-4. GIP = glucose-dependent insulinotropic peptide; GLP-1 = glucagon-like peptide-1.

reduces inappropriate secretion of glucagon. DPP-4 inhibitors may be used as monotherapy or in combination with sulfonylureas, *metformin*, TZDs, or insulin. Treatment guidelines do not recommend the combination of DPP-4 inhibitors with GLP-1 receptor agonists for management of diabetes due to overlapping mechanisms and toxicity. Unlike GLP-1 receptor agonists, these drugs do not cause satiety or fullness and are weight neutral.

2. **Pharmacokinetics:** The DPP-4 inhibitors are well absorbed after oral administration. Food does not affect the extent of absorption. *Alogliptin* and *sitagliptin* are mostly excreted unchanged in the urine. *Saxagliptin* is metabolized via CYP450 3A4/5 to an active metabolite. The primary route of elimination for *saxagliptin* and the metabolite is renal. *Linagliptin* is primarily eliminated via the enterohepatic system. All DPP-4 inhibitors except *linagliptin* require dosage adjustments in renal dysfunction.

3. **Adverse effects:** In general, DPP-4 inhibitors are well tolerated, with the most common adverse effects being nasopharyngitis and headache. Although infrequent, pancreatitis has occurred with the use of DPP-4 inhibitors. Agents in this class may also increase the risk of severe, disabling joint pain. *Alogliptin* and *saxagliptin* have also been shown to increase the risk of heart failure hospitalizations and should be used with caution in patients with or at risk for heart failure.

G. Sodium–glucose cotransporter 2 inhibitors

Canagliflozin [kan-a-gli-FLOE-zin], *dapagliflozin* [dap-a-gli-FLOE-zin], *empagliflozin* [em-pa-gli-FLOE-zin], and *ertugliflozin* [er-too-gli-FLOE-zin] are oral agents for the treatment of type 2 diabetes. *Empagliflozin* is also indicated to reduce the risk of cardiovascular death in patients with type 2 diabetes and cardiovascular disease.

1. **Mechanism of action:** The sodium–glucose cotransporter 2 (SGLT2) is responsible for reabsorbing filtered glucose in the tubular lumen of the kidney. By inhibiting SGLT2, these agents decrease reabsorption of glucose, increase urinary glucose excretion, and lower blood glucose. Inhibition of SGLT2 also decreases reabsorption of sodium and causes osmotic diuresis. Therefore, SGLT2 inhibitors may reduce systolic blood pressure. However, they are not indicated for the treatment of hypertension.

2. **Pharmacokinetics:** These agents are given once daily in the morning. *Canagliflozin* should be taken before the first meal of the day. All drugs are mainly metabolized by glucuronidation to inactive metabolites. These agents should be avoided in patients with renal dysfunction.

3. **Adverse effects:** The most common adverse effects with SGLT2 inhibitors are female genital mycotic infections (for example, vulvovaginal candidiasis), urinary tract infections, and urinary frequency. Hypotension has also occurred, particularly in the elderly or patients on diuretics. Thus, volume status should be evaluated prior to starting these agents. Ketoacidosis has been reported with use of SGLT2 inhibitors, and these agents should be used with caution in patients with risk factors that predispose to ketoacidosis (for example, alcohol abuse and caloric restriction related to surgery or illness).

DRUG CLASS	MECHANISM OF ACTION	EFFECT ON PLASMA INSULIN	RISK OF HYPO-GLYCEMIA	COMMENTS
Sulfonylureas *Glimepiride* *Glipizide* *Glyburide*	Stimulates insulin secretion	⬆	Yes	Well-established history of effectiveness. Weight gain can occur. Hypoglycemia most common with this class of oral agents.
Glinides *Nateglinide* *Repaglinide*	Stimulates insulin secretion	⬆	Yes (rarely)	Taken with meals. Short action with less hypoglycemia. Postprandial effect.
Biguanides *Metformin*	Decreases hepatic production of glucose	⬇	No	Preferred agent for type 2 diabetes. Well-established history of effectiveness. Weight loss may occur. Monitor renal function and vitamin B_{12} levels.
Thiazolidinediones *Pioglitazone* *Rosiglitazone*	Binds to peroxisome proliferator–activated receptor-γ in muscle, fat and liver to decrease insulin resistance	⬇⬇	No	Effective in highly insulin-resistant patients. Once-daily dosing for *pioglitazone*. Check liver function before initiation. Avoid in liver disease or heart failure.
α-Glucosidase inhibitors *Acarbose* *Miglitol*	Decreases glucose absorption	⬌	No	Taken with meals. Adverse gastro-intestinal effects. Not a preferred therapy. Reserve for patients unable to tolerate other agents.
DPP-4 inhibitors *Alogliptin* *Linagliptin* *Sitagliptin* *Saxagliptin*	Increases glucose-dependent insulin release; decreases secretion of glucagon	⬆	No	Once-daily dosing. May be taken with or without food. Well tolerated. Risk of pancreatitis.
SGLT2 inhibitors *Canagliflozin* *Dapagliflozin* *Empagliflozin* *Ertugliflozin*	Increases urinary glucose excretion	⬌	No	Once-daily dosing in the morning. Risk of hypotension, genitourinary infections. Avoid in severe renal impairment. *Empagliflozin* is approved to reduce cardiovascular events in patients with type 2 diabetes.
GLP-1 receptor agonists *Albiglutide* *Dulaglutide* *Exenatide* *Liraglutide* *Lixisenatide* *Semaglutide*	Increases glucose-dependent insulin release; decreases secretion of glucagon; slows gastric emptying; increases satiety	⬆	No	Injection formulation. *Liraglutide* and *lixisenatide* are dosed once daily. *Albiglutide*, *dulaglutide*, and *semaglutide* are dosed once weekly. *Exenatide* is dosed twice daily and extended-release *exenatide* is dosed once weekly. *Liraglutide* is approved to reduce cardiovascular events in patients with type 2 diabetes. Weight loss may occur. Risk of pancreatitis. Contraindicated in patients with a history of medullary thyroid carcinoma.

Figure 24.14
Summary of oral agents and GLP-1 receptor agonists used to treat diabetes. ⬌ = little or no change; DPP-4 = dipeptidyl peptidase-4; GLP-1 = glucagon-like peptide-1; SGLT2 = sodium–glucose cotransporter 2.

H. Other agents

Both the dopamine agonist *bromocriptine* and the bile acid sequestrant *colesevelam* produce modest reductions in HbA_{1c}. The mechanism of action of glucose lowering is unknown for both of these drugs. Although *bromocriptine* and *colesevelam* are indicated for the treatment of type 2 diabetes, their modest efficacy, adverse effects, and pill burden limit their use in clinical practice.

Figure 24.14 provides a summary of the oral antidiabetic agents and GLP-1 receptor agonists.

Figure 24.15 shows treatment guidelines for type 2 diabetes.

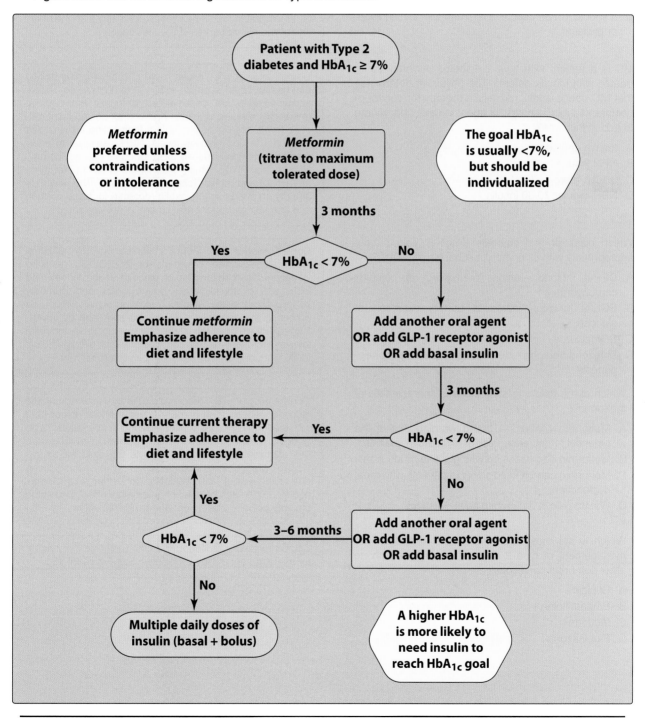

Figure 24.15
Treatment guidelines for type 2 diabetes.

Study Questions

Choose the ONE best answer.

24.1 Which of the following statements is correct regarding insulin glargine?

 A. It is primarily used to control postprandial hyperglycemia.

 B. It is a "peakless" insulin.

 C. The prolonged duration of activity is due to slow dissociation from albumin.

 D. It should not be used in a regimen with insulin *lispro* or glulisine.

Correct answer = B. Insulin glargine has a relatively flat, prolonged hypoglycemic effect. Because of this, it is used for basal glucose control, not postprandial. The prolonged duration is due to its low pH, which leads to precipitation at the injection site and resultant extended action. Insulin glargine is often used for basal control in a regimen where insulin lispro, glulisine, or aspart are used for mealtime glucose control. [Note: Glargine should not be combined with other insulins in the same syringe, as it may alter the pharmacodynamic properties of the medication.]

24.2 MC is a patient with type 2 diabetes currently being treated with insulin detemir. The physician determines that MC needs additional insulin therapy for control of postprandial glucose. Which agent is most appropriate to add at this time?

 A. Insulin degludec

 B. NPH insulin

 C. Insulin lispro

 D. NPH/regular 70/30 insulin

Correct answer = C. Insulin lispro is a rapid-acting insulin that has an onset of action within 15 to 30 minutes. Rapid-acting insulins are administered to mimic the prandial (mealtime) release of insulin and control postprandial glucose levels. Insulin degludec is a long-acting insulin used to control fasting glucose levels. NPH insulin is an intermediate-acting insulin also used for basal (fasting) control. NPH/regular 70/30 insulin is a mixture of NPH (intermediate-acting) and regular (short-acting) insulin. The patient is already on a long-acting insulin (detemir) for basal control, and another insulin for basal control is not warranted.

24.3 Which class of oral diabetes drugs is paired most appropriately with its primary mechanism of action?

 A. DPP-4 inhibitor—inhibits breakdown of complex carbohydrates

 B. SGLT2 inhibitor—increases urinary excretion of glucose

 C. Sulfonylurea—increases insulin sensitivity

 D. Thiazolidinedione—decreases hepatic gluconeogenesis

Correct answer = B. SGLT2 inhibitors work by inhibiting the sodium-glucose cotransporter 2 (SGLT2), resulting in decreased reabsorption of glucose in the kidney and increased urinary excretion. Sulfonylureas work primarily by increasing insulin secretion through stimulation of the β cells in the pancreas. DPP-4 inhibitors work by inhibiting breakdown of incretins, thereby increasing postprandial insulin secretion, decreasing postprandial glucagon, etc. TZDs work primarily by increasing insulin sensitivity.

24.4 Which of the following statements is characteristic of metformin?

 A. Metformin contains a boxed warning due to the potential for increased risk of myocardial infarction.

 B. Metformin decreases hepatic glucose production.

 C. Metformin can be used safely in patients with renal dysfunction.

 D. Weight gain is a common adverse effect.

Correct answer = B. Metformin works by inhibiting hepatic gluconeogenesis. The primary adverse effects associated with metformin are gastrointestinal and in rare cases, lactic acidosis. Metformin does not carry a warning for increased risk of myocardial infarction (this is the case for rosiglitazone). Metformin is contraindicated in renal dysfunction due to the risk of lactic acidosis. Unlike the sulfonylureas and insulin, weight gain is not an adverse effect, and some patients actually lose weight due to GI side effects.

24.5 Which is the most appropriate initial oral agent for management of type 2 diabetes in patients with no other comorbid conditions?

 A. Glipizide

 B. Empagliflozin

 C. Metformin

 D. Pioglitazone

Correct answer = C. Metformin is the preferred initial agent for management of type 2 diabetes. See Figure 24.15.

24.6 A 64-year-old woman with a history of type 2 diabetes is diagnosed with heart failure. Which of the following medications would be a poor choice for controlling her diabetes?

A. Exenatide
B. Glyburide
C. Pioglitazone
D. Insulin

Correct answer = C. The TZDs (pioglitazone and rosiglitazone) can cause fluid retention and lead to a worsening of heart failure. They should be used with caution and dose reduction, if at all, in patients with heart failure. Exenatide, glyburide, and insulin do not have precautions for use in heart failure patients.

24.7 KD is a 69-year-old male with type 2 diabetes and chronic pancreatitis. Which of the following diabetes medications is contraindicated in this patient?

A. Glipizide
B. Insulin lispro
C. Metformin
D. Dulaglutide

Correct answer = D. Dulaglutide is a GLP-1 receptor agonist. Although infrequent, GLP-1 receptor agonists have been associated with pancreatitis and should be avoided in patients with chronic pancreatitis. Glipizide, insulin lispro, and metformin have not been associated with an increased risk of pancreatitis.

24.8 Which of the following drugs for diabetes is LEAST likely to cause weight gain?

A. Liraglutide
B. Pioglitazone
C. Repaglinide
D. Insulin glulisine

Correct answer = A. GLP-1 receptor agonists are usually associated with weight loss due to their ability to enhance satiety. All of the other agents are associated with weight gain.

24.9 HB is a 55-year-old obese female who has had type 2 diabetes for 10 years. She is currently being treated with metformin, but her HbA$_{1c}$ is above goal. She has a history of heart failure and chronic obstructive pulmonary disorder. Her physician would like to add a medication that will not cause any weight gain. Which of the following would be most appropriate to control HB's diabetes?

A. Linagliptin
B. Glimepiride
C. Pioglitazone
D. Inhaled insulin

Correct answer = A. Linagliptin is a DPP-4 inhibitor, and this class of medications is effective in lowering HbA1c levels without causing weight gain (they are usually weight neutral). Sulfonylureas (glimepiride) are associated with weight gain and should be avoided in this obese patient. TZDs (pioglitazone) should be avoided in patients with heart failure. Because of the potential for bronchospasm associated with inhaled insulin, it should be avoided in patients with a history of chronic obstructive pulmonary disorder and asthma.

24.10 Which of the following diabetes medications is most appropriately paired with an adverse effect associated with its use?

A. Canagliflozin—urinary tract infections
B. Nateglinide—heart failure
C. Glipizide—weight loss
D. Liraglutide—lactic acidosis

Correct answer = A. Adverse effects of canagliflozin are genital mycotic infections, urinary tract infections, and urinary frequency. Nateglinide may cause hypoglycemia but has not been associated with heart failure. Sulfonylureas are associated with weight gain. Lactic acidosis is a rare but serious side effect of metformin (not liraglutide).

Estrogens and Androgens

Karen Whalen

25

I. OVERVIEW

Estrogens and androgens are sex hormones produced by the gonads. These hormones are necessary for conception, embryonic maturation, and development of primary and secondary sexual characteristics at puberty. The sex hormones are used therapeutically for contraception, management of menopausal symptoms, and replacement therapy in hormone deficiency. Several antagonists are effective in the treatment or prevention of hormone-responsive cancers. Sex hormones are synthesized from the precursor, cholesterol, in a series of steps that includes shortening of the hydrocarbon side chain and hydroxylation of the steroid nucleus. Aromatization is the last step in estrogen synthesis. Figure 25.1 lists the sex hormones discussed in this chapter.

II. ESTROGENS

Estradiol [ess-tra-DYE-ole] is the most potent estrogen produced and secreted by the ovary. It is the principal estrogen in premenopausal women. *Estrone* [ESS-trone] is a metabolite of *estradiol* that has approximately one-third the estrogenic potency of *estradiol*. *Estrone* is the primary circulating estrogen after menopause, and it is generated mainly from conversion of dehydroepiandrosterone [DHEA] in adipose tissue. *Estriol* [ess-TRI-ole], another metabolite of *estradiol*, is significantly less potent than is *estradiol*. It is present in significant amounts during pregnancy, because it is synthesized by the placenta. Synthetic estrogens, such as *ethinyl estradiol* [ETH-ih-nil ess-tra-DYE-ole], undergo less first-pass metabolism than do naturally occurring hormones and, thus, are effective when administered orally at lower doses.

ESTROGENS
Conjugated estrogens PREMARIN
Esterified estrogens MENEST
Estradiol (oral) ESTRACE
Estradiol (topical) DIVIGEL, ESTROGEL
Estradiol (transdermal) ALORA, CLIMARA, VIVELLE
Estradiol (vaginal) ESTRACE, ESTRING, FEMRING, VAGIFEM
Estropipate GENERIC ONLY
*Ethinyl estradiol**
SELECTIVE ESTROGEN-RECEPTOR MODULATORS (SERMs)
Clomiphene CLOMID
Ospemifene OSPHENA
Raloxifene EVISTA
Tamoxifen GENERIC ONLY
PROGESTOGENS
*Desogestrel*** DESOGEN
*Dienogest*** NATAZIA
*Drospirenone*** YASMIN, YAZ
Etonogestrel (subdermal) NEXPLANON
*Etonogestrel*** *(vaginal ring)* NUVARING
Levonorgestrel PLAN B ONE-STEP
Levonorgestrel (IUD) KYLEENA, LILETTA, MIRENA, SKYLA
Medroxyprogesterone DEPO-PROVERA, PROVERA
*Norelgestromin*** *(transdermal)* XULANE
Norethindrone MICRONOR
*Norethindrone*** ORTHO-NOVUM, TRI-NORINYL
Norethindrone acetate AYGESTIN
*Norethindrone acetate*** FEMHRT, LOESTRIN
*Norgestimate*** ORTHO TRI-CYCLEN, SPRINTEC
*Norgestrel*** LO/OVRAL
Progesterone PROMETRIUM
PROGESTERONE AGONIST/ANTAGONIST
Ulipristal acetate ELLA

Figure 25.1
Summary of sex hormones. *Available in many combinations with a progestin. **Available in combination with *ethinyl estradiol*. [Note: *Dienogest* is available in combination with *estradiol valerate*.] IUD = intrauterine device. (Figure continues on next page)

A. Mechanism of action

After dissociation from their binding sites on sex hormone–binding globulin or albumin in the plasma, steroid hormones (for example, *estradiol*) diffuse across the cell membrane and bind with high affinity to specific nuclear receptor proteins (Figure 25.2). The activated steroid–receptor complex interacts with nuclear chromatin to initiate hormone-specific RNA synthesis. This results in the synthesis of specific proteins that mediate a number of physiologic functions. [Note: The steroid hormones may elicit the synthesis of different RNA species in diverse target tissues and, therefore, are both receptor and tissue specific.] Other pathways that require these hormones have been identified that lead to more rapid actions.

B. Therapeutic uses

Estrogens are most frequently used for contraception and postmenopausal hormone therapy (HT). In the past, estrogens were widely used for prevention of osteoporosis; however, due to risks associated with estrogen therapy, current guidelines recommend use of other therapies, such as bisphosphonates (see Chapter 27).

1. **Postmenopausal HT:** The primary indication for estrogen therapy in postmenopausal women is menopausal symptoms, such as vasomotor instability (for example, "hot flashes" or "hot flushes") and vaginal atrophy (Figure 25.3). A common oral preparation used for the treatment of menopausal symptoms is *conjugated equine estrogens* (obtained from urine of pregnant mares), which primarily contains sulfate esters of *estrone* and *equilin*. Other *estrone*-based oral preparations include *esterified estrogens* and *estropipate* [ES-troe-PIP-ate]. Transdermal preparations of *estradiol* are also effective in treating menopausal symptoms. For women with an intact uterus, a progestogen is always included with the estrogen therapy, because the combination reduces the risk of endometrial carcinoma associated with unopposed

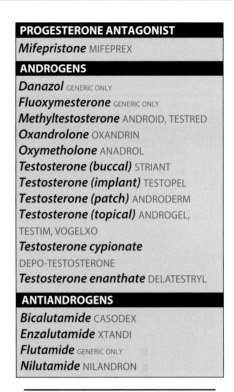

PROGESTERONE ANTAGONIST
Mifepristone MIFEPREX
ANDROGENS
Danazol GENERIC ONLY
Fluoxymesterone GENERIC ONLY
Methyltestosterone ANDROID, TESTRED
Oxandrolone OXANDRIN
Oxymetholone ANADROL
Testosterone (buccal) STRIANT
Testosterone (implant) TESTOPEL
Testosterone (patch) ANDRODERM
Testosterone (topical) ANDROGEL, TESTIM, VOGELXO
Testosterone cypionate DEPO-TESTOSTERONE
Testosterone enanthate DELATESTRYL
ANTIANDROGENS
Bicalutamide CASODEX
Enzalutamide XTANDI
Flutamide GENERIC ONLY
Nilutamide NILANDRON

Figure 25.1 (continued)

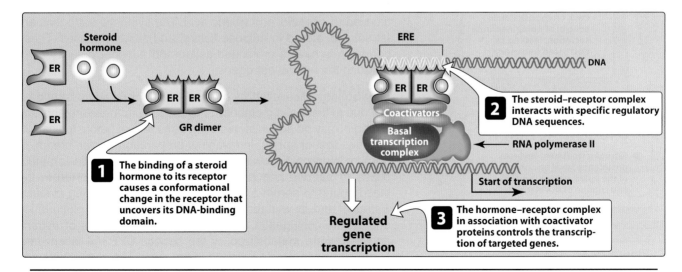

Figure 25.2
Transcriptional regulation by intracellular steroid hormone receptors. ERE = estrogen response element; ER = estrogen receptor; GR = glucocorticoid receptor.

Text within Figure 25.2:
- Steroid hormone
- ER
- ER ER GR dimer
- **1** The binding of a steroid hormone to its receptor causes a conformational change in the receptor that uncovers its DNA-binding domain.
- ERE
- ER ER
- DNA
- Coactivators
- Basal transcription complex
- **2** The steroid–receptor complex interacts with specific regulatory DNA sequences.
- RNA polymerase II
- Start of transcription
- Regulated gene transcription
- **3** The hormone–receptor complex in association with coactivator proteins controls the transcription of targeted genes.

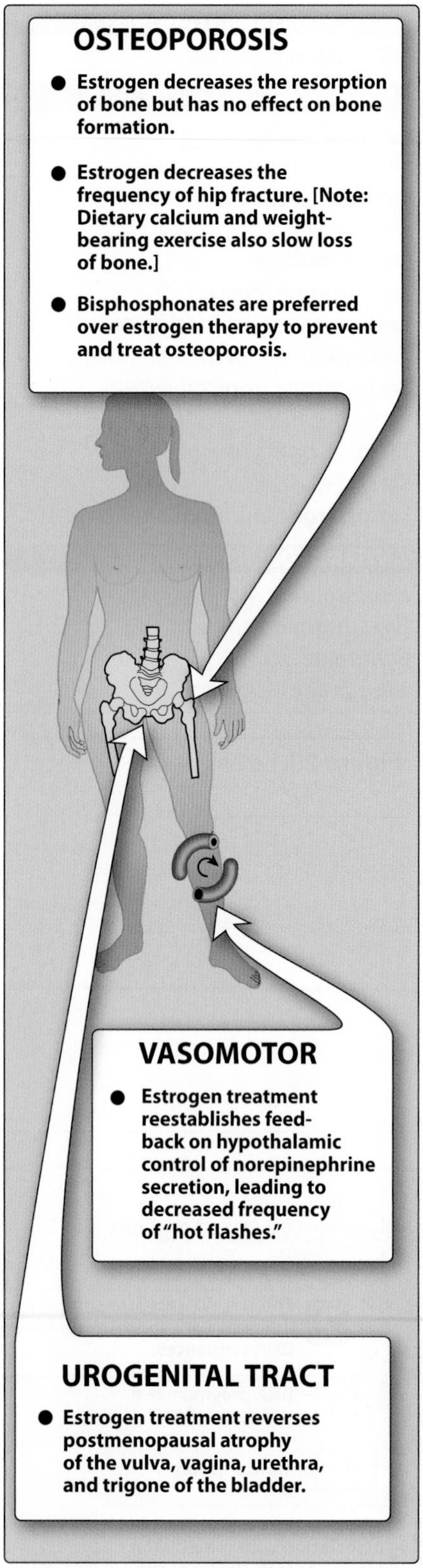

OSTEOPOROSIS

- Estrogen decreases the resorption of bone but has no effect on bone formation.

- Estrogen decreases the frequency of hip fracture. [Note: Dietary calcium and weight-bearing exercise also slow loss of bone.]

- Bisphosphonates are preferred over estrogen therapy to prevent and treat osteoporosis.

VASOMOTOR

- Estrogen treatment reestablishes feedback on hypothalamic control of norepinephrine secretion, leading to decreased frequency of "hot flashes."

UROGENITAL TRACT

- Estrogen treatment reverses postmenopausal atrophy of the vulva, vagina, urethra, and trigone of the bladder.

Figure 25.3
Benefits associated with postmenopausal estrogen replacement.

estrogen. Women who have undergone a hysterectomy may use estrogen alone. [Note: The potency of estrogen used in HT is substantially less than that of estrogens used in contraception. Thus, the adverse effects of estrogen replacement therapy are usually less pronounced than those seen in women taking estrogen for contraceptive purposes.] Use of HT has been associated with an increased risk of cardiovascular events and breast cancer. Thus, HT should be prescribed at the lowest effective dose for the shortest possible time to relieve menopausal symptoms. Women who only have urogenital symptoms, such as vaginal atrophy, should be treated with vaginal rather than systemic estrogen to minimize the risks of use.

2. **Contraception:** The combination of an estrogen and progestogen provides effective contraception via the oral, transdermal, or vaginal route.

3. **Other uses:** Estrogen therapy mimicking the natural cyclic pattern, and usually in combination with a progestogen, is instituted to stimulate development of secondary sex characteristics in young women with primary hypogonadism. Similarly, replacement therapy is used for women who have hormonal deficiencies due to surgical menopause or premature ovarian failure.

C. **Pharmacokinetics**

1. **Naturally occurring estrogens:** These agents and their esterified or conjugated derivatives are readily absorbed through the gastrointestinal tract, skin, and mucous membranes. Taken orally, *estradiol* is rapidly metabolized (and partially inactivated) by the microsomal enzymes of the liver. Micronized *estradiol* has better bioavailability. Although *estradiol* is subject to first-pass metabolism, it is still effective when taken orally.

2. **Synthetic estrogens:** These compounds, such as *ethinyl estradiol* and *estradiol valerate* are well absorbed after oral administration. *Estradiol valerate* is a prodrug of *estradiol* which is rapidly cleaved to *estradiol* and valeric acid. The synthetic estrogens are fat soluble, stored in adipose tissue, and slowly released. These compounds have a prolonged action and a higher potency compared to the natural estrogens.

3. **Metabolism:** Bioavailability of *estradiol* after oral administration is low due to first-pass metabolism. To reduce first-pass metabolism, *estradiol* may be administered via a transdermal patch, topical formulation (gel or spray), intravaginal preparation (tablet, cream, or ring), or injection. Following oral administration, *estradiol* is metabolized to *estrone* and *estriol*. Estrogens are transported in the blood bound to serum albumin or sex hormone–binding globulin. *Estradiol* and its metabolites subsequently undergo glucuronide and sulfate conjugation. In addition, smaller amounts of *estrone* and *estriol* are metabolized by the hepatic CYP3A4 isoenzyme. Metabolites are mainly excreted in the urine. The glucuronide and sulfate metabolites are also subject to enterohepatic recirculation. These compounds are secreted into the bile, hydrolyzed by gut bacteria, and then reabsorbed.

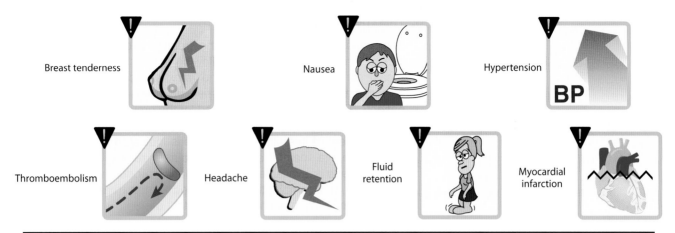

Figure 25.4
Some adverse effects associated with estrogen therapy. BP = blood pressure.

D. Adverse effects

Nausea and breast tenderness are among the most common adverse effects of estrogen therapy. In addition, the risk of thromboembolic events, myocardial infarction, and breast and endometrial cancer is increased with the use of estrogen therapy. [Note: The increased risk of endometrial cancer can be offset by including a progestogen along with the estrogen therapy.] Other effects of estrogen therapy are shown in Figure 25.4.

III. SELECTIVE ESTROGEN RECEPTOR MODULATORS

SERMs are a class of estrogen-related compounds that display selective agonism or antagonism for estrogen receptors depending on the tissue type. This category includes *tamoxifen*, *raloxifene*, *bazedoxifene*, *clomiphene*, and *ospemifene*.

A. Mechanism of action

Tamoxifen [tah-MOKS-ih-fen] and *raloxifene* [rah-LOX-ih-feen] compete with estrogen for binding to the estrogen receptor in breast tissue. [Note: Normal breast growth is stimulated by estrogens. Therefore, some hormone-responsive breast tumors regress following treatment with these agents.] In addition, *raloxifene* acts as an estrogen agonist in bone, leading to decreased bone resorption, increased bone density, and decreased vertebral fractures (Figure 25.5). Unlike estrogen and *tamoxifen*, *raloxifene* does not stimulate growth of the endometrium and, therefore, does not predispose to endometrial cancer. *Raloxifene* also lowers serum total cholesterol and low-density lipoprotein (LDL). Like *raloxifene*, *bazedoxifene* [BA-ze-DOX-i-feen] antagonizes the action of estrogen on the uterus. The drug reduces the risk of endometrial hyperplasia with estrogen use. *Clomiphene* [KLOE-mi-feen] acts as a partial estrogen agonist and interferes with the negative feedback of estrogens on the hypothalamus. This effect increases the secretion of gonadotropin-releasing hormone and gonadotropins, thereby leading to stimulation of ovulation.

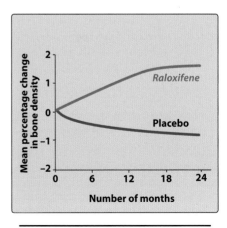

Figure 25.5
Hip bone density increases with *raloxifene* in postmenopausal women.

B. Therapeutic uses

Tamoxifen is currently used in the treatment of metastatic breast cancer, or as adjuvant therapy following mastectomy or radiation for breast cancer. Both *tamoxifen* and *raloxifene* can be used as prophylactic therapy to reduce the risk of breast cancer in high-risk patients. *Raloxifene* is also approved for the prevention and treatment of osteoporosis in postmenopausal women. *Clomiphene* is used in the treatment of infertility. *Ospemifene* is indicated for the treatment of dyspareunia (painful sexual intercourse) related to menopause. *Bazedoxifene* is available in a combination product with *conjugated estrogens*. The combination is indicated for the treatment of menopausal symptoms in women with an intact uterus.

C. Pharmacokinetics

The SERMs are rapidly absorbed after oral administration. *Tamoxifen* is extensively metabolized by cytochrome P450 system, including the formation of active metabolites via the CYP3A4/5 and CYP2D6 isoenzymes. [Note: Patients with a genetic polymorphism in CYP2D6 may produce less active metabolite, resulting in diminished activity of *tamoxifen*.] *Raloxifene* is rapidly converted to glucuronide conjugates through first-pass metabolism. These agents undergo enterohepatic cycling, and the primary route of excretion is through the bile into feces.

D. Adverse effects

The most frequent adverse effects of *tamoxifen* are hot flashes and nausea. Due to its estrogenic activity in the endometrium, endometrial hyperplasia and malignancies have been reported with *tamoxifen* therapy. This has led to recommendations for limiting the length of time on the drug for some indications. Because it is metabolized by various CYP450 isoenzymes, *tamoxifen* is subject to many drug interactions. [Note: *Tamoxifen* is also an inhibitor of P-glycoprotein.] Some CYP450 inhibitors may prevent the formation of active metabolites of *tamoxifen* and possibly reduce the efficacy (for example, *amiodarone, haloperidol, paroxetine*). Hot flashes and leg cramps are common adverse effects with *raloxifene*. In addition, there is an increased risk of deep vein thrombosis and pulmonary embolism. Women who have a past or active history of venous thromboembolic events should not take the drug. Adverse effects of *clomiphene* are dose-related and include headache, nausea, vasomotor flushes, visual disturbances, and ovarian enlargement. Use of *clomiphene* increases the risk of multiple gestation, usually twins. *Ospemifene* may stimulate endometrial growth, and addition of a progestogen in women with an intact uterus should be considered.

IV. PROGESTOGENS

Progesterone, the natural progestogen, is produced in response to luteinizing hormone (LH) by both females (secreted by the corpus luteum, primarily during the second half of the menstrual cycle, and by the placenta) and by males (secreted by the testes). It is also synthesized by the adrenal cortex in both sexes.

A. Mechanism of action

Progestogens exert their effects in a manner analogous to that of the other steroid hormones. In females, progesterone promotes the development of a secretory endometrium that can accommodate implantation of a newly forming embryo. The high levels of progesterone that are released during the second half of the menstrual cycle (the luteal phase) inhibit the production of gonadotropin and, therefore, prevent further ovulation. If conception takes place, progesterone continues to be secreted, maintaining the endometrium in a favorable state for the continuation of the pregnancy and reducing uterine contractions. If conception does not take place, the release of progesterone from the corpus luteum ceases abruptly. The decline in progesterone stimulates the onset of menstruation. Figure 25.6 summarizes the hormones produced during the menstrual cycle.

B. Therapeutic uses

The major clinical uses of progestogens are for contraception or hormone replacement therapy. For both contraception and HT, progestogens are often used in combination with estrogens. Progesterone is not used as a contraceptive therapy because of its rapid metabolism, resulting in low bioavailability. Synthetic progestogens (that is, progestins) used for contraception are more stable to first-pass metabolism, allowing lower doses when administered orally. These agents include *desogestrel* [des-oh-JES-trel], *dienogest* [dye-EN-oh-jest], *drospirenone* [droe-SPY-re-none], *levonorgestrel* [lee-voe-nor-JES-trel], *norethindrone* [nor-ETH-in-drone], *norethindrone acetate*, *norgestimate* [nor-JES-tih-mate], and *norgestrel* [nor-JES-trel]. *Medroxyprogesterone* [me-DROK-see-proe-JES-ter-one] *acetate* is an injectable contraceptive, and the oral form is a common progestin component of postmenopausal HT. Progestogens are also used for the control of dysfunctional uterine bleeding, treatment of dysmenorrhea, and management of endometriosis and infertility.

C. Pharmacokinetics

A micronized preparation of *progesterone* is rapidly absorbed after oral administration. It has a short half-life in the plasma and is metabolized by the liver to pregnanediol and glucuronide and sulfate conjugates. The metabolites are excreted primarily in the urine. Synthetic progestins are less rapidly metabolized. Oral *medroxyprogesterone acetate* has a half-life of 30 hours. When injected intramuscularly or subcutaneously, the drug has a half-life of about 40 to 50 days and provides contraception for approximately 3 months. The other progestins have half-lives of 7 to 30 hours, allowing for once-daily dosing.

D. Adverse effects

The major adverse effects associated with the use of progestins are headache, depression, weight gain, and changes in libido (Figure 25.7). Progestins that are derived from 19-nortestosterone (for example, *norethindrone*, *norethindrone acetate*, *norgestrel*, *levonorgestrel*) possess some androgenic activity because of their structural similarity to *testosterone* and can cause acne and hirsutism. Less androgenic progestins, such as *norgestimate* and *drospirenone*,

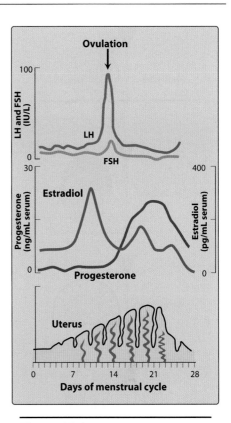

Figure 25.6
The menstrual cycle with plasma levels of pituitary and ovarian hormones and a schematic representation of changes in the morphology of the uterine lining. FSH = follicle-stimulating hormone; LH = luteinizing hormone.

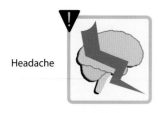

Headache

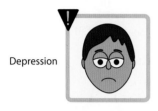

Depression

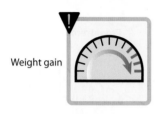

Weight gain

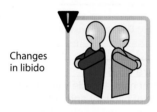

Changes
in libido

Figure 25.7
Some adverse effects
associated with
progestin therapy.

may be preferred in women with acne. *Drospirenone* may raise serum potassium due to antimineralocorticoid effects, and concurrent use with other drugs that increase potassium (for example, angiotensin-converting enzyme inhibitors) may increase the risk of hyperkalemia.

E. Antiprogestin

Mifepristone [mih-feh-PRIH-stone] (also designated as RU-486) is a progesterone antagonist. Administration of this drug results in termination of pregnancy due to interference with the progesterone needed to maintain pregnancy. *Mifepristone* is often combined with the prostaglandin analog *misoprostol* to induce uterine contractions. The major adverse effects are abdominal pain, uterine bleeding, and the possibility of an incomplete abortion.

V. CONTRACEPTIVES

Contraceptives may be hormonal or nonhormonal (for example, condom, diaphragm, contraceptive sponge, and copper intrauterine device). Figure 25.8 outlines the frequency of use for various hormonal and nonhormonal methods of contraception. An overview of the hormonal methods of contraception is provided below.

A. Types of hormonal contraceptives

1. **Combination oral contraceptives:** A combination of estrogen and progestin is the most common type of oral contraceptive. [Note: The most common estrogen in combination pills is *ethinyl estradiol*. The most common progestins are *norethindrone*, *norethindrone acetate*, *levonorgestrel*, *desogestrel*, *norgestimate*, and *drospirenone*.] These preparations are highly effective in achieving contraception (Figure 25.9). Monophasic combination pills contain a constant dose of estrogen and progestin given over 21 to 24 days.

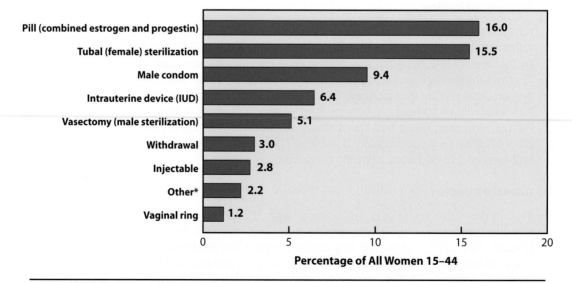

Figure 25.8
Comparison of contraceptive use among U.S. women ages 15 to 44 years. *Patch, implant, fertility awareness methods, and other barrier methods (for example, diaphragm).

Triphasic oral contraceptive products attempt to mimic the natural female cycle and usually contain a constant dose of estrogen with increasing doses of progestin given over 21 days. With most oral contraceptives, active pills are taken for 21 to 24 days, followed by 4 to 7 days of placebo, for a total regimen of 28 days. Withdrawal bleeding occurs during the hormone-free (placebo) interval. Use of extended-cycle contraception (84 active pills followed by 7 days of placebo) results in less frequent withdrawal bleeding. A continuous oral contraceptive product (active pills taken every day) is also available.

2. **Transdermal patch:** The contraceptive transdermal patch contains *ethinyl estradiol* and the progestin *norelgestromin*. During the 28-day cycle, one patch is applied each week for 3 weeks to the abdomen, upper torso, or buttock. No patch is worn during the 4th week, and withdrawal bleeding occurs. The transdermal patch has efficacy comparable to that of the oral contraceptives, but it is less effective in women weighing greater than 90 kg. Total estrogen exposure with the transdermal patch may be significantly greater than that seen with oral contraceptives.

3. **Vaginal ring:** The contraceptive vaginal ring contains *ethinyl estradiol* and *etonogestrel*. The ring is inserted into the vagina and left in place for 3 weeks. After 3 weeks, the ring is removed, and withdrawal bleeding occurs during the 4th week.

4. **Progestin-only pills:** Progestin-only pills (the "mini-pill") contain a progestin, usually *norethindrone*, and are administered daily to deliver a low, continuous dosage of drug. These preparations are less effective than combination oral contraceptives, and irregular menstrual cycles may be more frequent. Progestin-only pills may be used in patients who are breast-feeding (unlike estrogen, progestins do not have an effect on milk production) or who have intolerance or contraindications to estrogen-containing products.

5. **Injectable progestin:** *Medroxyprogesterone acetate* is a contraceptive that is administered via intramuscular or subcutaneous injection every 3 months. This product provides high sustained levels of progestin, and many women experience amenorrhea with *medroxyprogesterone acetate*. In addition, return to fertility may be delayed for several months after discontinuation. Weight gain is a common adverse effect. *Medroxyprogesterone acetate* may contribute to bone loss and predispose patients to osteoporosis and/or fractures. Therefore, the drug should not be continued for more than 2 years unless the patient is unable to tolerate other contraceptive options.

6. **Progestin implants:** After subdermal placement in the upper arm, the *etonogestrel* implant offers contraception for up to 3 years. The implant is as reliable as sterilization, and the contraceptive effect is reversible when removed. [Note: Progestin implants and intrauterine devices are known as long-acting reversible contraceptives (LARC).] Adverse effects include irregular menstrual bleeding and headaches. The *etonogestrel* implant has not been studied in women who weigh more than 130% of ideal body weight and may be less effective in this population.

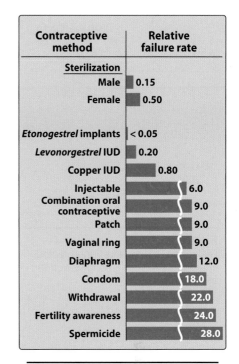

Contraceptive method	Relative failure rate
Sterilization	
Male	0.15
Female	0.50
Etonogestrel implants	< 0.05
Levonorgestrel IUD	0.20
Copper IUD	0.80
Injectable	6.0
Combination oral contraceptive	9.0
Patch	9.0
Vaginal ring	9.0
Diaphragm	12.0
Condom	18.0
Withdrawal	22.0
Fertility awareness	24.0
Spermicide	28.0

Figure 25.9
Comparison of failure rate for various methods of contraception with typical use. *Longer bars* indicate a higher failure rate—that is, more pregnancies.

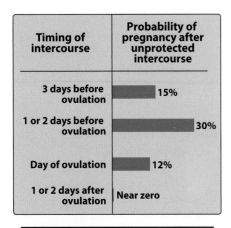

Timing of intercourse	Probability of pregnancy after unprotected intercourse
3 days before ovulation	15%
1 or 2 days before ovulation	30%
Day of ovulation	12%
1 or 2 days after ovulation	Near zero

Figure 25.10
Risk of pregnancy after unprotected intercourse in young couples in their mid-twenties.

7. **Progestin intrauterine device:** Various *levonorgestrel*-releasing intrauterine devices offer a highly effective method of contraception for 3 to 5 years. This is a suitable method of contraception for women who desire long-term contraception. It should be avoided in patients with pelvic inflammatory disease or a history of ectopic pregnancy. The *levonorgestrel* intrauterine device is a highly effective treatment for heavy menstrual bleeding. [Note: The nonhormonal copper intrauterine device provides contraception for up to 10 years.]

8. **Postcoital contraception:** Postcoital or emergency contraception reduces the probability of pregnancy after intercourse without effective contraception (Figure 25.10) to between 0.2% and 3%. The most common method of emergency contraception uses a single high dose of *levonorgestrel*. For maximum effectiveness, emergency contraception should be taken as soon as possible after unprotected intercourse and preferably within 72 hours. The *levonorgestrel* emergency contraceptive regimens are generally better tolerated than the estrogen–progestin combination regimens. An alternative emergency contraceptive is the progesterone agonist/antagonist *ulipristal* [ue-li-PRIS-tal]. It is indicated for emergency contraception within 5 days of unprotected intercourse.

B. Mechanism of action

Exogenously administered estrogen in contraceptives provides negative feedback which blunts release of follicle-stimulating hormone (FSH) by the pituitary gland and progestin inhibits LH secretion, thus preventing ovulation. Progestin also thickens the cervical mucus, thus hampering the transport of sperm. Withdrawal of the progestin stimulates menstrual bleeding during the placebo week.

C. Adverse effects

The incidence of adverse effects with contraceptives is determined by the specific compounds and combinations used. The most common adverse effects with estrogens are breast fullness, fluid retention, headache, and nausea. Increased blood pressure may also occur. Progestins may be associated with depression, changes in libido, hirsutism, and acne. Although rare, thromboembolism, thrombophlebitis, myocardial infarction, and stroke may occur with use of estrogen-containing contraceptives. These severe adverse effects are most common among women who are over age 35 and smoke, and estrogen-containing contraceptives should be avoided in this population. Progestin-only products are preferred in older women who are smokers, due to a lower risk of severe adverse effects. The incidence of cervical cancer may be increased with hormonal contraceptives, because women are less likely to use barrier methods of contraception that reduce exposure to human papillomavirus, the primary risk factor for cervical cancer. [Note: Oral contraceptives are associated with a decreased risk of endometrial and ovarian cancer.] Oral contraceptives are contraindicated in the presence of cerebrovascular and thromboembolic disease, estrogen-dependent neoplasms, liver disease, and pregnancy. Drugs that induce the CYP3A4 isoenzyme (for example, *rifampin* and *bosentan*) significantly reduce the efficacy of oral contraceptives. Concurrent use of these agents with oral contraceptives should be avoided, or an alternate barrier method of contraception should be utilized. Antibiotics that alter normal gastrointestinal flora may reduce enterohepatic recycling of estrogen, thereby diminishing effectiveness of oral contraceptives. Patients should be warned of the possible interaction between antibiotics and oral contraceptives, along with the potential need for an alternate method of contraception during antibiotic therapy.

VI. ANDROGENS

The androgens are a group of steroids that have anabolic and/or masculinizing effects in both males and females. *Testosterone* [tess-TOSS-te-rone], the most important androgen in humans, is synthesized by Leydig cells in the testes and, in smaller amounts, by thecal cells in the ovaries and by the adrenal gland in both sexes. Other androgens secreted by the testes are 5α-dihydrotestosterone (DHT), androstenedione, and DHEA in small amounts. In adult males, *testosterone* secretion by Leydig cells is controlled by gonadotropin-releasing hormone from the hypothalamus, which stimulates the anterior pituitary gland to secrete FSH and LH. *Testosterone* or its active metabolite, DHT, inhibits production of these specific trophic hormones through a negative feedback loop and, thus, regulates *testosterone* production (Figure 25.11). The androgens are required for 1) normal maturation in the male, 2) sperm production, 3) increased synthesis of muscle proteins and hemoglobin, and 4) decreased bone resorption. Synthetic modifications of the androgen structure modify solubility and susceptibility to metabolism (thus prolonging the half-life of the hormone), and separate anabolic and androgenic effects.

A. Mechanism of action

Like the estrogens and progestins, androgens bind to a specific nuclear receptor in a target cell. Although *testosterone* itself is the active ligand in muscle and liver, in other tissues, it must be metabolized to derivatives, such as DHT. For example, after diffusing into the cells of the prostate, seminal vesicles, epididymis, and skin, *testosterone* is converted by 5α-reductase to DHT, which binds to the receptor.

B. Therapeutic uses

Androgenic steroids are used for males with primary hypogonadism (caused by testicular dysfunction) or secondary hypogonadism (due to failure of the hypothalamus or pituitary). [Note: *Testosterone* replacement should only be used for males with hypogonadism related to medical conditions and not low *testosterone* associated with aging.] Anabolic steroids can be used to treat chronic wasting associated with human immunodeficiency virus or cancer. An unapproved use of anabolic steroids is to increase lean body mass, muscle strength, and endurance in athletes and body builders (see below). Because of the potential misuse of *testosterone* and its derivatives, these agents are classified as controlled substances. DHEA (a precursor of *testosterone* and estrogen) has been touted as an antiaging hormone as well as a "performance enhancer." There is no definitive evidence that

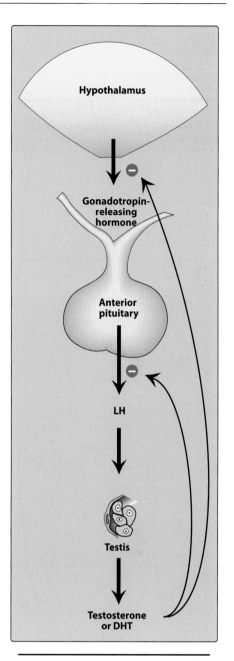

Figure 25.11
Regulation of secretion of *testosterone*.
DHT = 5-α-dihydrotestosterone;
LH = luteinizing hormone.

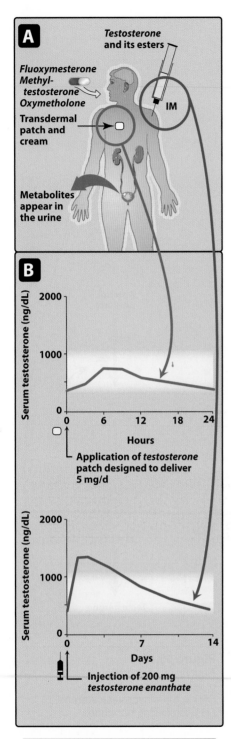

Figure 25.12
A. Administration and fate of androgens. IM = intramuscular.
B. Serum *testosterone* concentrations after administration by injection or transdermal patch to hypogonadal men. The *yellow band* indicates the upper and lower limits of normal.

it slows aging, however, or that it improves performance at normal therapeutic doses. Formulations of *testosterone* or its derivatives (for example, *methyltestosterone*) may be used in combination with estrogen for women with menopausal symptoms unresponsive to estrogen alone. *Danazol* [DAH-nah-zole], a weak androgen, is used in the treatment of endometriosis and fibrocystic breast disease. [Note: *Danazol* also possesses antiestrogenic activity.] Weight gain, acne, decreased breast size, deepening voice, increased libido, and increased hair growth are among the adverse effects.

C. Pharmacokinetics

1. **Testosterone:** This agent is ineffective orally because of inactivation by first-pass metabolism. Therefore, *testosterone* is administered via a transdermal patch, topical gel or solution, buccal tablet, or implantable pellet. Esters of *testosterone* (for example, *testosterone cypionate* or *enanthate*) are administered intramuscularly. The esterified formulations are more lipid soluble and have an increased duration of action up to several weeks. Figure 25.12 shows serum levels of *testosterone* achieved by injection and by a transdermal patch in hypogonadal men. Active metabolites of *testosterone* include DHT and *estradiol*, with activity related to the formation of DHT. Inactive metabolites are excreted primarily in the urine. *Testosterone* and its esters demonstrate a 1:1 relative ratio of androgenic to anabolic activity.

2. **Testosterone derivatives:** Alkylation of the 17α position of *testosterone* is associated with less hepatic metabolism and allows oral administration of the hormone. *Methyltestosterone* and *fluoxymesterone* [floo-oks-i-MES-te-rone] are examples of orally administered *testosterone* derivatives. *Oxandrolone* [ox-AN-droe-lone] and *oxymetholone* [OKS-ee-METH-oh-lone] are orally active 17α-alkylated derivatives of DHT. *Oxandrolone* has anabolic activity 3 to 13 times that of *testosterone*.

D. Adverse effects

1. **In females:** Androgens can cause masculinization, acne, growth of facial hair, deepening of the voice, male pattern baldness, and excessive muscle development. Menstrual irregularities may also occur. *Testosterone* should not be used by pregnant women because of possible virilization of the female fetus.

2. **In males:** Excess androgen can cause priapism, impotence, decreased spermatogenesis, gynecomastia, and cosmetic changes such as those described for females. Androgens can also stimulate growth of the prostate.

3. **In children:** Androgens can cause abnormal sexual maturation and growth disturbances resulting from premature closing of the epiphyseal plates.

4. **General effects:** Androgens can increase serum LDL and lower serum high-density lipoprotein levels. They may also cause fluid retention and peripheral edema. *Testosterone* replacement therapy has been associated with a possible increased risk of

myocardial infarction and stroke. Hepatic adverse effects have been associated with the 17α-alkylated androgens. Local skin irritation is a common adverse effect with topical formulations.

5. **In athletes:** Use of anabolic steroids (for example, DHEA) by athletes can cause premature closing of the epiphysis of the long bones, which stunts growth and interrupts development. High doses taken by young athletes may result in reduction of testicular size, hepatic abnormalities, increased aggression ("roid rage"), major mood disorders, and other adverse effects described above.

E. Antiandrogens

Antiandrogens counter male hormonal action by interfering with the synthesis of androgens or by blocking their receptors. Antiandrogens, such as *flutamide* [FLOO-tah-mide], *bicalutamide* [bye-ka-LOO-ta-mide], *enzalutamide* [enz-a-LOO-ta-mide], and *nilutamide* [nye-LOO-ta-mide], act as competitive inhibitors of androgens at the target cell and are effective orally for the treatment of prostate cancer (see Chapter 35). *Finasteride* [fin-AS-ter-ide] and *dutasteride* [doo-TAS-ter-ride] inhibit 5α-reductase, resulting in decreased formation of dihydrotestosterone. These agents are used for the treatment of benign prostatic hyperplasia (see Chapter 41).

Study Questions

Choose the ONE best answer.

25.1 A 53-year-old woman has severe vasomotor symptoms (hot flushes) associated with menopause. She has no pertinent past medical or surgical history. Which would be most appropriate for her symptoms?

A. Conjugated estrogens vaginal cream
B. Estradiol transdermal patch
C. Oral estradiol and medroxyprogesterone acetate
D. Injectable medroxyprogesterone acetate

Correct answer = C. Estrogen vaginal cream only treats vaginal symptoms of menopause such as vaginal atrophy and does not treat hot flushes. Since this patient has an intact uterus, a progestin such as medroxyprogesterone needs to be used along with the estrogen to prevent the development of endometrial hyperplasia. Unopposed estrogen (for example, the estradiol transdermal patch) should not be used. Injectable medroxyprogesterone acetate is used for contraception.

25.2 A 70-year-old woman is being treated with raloxifene for osteoporosis. Which is a concern with this therapy?

A. Breast cancer
B. Endometrial cancer
C. Venous thrombosis
D. Hypercholesterolemia

Correct answer = C. Raloxifene can increase the risk of venous thromboembolism. Unlike estrogen and tamoxifen, raloxifene does not result in an increased incidence of endometrial cancer. Raloxifene lowers the risk of breast cancer in high-risk women, and it also lowers LDL cholesterol.

25.3 Which is the most appropriate oral contraceptive for a patient with moderate acne?

A. Ethinyl estradiol/levonorgestrel
B. Ethinyl estradiol/norethindrone acetate
C. Ethinyl estradiol/norgestimate
D. Ulipristal

Correct answer = C. The progestins levonorgestrel and norethindrone acetate may have androgenic activity and contribute to acne. Norgestimate has less androgenic activity and is preferred for this patient. Ulipristal is an emergency contraceptive and should not be used as a regular method of contraception.

25.4 A 25-year-old woman is using injectable medroxyprogesterone acetate as a method of contraception. Which adverse effect is a concern if she wishes to use this therapy long-term?

A. Hyperkalemia
B. Male pattern baldness
C. Osteoporosis
D. Weight loss

Correct answer = C. Medroxyprogesterone acetate may contribute to bone loss and predispose patients to osteoporosis and/or fractures. Therefore, the drug should not be continued for more than 2 years if possible. The drug often causes weight gain, not weight loss. The other adverse effects are not associated with medroxyprogesterone.

25.5 Which contraceptive method provides long-acting reversible contraception (LARC)?

A. Contraceptive vaginal ring
B. Intrauterine device
C. Extended-cycle oral contraceptives
D. Transdermal contraceptive patch

Correct answer = B. The progestin-only intrauterine devices provide contraception for 3 to 5 years, depending on the device. The etonogestrel subdermal implant is another LARC that provides contraception for 3 years. The contraceptive vaginal ring is worn for 3 weeks at a time, and the transdermal patch for 1 week at a time. Extended cycle oral contraceptives must be administered daily.

25.6 Which is the most effective form of contraception with typical use?

A. Combined oral contraceptives
B. Progestin-only "mini-pill"
C. Depot medroxyprogesterone acetate injection
D. Subdermal progestin implant

Correct answer = D. See Figure 25.9. The subdermal implant has a very low failure rate, since it does not require adherence of the patient after implantation. Progestin-only pills are less effective than combined oral contraceptives and the depot medroxyprogesterone acetate injection.

25.7 A 36-year-old woman requests birth control. She has no medical conditions, and she smokes one pack of cigarettes per day. Which would be the most appropriate to recommend?

A. Vaginal contraceptive ring
B. Transdermal contraceptive patch
C. Progestin-only "mini-pill"
D. Combination oral contraceptive pill

Correct answer = C. Progestin-only products are preferred in older women who are smokers, due to a lower risk of severe adverse effects, such as myocardial infarction and stroke. Estrogen-containing contraceptives are not recommended in women over the age of 35 who are smokers. The vaginal contraceptive ring, transdermal contraceptive patch, and combination oral contraceptive pills all contain estrogen.

25.8 A 22-year-old woman requests emergency contraception after unprotected intercourse that occurred 1 day ago. She has no medical conditions. Which agent is most appropriate?

A. Ethinyl estradiol/norgestimate
B. Etonogestrel
C. Levonorgestrel
D. Mifepristone

Correct answer = C. A single dose of levonorgestrel is preferred for emergency contraception and should be administered within 72 hours of unprotected intercourse for best efficacy. Estrogen/progestin regimens are less used for emergency contraception due to a higher incidence of adverse effects such as nausea/vomiting. Etonogestrel is a progestin used in the contraceptive ring and implant. Mifepristone is a progesterone antagonist used to terminate pregnancy once it has occurred.

25.9 A 35-year-old woman is experiencing infertility due to anovulation. Which agent is most appropriate for this patient?

A. Clomiphene
B. Ospemifene
C. Raloxifene
D. Ulipristal

Correct answer = A. Clomiphene is a SERM that interferes with negative feedback of estrogens on the hypothalamus, thereby increasing the secretion of gonadotropin-releasing hormone and gonadotropins, and leading to stimulation of ovulation. Ospemifene is a SERM indicated for the treatment of dyspareunia. Raloxifene is a SERM used in the prevention of breast cancer and osteoporosis. Ulipristal is a progesterone agonist/antagonist used as an emergency contraceptive.

25.10 Use of testosterone is most appropriate in which patient?

   A. A 25-year-old competitive athlete
   B. A 30-year-old man with hypogonadism due to testicular injury
   C. A 50-year-old man with low testosterone related to aging
   D. A 65-year-old man with low testosterone and a history of myocardial infarction

Correct answer = B. Testosterone should only be used only for hypogonadism associated with documented medical conditions and not low testosterone associated with aging. Testosterone replacement may increase the risk of cardiovascular events and should be used with caution in patients with a history of myocardial infarction and heart disease.

Adrenal Hormones

26

Shannon Miller and Karen Whalen

I. OVERVIEW

The adrenal cortex secretes two types of corticosteroids (glucocorticoids and mineralocorticoids; Figure 26.1) and the adrenal androgens. The adrenal cortex has three zones, and each zone synthesizes a different type of steroid hormone from cholesterol (Figure 26.2). The outer zona glomerulosa produces mineralocorticoids (for example, aldosterone) that are responsible for regulating salt and water metabolism. The middle zona fasciculata synthesizes glucocorticoids (for example, cortisol) that are involved with metabolism and response to stress. The inner zona reticularis secretes adrenal androgens (see Chapter 25). Secretion by the two inner zones and, to a lesser extent, the outer zone is controlled by pituitary adrenocorticotropic hormone (ACTH; also called corticotropin), which is released in response to hypothalamic corticotropin-releasing hormone (CRH). Glucocorticoids serve as feedback inhibitors of ACTH and CRH secretion.

II. CORTICOSTEROIDS

Corticosteroids differ in their metabolic (glucocorticoid) and electrolyte-regulating (mineralocorticoid) activity. The corticosteroids bind to specific intracellular cytoplasmic receptors in target tissues. Glucocorticoid receptors are widely distributed throughout the body, whereas mineralocorticoid receptors are confined mainly to excretory organs, such as the kidney, colon, salivary glands, and sweat glands. Both types of receptors are found in the brain. After dimerizing, the receptor–hormone complex recruits coactivator (or corepressor) proteins and translocates into the nucleus, where it attaches to gene promoter elements. There it acts as a transcription factor to turn genes on (when complexed with coactivators) or off (when complexed with corepressors), depending on the tissue (Figure 26.3). Because of this mechanism, some effects of corticosteroids take hours to days to occur. This section describes normal actions and therapeutic uses of corticosteroids.

A. Glucocorticoids

Cortisol is the principal human glucocorticoid. Normally, its production is diurnal, with a peak in early morning followed by a decline and

CORTICOSTEROIDS
Betamethasone CELESTONE, DIPROLENE
Cortisone GENERIC ONLY
Dexamethasone DECADRON
Fludrocortisone GENERIC ONLY
Hydrocortisone CORTEF
Methylprednisolone MEDROL
Prednisolone ORAPRED, PEDIAPRED
Prednisone DELTASONE
Triamcinolone KENALOG, NASACORT, ARISTOSPAN
INHIBITORS OF ADRENOCORTICOID BIOSYNTHESIS OR FUNCTION
Eplerenone INSPRA
Ketoconazole NIZORAL
Spironolactone ALDACTONE

Figure 26.1
Summary of adrenal corticosteroids.

then a secondary, smaller peak in late afternoon. Stress and levels of the circulating steroid influence secretion. The effects of cortisol are many and diverse. In general, all glucocorticoids:

1. **Promote normal intermediary metabolism:** Glucocorticoids stimulate hepatic glucose production by enhancing expression of enzymes involved in gluconeogenesis. They mobilize amino acids and stimulate lipolysis, thereby providing the building blocks and energy for glucose synthesis.

2. **Increase resistance to stress:** By raising plasma glucose levels, glucocorticoids provide the body with energy to combat stress caused by trauma, fright, infection, bleeding, or debilitating disease. [Note: Glucocorticoid insufficiency may result in hypoglycemia (for example, during stressful periods or fasting).]

3. **Alter blood cell levels in plasma:** Glucocorticoids cause a decrease in eosinophils, basophils, monocytes, and lymphocytes by redistributing them from the circulation to lymphoid tissue. Glucocorticoids also increase hemoglobin, erythrocytes, platelets, and polymorphonuclear leukocytes.

4. **Possess anti-inflammatory action:** Potent anti-inflammatory and immunosuppressive activities are the most important therapeutic properties of glucocorticoids. Glucocorticoids lower circulating lymphocytes and inhibit the ability of leukocytes and macrophages to respond to mitogens and antigens. Glucocorticoids also decrease the production and release of proinflammatory cytokines. They inhibit phospholipase A_2, which blocks the release of arachidonic acid (the precursor of the prostaglandins and leukotrienes), resulting in anti-inflammatory actions. Lastly, these agents influence the inflammatory response by stabilizing mast cell and basophil membranes, thereby decreasing histamine release.

5. **Affect other systems:** High levels of glucocorticoids provide negative feedback to reduce ACTH production and affect the endocrine system by suppressing synthesis of glucocorticoids and thyroid-stimulating hormone. In addition, adequate cortisol levels are essential for normal glomerular filtration. Corticosteroids may adversely affect other systems (see Adverse Effects below).

B. Mineralocorticoids

Mineralocorticoids help to control fluid status and concentration of electrolytes, especially sodium and potassium. Aldosterone acts on mineralocorticoid receptors in the distal tubules and collecting ducts in the kidney, causing reabsorption of sodium, bicarbonate, and water. Conversely, aldosterone decreases reabsorption of potassium, which, with H^+, is lost in the urine. Enhancement of sodium reabsorption by aldosterone also occurs in gastrointestinal mucosa and in sweat and salivary glands. [Note: Elevated aldosterone levels may cause alkalosis and hypokalemia, retention of sodium and water, and increased blood volume and blood pressure. Hyperaldosteronism is treated with *spironolactone.*]

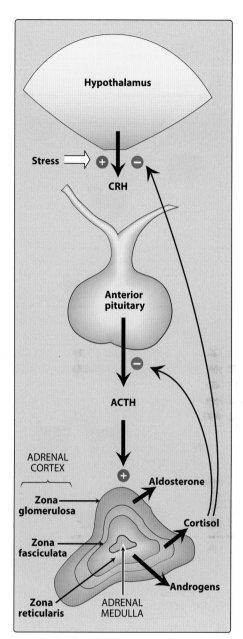

Figure 26.2
Regulation of corticosteroid secretion.
ACTH = adrenocorticotropic hormone;
CRH = corticotropin-releasing hormone.

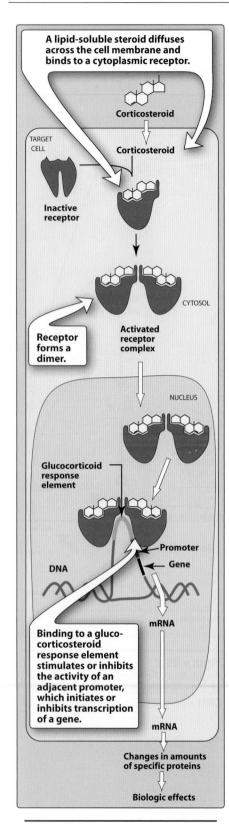

A lipid-soluble steroid diffuses across the cell membrane and binds to a cytoplasmic receptor.

Corticosteroid

TARGET CELL

Corticosteroid

Inactive receptor

CYTOSOL

Receptor forms a dimer.

Activated receptor complex

NUCLEUS

Glucocorticoid response element

DNA

Promoter

Gene

mRNA

Binding to a gluco-corticosteroid response element stimulates or inhibits the activity of an adjacent promoter, which initiates or inhibits transcription of a gene.

mRNA

Changes in amounts of specific proteins

Biologic effects

Figure 26.3
Gene regulation by glucocorticoids.

C. Therapeutic uses of the corticosteroids

Semisynthetic derivatives of corticosteroids vary in anti-inflammatory potency, mineralocorticoid activity, and duration of action (Figure 26.4). These agents are used in replacement therapy and in the treatment of severe allergic reactions, asthma, rheumatoid arthritis, other inflammatory disorders, and some cancers.

1. **Replacement therapy for primary adrenocortical insufficiency (Addison disease):** Addison disease is caused by adrenal cortex dysfunction (diagnosed by lack of response to ACTH administration). *Hydrocortisone* [hye-droe-KOR-tih-sone], which is identical to natural cortisol, is given to correct the deficiency. Failure to do so results in death. Two-thirds of the daily dosage of *hydrocortisone* is administered in the morning and one-third in the afternoon, mimicking the normal diurnal variation in cortisol levels. Administration of *fludrocortisone* [floo-droe-KOR-tih-sone], a potent synthetic mineralocorticoid, may also be necessary to correct mineralocorticoid deficiency.

2. **Replacement therapy for secondary or tertiary adrenocortical insufficiency:** These disorders are caused by a defect in CRH production by the hypothalamus or in ACTH production by the pituitary. *Hydrocortisone* is used for treatment of these deficiencies.

3. **Diagnosis of Cushing syndrome:** Cushing syndrome is caused by hypersecretion of glucocorticoids (hypercortisolism) that results from excessive release of ACTH by the anterior pituitary or an adrenal tumor. [Note: Chronic treatment with high doses of glucocorticoids is a frequent cause of iatrogenic Cushing syndrome.] Cortisol levels (urine, plasma, and saliva) and the *dexamethasone* [dex-a-METH-a-sone] suppression test are used to diagnose Cushing syndrome. The synthetic glucocorticoid *dexamethasone* suppresses cortisol release in normal individuals, but not those with Cushing syndrome.

4. **Replacement therapy for congenital adrenal hyperplasia (CAH):** CAH is a group of diseases resulting from an enzyme defect in the synthesis of one or more of the adrenal steroid hormones. CAH may lead to virilization in females due to overproduction of adrenal androgens. Treatment requires administration of sufficient corticosteroids to suppress release of CRH and ACTH and normalize hormone levels. This decreases production of adrenal androgens. The choice of replacement hormone depends on the specific enzyme defect.

5. **Relief of inflammatory symptoms:** Corticosteroids significantly reduce inflammation associated with rheumatoid arthritis and inflammatory skin conditions, including redness, swelling, heat, and tenderness. These agents are important for symptom control in persistent asthma, as well as treatment of exacerbations of asthma and inflammatory bowel disease. In osteoarthritis, intraarticular corticosteroids may be used for treatment of a disease flare. Corticosteroids are not curative in these disorders.

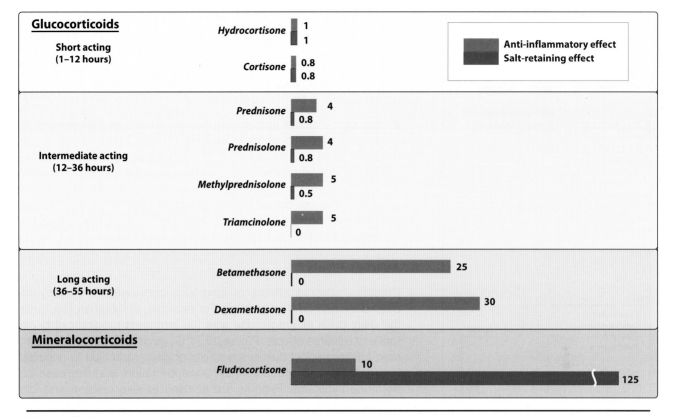

Figure 26.4
Pharmacologic effects and duration of action of some commonly used natural and synthetic corticosteroids. Activities are all relative to that of *hydrocortisone*, which is considered to be 1.

6. **Treatment of allergies:** Corticosteroids are beneficial in the treatment of allergic rhinitis, as well as drug, serum, and transfusion allergic reactions. In the treatment of allergic rhinitis and asthma, *fluticasone* [floo-TIK-a-sone] and others (see Figure 26.5) are inhaled into the respiratory tract from a metered dose dispenser. This minimizes systemic effects, reducing or eliminating the use of oral corticosteroids.

7. **Acceleration of lung maturation:** Fetal cortisol is a regulator of lung maturation. Consequently, a regimen of *betamethasone* or *dexamethasone* administered intramuscularly to the mother within 48 hours proceeding premature delivery can accelerate lung maturation in the fetus and prevent respiratory distress syndrome.

D. Pharmacokinetics

1. **Absorption and fate:** Corticosteroids are readily absorbed after oral administration. Selected compounds may be administered intravenously, intramuscularly, intra-articularly, topically, or via inhalation or intranasal delivery (Figure 26.5). All topical and inhaled glucocorticoids are absorbed to some extent and, therefore, have the potential to suppress the hypothalamic–pituitary–adrenal (HPA) axis. After absorption, glucocorticoids are greater than 90% bound to plasma proteins, mostly corticosteroid-binding globulin or albumin. Corticosteroids are metabolized by the liver microsomal oxidizing enzymes. The metabolites are conjugated to glucuronic acid or sulfate and excreted by the kidney. [Note: The

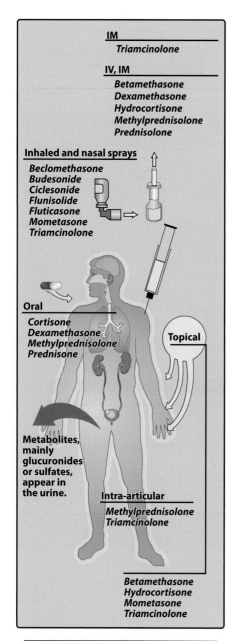

IM

Triamcinolone

IV, IM

Betamethasone
Dexamethasone
Hydrocortisone
Methylprednisolone
Prednisolone

Inhaled and nasal sprays

Beclomethasone
Budesonide
Ciclesonide
Flunisolide
Fluticasone
Mometasone
Triamcinolone

Oral

Cortisone
Dexamethasone
Methylprednisolone
Prednisone

Topical

Metabolites, mainly glucuronides or sulfates, appear in the urine.

Intra-articular

Methylprednisolone
Triamcinolone

Betamethasone
Hydrocortisone
Mometasone
Triamcinolone

Figure 26.5
Routes of administration and elimination of corticosteroids.
(IM = intramuscular; IV = intravenous.)

half-life of corticosteroids may increase substantially in hepatic dysfunction.] *Prednisone* [PRED-nih-sone] is preferred in pregnancy because it minimizes steroid effects on the fetus. It is a prodrug that is not converted to the active compound, *prednisolone* [pred-NIH-so-lone], in the fetal liver. Any *prednisolone* formed in the mother is biotransformed to *prednisone* by placental enzymes.

2. **Dosage:** Factors that should be considered in determining the dosage of corticosteroids include glucocorticoid versus mineralocorticoid activity, duration of action, type of preparation, and time of day when the drug is administered. When large doses of corticosteroids are required for more than 2 weeks, suppression of the HPA axis occurs. Alternate-day administration of corticosteroids may prevent this adverse effect by allowing the HPA axis to recover/function on days the hormone is not taken.

E. Adverse effects

Common adverse effects of long-term corticosteroid therapy are often dose related (Figure 26.6). For example, in rheumatoid arthritis, the daily dose of *prednisone* was the strongest predictor of occurrence of adverse effects (Figure 26.7). Osteoporosis is the most common adverse effect due to the ability of glucocorticoids to suppress intestinal Ca^{2+} absorption, inhibit bone formation, and decrease sex hormone synthesis. Patients are advised to take calcium and vitamin D supplements. Bisphosphonates may also be useful in the treatment of glucocorticoid-induced osteoporosis. [Note: Increased appetite is not necessarily an adverse effect. In fact, it is one of the reasons for the use of *prednisone* in cancer chemotherapy.] The classic Cushing-like syndrome (redistribution of body fat, puffy face, hirsutism, and increased appetite) is observed in excess corticosteroid replacement. Cataracts may also occur with long-term corticosteroid therapy. Hyperglycemia may develop and lead to diabetes mellitus. Diabetic patients should monitor blood glucose and adjust medications accordingly if taking corticosteroids. Topical therapy can cause skin atrophy, ecchymosis, and purple striae.

F. Discontinuation

Sudden discontinuation of these drugs can cause serious consequences if the patient has suppression of the HPA axis. In this case, abrupt removal of corticosteroids causes acute adrenal insufficiency that can be fatal. This risk, coupled with the possibility that withdrawal could exacerbate the disease, means that the dose must be tapered slowly according to individual tolerance. The patient must be monitored carefully.

G. Inhibitors of adrenocorticoid biosynthesis or function

Several substances are therapeutically useful as inhibitors of the synthesis or function of adrenal steroids: *ketoconazole*, *spironolactone*, and *eplerenone*.

1. **Ketoconazole:** *Ketoconazole* [kee-toe-KON-ah-zole] is an antifungal agent that strongly inhibits all gonadal and adrenal steroid hormone synthesis. It is used in the treatment of patients with Cushing syndrome.

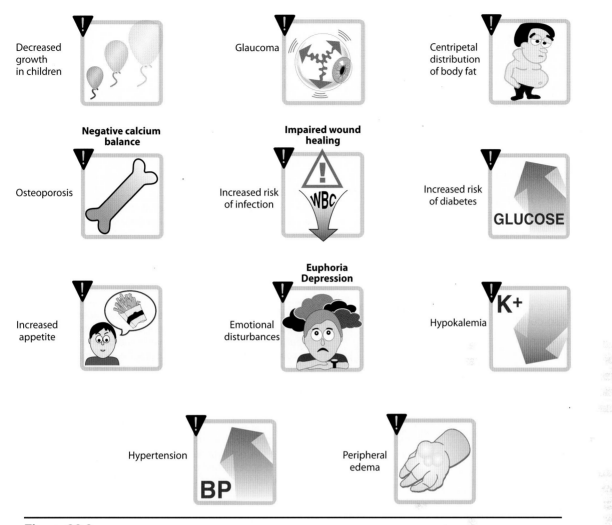

Figure 26.6
Some commonly observed effects of long-term corticosteroid therapy. BP = blood pressure.

2. **Spironolactone:** This antihypertensive drug competes for the mineralocorticoid receptor and, thus, inhibits sodium reabsorption in the kidney. *Spironolactone* [speer-oh-no-LAK-tone] also antagonizes aldosterone and testosterone synthesis. It is effective for hyperaldosteronism and hepatic cirrhosis, and is used with other standard therapies for treatment of heart failure with reduced ejection fraction. It is also useful in the management of hirsutism in women, probably due to antiandrogen activity on the hair follicle. Adverse effects include hyperkalemia, gynecomastia, menstrual irregularities, and skin rashes.

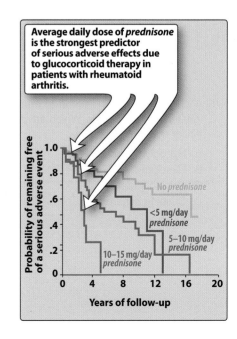

Figure 26.7
Probability of remaining free of a serious adverse event in patients with rheumatoid arthritis treated with no or different doses of *prednisone*.

3. Eplerenone: *Eplerenone* [e-PLER-ih-none] specifically binds to the mineralocorticoid receptor, where it acts as an aldosterone antagonist. This specificity avoids the adverse effect of gynecomastia that is associated with *spironolactone.* It is approved for the treatment of hypertension and for heart failure with reduced ejection fraction.

Study Questions

Choose the ONE best answer.

26.1 Which part of the adrenal gland is correctly paired with the type of substance it secretes?

A. Adrenal medulla—corticotropin

B. Zona fasciculata—cortisol

C. Zona glomerulosa—androgens

D. Zona reticularis—catecholamines

> Correct answer = B. The adrenal medulla secretes catecholamines. Corticotropin is secreted by the anterior pituitary. The zona glomerulosa secretes aldosterone, and the zona reticularis secretes androgens.

26.2 Corticosteroids are useful in the treatment of which of the following disorders?

A. Cushing syndrome

B. Diabetes

C. Hypertension

D. Inflammatory bowel disease

> Correct answer = D. Corticosteroids can increase blood pressure and glucose and are not used in the treatment of hypertension or diabetes. Cushing syndrome is an excess secretion of glucocorticoids. Dexamethasone may be used in the diagnosis of Cushing syndrome, but not its treatment. Corticosteroids reduce inflammation and can be used in the management of inflammatory bowel disease.

26.3 Which adverse effect commonly occurs with glucocorticoid therapy?

A. Glaucoma

B. Hyperkalemia

C. Weight loss

D. Osteoarthritis

> Correct answer = A. Glucocorticoid therapy may cause hypokalemia, not hyperkalemia. Glucocorticoids also cause increased appetite and osteoporosis. Glaucoma is a known potential adverse effect of this class.

26.4 Which contributes to osteoporosis with long-term use of glucocorticoids?

A. Increased excretion of calcium

B. Inhibition of calcium absorption

C. Stimulation of the hypothalamic–pituitary–adrenal axis

D. Decreased production of prostaglandins

> Correct answer = B. Glucocorticoid-induced osteoporosis is attributed to inhibition of calcium absorption and bone formation. Increased intake of calcium plus vitamin D and use of bisphosphonates may be indicated. Glucocorticoids suppress rather than stimulate the hypothalamic–pituitary–adrenal axis. The decreased production of prostaglandins does not play a role in bone formation.

26.5 A child with severe asthma is treated with high-dose inhaled corticosteroids. Which adverse effect is of particular concern?

A. Hypoglycemia

B. Hirsutism

C. Growth suppression

D. Cushing syndrome

> Correct answer = C. Corticosteroids may retard bone growth. Chronic use of the medication may lead to growth suppression, so linear growth should be monitored periodically. Hyperglycemia, not hypoglycemia, is a possible adverse effect. Hirsutism and Cushing syndrome are unlikely with the dose that the child receives via inhalation.

26.6 Which is appropriate for treatment of congenital adrenal hyperplasia in a child?

    A. Adrenocorticotropic hormone (ACTH)

    B. Ketoconazole

    C. Prednisone

    D. Spironolactone

Correct answer = C. Congenital adrenal hyperplasia is seen in infancy and childhood. Because cortisol synthesis is decreased, feedback inhibition of adrenocorticotropic hormone (ACTH) formation and release is also decreased, resulting in enhanced ACTH formation. This in turn leads to increased levels of adrenal androgens and/or mineralocorticoids. The treatment is to administer a glucocorticoid, such as hydrocortisone (in infants) or prednisone, which restores the feedback inhibition. The other options are inappropriate.

26.7 A patient with Addison disease treated with hydrocortisone is experiencing dehydration and hyponatremia. Which drug is best to add to the patient's therapy?

    A. Dexamethasone

    B. Fludrocortisone

    C. Prednisone

    D. Triamcinolone

Correct answer = B. To combat dehydration and hyponatremia, a corticosteroid with high mineralocorticoid activity is needed. Fludrocortisone has the greatest mineralocorticoid activity of the agents provided. The other drugs have little or no mineralocorticoid activity.

26.8 Which strategy is effective to minimize development of HPA axis suppression in a patient with rheumatoid arthritis on long-term high-dose corticosteroid therapy?

    A. Alternate-day administration

    B. Administration via topical or inhalation route when possible

    C. Immediate cessation of the corticosteroid

    D. Administration of two-thirds of the daily dose in the morning and one-third in the afternoon

Correct answer = A. Topical or inhaled corticosteroids may minimize HPA axis suppression, but are unlikely to be effective in rheumatoid arthritis. Since the patient has been on long-term therapy, a taper would be necessary. Administration of two-thirds of the dose in the morning and one-third in the afternoon is a strategy to mimic the normal diurnal variation of cortisol secretion, but it does not prevent suppression of the HPA axis. Alternate-day administration is beneficial.

26.9 Which patient is most likely to have suppression of the HPA axis and require a slow taper of corticosteroid therapy?

    A. A patient taking 40 mg of prednisone daily for 7 days to treat an asthma exacerbation.

    B. A patient taking 10 mg of prednisone daily for 3 months for rheumatoid arthritis.

    C. A patient using mometasone nasal spray daily for 6 months for allergic rhinitis.

    D. A patient receiving an intraarticular injection of methylprednisolone for osteoarthritis.

Correct answer = B. Suppression of the HPA axis usually occurs with higher doses of corticosteroids when used for a duration of 2 weeks or more. Although the dose of prednisone is higher in the asthma patient, the duration of therapy is short, so the risk of HPA axis suppression is lower. The risk of HPA axis suppression is low with topical therapies like intranasal mometasone and with one-time joint injections.

26.10 Which corticosteroid is most appropriate to administer to a woman in preterm labor to accelerate fetal lung maturation?

    A. Betamethasone

    B. Fludrocortisone

    C. Hydrocortisone

    D. Prednisone

Correct answer = A. A corticosteroid with high glucocorticoid activity is needed to speed fetal lung maturation prior to delivery. Betamethasone has high glucocorticoid activity and is one of the recommended drugs in this context. Dexamethasone is the other. Fludrocortisone mainly has mineralocorticoid activity and is not useful in this situation. Hydrocortisone has much lower glucocorticoid activity. Prednisone has a higher glucocorticoid activity than hydrocortisone, but the fetus is not able to convert it to prednisolone, the active form.

Drugs Affecting Bone Metabolism

Karen Whalen

27

I. OVERVIEW

Osteoporosis, Paget disease, and osteomalacia are disorders of the bone. Osteoporosis is characterized by progressive loss of bone mass and skeletal fragility. Patients with osteoporosis have an increased risk of fractures, which can cause significant morbidity. Osteoporosis occurs most frequently in postmenopausal women and older adults of both sexes. Paget disease is a disorder of bone remodeling that results in disorganized bone formation and enlarged or misshapen bones. Unlike osteoporosis, Paget disease is usually limited to one or a few bones. Patients may experience bone pain, bone deformities, or fractures. Osteomalacia is softening of the bones that is most often attributed to vitamin D deficiency. [Note: Osteomalacia in children is referred to as rickets]. As osteoporosis is more common, drug therapy for osteoporosis is the focus of this chapter (Figure 27.1).

II. BONE REMODELING

Throughout life, bone undergoes continuous remodeling, with about 10% of the skeleton replaced each year. Bone remodeling serves to remove and replace damaged bone and to maintain calcium homeostasis. Osteoclasts are cells that break down bone, a process known as bone resorption. Following bone resorption, osteoblasts or bone-building cells synthesize new bone. Crystals of calcium phosphate known as hydroxyapatite are deposited in the new bone matrix during the process of bone mineralization. Bone mineralization is essential for bone strength. Lastly, bone enters a resting phase until remodeling begins again. Bone loss occurs when bone resorption exceeds bone formation during the remodeling process. Figure 27.2 shows changes in bone morphology seen in osteoporosis.

III. PREVENTION OF OSTEOPOROSIS

Strategies to reduce bone loss in postmenopausal women include adequate dietary intake of calcium and vitamin D, weight-bearing exercise, smoking cessation, and avoidance of excessive alcohol intake. Patients with inadequate dietary intake of calcium should receive calcium supplementation. *Calcium carbonate* is an inexpensive and commonly used calcium supplement. It contains 40% elemental calcium and should be taken

DRUGS FOR OSTEOPOROSIS
Abaloparatide TYMLOS
Alendronate FOSAMAX, BINOSTO
Calcitonin MIACALCIN
Denosumab PROLIA
Ibandronate BONIVA
Raloxifene EVISTA
Risedronate ACTONEL, ATELVIA
Teriparatide FORTEO
Zoledronic acid RECLAST, ZOMETA

DRUGS FOR DISORDERS OF BONE REMODELING
Etidronate GENERIC ONLY
Pamidronate AREDIA
Tiludronate SKELID

Figure 27.1
Summary of drugs used in the treatment of osteoporosis and other bone disorders.

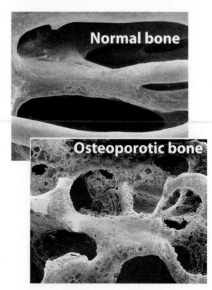

Figure 27.2
Changes in bone morphology seen in osteoporosis.

with meals for best absorption. *Calcium citrate* (21% elemental calcium) is better tolerated and may be taken with or without food. Adverse effects of calcium supplementation include gas and bloating. Calcium may interfere with absorption of iron preparations, thyroid replacement, and fluoroquinolone and tetracycline antibiotics, and administration of these drugs should be separated by several hours. Vitamin D is essential for absorption of calcium and bone health, and older patients are often at risk for vitamin D deficiency. Supplementation with vitamin D_2 (*ergocalciferol*) or vitamin D_3 (*cholecalciferol*) is used for treatment. In addition, patients at risk for osteoporosis should avoid drugs that increase bone loss such as glucocorticoids (Figure 27.3). [Note: Use of glucocorticoids (for example, *prednisone* 5 mg/d or equivalent) for 3 months or more is a significant risk factor for osteoporosis.]

IV. TREATMENT OF OSTEOPOROSIS

Pharmacologic therapy for osteoporosis is warranted in postmenopausal women and men aged 50 years or over who have a previous osteoporotic fracture, a bone mineral density that is 2.5 standard deviations or more below that of a healthy young adult, or a low bone mass (osteopenia) with a high probability of future fractures.

A. Bisphosphonates

Bisphosphonates including *alendronate* [a-LEND-row-nate], *risedronate* [rih-SED-row-nate], and *zoledronic* [zole-DROE-nick] *acid* are preferred agents for treatment of postmenopausal osteoporosis. These bisphosphonates, along with *etidronate* [e-TID-row-nate], *ibandronate* [eye-BAN-dro-nate], *pamidronate* [pah-MID-row-nate], and *tiludronate* [till-UH-droe-nate], comprise an important drug group used for the treatment of bone disorders such as osteoporosis and Paget disease, as well as for treatment of bone metastases and hypercalcemia of malignancy.

1. **Mechanism of action:** Bisphosphonates bind to hydroxyapatite crystals in the bone and decrease osteoclastic bone resorption, resulting in a small increase in bone mass and a decreased risk of fractures in patients with osteoporosis. The beneficial effects of *alendronate* persist over several years of therapy (Figure 27.4), but discontinuation results in a gradual loss of effects.

2. **Pharmacokinetics:** The oral bisphosphonates *alendronate*, *risedronate*, and *ibandronate* are dosed on a daily, weekly, or monthly basis depending on the drug (Figure 27.5). Absorption after oral administration is poor, with less than 1% of the dose absorbed. Food and other medications significantly interfere with absorption of oral bisphosphonates, and guidelines for administration should be followed to maximize absorption (Figure 27.5). Bisphosphonates are rapidly cleared from the plasma, primarily because they avidly bind to hydroxyapatite in the bone. Once bound to bone, they are cleared over a period of hours to years. Elimination is predominantly via the kidney, and bisphosphonates should be avoided in severe renal impairment. For patients unable to tolerate oral bisphosphonates, intravenous *ibandronate* and *zoledronic acid* are alternatives.

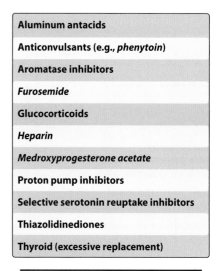

| Aluminum antacids |
| Anticonvulsants (e.g., *phenytoin*) |
| Aromatase inhibitors |
| *Furosemide* |
| Glucocorticoids |
| *Heparin* |
| *Medroxyprogesterone acetate* |
| Proton pump inhibitors |
| Selective serotonin reuptake inhibitors |
| Thiazolidinediones |
| Thyroid (excessive replacement) |

Figure 27.3
Drugs that can contribute to bone loss or increased fracture risk.

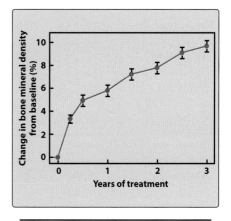

Figure 27.4
Effect of *alendronate* therapy on the bone mineral density of the lumbar spine.

BISPHOSPHONATE	FORMULATION	DOSING FREQUENCY*
Alendronate	Oral tablet Effervescent tablet	Daily or weekly Weekly
Ibandronate	Oral tablet Intravenous	Daily or monthly Every 3 months
Risedronate	Oral tablet Oral delayed-release tablet	Daily, weekly, or monthly Weekly
Zoledronic acid	Intravenous	Yearly

DOSING INSTRUCTIONS FOR ORAL BISPHOSPHONATES

- Take with 6 to 8 ounces of plain water only
  [Note: Take *risedronate* delayed-release tablet with at least 4 ounces of plain water]

- Take at least 30 minutes (60 minutes for *ibandronate*) BEFORE other food, drink, or medications
  [Note: Take *risedronate* delayed-release tablet immediately AFTER breakfast]

- Remain upright and do not lie down or recline for at least 30 minutes (60 minutes for *ibandronate*) after taking

Figure 27.5
Dosage formulations and instructions for administration of bisphosphonates for the treatment of osteoporosis. *Frequency of administration for individual agents varies with dosage, with higher doses administered less frequently.

3. **Adverse effects:** These include diarrhea, abdominal pain, and musculoskeletal pain. *Alendronate*, *risedronate*, and *ibandronate* are associated with esophagitis and esophageal ulcers. To minimize esophageal irritation, patients should remain upright after taking oral bisphosphonates. Although uncommon, osteonecrosis of the jaw and atypical femur fractures may occur with use of bisphosphonates. The risk of atypical fractures seems to increase with long-term use of bisphosphonates. Therefore, current guidelines recommend a drug holiday for some patients after 5 years of oral bisphosphonates or 3 years of *zoledronic acid*. Figure 27.6 shows relative potencies of the bisphosphonates.

B. Denosumab

Denosumab [den-OH-sue-mab] is a monoclonal antibody that targets receptor activator of nuclear factor kappa-B ligand (RANKL) and inhibits osteoclast formation and function. *Denosumab* is approved for the treatment of postmenopausal osteoporosis in women at high risk of fracture. It is administered via subcutaneous injection every 6 months. *Denosumab* is considered a first-line agent for osteoporosis, particularly in patients at higher risk of fractures. The drug has been associated with an increased risk of infections, dermatological reactions, hypocalcemia, and rarely, osteonecrosis of the jaw, and atypical fractures.

C. Parathyroid agents

Teriparatide [ter-ih-PAR-a-tide] is a recombinant form of human parathyroid hormone and *abaloparatide* [a-bal-oh-PAR-a-tide] is an analog of parathyroid hormone-related peptide. These drugs act as agonists at the parathyroid hormone receptor, and once-daily subcutaneous administration results in stimulation of osteoblastic activity and increased bone formation and bone strength. By contrast, other drugs for osteoporosis inhibit bone resorption. These agents should

Bisphosphonate	Antiresorptive activity
Etidronate	1
Tiludronate	10
Pamidronate	100
Alendronate	1000
Risedronate	5000
Ibandronate	10,000
Zoledronic acid	10,000

Figure 27.6
Antiresorptive activity of some bisphosphonates.

be reserved for patients at high risk of fractures and those who have failed or cannot tolerate other osteoporosis therapies. Both drugs have been associated with hypercalcemia, orthostatic hypotension, and an increased risk of osteosarcoma in rats. Cumulative lifetime use of either agent for more than 2 years is not recommended.

D. Selective estrogen receptor modulators

Lower estrogen levels after menopause promote proliferation and activation of osteoclasts, and bone mass can decline rapidly. Estrogen replacement is effective for the prevention of postmenopausal bone loss. However, since estrogen may increase the risk of endometrial cancer (when used without a progestin in women with an intact uterus), breast cancer, stroke, venous thromboembolism, and coronary events, it is no longer recommended as a preventive therapy for osteoporosis. *Raloxifene* [rah-LOX-ih-feen] is a selective estrogen receptor modulator approved for the prevention and treatment of osteoporosis. It has estrogen-like effects on bone and estrogen antagonist effects on breast and endometrial tissue. Therefore, *raloxifene* increases bone density without increasing the risk of endometrial cancer, and it decreases the risk of invasive breast cancer. Because it has not been shown to reduce nonvertebral or hip fractures, *raloxifene* should be used as an alternative to bisphosphonates or *denosumab* in the treatment of postmenopausal osteoporosis. Adverse effects include hot flashes, leg cramps, and increased risk of venous thromboembolism.

E. Calcitonin

Salmon *calcitonin* [cal-SIH-toe-nin] is indicated for the treatment of osteoporosis in women who are at least 5 years postmenopausal. The drug reduces bone resorption, but it is less effective than other agents, and is no longer routinely recommended for the treatment of osteoporosis. A unique property of *calcitonin* is relief of pain associated with osteoporotic fracture. Therefore, *calcitonin* is sometimes prescribed for the short-term treatment of patients with a recent painful vertebral fracture. The intranasal formulation is most commonly used in osteoporosis, and adverse effects include rhinitis and other nasal symptoms.

Study Questions

Choose the ONE best answer.

27.1 Which is correct regarding the pharmacokinetics of the bisphosphonates?

    A. Bisphosphonates are well absorbed after oral administration.

    B. Food or other medications greatly impair absorption of bisphosphonates.

    C. Bisphosphonates are mainly metabolized via the cytochrome P450 system.

    D. Elimination half-life of bisphosphonates ranges from 4 to 6 hours.

Correct answer = B. Food and other medications decrease absorption of bisphosphonates, which are already poorly absorbed (less than 1%) after oral administration. Bisphosphonates are cleared from the plasma by binding to bone and being cleared by the kidney (not metabolized by the CYP450 system). The elimination half-life may be years.

27.2 Which agent is administered once yearly to treat osteoporosis?

A. Abaloparatide
B. Denosumab
C. Risedronate
D. Zoledronic acid

Correct answer = D. Zoledronic acid is administered intravenously once per year. Abaloparatide is a daily subcutaneous injection. Denosumab is administered every 6 months, and risedronate is administered daily, weekly, or monthly.

27.3 Which osteoporosis medication works by preferentially stimulating activity of osteoblasts?

A. Denosumab
B. Ibandronate
C. Raloxifene
D. Teriparatide

Correct answer = D. Teriparatide is a parathyroid hormone analog that has anabolic effects on bone through stimulation of osteoblast activity. The other medications work primarily by inhibiting osteoclast activity (inhibition of bone resorption).

27.4 Which best describes the mechanism of action of denosumab in the treatment of osteoporosis?

A. Parathyroid hormone analog
B. RANKL inhibitor
C. Selective estrogen receptor modulator
D. Vitamin D analog

Correct answer = B. Denosumab is a monoclonal antibody that targets receptor activator of nuclear factor kappa-B ligand (RANKL) and inhibits osteoclast formation and function.

27.5 A 52-year-old woman has a history of rheumatoid arthritis, diabetes, hypertension, and heartburn. Her daily medications include methotrexate, prednisone, metformin, hydrochlorothiazide, and lisinopril, and calcium carbonate as needed for heartburn symptoms. She is worried about the risk of osteoporosis as she approaches menopause. Which of her medications is most likely to contribute to the risk of developing osteoporosis?

A. Calcium carbonate
B. Hydrochlorothiazide
C. Lisinopril
D. Prednisone

Correct answer = D. Glucocorticoids (for example, prednisone at a dose of ≥ 5 mg per day for greater than 3 months) are a significant risk factor for osteoporosis. The other medications have not been shown to increase the risk of osteoporosis, and calcium carbonate and hydrochlorothiazide (diuretic that increases calcium retention) may be beneficial for patients at risk of osteoporosis.

27.6 A 65-year-old woman who has been diagnosed with postmenopausal osteoporosis has no history of fractures and no other pertinent medical conditions. Which is most appropriate for management of her osteoporosis?

A. Alendronate
B. Calcitonin
C. Denosumab
D. Raloxifene

Correct answer = A. Bisphosphonates are first-line therapy for osteoporosis in postmenopausal women without contraindications. Raloxifene is an alternative that may be less efficacious (especially for nonvertebral and hip fractures), and calcitonin is not recommended. Denosumab is best used for patients at high risk of fractures.

27.7 A 55-year-old woman with postmenopausal osteoporosis has a past medical history of ethanol abuse, alcoholic liver disease, erosive esophagitis, and hypothyroidism. Which is the primary reason oral bisphosphonates should be used with caution in this patient?

A. Age
B. Erosive esophagitis
C. Liver disease
D. Thyroid disease

Correct answer = B. Bisphosphonates are known to cause esophageal irritation and should be used with caution in a patient with a history of erosive esophagitis. Age is not a factor for consideration in bisphosphonate use. Liver disease is not a contraindication to bisphosphonate use, since bisphosphonates are mainly cleared via the kidney. Thyroid disease is not a contraindication to bisphosphonate use, although overaggressive replacement of thyroid may contribute to osteoporosis.

27.8 A 70-year-old woman is being started on ibandronate once monthly for the treatment of osteoporosis. Which is important to communicate to this patient?

   A. Take this medication with orange juice to increase absorption.

   B. Take this medication after meals to minimize stomach upset.

   C. Remain upright for at least 60 minutes after taking this medication.

   D. Adverse effects may include blood clots and leg cramps.

Correct answer = C. Patients need to remain upright for 60 minutes after ibandronate (30 minutes for other bisphosphonates). Ibandronate should be given on an empty stomach with plain water only. Bisphosphonates, unlike raloxifene, are not associated with blood clots and leg cramps.

27.9 Use of which agent for osteoporosis should be limited to no more than 2 years?

   A. Calcitonin

   B. Denosumab

   C. Teriparatide

   D. Zoledronic acid

Correct answer = C. Use of the recombinant parathyroid hormone teriparatide should be limited to 2 years. Use beyond 2 years has not been studied, and is not recommended. The other agents do not have such limitations.

27.10 A patient has been taking alendronate for postmenopausal osteoporosis for 5 years with a slight increase in bone mineral density and no occurrence of fractures. Risk of which adverse effect might warrant consideration of a drug holiday from alendronate in this patient?

   A. Atypical femur fractures

   B. Esophagitis

   C. Osteosarcoma

   D. Rhinitis

Correct answer = A. Atypical femur fractures are associated with long-term use of bisphosphonates (greater than 5 years). Therefore, a drug holiday might be considered since the patient has had no fractures. Esophagitis, while a side effect of bisphosphonate therapy, can be prevented with appropriate administration. Osteosarcoma is associated with the parathyroid hormone analogs, and rhinitis is associated with intranasal calcitonin.

Principles of Antimicrobial Therapy

Jamie Kisgen

28

I. OVERVIEW

Antimicrobial therapy takes advantage of the biochemical differences that exist between microorganisms and human beings. Antimicrobial drugs are effective in the treatment of infections because of their selective toxicity; that is, they have the ability to injure or kill an invading microorganism without harming the cells of the host. In most instances, the selective toxicity is relative rather than absolute, requiring that the concentration of the drug be carefully controlled to attack the microorganism, while still being tolerated by the host.

II. SELECTION OF ANTIMICROBIAL AGENTS

Selection of the most appropriate antimicrobial agent requires knowledge of 1) the identity of the organism, 2) the susceptibility of the organism to a particular agent, 3) the site of the infection, 4) patient factors, 5) the safety and efficacy of the agent, and 6) the cost of therapy. However, most patients require empiric therapy (immediate administration of drug(s) prior to bacterial identification and susceptibility testing).

A. Identification of the infecting organism

Characterizing the organism is central to selection of appropriate therapy. A rapid assessment of the nature of the pathogen can sometimes be made on the basis of the Gram stain, which is particularly useful in identifying the presence and morphologic features of microorganisms in body fluids that are normally sterile (blood, cerebrospinal

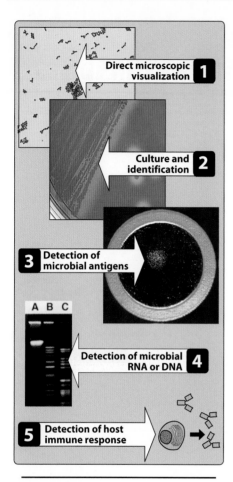

Figure 28.1
Some laboratory techniques that are useful in the diagnosis of microbial diseases.

fluid [CSF], pleural fluid, synovial fluid, peritoneal fluid, and urine). However, it is generally necessary to culture the infective organism to arrive at a conclusive diagnosis and determine the susceptibility to antimicrobial agents. Thus, it is essential to obtain a sample culture of the organism prior to initiating treatment. Otherwise, it is impossible to differentiate whether a negative culture is due to the absence of organisms or is a result of antimicrobial effects of administered antibiotic. Definitive identification of the infecting organism may require other laboratory techniques, such as detection of microbial antigens, DNA, or RNA, or an inflammatory or host immune response to the microorganism (Figure 28.1). Newer techniques such as rapid polymerase chain reaction (PCR) and matrix-assisted laser desorption/ionization time-of-flight (MALDI-TOF) mass spectrometry offer accurate, rapid, and cost-effective identification of the infecting organism(s).

B. Empiric antimicrobial therapy

Ideally, the antimicrobial agent used to treat an infection is selected after the organism has been identified and its susceptibility to antimicrobial agents established. However, in the critically ill patient, such a delay could prove fatal, and immediate empiric therapy is indicated.

1. **Timing:** Acutely ill patients with infections of unknown origin—for example, a neutropenic patient (one who is at risk for infections due to a reduction in neutrophils) or a patient with meningitis (acute inflammation of the membranes covering the brain and spinal cord)—require immediate treatment. If possible, therapy should be initiated after specimens for laboratory analysis have been obtained but before the results of the culture and sensitivity are available.

2. **Selecting a drug:** Drug choice in the absence of susceptibility data is influenced by the site of infection, the patient history (for example, previous infections, age, recent travel history, recent antimicrobial therapy, immune status, whether the infection was hospital- or community-acquired), and local susceptibility data. Broad-spectrum therapy may be indicated initially when the organism is unknown or polymicrobial infections are likely. The choice of agent(s) may also be guided by known association of particular organisms in a given clinical setting. For example, gram-positive cocci in the spinal fluid of a newborn is unlikely to be <u>Streptococcus pneumoniae</u> and most likely to be <u>Streptococcus agalactiae</u> (a group B streptococci), which is sensitive to *penicillin G*. By contrast, gram-positive cocci in the spinal fluid of a 40-year-old patient are most likely to be <u>S. pneumoniae</u>. This organism is frequently resistant to *penicillin G* and often requires treatment with a high-dose third-generation cephalosporin (such as *ceftriaxone*) or *vancomycin*.

C. Determination of antimicrobial susceptibility

After a pathogen is cultured, its susceptibility to specific antibiotics serves as a guide in selection of antimicrobial therapy. Some pathogens, such as <u>Streptococcus pyogenes</u> and <u>Neisseria meningitidis</u>, usually have predictable susceptibility patterns to certain antibiotics. In contrast, most gram-negative bacilli, enterococci, and staphylococcal species often show unpredictable susceptibility patterns and require susceptibility testing to determine appropriate antimicrobial therapy. The minimum inhibitory and bactericidal concentrations are used in determining susceptibility of a drug and can be experimentally determined (Figure 28.2).

1. **Bacteriostatic versus bactericidal drugs:** Antimicrobial drugs are commonly classified as either bacteriostatic or bactericidal. Historically, bacteriostatic drugs were thought to only arrest the growth and replication of bacteria at drug levels achievable in the patient, whereas bactericidal drugs were able to effectively kill ≥99.9% (3-log reduction) within 18 to 24 hours of incubation under specific laboratory conditions. There is a growing consensus that this classification may be too simplistic, as most bacteriostatic agents are able to effectively kill organisms; however, they are unable to meet the arbitrary cutoff value in the bactericidal definition. Figure 28.3 shows a laboratory experiment in which a bactericidal agent is compared to a bacteriostatic agent and a control. Note that the rate of in vitro killing is greater with bactericidal agents, but both agents are able to effectively kill the organism. It is also possible for an antibiotic to be bacteriostatic for one organism and bactericidal for another. For example, *linezolid* is bacteriostatic against S<u>taphylococcus aureus</u> and enterococci, but is bactericidal against most strains of <u>S. pneumoniae</u>. In addition, recent data have demonstrated that bactericidal and bacteriostatic agents have similar efficacy for treating common clinical infections. In the end, other factors may have a greater impact, including the host immune system, drug concentration at the site of infection, and underlying severity of the illness.

2. **Minimum inhibitory concentration:** The minimum inhibitory concentration (MIC) is the lowest antimicrobial concentration that prevents visible growth of an organism after 24 hours of incubation. This serves as a quantitative measure of in vitro susceptibility and is commonly used in practice to streamline therapy. Computer automation has improved the accuracy and decreased the turnaround time for determining MIC results and is the most common approach used by clinical laboratories.

3. **Minimum bactericidal concentration:** The minimum bactericidal concentration (MBC) is the lowest concentration of antimicrobial agent that results in a 99.9% decline in colony count after overnight broth dilution incubations (Figure 28.2). [Note: The MBC is rarely determined in clinical practice due to the time and labor requirements.]

D. **Effect of the site of infection on therapy: the blood–brain barrier**

Adequate levels of an antibiotic must reach the site of infection for the invading microorganisms to be effectively eradicated. Capillaries with varying degrees of permeability carry drugs to the body tissues. Natural barriers to drug delivery are created by the structures of the capillaries of some tissues, such as the prostate, testes, placenta, the vitreous body of the eye, and the central nervous system (CNS). Of particular significance are the capillaries in the brain, which help to create and maintain the blood–brain barrier. This barrier is formed by the single layer of endothelial cells fused by tight junctions that impede entry from the blood to the brain of virtually all molecules, except those that are small and lipophilic. The penetration and concentration

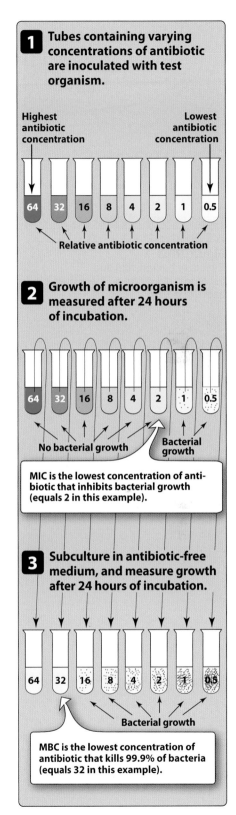

Figure 28.2
Determination of minimum inhibitory concentration (MIC) and minimum bactericidal concentration (MBC) of an antibiotic.

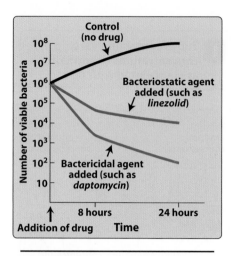

Figure 28.3
Effects of bactericidal and bacteriostatic drugs on the growth of bacteria in vitro.

of an antibacterial agent in the CSF are particularly influenced by the following:

1. **Lipid solubility:** The lipid solubility of a drug is a major determinant of its ability to penetrate the blood–brain barrier. Lipid-soluble drugs, such as *chloramphenicol* and *metronidazole*, have significant penetration into the CNS, whereas β-lactam antibiotics, such as *penicillin*, are ionized at physiologic pH and have low lipid solubility. Therefore, they have limited penetration through the intact blood–brain barrier under normal circumstances. In infections such as meningitis in which the brain becomes inflamed, the barrier does not function as effectively, and local permeability is increased. Some β-lactam antibiotics can enter the CSF in therapeutic amounts when the meninges are inflamed.

2. **Molecular weight:** A drug with a low molecular weight has an enhanced ability to cross the blood–brain barrier, whereas compounds with a high molecular weight (for example, *vancomycin*) penetrate poorly, even in the presence of meningeal inflammation.

3. **Protein binding:** A high degree of protein binding of a drug restricts its entry into the CSF. Therefore, the amount of free (unbound) drug in serum, rather than the total amount of drug present, is important for CSF penetration.

4. **Susceptibility to transporters or efflux pumps:** Antibiotics that have an affinity for transporter mechanisms or do not have an affinity for efflux pumps have better CNS penetration.

E. Patient factors

In selecting an antibiotic, attention must be paid to the condition of the patient. For example, the status of the immune system, kidneys, liver, circulation, and age must be considered. In women, pregnancy or breast-feeding also affects selection of the antimicrobial agent.

1. **Immune system:** Elimination of infecting organisms from the body is highly dependent on an intact immune system, and the host defense system must ultimately eliminate the invading organisms. Alcoholism, diabetes, HIV infection, malnutrition, autoimmune diseases, pregnancy, advanced age, and immunosuppressive drugs can affect immunocompetence. High doses of bactericidal agents or longer courses of treatment may be required to eliminate infective organisms in these individuals.

2. **Renal dysfunction:** Poor kidney function may cause accumulation of certain antibiotics. Dosage adjustment prevents drug accumulation and adverse effects. Serum creatinine levels are frequently used as an index of renal function for adjustment of drug regimens. However, direct monitoring of serum levels of some antibiotics (for example, *vancomycin*, aminoglycosides) is preferred to identify maximum and/or minimum values and prevent potential toxicities. [Note: The number of functional nephrons decreases with age. Thus, elderly patients are particularly vulnerable to accumulation of drugs eliminated by the kidneys, even with normal serum creatinine levels.]

3. **Hepatic dysfunction:** Antibiotics that are concentrated or eliminated by the liver (for example, *erythromycin* and *doxycycline*) must be used with caution when treating patients with liver dysfunction.

4. **Poor perfusion:** Decreased circulation to an anatomic area, such as the lower limbs of a diabetic patient, reduces the amount of antibiotic that reaches that site of infection, making it more difficult to treat. Decreased perfusion of the gastrointestinal tract may result in reduced absorption, making attainment of therapeutic concentrations more difficult with enteral routes.

5. **Age:** Renal or hepatic elimination processes are often poorly developed in newborns, making neonates particularly vulnerable to the toxic effects of agents such as *chloramphenicol* and sulfonamides. Young children should not be treated with tetracyclines or quinolones, which affect bone growth and joints, respectively. Elderly patients may have decreased renal or liver function, which may alter the pharmacokinetics of certain antibiotics.

6. **Pregnancy and lactation:** Many antibiotics cross the placental barrier or enter the nursing infant via the breast milk. Prescribers should consult the product labeling of an antibiotic to review the risk summary and clinical considerations for use in pregnancy and lactation. Although the concentration of an antibiotic in fetal circulation or in breast milk is usually low, the total dose to the infant may be sufficient to produce detrimental effects. For example, congenital abnormalities have been reported after administration of tetracyclines to pregnant women, and these agents should be generally be avoided in pregnancy due to the risk to the fetus.

7. **Risk factors for multidrug-resistant organisms:** Infections with multidrug-resistant pathogens need broader antibiotic coverage when initiating empiric therapy. Common risk factors for infection with these pathogens include prior antimicrobial therapy in the preceding 90 days, hospitalization for greater than 2 days within the preceding 90 days, current hospitalization exceeding 5 days, admission from a nursing home, high frequency of resistance in the community or local hospital unit (assessed using hospital antibiograms), and immunosuppressive diseases and/or therapies.

F. Safety of the agent

Penicillins are among the least toxic of all antimicrobial drugs because they interfere with a site or function unique to the growth of microorganisms. Other antimicrobial agents (for example, *chloramphenicol*) have less specificity and are reserved for life-threatening infections because of the potential for serious toxicity to the patient. [Note: Safety is related not only to the inherent nature of the drug but also to the patient factors described above that can predispose to toxicity.]

G. Cost of therapy

It is common for several drugs to show similar efficacy in treating an infection but vary widely in cost. For example, treatment of *methicillin*-resistant <u>Staphylococcus aureus</u> (MRSA) generally includes one of the following: *vancomycin, clindamycin, daptomycin,* or *linezolid.* Although choice of therapy usually centers on the site of infection, severity of the illness, and ability to take oral medications, it is also important to consider cost of the medication. Figure 28.4 illustrates the relative cost of commonly used drugs for staphylococcal infections.

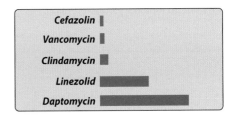

Figure 28.4
Relative cost of some drugs used for the treatment of <u>Staphylococcus aureus</u>.

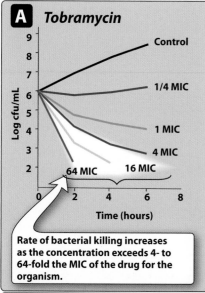

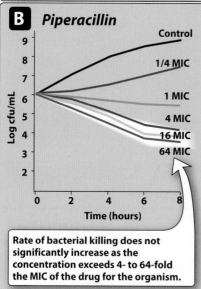

Figure 28.5
A. Significant dose-dependent killing effect shown by *tobramycin.*
B. Nonsignificant dose-dependent killing effect shown by *piperacillin.*
cfu = colony-forming units; MIC = minimum inhibitory concentration.

III. ROUTE OF ADMINISTRATION

The oral route of administration is appropriate for mild infections that can be treated on an outpatient basis. Parenteral administration is used for drugs that are poorly absorbed from the GI tract and for treatment of patients with serious infections who require maintenance of higher serum concentrations of antimicrobial agents. In hospitalized patients requiring intravenous (IV) therapy, the switch to oral agents should occur as soon as possible. Switching patients from IV to oral therapy when clinically stable has been shown to decrease health care costs, shorten length of stay, and decrease complications from IV catheters. However, some antibiotics, such as *vancomycin* and aminoglycosides, are poorly absorbed from the gastrointestinal (GI) tract and do not achieve adequate serum levels via oral administration.

IV. DETERMINANTS OF RATIONAL DOSING

Rational dosing of antimicrobial agents is based on pharmacodynamics (the relationship of drug concentrations to antimicrobial effects) and pharmacokinetic properties (the absorption, distribution, metabolism, and elimination of the drug). Three important properties that have a significant influence on the frequency of dosing are concentration-dependent killing, time-dependent (concentration-independent) killing, and postantibiotic effect (PAE). Utilizing these properties to optimize antibiotic dosing regimens can improve clinical outcomes and possibly decrease the development of resistance.

A. Concentration-dependent killing

Certain antimicrobial agents, including aminoglycosides and *daptomycin*, show a significant increase in the rate of bacterial killing as the concentration of antibiotic increases from 4- to 64-fold the MIC of the drug for the infecting organism (Figure 28.5A). Giving drugs that exhibit this concentration-dependent killing by a once-a-day bolus infusion achieves high peak levels, favoring rapid killing of the infecting pathogen.

B. Time-dependent (concentration-independent) killing

In contrast, β-lactams, glycopeptides, macrolides, *clindamycin*, and *linezolid* do not exhibit concentration-dependent killing (Figure 28.5B). The clinical efficacy of these antimicrobials is best predicted by the percentage of time that blood concentrations of a drug remain above the MIC. This effect is sometimes called time-dependent (or concentration-independent) killing. For example, dosing schedules for the penicillins and cephalosporins that ensure blood levels greater than the MIC for 50% and 60% of the time, respectively, provide the most clinical efficacy. Therefore, extended (generally 3 to 4 hours) or continuous (24 hours) infusions can be utilized instead of intermittent dosing (generally 30 minutes) to achieve prolonged time above the MIC and kill more bacteria. Other drugs, such as fluoroquinolones and *vancomycin*, work best by optimizing the ratio of the 24-hour area under the concentration–time curve to MIC (AUC_{24}/MIC). The AUC_{24} is the overall exposure of a drug during the dosing interval and takes into account the concentration as well as the time.

C. Postantibiotic effect

The PAE is a persistent suppression of microbial growth that occurs after levels of antibiotic have fallen below the MIC. Antimicrobial drugs exhibiting a long PAE (for example, aminoglycosides and fluoroquinolones) often require only one dose per day, particularly against gram-negative bacteria.

V. CHEMOTHERAPEUTIC SPECTRA

In this book, the clinically important bacteria have been organized into eight groups based on Gram stain, morphology, and biochemical or other characteristics. They are represented as a color-coded list (Figure 28.6A). The ninth section of the list is labeled "Other," and it is used to represent any organism not included in one of the other eight categories. In Figure 28.6B–D, the list is used to illustrate the spectra of bacteria for which a particular class of antibiotics is therapeutically effective.

A. Narrow-spectrum antibiotics

Chemotherapeutic agents acting only on a single or a limited group of microorganisms are said to have a narrow spectrum. For example, isoniazid is active only against <u>Mycobacterium tuberculosis</u> (Figure 28.6B).

B. Extended-spectrum antibiotics

Extended spectrum is the term applied to antibiotics that are modified to be effective against gram-positive organisms and also against a significant number of gram-negative bacteria. For example, ampicillin is considered to have an extended spectrum because it acts against gram-positive and some gram-negative bacteria (Figure 28.6C).

C. Broad-spectrum antibiotics

Drugs such as tetracycline, fluoroquinolones and carbapenems affect a wide variety of microbial species and are referred to as broad-spectrum antibiotics (Figure 28.6D). Administration of broad-spectrum antibiotics can drastically alter the nature of the normal bacterial flora and precipitate a superinfection due to organisms such as <u>Clostridium difficile</u>, the growth of which is normally kept in check by the presence of other colonizing microorganisms.

VI. COMBINATIONS OF ANTIMICROBIAL DRUGS

It is therapeutically advisable to treat patients with a single agent that is most specific to the infecting organism. This strategy reduces the possibility of superinfections, decreases the emergence of resistant organisms, and minimizes toxicity. However, in some situations, combinations of antimicrobial drugs are advantageous or even required.

A. Advantages of drug combinations

Certain combinations of antibiotics, such as β-lactams and aminoglycosides, show synergism; that is, the combination is more effective

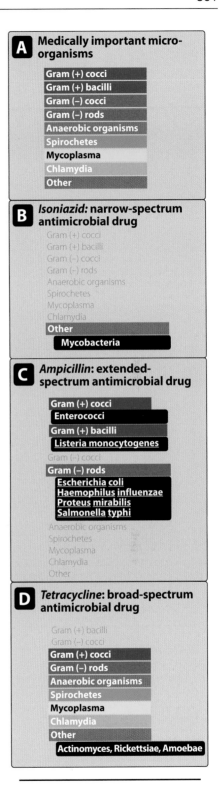

Figure 28.6
A. Color-coded representation of medically important microorganisms. **B.** Isoniazid, narrow-spectrum antimicrobial agent. **C.** Ampicillin, an extended-spectrum antimicrobial agent. **D.** Tetracycline, a broad-spectrum antimicrobial agent.

than either of the drugs used separately. Because such synergism among antimicrobial agents is rare, synergistic combinations are only indicated in special situations (for example, in the treatment of entero-coccal endocarditis). Combinations may also be used when an infection is of unknown origin or when there are organisms with variable sensitivity, such as when treating tuberculosis.

B. Disadvantages of drug combinations

A number of antibiotics act only when organisms are multiplying. Thus, coadministration of an agent that causes bacteriostasis plus a second agent that is bactericidal may result in the first drug interfering with the action of the second. For example, bacteriostatic tetracycline drugs may interfere with the bactericidal effects of penicillins and cephalosporins. Another concern is the risk of selection pressure and the development of antibiotic resistance by giving unnecessary combination therapy.

VII. DRUG RESISTANCE

Bacteria are considered resistant to an antibiotic if the maximal level of that antibiotic that can be tolerated by the host does not halt bacterial growth. Some organisms are inherently resistant to an antibiotic. For example, most gram-negative organisms are inherently resistant to *vancomycin*. However, microbial species that are normally responsive to a particular drug may develop more virulent or resistant strains through spontaneous mutation or acquired resistance and selection. Some of these strains may even become resistant to more than one antibiotic.

A. Genetic alterations leading to drug resistance

Acquired antibiotic resistance requires the temporary or permanent gain or alteration of bacterial genetic information. Resistance develops due to the ability of DNA to undergo spontaneous mutation or to move from one organism to another (Figure 28.7).

B. Altered expression of proteins in drug-resistant organisms

Drug resistance is mediated by a variety of mechanisms, such as an alteration in an antibiotic target site, decreased penetration of the drug due to lower permeability, increased efflux of the drug, or presence of antibiotic-inactivating enzymes (Figure 28.7).

1. **Modification of target sites:** Alteration of the target site of an antibiotic through mutation can confer resistance to one or more related antibiotics. For example, S. pneumoniae resistance to β-lactam antibiotics involves alterations in one or more of the major bacterial penicillin-binding proteins, resulting in decreased binding of the antibiotic to its target.

2. **Decreased accumulation:** Decreased uptake or increased efflux of an antibiotic can confer resistance because the drug is unable to attain access to the site of its action in sufficient concentrations to injure or kill the organism. For example, gram-negative

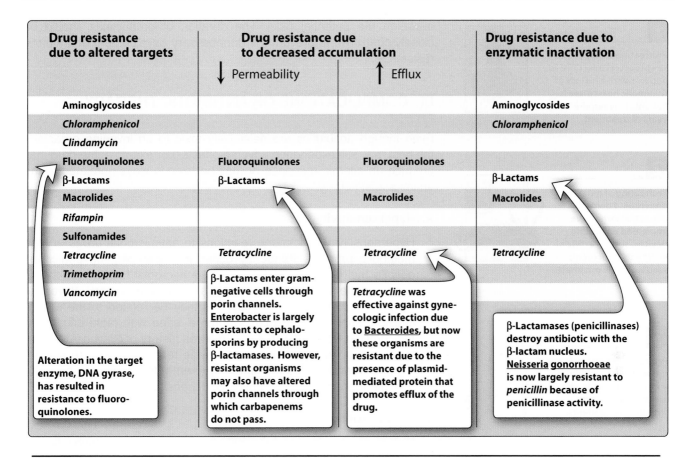

Drug resistance due to altered targets	Drug resistance due to decreased accumulation		Drug resistance due to enzymatic inactivation
	↓ Permeability	↑ Efflux	
Aminoglycosides			Aminoglycosides
Chloramphenicol			*Chloramphenicol*
Clindamycin			
Fluoroquinolones	Fluoroquinolones	Fluoroquinolones	
β-Lactams	β-Lactams		β-Lactams
Macrolides		Macrolides	Macrolides
Rifampin			
Sulfonamides			
Tetracycline	*Tetracycline*	*Tetracycline*	*Tetracycline*
Trimethoprim			
Vancomycin			

Alteration in the target enzyme, DNA gyrase, has resulted in resistance to fluoroquinolones.

β-Lactams enter gram-negative cells through porin channels. <u>Enterobacter</u> is largely resistant to cephalosporins by producing β-lactamases. However, resistant organisms may also have altered porin channels through which carbapenems do not pass.

Tetracycline was effective against gynecologic infection due to <u>Bacteroides</u>, but now these organisms are resistant due to the presence of plasmid-mediated protein that promotes efflux of the drug.

β-Lactamases (penicillinases) destroy antibiotic with the β-lactam nucleus. <u>Neisseria gonorrhoeae</u> is now largely resistant to *penicillin* because of penicillinase activity.

Figure 28.7
Some mechanisms of resistance to antibiotics.

organisms can limit the penetration of certain agents, including β-lactam antibiotics, as a result of an alteration in the number and structure of porins (channels) in the outer membrane. Also, the presence of an efflux pump can limit levels of a drug in an organism, as seen with tetracyclines.

3. **Enzymatic inactivation:** The ability to destroy or inactivate the antimicrobial agent can also confer resistance on microorganisms. Examples of antibiotic-inactivating enzymes include 1) β-lactamases ("penicillinases") that hydrolytically inactivate the β-lactam ring of penicillins, cephalosporins, and related drugs; 2) acetyltransferases that transfer an acetyl group to the antibiotic, inactivating *chloramphenicol* or aminoglycosides; and 3) esterases that hydrolyze the lactone ring of macrolides.

VIII. PROPHYLACTIC USE OF ANTIBIOTICS

Certain clinical situations, such as dental procedures and surgeries, require the use of antibiotics for the prevention rather than for the treatment of infections (Figure 28.8). Because the indiscriminate use of antimicrobial agents can result in bacterial resistance and superinfection, prophylactic use is restricted to clinical situations in which the benefits

1

Pretreatment may prevent streptococcal infections in patients with a history of rheumatic heart disease. Patients may require years of treatment.

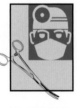

2

Pretreating of patients undergoing dental extractions who have implanted prosthetic devices, such as artificial heart valves, prevents seeding of the prosthesis.

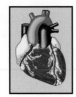

3

Pretreatment may prevent tuberculosis or meningitis among individuals who are in close contact with infected patients.

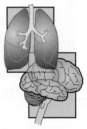

4

Treatment prior to most surgical procedures can decrease the incidence of infection afterwards. Effective prophylaxis is directed against the most likely organism, not eradication of every potential pathogen.

Figure 28.8
Some clinical situations in which prophylactic antibiotics are indicated.

outweigh the potential risks. The duration of prophylaxis should be closely controlled to prevent the unnecessary development of antibiotic resistance.

IX. COMPLICATIONS OF ANTIBIOTIC THERAPY

Even though antibiotics are selectively toxic to an invading organism, the host may still experience adverse effects. For example, the drug may produce an allergic response or may be toxic in ways unrelated to the antimicrobial activity.

A. Hypersensitivity

Hypersensitivity or immune reactions to antimicrobial drugs or their metabolic products frequently occur. For example, the penicillins, despite their almost absolute selective microbial toxicity, can cause serious hypersensitivity problems, ranging from urticaria (hives) to anaphylactic shock. Some reactions may be related to the rate of infusion, such as "Red man syndrome" seen with rapid infusion of *vancomycin*. Patients with a documented history of Stevens-Johnson syndrome or toxic epidermal necrolysis reaction (a severe slough-ing of skin and mucus membranes) to an antibiotic should *never* be rechallenged, not even for antibiotic desensitization.

B. Direct toxicity

High serum levels of certain antibiotics may cause toxicity by directly affecting cellular processes in the host. For example, aminogly-cosides can cause ototoxicity by interfering with membrane func-tion in the auditory hair cells. *Chloramphenicol* can have a direct toxic effect on mitochondria, leading to bone marrow suppression. Fluoroquinolones can have effects on cartilage and tendons, and tet-racyclines have direct effects on bones. A number of antibiotics can cause photosensitivity.

C. Superinfections

Drug therapy, particularly with broad-spectrum antimicrobials or com-binations of agents, can lead to alterations of the normal microbial flora of the upper respiratory, oral, intestinal, and genitourinary tracts, permitting the overgrowth of opportunistic organisms, especially fungi or resistant bacteria. These infections usually require secondary treat-ments using specific anti-infective agents.

X. SITES OF ANTIMICROBIAL ACTION

Antimicrobial drugs can be classified in a number of ways: 1) by their chemical structure (for example, β-lactams or aminoglycosides), 2) by their mechanism of action (for example, cell wall synthesis inhibitors), or 3) by their activity against particular types of organisms (for example, bacteria, fungi, or viruses). Chapters 29 through 31 are organized by the mechanisms of action of the drug (Figure 28.9), and Chapters 32 through 34 are organized according to the type of organisms affected by the drug.

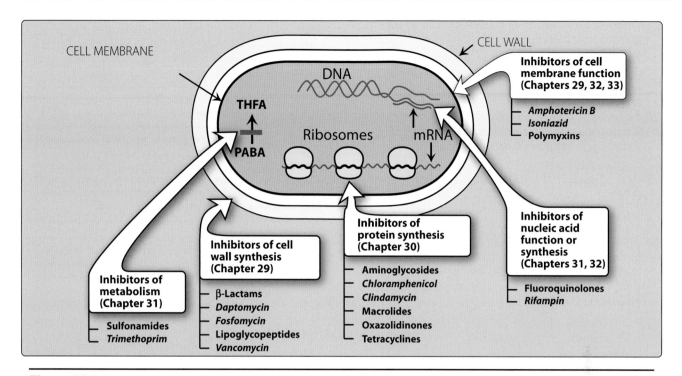

Figure 28.9
Classification of some antimicrobial agents by their sites of action. THFA = tetrahydrofolic acid; PABA = *p*-aminobenzoic acid.

Study Questions

Choose the ONE best answer.

28.1 A 24-year-old pregnant woman presents to the urgent care clinic with fever and urinary frequency and urgency. She is diagnosed with a urinary tract infection (UTI). Based on potential harm to the fetus, which of the following medications should be avoided in treating her UTI?

A. Nitrofurantoin
B. Amoxicillin
C. Cephalexin
D. Doxycycline

> Correct answer = D. Doxycycline (a tetracycline) should be avoided due to the potential harm to the fetus. Nitrofurantoin, amoxicillin (a penicillin), and cephalexin (a cephalosporin) are generally considered safe.

28.2 Which of the following is the primary method of β-lactam resistance with Streptococcus pneumoniae?

A. Modification of target site
B. Decreased drug levels due to changes in permeability
C. Decreased drug levels due to an efflux pump
D. Enzymatic inactivation

> Correct answer = A. S. pneumoniae resistance to β-lactam antibiotics involves alteration in one or more of the major penicillin-binding proteins.

28.3 Which of the following agents is considered a narrow-spectrum antibiotic?

A. Ceftriaxone
B. Ciprofloxacin
C. Isoniazid
D. Imipenem

> Correct answer = C. Isoniazid is only active against Mycobacterium tuberculosis, while ceftriaxone, ciprofloxacin, and imipenem are considered broad spectrum due to their activity against multiple types of bacteria and increased risk for contributing to the development of a superinfection.

28.4 Which of the following antibiotics exhibits concentration-dependent killing?

    A. Clindamycin

    B. Linezolid

    C. Vancomycin

    D. Daptomycin

> Correct answer = D. Clindamycin, linezolid, and vancomycin exhibit time-dependent killing, while daptomycin works best when administered in a fashion that optimizes concentration-dependent killing.

28.5 Which of the following antibiotics exhibits a long postantibiotic effect that permits once-daily dosing?

    A. Gentamicin

    B. Penicillin G

    C. Vancomycin

    D. Aztreonam

> Correct answer = A. Aminoglycosides, including gentamicin, possess a long postantibiotic effect, especially when given as a high dose every 24 hours. Penicillin G, clindamycin, and vancomycin have a relatively short postantibiotic effect and require dosing that maintains concentrations above the MIC for a longer portion of the dosing interval.

28.6 A 58-year-old man with a history of hepatitis C, cirrhosis, and ascites presents with spontaneous bacterial peritonitis. Which of the following antibiotics requires close monitoring and dosing adjustment in this patient given his liver disease?

    A. Penicillin G.

    B. Tobramycin.

    C. Erythromycin.

    D. Vancomycin.

> Correct answer = C. Erythromycin is metabolized by the liver and should be used with caution in patients with hepatic impairment. Penicillin G, tobramycin, and vancomycin are primarily eliminated by the kidneys.

28.7 JS is a 3-day-old neonate, born at 37 weeks' gestation, who presents with new onset fever, lethargy, and decreased desire to feed. Based on JS's age, which of the following antibiotics is considered safe to use in neonates?

    A. Chloramphenicol

    B. Sulfamethoxazole/trimethoprim

    C. Tetracycline

    D. Ampicillin

> Correct answer = D. Chloramphenicol and sulfonamides (sulfamethoxazole) can cause toxic effects in newborns due to poorly developed renal and hepatic elimination processes. Tetracycline can have effects on bone growth and development and should be avoided in newborns and young children. Ampicillin is safe and effective in this population.

28.8 When evaluating drug therapy for meningitis, which of the following factors is expected to have the LEAST influence on the penetration and concentration of an antibacterial agent in the cerebrospinal fluid?

    A. Lipid solubility of the drug

    B. Minimum inhibitory concentration of the drug

    C. Protein binding of the drug

    D. Molecular weight of the drug

> Correct answer = B. Although the minimum inhibitory concentration impacts the effectiveness of the drug against a given bacteria, it does not affect the ability of a drug to penetrate into the brain. Lipid solubility, protein binding, and molecular weight all determine the likelihood of a drug to penetrate the blood–brain barrier and concentrate in the brain.

28.9 A 72-year-old male presents with fever, cough, malaise, and shortness of breath. His chest x-ray shows bilateral infiltrates consistent with pneumonia. Bronchial wash cultures reveal Pseudomonas aeruginosa sensitive to cefepime. Which of the following is the best dosing scheme for cefepime based on the drug's time-dependent bactericidal activity?

    A. 1 g every 6 hours given over 30 minutes

    B. 2 g every 12 hours given over 3 hours

    C. 4 g every 24 hours given over 30 minutes

    D. 4 g given as continuous infusion over 24 hours

> Correct answer = D. The clinical efficacy of cefepime is based on the percentage of time that the drug concentration remains above the MIC. A continuous infusion would allow for the greatest amount of time above the MIC compared to intermittent (30 minutes) and prolonged infusions (3 to 4 hours).

28.10 Which of the following adverse drug reactions precludes a patient from being rechallenged with that drug in the future?

  A. Itching/rash from penicillin
  B. Stevens-Johnson syndrome from sulfamethoxazole–trimethoprim
  C. Gastrointestinal (GI) upset from clarithromycin
  D. Clostridium difficile superinfection from moxifloxacin

Correct answer = B. Stevens-Johnson syndrome is a severe idiosyncratic reaction that can be life threatening, and these patients should never be rechallenged with the offending agent. Itching/rash is a commonly reported reaction in patients receiving penicillins but is not life threatening. A patient may be rechallenged if the benefits outweigh the risk (for example, pregnant patient with syphilis) or the patient could be exposed through a desensitization procedure. GI upset is a common side effect of clarithromycin but is not due to an allergic reaction. Moxifloxacin is a broad-spectrum antibiotic that can inhibit the normal flora of the GI tract, increasing the risk for the development of superinfections like C. difficile. This is not an allergic reaction, and the patient can be rechallenged; however, the patient might be at risk for developing C. difficile infection again.

Cell Wall Inhibitors

29

Veena Venugopalan and Kenneth P. Klinker

I. OVERVIEW

Some antimicrobial drugs selectively interfere with synthesis of the bacterial cell wall—a structure that mammalian cells do not possess. The cell wall is composed of a polymer called peptidoglycan that consists of glycan units joined to each other by peptide cross-links. To be maximally effective, inhibitors of cell wall synthesis require actively proliferating microorganisms. Figure 29.1 shows the classification of agents affecting cell wall synthesis.

II. PENICILLINS

The basic structure of penicillins consists of a core four-membered β-lactam ring, which is attached to a thiazolidine ring and an R side chain. Members of this family differ from one another in the R substituent attached to the 6-aminopenicillanic acid residue (Figure 29.2). The nature of this side chain affects the antimicrobial spectrum, stability to stomach acid, cross-hypersensitivity, and susceptibility to bacterial degradative enzymes (β-lactamases).

A. Mechanism of action

Penicillins interfere with the last step of bacterial cell wall synthesis, which is the cross-linking of adjacent peptidoglycan strands by a process known as transpeptidation. Since penicillins structurally resemble the terminal portion of the peptidoglycan strand, they compete for and bind to enzymes called penicillin-binding proteins (PBPs), which catalyze transpeptidase and facilitate cross-linking of the cell wall (Figure 29.3). The result is the formation of a weakened cell wall and ultimately cell death. For this reason, penicillins are regarded as bactericidal and work in a time-dependent fashion.

B. Antibacterial spectrum

The antibacterial spectrum of the various penicillins is determined, in part, by their ability to cross the bacterial peptidoglycan cell wall to reach the PBPs in the periplasmic space. Factors determining PBP susceptibility to these antibiotics include size, charge, and hydrophobicity

PENICILLINS
Amoxicillin* AMOXIL
Ampicillin** GENERIC ONLY
Dicloxacillin* GENERIC ONLY
Nafcillin GENERIC ONLY
Oxacillin GENERIC ONLY
Penicillin G PFIZERPEN
Penicillin G benzathine BICILLIN L-A
Penicillin G benzathine and penicillin G procaine BICILLIN C-R
Penicillin V* GENERIC ONLY

CEPHALOSPORINS
Cefaclor* GENERIC ONLY
Cefadroxil* GENERIC ONLY
Cefazolin ANCEF, KEFZOL
Cefdinir* OMNICEF
Cefepime MAXIPIME
Cefixime* SUPRAX
Cefotetan CEFOTAN
Cefoxitin MEFOXIN
Cefprozil* CEFZIL
Ceftaroline TEFLARO
Ceftazidime FORTAZ
Ceftriaxone GENERIC ONLY
Cefuroxime** CEFTIN, ZINACEF
Cephalexin* KEFLEX

CARBAPENEMS
Doripenem DORIBAX
Ertapenem INVANZ
Imipenem/cilastatin PRIMAXIN
Meropenem MERREM

MONOBACTAMS
Aztreonam AZACTAM

Figure 29.1
Summary of antimicrobial agents affecting cell wall synthesis.
(Figure continues on next page.)

of the particular β-lactam antibiotic. In general, gram-positive microorganisms have cell walls that are easily traversed by penicillins, and, therefore, in the absence of resistance, they are susceptible to these drugs. Gram-negative microorganisms have an outer lipopolysaccharide membrane surrounding the cell wall that presents a barrier to the water-soluble penicillins. However, gram-negative bacteria have proteins inserted in the lipopolysaccharide layer that act as water-filled channels (called porins) to permit transmembrane entry.

1. **Natural penicillins:** *Penicillin G* and *penicillin V* are obtained from fermentations of the fungus <u>Penicillium chrysogenum</u>. *Penicillin* [pen-i-SILL-in] *G* (*benzylpenicillin*) has activity against a variety of gram-positive organisms, gram-negative organisms, and spirochetes (Figure 29.4). The potency of *penicillin G* is five to ten times greater than that of *penicillin V* against both <u>Neisseria</u> spp. and certain anaerobes. Most streptococci are very sensitive to *penicillin G*, but *penicillin*-resistant viridans streptococci and <u>Streptococcus pneumoniae</u> isolates are emerging. The vast majority of <u>Staphylococcus aureus</u> (greater than 90%) are now penicillinase producing and therefore resistant to *penicillin G*. Despite widespread use and increasing resistance in many types of bacteria, *penicillin* remains the drug of choice for the treatment of gas gangrene (<u>Clostridium perfringens</u>) and syphilis (<u>Treponema pallidum</u>). *Penicillin V*, only available in oral formulation, has a spectrum similar to that of *penicillin G*, but it is not used for treatment of severe infections because of its limited oral absorption. *Penicillin V* is more acid stable than is *penicillin G* and is the oral agent employed in the treatment of less severe infections.

2. **Semisynthetic penicillins:** *Ampicillin* [am-pi-SILL-in] and *amoxicillin* [a-mox-i-SILL-in] (also known as aminopenicillins or extended-spectrum penicillins) are created by chemically attaching different R groups to the 6-aminopenicillanic acid nucleus. Addition of R groups extends the gram-negative antimicrobial activity of aminopenicillins to include <u>Haemophilus influenzae</u>, <u>Escherichia coli,</u> and <u>Proteus mirabilis</u> (Figure 29.5A). *Ampicillin* (with or without the addition of *gentamicin*) is the drug of choice for the gram-positive bacillus <u>Listeria monocytogenes</u> and susceptible enterococcal species. These extended-spectrum agents are also widely used in the treatment of respiratory infections, and *amoxicillin* is employed prophylactically by dentists in high-risk patients for the prevention of bacterial endocarditis. These drugs are coformulated with β-lactamase inhibitors, such as *clavulanic acid* or *sulbactam*, to combat infections caused by β-lactamase–producing organisms. For example, without the β-lactamase inhibitor, *methicillin*-sensitive <u>Staphylococcus aureus</u> (MSSA) is resistant to *ampicillin* and *amoxicillin*. Resistance in the form of plasmid-mediated penicillinases is a major clinical problem, which limits use of aminopenicillins with some gram-negative organisms.

3. **Antistaphylococcal penicillins:** *Methicillin* [meth-i-SILL-in], *nafcillin* [naf-SILL-in], *oxacillin* [ox-a-SILL-in], and *dicloxacillin* [dye-klox-a-SILL-in] are β-lactamase (penicillinase)-resistant penicillins. Their use is restricted to the treatment of infections caused by penicillinase-producing staphylococci, including MSSA. [Note:

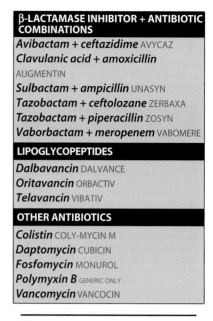

β-LACTAMASE INHIBITOR + ANTIBIOTIC COMBINATIONS

Avibactam + ceftazidime AVYCAZ
Clavulanic acid + amoxicillin AUGMENTIN
Sulbactam + ampicillin UNASYN
Tazobactam + ceftolozane ZERBAXA
Tazobactam + piperacillin ZOSYN
Vaborbactam + meropenem VABOMERE

LIPOGLYCOPEPTIDES

Dalbavancin DALVANCE
Oritavancin ORBACTIV
Telavancin VIBATIV

OTHER ANTIBIOTICS

Colistin COLY-MYCIN M
Daptomycin CUBICIN
Fosfomycin MONUROL
Polymyxin B GENERIC ONLY
Vancomycin VANCOCIN

Figure 29.1 (continued)
*Only available in oral formulation.
**Available in oral and intravenous formulations.

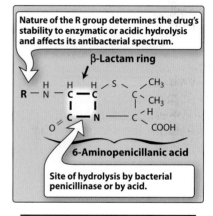

Nature of the R group determines the drug's stability to enzymatic or acidic hydrolysis and affects its antibacterial spectrum.

β-Lactam ring

6-Aminopenicillanic acid

Site of hydrolysis by bacterial penicillinase or by acid.

Figure 29.2
Structure of β-lactam antibiotics.

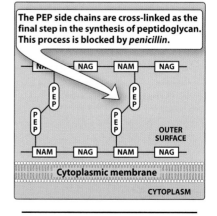

The PEP side chains are cross-linked as the final step in the synthesis of peptidoglycan. This process is blocked by *penicillin*.

NAG NAM NAG

PEP PEP

PEP PEP

OUTER SURFACE

NAM NAG NAM NAG

Cytoplasmic membrane

CYTOPLASM

Figure 29.3
Bacterial cell wall of gram-positive bacteria. NAM = *N*-acetylmuramic acid; NAG = *N*-acetylglucosamine; PEP = cross-linking peptide.

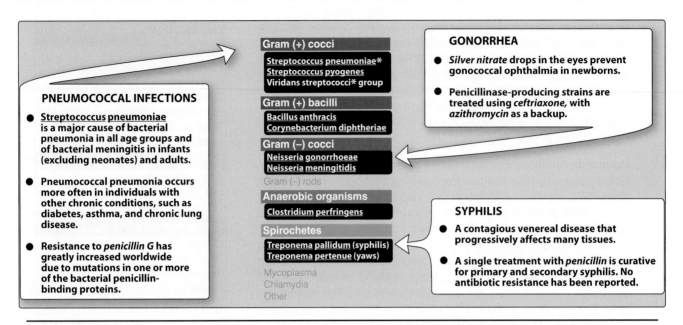

PNEUMOCOCCAL INFECTIONS

- <u>Streptococcus pneumoniae</u> is a major cause of bacterial pneumonia in all age groups and of bacterial meningitis in infants (excluding neonates) and adults.

- Pneumococcal pneumonia occurs more often in individuals with other chronic conditions, such as diabetes, asthma, and chronic lung disease.

- Resistance to *penicillin G* has greatly increased worldwide due to mutations in one or more of the bacterial penicillin-binding proteins.

Gram (+) cocci

<u>Streptococcus pneumoniae</u>*
<u>Streptococcus pyogenes</u>
Viridans streptococci* group

Gram (+) bacilli

<u>Bacillus anthracis</u>
<u>Corynebacterium diphtheriae</u>

Gram (–) cocci

<u>Neisseria gonorrhoeae</u>
<u>Neisseria meningitidis</u>

Gram (–) rods

Anaerobic organisms

<u>Clostridium perfringens</u>

Spirochetes

<u>Treponema pallidum</u> (syphilis)
<u>Treponema pertenue</u> (yaws)

Mycoplasma
Chlamydia
Other

GONORRHEA

- *Silver nitrate* drops in the eyes prevent gonococcal ophthalmia in newborns.

- Penicillinase-producing strains are treated using *ceftriaxone,* with *azithromycin* as a backup.

SYPHILIS

- A contagious venereal disease that progressively affects many tissues.

- A single treatment with *penicillin* is curative for primary and secondary syphilis. No antibiotic resistance has been reported.

Figure 29.4
Typical therapeutic applications of *penicillin G.* *Resistant strains are increasingly seen.

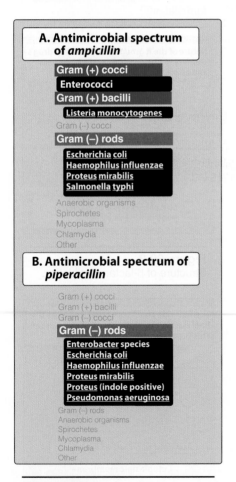

A. Antimicrobial spectrum of *ampicillin*

Gram (+) cocci

Enterococci

Gram (+) bacilli

<u>Listeria monocytogenes</u>

Gram (–) cocci

Gram (–) rods

<u>Escherichia coli</u>
<u>Haemophilus influenzae</u>
<u>Proteus mirabilis</u>
<u>Salmonella typhi</u>

Anaerobic organisms
Spirochetes
Mycoplasma
Chlamydia
Other

B. Antimicrobial spectrum of *piperacillin*

Gram (+) cocci
Gram (+) bacilli
Gram (–) cocci

Gram (–) rods

<u>Enterobacter</u> species
<u>Escherichia coli</u>
<u>Haemophilus influenzae</u>
<u>Proteus mirabilis</u>
<u>Proteus</u> (indole positive)
<u>Pseudomonas aeruginosa</u>

Gram (–) rods
Anaerobic organisms
Spirochetes
Mycoplasma
Chlamydia
Other

Figure 29.5
Antimicrobial activity of *ampicillin* **(A)** and *piperacillin* **(B)**.

Because of its toxicity (interstitial nephritis), *methicillin* is not used clinically in the United States except in laboratory tests to identify resistant strains of <u>Staphylococcus aureus</u>. *Methicillin*-resistant <u>Staphylococcus aureus</u> (MRSA) is currently a source of serious community and nosocomial (hospital-acquired) infections and is resistant to most commercially available β-lactam antibiotics.] The penicillinase-resistant penicillins have minimal to no activity against gram-negative infections.

4. **Antipseudomonal penicillin:** *Piperacillin* [pip-er-a-SILL-in] is also referred to as an antipseudomonal penicillin because of its activity against <u>Pseudomonas aeruginosa</u> (Figure 29.5B). Formulation of *piperacillin* with *tazobactam* extends the antimicrobial spectrum to include penicillinase-producing organisms (for example, most Enterobacteriaceae and <u>Bacteroides</u> species). Figure 29.6 summarizes the stability of the penicillins to acid or the action of penicillinase.

C. Resistance

Survival of bacteria in the presence of β-lactam antibiotics occurs due to the following:

1. **β-Lactamase production:** This family of enzymes hydrolyzes the cyclic amide bond of the β-lactam ring, which results in loss of bactericidal activity (Figure 29.2). They are the major cause of resistance to the penicillins and are an increasing problem. β-Lactamases either are constitutive, mostly produced by the bacterial chromosome or, more commonly, are acquired by the transfer of plasmids. Some of the β-lactam antibiotics are poor substrates for β-lactamases and resist hydrolysis, thus retaining their activity against β-lactamase–producing organisms. [Note: Certain organisms may have chromosome-associated β-lactamases that are

inducible by β-lactam antibiotics (for example, second- and third-generation cephalosporins).] Gram-positive organisms secrete β-lactamases extracellularly, whereas gram-negative bacteria inactivate β-lactam drugs in the periplasmic space.

2. **Decreased permeability to the drug:** Decreased penetration of the antibiotic through the outer cell membrane of the bacteria prevents the drug from reaching the target PBPs. In gram-positive bacteria, the peptidoglycan layer is near the surface of the bacteria and there are few barriers for the drug to reach its target. Reduced penetration of drug into the cell is a greater concern in gram-negative organisms, which have a complex cell wall that includes aqueous channels called porins. An excellent example of a pathogen lacking high permeability porins is <u>Pseudomonas aeruginosa</u>. The presence of an efflux pump, which actively removes antibiotics from the site of action, can also reduce the amount of intracellular drug (for example, <u>Klebsiella pneumoniae</u>).

3. **Altered PBPs:** These are bacterial enzymes involved in the synthesis of the cell wall and in the maintenance of morphologic features of the bacterium. Antibiotic exposure can prevent cell wall synthesis and can lead to morphologic changes or lysis of susceptible bacteria. The number of PBPs varies with the type of organism. Modified PBPs have a lower affinity for β-lactam antibiotics, requiring clinically unattainable concentrations of the drug to effect inhibition of bacterial growth. This explains MRSA resistance to most commercially available β-lactams.

D. Pharmacokinetics

1. **Administration:** The route of administration of a β-lactam antibiotic is determined by the stability of the drug to gastric acid and by the severity of the infection.

2. **Routes of administration:** The combination of *ampicillin* with *sulbactam*, *piperacillin* with *tazobactam*, and the antistaphylococcal penicillins *nafcillin* and *oxacillin* must be administered intravenously (IV) or intramuscularly (IM). *Penicillin V*, *amoxicillin*, and *dicloxacillin* are available only as oral preparations. Others are effective by the oral, IV, or IM routes (Figure 29.6). [Note: The combination of *amoxicillin* with *clavulanic acid* is only available in an oral formulation in the United States.]

3. **Depot forms:** *Procaine penicillin G* and *benzathine penicillin G* are administered IM and serve as depot forms. They are slowly absorbed into the circulation and persist at low levels over a long time period.

4. **Absorption:** The acidic environment within the intestinal tract is unfavorable for the absorption of penicillins. In the case of *penicillin V*, only one-third of an oral dose is absorbed under the best of conditions. Food decreases the absorption of the penicillinase-resistant penicillin *dicloxacillin* because as gastric emptying time increases, the drug is destroyed by stomach acid. Therefore, it

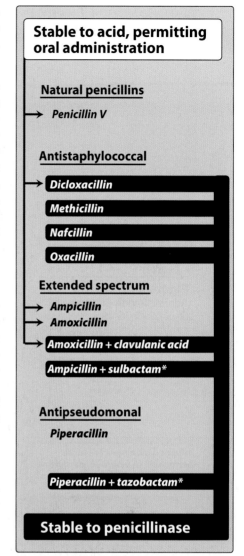

Figure 29.6
Stability of the penicillins to acid or the action of penicillinase. *Available only as parenteral preparation.

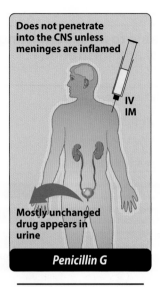

Figure 29.7
Administration and fate
of *penicillin*. CNS =
central nervous system.

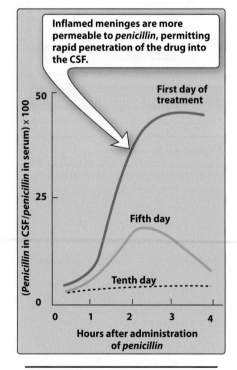

Figure 29.8
Enhanced penetration of *penicillin*
into the cerebral spinal fluid (CSF)
during inflammation.

should be taken on an empty stomach. Conversely, *amoxicillin* is
stable in acid and is readily absorbed from the gastrointestinal (GI)
tract.

5. **Distribution:** The β-lactam antibiotics distribute well throughout
the body. All the penicillins cross the placental barrier, but none
have been shown to have teratogenic effects. However, penetration into bone or cerebrospinal fluid (CSF) is insufficient for therapy unless these sites are inflamed (Figures 29.7 and 29.8). [Note:
Inflamed meninges are more permeable to the penicillins, resulting in an increased ratio of the drug in the CSF compared to the
serum.] *Penicillin* levels in the prostate are insufficient to be effective against infections.

6. **Metabolism:** Host metabolism of the β-lactam antibiotics is usually insignificant, but some metabolism of *penicillin G* may occur
in patients with impaired renal function. *Nafcillin* and *oxacillin*
are exceptions to the rule and are primarily metabolized in the
liver.

7. **Excretion:** The primary route of excretion is through the organic
acid (tubular) secretory system of the kidney as well as by glomerular filtration. Patients with impaired renal function must have
dosage regimens adjusted. Because *nafcillin* and *oxacillin* are primarily metabolized in the liver, they do not require dose adjustment for renal insufficiency. *Probenecid* inhibits the secretion of
penicillins by competing for active tubular secretion via the organic
acid transporter and, thus, can increase blood levels. The penicillins are also excreted in breast milk.

E. Adverse reactions

Penicillins are among the safest drugs. However, adverse reactions
may occur (Figure 29.9).

1. **Hypersensitivity:** Approximately 10% of patients self-report
allergy to penicillin. Reactions range from rashes to angioedema
(marked swelling of the lips, tongue, and periorbital area) and
anaphylaxis. Cross-allergic reactions occur among the β-lactam
antibiotics. To determine whether treatment with a β-lactam is safe
when an allergy is noted, patient history regarding severity of previous reaction is essential.

2. **Diarrhea:** Diarrhea is a common problem that is caused by a
disruption of the normal balance of intestinal microorganisms.
It occurs to a greater extent with those agents that are incompletely absorbed and have an extended antibacterial spectrum.
Pseudomembranous colitis from <u>Clostridium difficile</u> and other
organisms may occur with penicillin use.

3. **Nephritis:** Penicillins, particularly *methicillin*, have the potential to
cause acute interstitial nephritis. [Note: *Methicillin* is therefore no
longer used clinically.]

4. **Neurotoxicity:** The penicillins are irritating to neuronal tissue, and
they can provoke seizures if injected intrathecally or if very high

blood levels are reached. Epileptic patients are particularly at risk due to the ability of penicillins to cause GABAergic inhibition.

5. **Hematologic toxicities:** Decreased coagulation may be observed with high doses of *piperacillin* and *nafcillin* (and, to some extent, with *penicillin G*). Cytopenias have been associated with therapy of greater than 2 weeks, and therefore, blood counts should be monitored weekly for such patients.

III. CEPHALOSPORINS

The cephalosporins are β-lactam antibiotics closely related both structurally and functionally to penicillins. Most cephalosporins are produced semisynthetically by the chemical attachment of side chains to 7-aminocephalosporanic acid. Structural changes on the acyl side chain at the 7-position alter antibacterial activity and variations at the 3-position modify the pharmacokinetic profile (Figure 29.10). Cephalosporins have the same mode of action as penicillins, and they are affected by the same resistance mechanisms. However, they tend to be more resistant than the penicillins to certain β-lactamases.

A. Antibacterial spectrum

Cephalosporins have been classified as first, second, third, fourth, and advanced generation, based largely on their bacterial susceptibility patterns and resistance to β-lactamases (Figure 29.11). [Note: Commercially available cephalosporins are ineffective against L. monocytogenes, C. difficile, and the enterococci.]

1. **First generation:** The first-generation cephalosporins act as *penicillin G* substitutes. They are resistant to the staphylococcal penicillinase (that is, they cover MSSA). Isolates of S. pneumoniae resistant to *penicillin* are also resistant to first-generation cephalosporins. Agents in this generation also have modest activity against Proteus mirabilis, E. coli, and K. pneumoniae. Most oral cavity anaerobes like Peptostreptococcus are sensitive, but the Bacteroides fragilis group is resistant.

2. **Second generation:** The second-generation cephalosporins display greater activity against gram-negative organisms, such as H. influenzae, Klebsiella species, Proteus species, Escherichia coli, and Moraxella catarrhalis, whereas activity against gram-positive organisms is weaker. Antimicrobial coverage of the cephamycins (*cefotetan* [sef-oh-TEE-tan] and *cefoxitin* [sef-OX-i-tin]) also includes anaerobes (for example, Bacteroides fragilis). They are the only cephalosporins commercially available with appreciable activity against gram-negative anaerobic bacteria. However, neither drug is first line because of the increasing prevalence of resistance among B. fragilis.

3. **Third generation:** These cephalosporins have assumed an important role in the treatment of infectious diseases. Although they are less potent than first-generation cephalosporins against

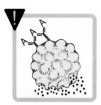
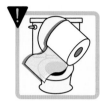
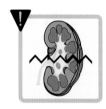

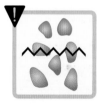

Figure 29.9
Summary of the adverse effects of penicillins.

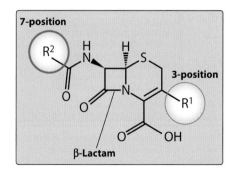

Figure 29.10
Structural features of cephalosporin antibiotics.

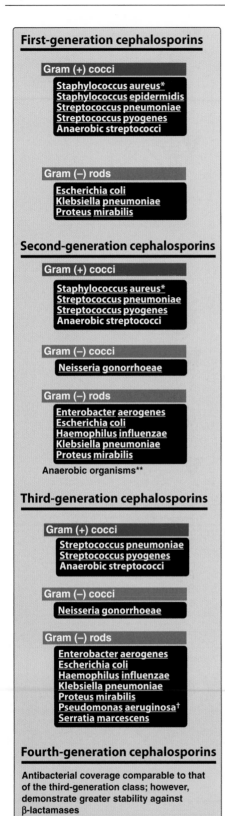

Figure 29.11
Summary of therapeutic applications of cephalosporins. *Methicillin-resistant staphylococci are resistant. **Cefoxitin and cefotetan have anaerobic coverage. †Ceftazidime only.

MSSA, the third-generation cephalosporins have enhanced activity against gram-negative bacilli, including β-lactamase producing strains of H. influenzae and Neisseria gonorrhoeae. The spectrum of activity of this class includes enteric organisms, such as Serratia marcescens and Providencia species. Ceftriaxone [sef-trye-AKS-own] and cefotaxime [sef-oh-TAKS-eem] have become agents of choice in the treatment of meningitis. Ceftazidime [sef-TA-zi-deem] has activity against P. aeruginosa; however, resistance is increasing and use should be evaluated on a case-by-case basis. Third-generation cephalosporins must be used with caution, as they are associated with significant "collateral damage," including the induction of antimicrobial resistance and development of Clostridium difficile infection. [Note: Fluoroquinolone use is also associated with collateral damage.]

4. **Fourth generation:** Cefepime [SEF-eh-peem] is classified as a fourth-generation cephalosporin and must be administered parenterally. Cefepime has a wide antibacterial spectrum, with activity against streptococci and staphylococci (but only those that are methicillin susceptible). Cefepime is also effective against aerobic gram-negative organisms, such as Enterobacter species, E. coli, K. pneumoniae, P. mirabilis, and P. aeruginosa. When selecting an antibiotic that is active against P. aeruginosa, clinicians should refer to their local antibiograms (laboratory testing for the sensitivity of an isolated bacterial strain to different antibiotics) for direction.

5. **Advanced generation:** Ceftaroline [sef-TAR-oh-leen] is a broad-spectrum, advanced-generation cephalosporin. It is the only β-lactam in the United States with activity against MRSA, and it is indicated for the treatment of complicated skin and skin structure infections and community-acquired pneumonia. The unique structure allows ceftaroline to bind to PBPs found in MRSA and penicillin-resistant Streptococcus pneumoniae. In addition to its broad gram-positive activity, it also has similar gram-negative activity to the third-generation cephalosporin ceftriaxone. Important gaps in coverage include P. aeruginosa, extended-spectrum β-lactamase (ESBL)-producing Enterobacteriaceae, and Acinetobacter baumannii. The twice-daily dosing regimen also limits use outside of an institutional setting.

B. Resistance

Resistance to the cephalosporins is either due to the hydrolysis of the beta-lactam ring by β-lactamases or reduced affinity for PBPs.

C. Pharmacokinetics

1. **Administration:** Many of the cephalosporins must be administered IV or IM (Figure 29.12) because of their poor oral absorption. Exceptions are noted in Figure 29.13.

2. **Distribution:** All cephalosporins distribute very well into body fluids. However, adequate therapeutic levels in the CSF, regardless of inflammation, are achieved with only a few cephalosporins.

For example, *ceftriaxone* and *cefotaxime* are effective in the treatment of neonatal and childhood meningitis caused by H̲. influenzae. *Cefazolin* [se-FA-zo-lin] is commonly used for surgical prophylaxis due to its activity against penicillinase-producing S̲. aureus, along with its good tissue and fluid penetration.

3. **Elimination:** Cephalosporins are eliminated through tubular secretion and/or glomerular filtration (Figure 29.12). Therefore, doses must be adjusted in renal dysfunction to guard against accumulation and toxicity. One exception is *ceftriaxone*, which is excreted through the bile into the feces and, therefore, is frequently employed in patients with renal insufficiency.

D. Adverse effects

Like the penicillins, the cephalosporins are generally well tolerated. However, allergic reactions are a concern. Patients who have had an anaphylactic response, Stevens-Johnson syndrome, or toxic epidermal necrolysis to penicillins should not receive cephalosporins. Cephalosporins should be avoided or used with caution in individuals with penicillin allergy. Current data suggest that the cross-reactivity between penicillin and cephalosporins is around 3% to 5% and is determined by the similarity in the side chain, not the β-lactam

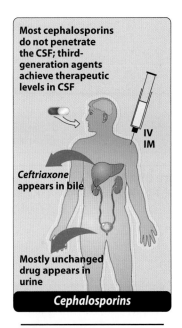

Figure 29.12
Administration and fate of the cephalosporins. CSF = cerebrospinal fluid.

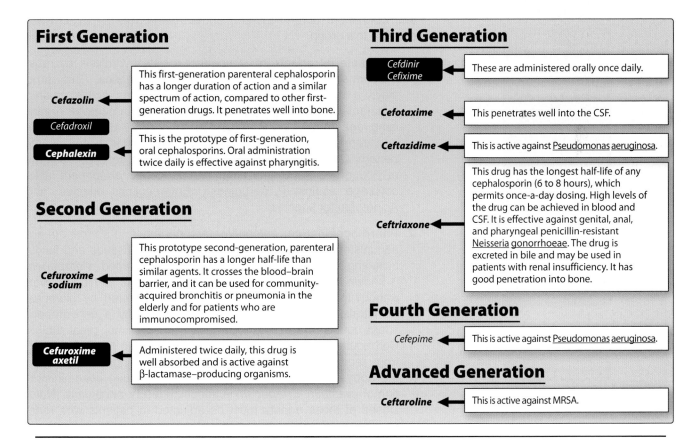

First Generation

Cefazolin ← This first-generation parenteral cephalosporin has a longer duration of action and a similar spectrum of action, compared to other first-generation drugs. It penetrates well into bone.

Cefadroxil

Cephalexin ← This is the prototype of first-generation, oral cephalosporins. Oral administration twice daily is effective against pharyngitis.

Second Generation

Cefuroxime sodium ← This prototype second-generation, parenteral cephalosporin has a longer half-life than similar agents. It crosses the blood–brain barrier, and it can be used for community-acquired bronchitis or pneumonia in the elderly and for patients who are immunocompromised.

Cefuroxime axetil ← Administered twice daily, this drug is well absorbed and is active against β-lactamase–producing organisms.

Third Generation

Cefdinir
Cefixime ← These are administered orally once daily.

Cefotaxime ← This penetrates well into the CSF.

Ceftazidime ← This is active against Pseudomonas aeruginosa.

Ceftriaxone ← This drug has the longest half-life of any cephalosporin (6 to 8 hours), which permits once-a-day dosing. High levels of the drug can be achieved in blood and CSF. It is effective against genital, anal, and pharyngeal penicillin-resistant Neisseria gonorrhoeae. The drug is excreted in bile and may be used in patients with renal insufficiency. It has good penetration into bone.

Fourth Generation

Cefepime ← This is active against Pseudomonas aeruginosa.

Advanced Generation

Ceftaroline ← This is active against MRSA.

Figure 29.13
Therapeutic advantages of some clinically useful cephalosporins. [Note: Drugs that can be administered orally are shown in reverse type. More useful drugs shown in bold.]. CSF = cerebrospinal fluid; MRSA = *methicillin*-resistant Staphylococcus aureus.

β-Lactam ring

Imipenem
(a carbapenem)

β-Lactam ring

Aztreonam
(a monobactam)

Figure 29.14
Structural features of *imipenem* and *aztreonam*.

structure. The highest rate of allergic cross-sensitivity is between *penicillin* and first-generation cephalosporins.

IV. OTHER β-LACTAM ANTIBIOTICS

A. Carbapenems

Carbapenems are synthetic β-lactam antibiotics that differ in structure from the penicillins in that the sulfur atom of the thiazolidine ring (Figure 29.2) has been externalized and replaced by a carbon atom (Figure 29.14). *Imipenem* [i-mi-PEN-em], *meropenem* [mer-oh-PEN-em], *doripenem* [dore-i-PEN-em], and *ertapenem* [er-ta-PEN-em] are drugs in this group.

1. **Antibacterial spectrum:** *Imipenem* resists hydrolysis by most β-lactamases, but not the metallo-β-lactamases. This drug plays a role in empiric therapy because it is active against β-lactamase–producing gram-positive and gram-negative organisms, anaerobes, and P. aeruginosa (Figure 29.15). *Meropenem* and *doripenem* have antibacterial activity similar to that of *imipenem*. *Doripenem* may retain activity against resistant isolates of Pseudomonas. Unlike other carbapenems, *ertapenem* lacks coverage against P. aeruginosa, Enterococcus species, and Acinetobacter species.

2. **Pharmacokinetics:** *Imipenem*, *meropenem*, and *doripenem* are administered IV and penetrate well into body tissues and fluids, including the CSF when the meninges are inflamed. *Meropenem* is known to reach therapeutic levels in bacterial meningitis even without inflammation. These agents are excreted by glomerular filtration. *Imipenem* undergoes cleavage by a dehydropeptidase found in the brush border of the proximal renal tubule. Compounding *imipenem* with *cilastatin* protects the parent drug from renal dehydropeptidase and, thus, prolongs its activity in the body. The other carbapenems do not require coadministration of *cilastatin*. *Ertapenem* is administered IV once daily. [Note: Doses of these agents must be adjusted in patients with renal insufficiency.]

3. **Adverse effects:** *Imipenem/cilastatin* can cause nausea, vomiting, and diarrhea. Eosinophilia and neutropenia are less common

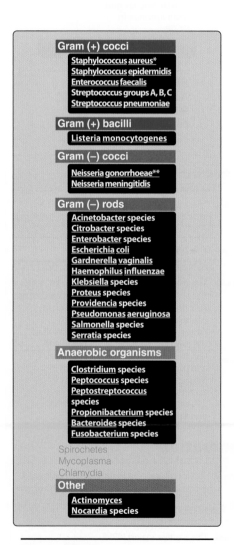

Figure 29.15
Antimicrobial spectrum of *imipenem*.
Methicillin-resistant staphylococci are resistant. **Includes penicillinase-producing strains.

than with other β-lactams. High levels of *imipenem* may provoke seizures; however, the other carbapenems are less likely to do so. Carbapenems and *penicillin* share a common bicyclic core. Structural similarity may confer cross-reactivity between classes. While those with true *penicillin* allergy should use carbapenems cautiously, the cross-reactivity rate seen in studies is very low (less than 1%).

B. Monobactams

The monobactams, which also disrupt bacterial cell wall synthesis, are unique because the β-lactam ring is not fused to another ring (Figure 29.14). *Aztreonam* [az-TREE-oh-nam], which is the only commercially available monobactam, has antimicrobial activity directed primarily against gram-negative pathogens, including the Enterobacteriaceae and P. aeruginosa. It lacks activity against gram-positive organisms and anaerobes. *Aztreonam* is administered either IV or IM and can accumulate in patients with renal failure. *Aztreonam* is relatively nontoxic, but it may cause phlebitis, skin rash, and, occasionally, abnormal liver function tests. This drug has a low immunogenic potential, and it shows little cross-reactivity with antibodies induced by other β-lactams. Thus, this drug may offer a safe alternative for treating patients who are allergic to other penicillins, cephalosporins, or carbapenems.

V. β-LACTAMASE INHIBITORS

Hydrolysis of the β-lactam ring, either by enzymatic cleavage with a β-lactamase or by acid, destroys the antimicrobial activity of a β-lactam antibiotic. β-Lactamase inhibitors, such as *clavulanic* [cla-vue-LAN-ick] *acid*, *sulbactam* [sul-BACK-tam], and *tazobactam* [ta-zoh-BACK-tam], contain a β-lactam ring but, by themselves, do not have significant antibacterial activity or cause any significant adverse effects. *Avibactam* [av-ee-BACK-tam] and *vaborbactam* [vay-bor-BACK-tam] are also β-lactamase inhibitors; however, their structures lack the core β-lactam ring. β-Lactamase inhibitors function by inactivating β-lactamases, thereby protecting the antibiotics that are normally substrates for these enzymes. The β-lactamase inhibitors are, therefore, formulated in combination with β-lactamase–sensitive antibiotics, such as *amoxicillin*, *ampicillin*, and *piperacillin* (Figure 29.1). Figure 29.16 shows the effect of *clavulanic acid* and *amoxicillin* on the growth of β-lactamase–producing E. coli. [Note: *Clavulanic acid* is nearly devoid of any antibacterial activity.]

A. Cephalosporin and β-lactamase inhibitor combinations

Ceftolozane [sef-TOL-oh-zane] is a third-generation cephalosporin combined with the β-lactamase inhibitor, *tazobactam*. *Ceftolozane-tazobactam* is available only in an IV formulation. Its niche for use is in the treatment of resistant Enterobacteriaceae and multidrug-resistant Pseudomonas aeruginosa. *Ceftolozane-tazobactam* has activity against some β-lactamase–producing bacteria (for example, select strains of ESBLs). This combination has narrow gram-positive and very limited anaerobic activity. *Ceftazidime*, a third-generation

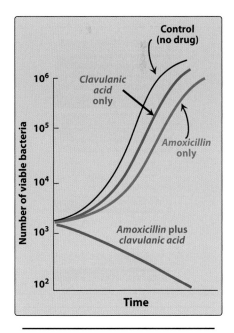

Figure 29.16
The in vitro growth of Escherichia coli in the presence of *amoxicillin*, with and without *clavulanic acid*.

cephalosporin is combined with the β-lactamase inhibitor *avibactam* [AV-i-BAK-tam]. *Ceftazidime-avibactam*, available only in IV formulation, has broad gram-negative activity including Enterobacteriaceae and P. aeruginosa. Addition of *avibactam* allows the drug to resist hydrolysis against broad spectrum β-lactamases (AmpC, ESBL, carbapenemases) with the exception of metallo-β-lactamases. *Ceftazidime-avibactam* has minimal activity against Acinetobacter as well as anaerobic and gram-positive organisms. Both of these combinations are indicated for the treatment of intra-abdominal infections (in combination with *metronidazole*) and for the management of complicated urinary tract infections. Given the extensive antimicrobial activity, *ceftolozane–tazobactam* and *ceftazidime–avibactam* are reserved for the treatment of infections due to multidrug-resistant pathogens.

B. Carbapenem/β-lactamase inhibitor combination

Meropenem-vaborbactam is a combination of a carbapenem and a β-lactamase inhibitor. It is approved for the treatment of complicated urinary tract infections including pyelonephritis. This combination agent has activity against Enterobacteriaceae producing a broad spectrum of β-lactamases, except metallo-β-lactamases.

VI. VANCOMYCIN

Vancomycin [van-koe-MYE-sin] is a tricyclic glycopeptide active against aerobic and anaerobic gram-positive bacteria, including MRSA, *methicillin*-resistant Staphylococcus epidermidis (MRSE), Enterococcus spp., and Clostridium difficile (Figure 29.17). Following cell entry, it binds to peptidoglycan precursors, disrupting polymerization and cross-linking required for maintenance of cell wall integrity. This interaction results in bactericidal activity. Due to an increase in MRSA, *vancomycin* is commonly used in patients with skin and soft tissue infections, infective endocarditis, and nosocomial pneumonia. Frequency of administration is dependent on renal function. Therefore, monitoring of creatinine clearance is required to optimize exposure and minimize toxicity. Optimal cure rates are observed when trough concentrations are maintained between 10 and 20 mcg/mL. [Note: The area under the curve/minimum inhibitory concentration ratio (AUC/MIC) is the best predictor of *vancomycin* activity against S. aureus, with an AUC/MIC of greater than or equal to 400 associated with treatment success.] Initial trough concentrations are attained prior to the fourth or fifth *vancomycin* dose to ensure appropriate dosing. Common adverse events include nephrotoxicity, infusion-related reactions (red man syndrome and phlebitis), and ototoxicity. Emergence of resistance is uncommon within Streptococcus and Staphylococcus spp., but frequently observed in Enterococcus faecium infections. Resistance is driven by alterations in binding affinity to peptidoglycan precursors. Due to the prevalence of resistance, prudent use of *vancomycin* is warranted. Lastly, *vancomycin* has poor absorption after oral administration, so use of the oral formulation is limited to the management of Clostridium difficile infection in the colon.

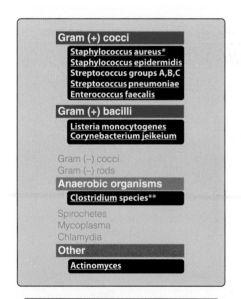

Figure 29.17
Antimicrobial spectrum of *vancomycin*. *Includes *methicillin*-resistant strains. **Oral *vancomycin* only for C. difficile.

VII. LIPOGLYCOPEPTIDES

Telavancin [tel-a-VAN-sin], *oritavancin* [or-IT-a-VAN-sin], and *dalba-vancin* [dal-ba-VAN-sin] are bactericidal concentration-dependent semi-synthetic lipoglycopeptide antibiotics with activity against gram-positive bacteria. The lipoglycopeptides maintain a spectrum of activity similar to *vancomycin*, affecting primarily staphylococci, streptococci, and enterococci. Because of structural differences, they are more potent than *vancomycin* and may have activity against *vancomycin*-resistant isolates. Like *vancomycin*, these agents inhibit bacterial cell wall synthesis. The lipid tail is essential in anchoring the drug to the cell walls to improve target site binding. Additionally, *telavancin* and *oritavancin* disrupt membrane potential. In combination, these actions improve activity and minimize selection of resistance. *Telavancin* is considered an alternative to *vancomycin* in treating acute bacterial skin and skin structure infections (ABSSSIs) and hospital-acquired pneumonia caused by resistant gram-positive organisms, including MRSA. The use of *telavancin* in clinical practice may be limited by its adverse effect profile, which includes nephrotoxicity, risk of fetal harm, and interactions with medications known to prolong the QT_c interval (for example, fluoroquinolones, macrolides). Prior to initiation, assessment of renal function, pregnancy status, and current medications is needed to ensure safe administration.

In contrast to *telavancin*, *oritavancin* and *dalbavancin* have prolonged half-lives (245 and 187 hours, respectively), allowing for single-dose administration for the management of ABSSSI. Stable patients with ABSSSI may be treated as outpatients, eliminating the need for inpatient admission, central catheter placement, and/or daily outpatient parenteral antibiotic therapy. Consistent with other glycopeptides, infusion-related reactions may occur. *Oritavancin* and *telavancin* are known to interfere with phospholipid reagents used in assessing coagulation. Alternative therapy should be considered with concomitant *heparin* use.

VIII. DAPTOMYCIN

Daptomycin [DAP-toe-mye-sin] is a bactericidal concentration-dependent cyclic lipopeptide antibiotic that is an alternative to other agents, such as *vancomycin or linezolid*, for treating infections caused by resistant gram-positive organisms, including MRSA and *vancomycin*-resistant enterococci (VRE) (Figure 29.18). *Daptomycin* is indicated for the treatment of complicated skin and skin structure infections and bacteremia caused by <u>S</u>. <u>aureus</u>, including those with right-sided infective endocarditis. Efficacy of treatment with *daptomycin* in left-sided endocarditis has not been demonstrated. Additionally, *daptomycin* is inactivated by pulmonary surfactants; thus, it should *never* be used in the treatment of pneumonia. *Daptomycin* is dosed IV once daily. Figure 29.19 provides a comparison of important characteristics of *vancomycin, daptomycin*, and lipoglycopeptides.

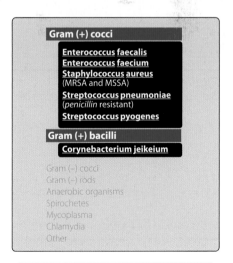

Figure 29.18
Antimicrobial spectrum of *daptomycin*. MRSA = *methicillin*-resistant <u>S</u>. <u>aureus</u>; MSSA = *methicillin*-susceptible <u>S</u>. <u>aureus</u>.

	VANCOMYCIN	DAPTOMYCIN	TELAVANCIN
Mechanism of Action	Inhibits bacterial cell wall synthesis	Causes rapid depolarization of the cell membrane, inhibits intracellular synthesis of DNA, RNA, and protein	Inhibits bacterial cell wall synthesis; disrupts cell membrane
Pharmacodynamics	Combination of time and concentration-dependent Bactericidal	Concentration-dependent Bactericidal	Concentration-dependent Bactericidal
Common Antibacterial Spectrum	Activity limited to gram-positive organisms: Staphylococcus aureus (including MRSA), Streptococcus pyogenes, S. agalactiae, penicillin-resistant S. pneumoniae, Corynebacterium jeikeium, vancomycin-susceptible Enterococcus faecalis, and E. faecium		
Unique Antibacterial Spectrum	Clostridium difficile (oral only)	Vancomycin-resistant E. faecalis and E. faecium (VRE)	Some isolates of vancomycin-resistant enterococci (VRE)
Route	IV/PO	IV	IV
Administration Time	60- to 90-min IV infusion	2-min IV push 30-min IV infusion	60-min IV infusion
Pharmacokinetics	Renal elimination Half-life: 6–10 h Dose is adjusted based on renal function and serum trough levels	Renal elimination Half-life: 7–8 h Dose is adjusted based on renal function	Renal elimination Half-life: 7–9 h Dose is adjusted based on renal function
Unique Adverse Effects	Infusion-related reactions due to histamine release: Fever, chills, phlebitis, flushing (red man syndrome); dose-related ototoxicity and nephrotoxicity	Elevated hepatic transaminases and creatine phosphokinase (check weekly), myalgias and rhabdomyolysis (consider holding HMG-CoA reductase inhibitors [statins] while receiving therapy)	Taste disturbances, foamy urine, QTc prolongation, interferes with coagulation labs (PT/INR, aPTT, ACT), not recommended in pregnancy (box warning recommends pregnancy test prior to initiation)
Key Learning Points	Drug of choice for severe MRSA infections; oral form only used for C. difficile infection; monitor serum trough concentrations for safety and efficacy	Daptomycin is inactivated by pulmonary surfactants and should never be used in the treatment of pneumonia	Use with caution in patients with baseline renal dysfunction (CrCl < 50 mL/min) due to higher rates of treatment failure and mortality in clinical studies; any necessary coagulation labs should be drawn just prior to the telavancin dose to avoid interaction

Figure 29.19
Side-by-side comparison of *vancomycin*, *daptomycin*, and *telavancin*.

IX. FOSFOMYCIN

Fosfomycin [fos-foe-MYE-sin] is a bactericidal synthetic derivative of phosphonic acid. It blocks cell wall synthesis by inhibiting the enzyme enolpyruvyl transferase, a key step in peptidoglycan synthesis. It is indicated for urinary tract infections caused by E. coli or E. faecalis and is considered first-line therapy for acute cystitis. Due to its unique structure and mechanism of action, cross-resistance with other antimicrobial agents is unlikely. *Fosfomycin* is rapidly absorbed after oral administration and distributes well to the kidneys, bladder, and prostate. The drug is excreted in its active form in the urine and maintains high concentrations over several days, allowing for a one-time dose. [Note: A parenteral formulation is available in select countries and has been used for the treatment of systemic infections.] The most commonly reported adverse effects include diarrhea, vaginitis, nausea, and headache.

X. POLYMYXINS

The polymyxins are cation polypeptides that bind to phospholipids on the bacterial cell membrane of gram-negative bacteria. They have a detergent-like effect that disrupts cell membrane integrity, leading to leakage of cellular components and cell death. Polymyxins are concentration-dependent bactericidal agents with activity against most clinically important gram-negative bacteria, including P. aeruginosa, E. coli, K. pneumoniae, Acinetobacter spp., and Enterobacter spp. However, alterations in the cell membrane, lipid polysaccharides allow many species of Proteus and Serratia to be intrinsically resistant. Only two forms of polymyxin are in clinical use today, *polymyxin B* and *colistin* (*polymyxin E*). *Polymyxin B* is available in parenteral, ophthalmic, otic, and topical preparations. *Colistin* is only available as a prodrug, *colistimethate sodium*, which is administered IV or inhaled via a nebulizer. The use of these drugs has been limited due to the increased risk of nephrotoxicity and neurotoxicity (for example, slurred speech, muscle weakness) when used systemically. However, with increasing gram-negative resistance, they are now commonly used as salvage therapy for patients with multidrug-resistant infections. Careful dosing and monitoring of adverse effects are important to maximize the safety and efficacy of these agents.

Study Questions

Choose the ONE best answer.

29.1 A 45-year-old man presented to the hospital 3 days ago with severe cellulitis and a large abscess on his left leg. Incision and drainage were performed on the abscess, and cultures revealed methicillin-resistant Staphylococcus aureus. Which is the most appropriate treatment option for once-daily outpatient intravenous therapy in this patient?

A. Ertapenem
B. Ceftaroline
C. Daptomycin
D. Piperacillin/tazobactam

> Correct answer = C. Daptomycin is approved for skin and skin structure infections caused by MRSA and is given once daily. A and D are incorrect because they do not cover MRSA. Ceftaroline covers MRSA, but it must be given twice daily.

29.2 Which of the following adverse effects is associated with daptomycin?

A. Ototoxicity
B. Red man syndrome
C. QT$_c$ prolongation
D. Rhabdomyolysis

> Correct answer = D. Ototoxicity and red man syndrome are associated with vancomycin. QTc prolongation is associated with telavancin. Myalgias and rhabdomyolysis have been reported with daptomycin therapy and require patient education and monitoring.

29.3 A 72-year-old man is admitted to the hospital from a nursing home with severe pneumonia. He was discharged from the hospital 1 week ago after open heart surgery. The patient has no known allergies. Which of the following regimens is most appropriate for empiric coverage of methicillin-resistant Staphylococcus aureus and Pseudomonas aeruginosa in this patient?

A. Vancomycin + cefepime + ciprofloxacin
B. Vancomycin + cefazolin + ciprofloxacin
C. Telavancin + cefepime + ciprofloxacin
D. Daptomycin + cefepime + ciprofloxacin

> Correct answer = A. Vancomycin provides adequate coverage against MRSA, and cefepime and ciprofloxacin provide adequate empiric coverage of Pseudomonas. B is incorrect because cefazolin does not have activity against Pseudomonas. C is incorrect because telavancin should be avoided if possible with drugs that prolong the QTc interval, in this case ciprofloxacin. Daptomycin is inactivated by pulmonary surfactant and should not be used for pneumonia.

29.4 A 23-year-old man presents with acute appendicitis that ruptures shortly after admission. He is taken to the operating room for surgery, and postsurgical cultures reveal Escherichia coli and Bacteroides fragilis, susceptibilities pending. Which of the following provides adequate empiric coverage of these two pathogens?

A. Cefepime

B. Piperacillin/tazobactam

C. Aztreonam

D. Ceftaroline

Correct answer = B. While all of these agents cover most strains of E. coli, piperacillin/tazobactam is the only drug on this list that provides coverage against Bacteroides species.

29.5 A 68-year-old man presents from a nursing home with fever, increased urinary frequency and urgency, and mental status changes. He has a penicillin allergy of anaphylaxis. Which of the following β-lactams is the most appropriate choice for gram-negative coverage of this patient's urinary tract infection?

A. Cefepime

B. Ertapenem

C. Aztreonam

D. Ceftaroline

Correct answer = C. Based on the severity of the allergic reaction, aztreonam is the choice of all the β-lactams. Although cross-reactivity with cephalosporins and carbapenems is low, the risk rarely outweighs the benefit in these cases.

29.6 A 25-year-old man presents to the urgent care center with a painless sore on his genitals that started 2 weeks ago. He reports unprotected sex with a new partner about a month ago. A blood test confirms the patient has Treponema pallidum. Which is the drug of choice for the treatment of this patient's infection as a single dose?

A. Benzathine penicillin G

B. Ceftriaxone

C. Aztreonam

D. Vancomycin

Correct answer = A. A single treatment with penicillin is curative for primary and secondary syphilis. No antibiotic resistance has been reported, and it remains the drug of choice unless the patient has a severe allergic reaction.

29.7 A 20-year-old woman presents to the emergency room with headache, stiff neck, and fever for 2 days and is diagnosed with meningitis. Which is the best agent for the treatment of meningitis in this patient?

A. Cefazolin

B. Cefdinir

C. Cefotaxime

D. Cefuroxime axetil

Correct answer = C. Cefotaxime is the only drug on this list with adequate CSF penetration to treat meningitis. Cefdinir and cefuroxime axetil are only available orally, and cefazolin's CSF penetration and spectrum of coverage against S. pneumoniae are likely inadequate to treat meningitis.

29.8 Which of the following cephalosporins has activity against gram-negative anaerobic pathogens like Bacteroides fragilis?

A. Cefoxitin

B. Cefepime

C. Ceftriaxone

D. Cefazolin

Correct answer = A. The cephamycins (cefoxitin and cefotetan) are the only cephalosporins with in vitro activity against anaerobic gram-negative pathogens. Cefepime, ceftriaxone, and cefazolin have no appreciable activity against Bacteroides fragilis.

29.9 In which of the following cases would it be appropriate to use telavancin?

A. A 29-year-old pregnant woman with ventilator-associated pneumonia

B. A 76-year-old man with hospital-acquired pneumonia also receiving amiodarone for atrial fibrillation

C. A 36-year-old man with cellulitis and abscess growing MRSA

D. A 72-year-old woman with a diabetic foot infection growing MRSA who has moderate renal dysfunction

Correct answer = C. A is not a good option due to the potential of telavancin harming the fetus. Option B is not a good choice because the patient is on amiodarone, and telavancin can cause QT_c prolongation. Option D is not an appropriate choice because the patient has baseline renal dysfunction and telavancin should be avoided unless benefit outweighs the risk. Option C is the best choice since telavancin is approved for skin and skin structure infections, and the patient has no apparent contraindication.

29.10 An 18-year-old woman presents to the urgent care clinic with symptoms of a urinary tract infection. Cultures reveal <u>Enterococcus faecalis</u> that is pan sensitive. Which of the following is an appropriate oral option to treat the urinary tract infection in this patient?

A. *Cephalexin*

B. *Vancomycin*

C. *Cefdinir*

D. *Amoxicillin*

Correct answer = D. Option A and C are incorrect because enterococci are inherently resistant to all cephalosporins. Option B is incorrect because oral vancomycin is not absorbed and would not reach the urinary tract in sufficient quantities to treat a urinary tract infection. Option D is the best choice, as amoxicillin is well absorbed orally and concentrates in the urine.

Protein Synthesis Inhibitors

Jacqueline Jourjy

30

I. OVERVIEW

A number of antibiotics exert their antimicrobial effects by targeting bacterial ribosomes and inhibiting bacterial protein synthesis. Most of these agents exhibit bacteriostatic activity. Bacterial ribosomes differ structurally from mammalian cytoplasmic ribosomes and are composed of 30S and 50S subunits (mammalian ribosomes have 40S and 60S subunits). In general, selectivity for bacterial ribosomes minimizes potential adverse consequences encountered with the disruption of protein synthesis in mammalian host cells. However, high concentrations of drugs such as *chloramphenicol* or the tetracyclines may cause toxic effects as a result of interaction with mitochondrial mammalian ribosomes, because the structure of mitochondrial ribosomes more closely resembles bacterial ribosomes. Figure 30.1 summarizes the antimicrobial protein synthesis inhibitors discussed in this chapter.

II. TETRACYCLINES

Tetracyclines consist of four fused rings with a system of conjugated double bonds. Substitutions on these rings alter the individual pharmacokinetics and spectrum of antimicrobial activity.

A. Mechanism of action

Tetracyclines enter susceptible organisms via passive diffusion and by an energy-dependent transport protein mechanism unique to the bacterial inner cytoplasmic membrane. Tetracyclines concentrate intracellularly in susceptible organisms. The drugs bind reversibly to the 30S subunit of the bacterial ribosome. This action prevents binding of tRNA to the mRNA–ribosome complex, thereby inhibiting bacterial protein synthesis (Figure 30.2).

B. Antibacterial spectrum

The tetracyclines are bacteriostatic antibiotics effective against a wide variety of organisms, including gram-positive and gram-negative bacteria, protozoa, spirochetes, mycobacteria, and atypical species. They are commonly used in the treatment of acne and <u>Chlamydia</u> infections (Figure 30.3).

TETRACYCLINES
Demeclocycline DECLOMYCIN
Doxycycline DORYX, VIBRAMYCIN
Minocycline MINOCIN
Tetracycline GENERIC ONLY
GLYCYLCYCLINES
Tigecycline TYGACIL
AMINOGLYCOSIDES
Amikacin GENERIC ONLY
Gentamicin GENERIC ONLY
Neomycin GENERIC ONLY
Streptomycin GENERIC ONLY
Tobramycin TOBI, TOBREX
MACROLIDES/KETOLIDES
Azithromycin ZITHROMAX
Clarithromycin BIAXIN
Erythromycin E.E.S., ERY-TAB
Telithromycin GENERIC ONLY
MACROCYCLIC
Fidaxomicin DIFICID
LINCOSAMIDES
Clindamycin CLEOCIN
OXAZOLIDINONES
Linezolid ZYVOX
Tedizolid SIVEXTRO
OTHERS
Chloramphenicol GENERIC ONLY
Quinupristin/Dalfopristin SYNERCID

Figure 30.1
Summary of protein synthesis inhibitors.

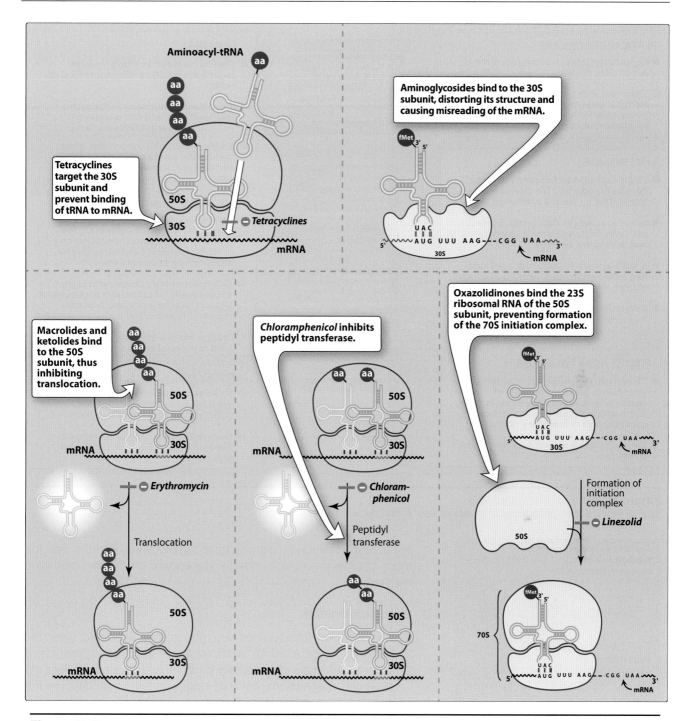

Figure 30.2
Mechanisms of action of the various protein synthesis inhibitors. aa = amino acid.

C. Resistance

The most commonly encountered naturally occurring resistance to tetracyclines is an efflux pump that expels drug out of the cell, thus preventing intracellular accumulation. Other mechanisms of bacterial resistance to tetracyclines include enzymatic inactivation of the drug and production of bacterial proteins that prevent tetracyclines from binding to the ribosome. Resistance to one tetracycline does

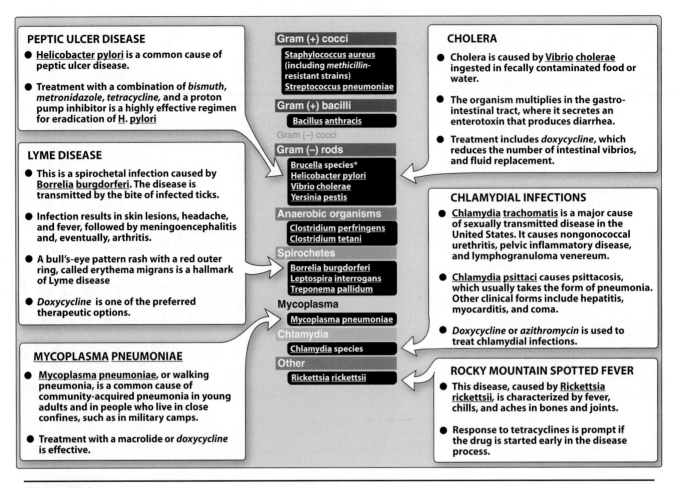

PEPTIC ULCER DISEASE

● <u>Helicobacter</u> <u>pylori</u> is a common cause of peptic ulcer disease.

● Treatment with a combination of *bismuth*, *metronidazole*, *tetracycline*, and a proton pump inhibitor is a highly effective regimen for eradication of <u>H</u>. <u>pylori</u>

LYME DISEASE

● This is a spirochetal infection caused by <u>Borrelia</u> <u>burgdorferi</u>. The disease is transmitted by the bite of infected ticks.

● Infection results in skin lesions, headache, and fever, followed by meningoencephalitis and, eventually, arthritis.

● A bull's-eye pattern rash with a red outer ring, called erythema migrans is a hallmark of Lyme disease

● *Doxycycline* is one of the preferred therapeutic options.

<u>MYCOPLASMA</u> <u>PNEUMONIAE</u>

● <u>Mycoplasma</u> <u>pneumoniae</u>, or walking pneumonia, is a common cause of community-acquired pneumonia in young adults and in people who live in close confines, such as in military camps.

● Treatment with a macrolide or *doxycycline* is effective.

Gram (+) cocci
<u>Staphylococcus</u> <u>aureus</u> (including *methicillin-resistant strains*)
<u>Streptococcus</u> <u>pneumoniae</u>

Gram (+) bacilli
<u>Bacillus</u> <u>anthracis</u>

Gram (–) cocci

Gram (–) rods
<u>Brucella</u> species*
<u>Helicobacter</u> <u>pylori</u>
<u>Vibrio</u> <u>cholerae</u>
<u>Yersinia</u> <u>pestis</u>

Anaerobic organisms
<u>Clostridium</u> <u>perfringens</u>
<u>Clostridium</u> <u>tetani</u>

Spirochetes
<u>Borrelia</u> <u>burgdorferi</u>
<u>Leptospira</u> <u>interrogans</u>
<u>Treponema</u> <u>pallidum</u>

Mycoplasma
<u>Mycoplasma</u> <u>pneumoniae</u>

Chlamydia
<u>Chlamydia</u> species

Other
<u>Rickettsia</u> <u>rickettsii</u>

CHOLERA

● Cholera is caused by <u>Vibrio</u> <u>cholerae</u> ingested in fecally contaminated food or water.

● The organism multiplies in the gastro-intestinal tract, where it secretes an enterotoxin that produces diarrhea.

● Treatment includes *doxycycline*, which reduces the number of intestinal vibrios, and fluid replacement.

CHLAMYDIAL INFECTIONS

● <u>Chlamydia</u> <u>trachomatis</u> is a major cause of sexually transmitted disease in the United States. It causes nongonococcal urethritis, pelvic inflammatory disease, and lymphogranuloma venereum.

● <u>Chlamydia</u> <u>psittaci</u> causes psittacosis, which usually takes the form of pneumonia. Other clinical forms include hepatitis, myocarditis, and coma.

● *Doxycycline* or *azithromycin* is used to treat chlamydial infections.

ROCKY MOUNTAIN SPOTTED FEVER

● This disease, caused by <u>Rickettsia</u> <u>rickettsii</u>, is characterized by fever, chills, and aches in bones and joints.

● Response to tetracyclines is prompt if the drug is started early in the disease process.

Figure 30.3
Typical therapeutic applications of tetracyclines. *A *tetracycline* + *gentamicin*.

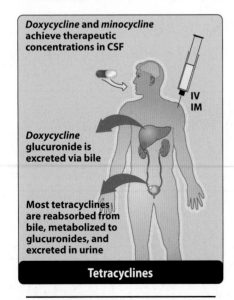

Doxycycline and *minocycline* achieve therapeutic concentrations in CSF

Doxycycline glucuronide is excreted via bile

Most tetracyclines are reabsorbed from bile, metabolized to glucuronides, and excreted in urine

Tetracyclines

Figure 30.4
Administration and fate of tetracyclines. CSF = cerebrospinal fluid.

not confer universal resistance to all tetracyclines, and the development of cross-resistance may be dependent on the mechanism of resistance.

D. Pharmacokinetics

1. **Absorption:** Tetracyclines are adequately absorbed after oral ingestion (Figure 30.4). Administration with dairy products or other substances that contain divalent and trivalent cations (for example, magnesium, calcium and aluminum antacids, or iron supplements) decreases absorption, particularly for *tetracycline* [tet-rah-SYE-kleen], due to the formation of nonabsorbable chelates (Figure 30.5). Both *doxycycline* [dox-i-SYE-kleen] and *minocycline* [min-oh-SYE-kleen] are available as oral and intravenous (IV) preparations.

2. **Distribution:** The tetracyclines concentrate well in the bile, liver, kidney, gingival fluid, and skin. Moreover, they bind to tissues undergoing calcification (for example, teeth and bones) or to tumors that have high calcium content. Penetration into most body fluids is adequate. Only *minocycline* and *doxycycline* achieve therapeutic levels in the cerebrospinal fluid (CSF). *Minocycline* also achieves

high concentrations in saliva and tears, rendering it useful in eradicating the meningococcal carrier state. All *tetracyclines* cross the placental barrier and concentrate in fetal bones and dentition.

3. **Elimination:** *Tetracycline* is primarily eliminated unchanged in the urine, whereas *minocycline* undergoes hepatic metabolism and is eliminated to a lesser extent via the kidney. *Doxycycline* is preferred in patients with renal dysfunction, as it is primarily eliminated via the bile into the feces.

E. Adverse effects

1. **Gastric discomfort:** Epigastric distress commonly results from irritation of the gastric mucosa (Figure 30.6) and is often responsible for noncompliance with tetracyclines. Esophagitis may be minimized through coadministration with food (other than dairy products) or fluids and the use of capsules rather than tablets. [Note: *Tetracycline* should be taken on an empty stomach.]

2. **Effects on calcified tissues:** Deposition in the bone and primary dentition occurs during the calcification process in growing children. This may cause discoloration and hypoplasia of teeth and a temporary stunting of growth. For this reason, the use of tetracyclines is limited in pediatrics.

3. **Hepatotoxicity:** Rarely hepatotoxicity may occur with high doses, particularly in pregnant women and those with preexisting hepatic dysfunction or renal impairment.

4. **Phototoxicity:** Severe sunburn may occur in patients receiving a tetracycline who are exposed to sun or ultraviolet rays. This toxicity is encountered with any tetracycline, but more frequently with *tetracycline* and *demeclocycline* [dem-e-kloe-SYE-kleen]. Patients should be advised to wear adequate sun protection.

5. **Vestibular dysfunction:** Dizziness, vertigo, and tinnitus may occur particularly with *minocycline*, which concentrates in the endolymph of the ear and affects function.

6. **Pseudotumor cerebri:** Benign, intracranial hypertension characterized by headache and blurred vision may occur rarely in adults. Although discontinuation of the drug reverses this condition, it is not clear whether permanent sequelae may occur.

7. **Contraindications:** The tetracyclines should not be used in pregnant or breast-feeding women or in children less than 8 years of age.

III. GLYCYLCYCLINES

Tigecycline [tye-ge-SYE-kleen], a derivative of *minocycline*, is the first member of the glycylcycline antimicrobial class. It is indicated for the treatment of complicated skin and soft tissue infections, complicated intra-abdominal infections, and community-acquired pneumonia.

A. Mechanism of action

Tigecycline exhibits bacteriostatic action by reversibly binding to the 30S ribosomal subunit and inhibiting bacterial protein synthesis.

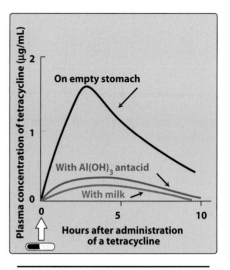

Figure 30.5
Effect of antacids and milk on the absorption of tetracyclines.

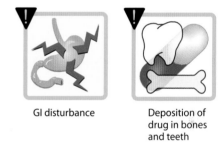

GI disturbance

Deposition of drug in bones and teeth

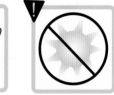

Liver failure

Phototoxicity

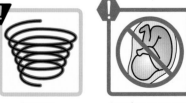

Vertigo

Avoid in pregnancy

Figure 30.6
Some adverse effects of tetracyclines. GI = gastrointestinal.

B. Antibacterial spectrum

Tigecycline exhibits broad-spectrum activity that includes *methicillin*-resistant staphylococci (MRSA), multidrug-resistant streptococci, *vancomycin*-resistant enterococci (VRE), extended-spectrum β-lactamase–producing gram-negative bacteria, Acinetobacter baumannii, and many anaerobic organisms. *Tigecycline* is not active against Morganella, Proteus, Providencia, or Pseudomonas species.

C. Resistance

Tigecycline was developed to overcome the emergence of tetracycline class–resistant organisms that utilize efflux pumps and ribosomal protection to confer resistance. Resistance to *tigecycline* has been observed and is primarily attributed to overexpression of efflux pumps.

D. Pharmacokinetics

Following IV infusion, *tigecycline* exhibits a large volume of distribution. It penetrates tissues well but achieves low plasma concentrations. Consequently, *tigecycline* is a poor option for bloodstream infections. The primary route of elimination is biliary/fecal. No dosage adjustments are necessary for patients with renal impairment; however, a dose reduction is recommended in severe hepatic dysfunction.

E. Adverse effects

Tigecycline is associated with significant nausea and vomiting. Acute pancreatitis, including fatality, has been reported with therapy. Elevations in liver enzymes and serum creatinine may also occur. All-cause mortality in patients treated with *tigecycline* is higher than with other agents. A boxed warning states that *tigecycline* should be reserved for use in situations when alternative treatments are not suitable. Other adverse effects are similar to those of the tetracyclines and include photosensitivity, pseudotumor cerebri, discoloration of permanent teeth when used during tooth development, and fetal harm when administered in pregnancy. *Tigecycline* may decrease the clearance of *warfarin*. Therefore, the international normalized ratio should be monitored closely when *tigecycline* is coadministered with *warfarin*.

IV. AMINOGLYCOSIDES

Aminoglycosides are used for the treatment of serious infections due to aerobic gram-negative bacilli; however, their clinical utility is limited due to serious toxicities.

A. Mechanism of action

Aminoglycosides diffuse through porin channels in the outer membrane of susceptible organisms. These organisms also have an oxygen-dependent system that transports the drug across the cytoplasmic membrane. Inside the cell, they bind the 30S ribosomal subunit, where they interfere with assembly of the functional ribosomal apparatus and/or cause the 30S subunit of the completed ribosome to misread the genetic code (Figure 30.2). Aminoglycosides have concentration-dependent bactericidal activity; that is, their efficacy is dependent on the maximum concentration (C_{max}) of drug above the minimum inhibitory concentration (MIC) of the organism. For aminoglycosides, the target C_{max} is eight to ten times the MIC. They also exhibit a postantibiotic effect (PAE), which is continued bacterial suppression after drug concentrations fall below the MIC. The larger the dose, the longer the PAE. Because of these properties, high-dose extended-interval dosing is commonly utilized. This dosing strategy also reduces the risk of nephrotoxicity and increases convenience.

B. Antibacterial spectrum

The aminoglycosides are effective for the majority of aerobic gram-negative bacilli, including those that may be multidrug resistant, such as Pseudomonas aeruginosa, Klebsiella pneumoniae, and Enterobacter sp. Additionally, aminoglycosides are often combined with a β-lactam antibiotic to employ a synergistic effect, particularly in the treatment of Enterococcus faecalis and Enterococcus faecium infective endocarditis. Some therapeutic applications of four commonly used aminoglycosides—amikacin [am-i-KAY-sin], gentamicin [jen-ta-MYE-sin], tobramycin [toe-bra-MYE-sin], and streptomycin [strep-toe-MYE-sin]—are shown in Figure 30.7.

C. Resistance

Resistance to aminoglycosides occurs via: 1) efflux pumps, 2) decreased uptake, and/or 3) modification and inactivation by plasmid-associated synthesis of enzymes. Each of these enzymes has its own aminoglycoside specificity; therefore, cross-resistance cannot be presumed. [Note: Amikacin is less vulnerable to these enzymes than other antibiotics in this group.]

D. Pharmacokinetics

1. **Absorption:** The highly polar, polycationic structure of the aminoglycosides prevents adequate absorption after oral administration; therefore, all aminoglycosides (except neomycin [nee-oh-MYE-sin]) must be given parenterally to achieve adequate serum concentrations (Figure 30.8). [Note: Neomycin is not given parenterally due to severe nephrotoxicity. It is administered topically for skin infections or orally to decontaminate the gastrointestinal tract prior to colorectal surgery.]

2. **Distribution:** Because of their hydrophilicity, aminoglycoside tissue concentrations may be subtherapeutic, and penetration into most body fluids is variable. Concentrations achieved in CSF are inadequate, even in the presence of inflamed meninges. For central nervous system infections, the intrathecal or intraventricular routes may be utilized. All aminoglycosides cross the placental barrier and may accumulate in fetal plasma and amniotic fluid.

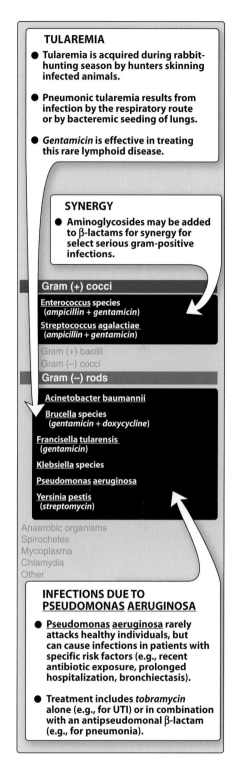

Figure 30.7
Typical therapeutic applications of aminoglycosides. UTI = urinary tract infection.

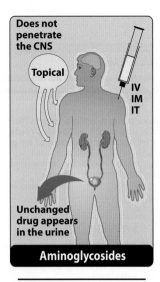

Figure 30.8
Administration and fate
of aminoglycosides.
CNS = central nervous
system.

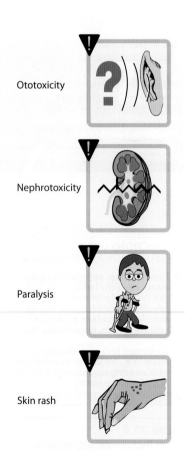

Figure 30.9
Some adverse effects of
aminoglycosides.

3. **Elimination:** More than 90% of the parenteral aminoglycosides are excreted unchanged in the urine (Figure 30.8). Accumulation occurs in patients with renal dysfunction; thus, dose adjustments are required. *Neomycin* is primarily excreted unchanged in the feces.

E. Adverse effects

Therapeutic drug monitoring of *gentamicin*, *tobramycin*, and *amikacin* plasma concentrations is imperative to ensure appropriateness of dosing and to minimize dose-related toxicities (Figure 30.9). The elderly are particularly susceptible to nephrotoxicity and ototoxicity.

1. **Ototoxicity:** Ototoxicity (vestibular and auditory) is directly related to high peak plasma concentrations and the duration of treatment. Aminoglycosides accumulate in the endolymph and perilymph of the inner ear. Deafness may be irreversible and has been known to affect developing fetuses. Patients simultaneously receiving concomitant ototoxic drugs, such as *cisplatin* or loop diuretics, are particularly at risk. Vertigo (especially in patients receiving *streptomycin*) may also occur.

2. **Nephrotoxicity:** Retention of the aminoglycosides by the proximal tubular cells disrupts calcium-mediated transport processes. This results in kidney damage ranging from mild, reversible renal impairment to severe, potentially irreversible acute tubular necrosis.

3. **Neuromuscular paralysis:** This adverse effect is associated with a rapid increase in concentration (for example, high doses infused over a short period) or concurrent administration with neuromuscular blockers. Patients with myasthenia gravis are particularly at risk. Prompt administration of *calcium gluconate* or *neostigmine* can reverse the block that causes neuromuscular paralysis.

4. **Allergic reactions:** Contact dermatitis is a common reaction to topically applied *neomycin.*

V. MACROLIDES AND KETOLIDES

The macrolides are a group of antibiotics with a macrocyclic lactone structure to which one or more deoxy sugars are attached. *Erythromycin* [er-ith-roe-MYE-sin] was the first of these drugs to have clinical application, both as a drug of first choice and as an alternative to *penicillin* in individuals with an allergy to β-lactam antibiotics. *Clarithromycin* [kla-rith-roe-MYE-sin] (a methylated form of *erythromycin*) and *azithromycin* [a-zith-roe-MYE-sin] (having a larger lactone ring) have some features in common with, and others that improve upon, *erythromycin*. *Telithromycin* [tel-ith-roe-MYE-sin], a semisynthetic derivative of *erythromycin*, is a "ketolide" antimicrobial agent (no longer used in the United States).

A. Mechanism of action

The macrolides and ketolides bind irreversibly to a site on the 50S subunit of the bacterial ribosome, thus inhibiting translocation steps of protein synthesis (Figure 30.2). They may also interfere with other steps, such as transpeptidation. Generally considered to be bacteriostatic, they may be bactericidal at higher doses. Their binding site is either identical to or in close proximity to that for *clindamycin* and *chloramphenicol.*

B. Antibacterial spectrum

1. **Erythromycin:** This drug is effective against many of the same organisms as *penicillin G* (Figure 30.10); therefore, it may be considered as an alternative in patients with *penicillin* allergy.

2. **Clarithromycin:** *Clarithromycin* has activity similar to *erythromycin,* but it is also effective against <u>Haemophilus influenzae</u> and has greater activity against intracellular pathogens such as <u>Chlamydia</u>, <u>Legionella</u>, <u>Moraxella</u>, <u>Ureaplasma</u> species, and <u>Helicobacter pylori</u>.

3. **Azithromycin:** Although less active than *erythromycin* against streptococci and staphylococci, *azithromycin* is far more active against respiratory pathogens such as <u>H. influenzae</u> and <u>Moraxella catarrhalis</u>. Extensive use of *azithromycin* has resulted in growing <u>Streptococcus pneumoniae</u> resistance.

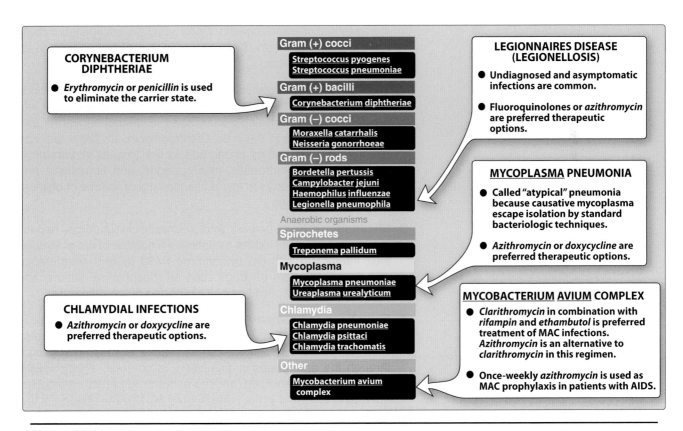

Figure 30.10
Typical therapeutic applications of macrolides.

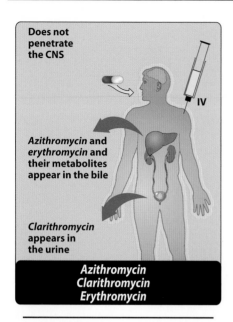

Figure 30.11
Administration and fate of the
macrolide antibiotics. CNS = central
nervous system.

	Erythro-mycin	Clarithro-mycin	Azithro-mycin	Telithro-mycin
Oral absorption	Yes	Yes	Yes	Yes
Half-life (hours)	2	3.5	68	10
Conversion to an active metabolite	No	Yes	No	Yes
Percent excretion in urine	< 15	30–50	< 10	13

Figure 30.12
Some properties of the macrolide
antibiotics.

4. **Telithromycin:** *Telithromycin* has an antimicrobial spectrum similar to that of *azithromycin*. Moreover, the structural modification within ketolides neutralizes the most common resistance mechanisms that render *macrolides* ineffective.

C. Resistance

Resistance to macrolides is associated with: 1) the inability of the organism to take up the antibiotic, 2) the presence of efflux pumps, 3) a decreased affinity of the 50S ribosomal subunit for the antibiotic due to methylation of an adenine in the 23S bacterial ribosomal RNA in gram-positive organisms, and 4) the presence of plasmid- associated *erythromycin* esterases in gram-negative organisms such as the Enterobacteriaceae. *Erythromycin* has limited clinical use due to increasing resistance. Both *clarithromycin* and *azithromycin* share some cross-resistance with *erythromycin*. *Telithromycin* may be effective against macrolide-resistant organisms.

D. Pharmacokinetics

1. **Absorption:** The *erythromycin* base is destroyed by gastric acid; thus, either enteric-coated tablets or esterified forms of the antibiotic are administered and all have adequate oral absorption (Figure 30.11). *Clarithromycin, azithromycin,* and *telithromycin* are stable in stomach acid and are readily absorbed. Food interferes with the absorption of *erythromycin* and *azithromycin* but can increase that of *clarithromycin*. *Telithromycin* is administered orally without regard to meals. *Erythromycin* and *azithromycin* are available in IV formulations.

2. **Distribution:** *Erythromycin* distributes well to all body fluids except the CSF. It is one of the few antibiotics that diffuse into prostatic fluid, and it also accumulates in macrophages. All four drugs concentrate in the liver. *Clarithromycin, azithromycin,* and *telithromycin* are widely distributed in the tissues. *Azithromycin* concentrates in neutrophils, macrophages, and fibroblasts, and serum concentrations are low. It has the largest volume of distribution of the four drugs

3. **Elimination:** *Erythromycin* and *telithromycin* undergo hepatic metabolism. They inhibit the oxidation of a number of drugs through their interaction with the cytochrome P450 system. Interference with the metabolism of drugs such as *theophylline,* statins, and numerous antiepileptics has been reported for *clarithromycin*.

4. **Excretion:** *Azithromycin* is primarily concentrated and excreted in the bile as active drug. *Erythromycin* and its metabolites are also excreted in the bile (Figure 30.11). Partial reabsorption occurs through the enterohepatic circulation. In contrast, *clarithromycin* is hepatically metabolized, and the active drug and its metabolites are mainly excreted in the urine (Figure 30.12). The dosage of this drug should be adjusted in patients with renal impairment.

E. Adverse effects

1. **Gastric distress and motility:** Gastrointestinal upset is the most common adverse effect of the macrolides and may lead to poor

patient compliance (especially with *erythromycin*). The other macrolides seem to be better tolerated (Figure 30.13). Higher doses of *erythromycin* lead to smooth muscle contractions that result in the movement of gastric contents to the duodenum, an adverse effect sometimes employed for the treatment of gastroparesis or postoperative ileus.

2. **Cholestatic jaundice:** This adverse effect occurs most commonly with the estolate form of *erythromycin* (not used in the United States); however, it has been reported with other formulations and other agents in this class.

3. **Ototoxicity:** Transient deafness has been associated with *erythromycin,* especially at high dosages. *Azithromycin* has also been associated with irreversible sensorineural hearing loss.

4. **QT$_c$ prolongation:** Macrolides and ketolides may prolong the QT$_c$ interval and should be used with caution in those patients with pro-arrhythmic conditions or concomitant use of proarrhythmic agents.

5. **Contraindications:** Patients with hepatic dysfunction should be treated cautiously with *erythromycin*, *telithromycin*, or *azithromycin*, because these drugs accumulate in the liver. Severe hepatotoxicity with *telithromycin* has limited its use, given the availability of alternative therapies.

6. **Drug Interactions:** *Erythromycin*, *telithromycin*, and *clarithromycin* inhibit the hepatic metabolism of a number of drugs, which can lead to toxic accumulation of these compounds (Figure 30.14). An interaction with *digoxin* may occur. One theory to explain this interaction is that the antibiotic eliminates a species of intestinal flora that ordinarily inactivates *digoxin*, leading to greater reabsorption of *digoxin* from the enterohepatic circulation.

Figure 30.13
Some adverse effects of macrolide antibiotics.

GI disturbance

Jaundice

Ototoxicity

QTc prolongation

VI. FIDAXOMICIN

Fidaxomicin [fye-DAX-oh-MYE-sin] is a macrocyclic antibiotic with a structure similar to the macrolides; however, it has a unique mechanism of action. *Fidaxomicin* acts on the sigma subunit of RNA polymerase, thereby disrupting bacterial transcription, terminating protein synthesis and resulting in cell death in susceptible organisms. *Fidaxomicin* has a very narrow spectrum of activity limited to gram-positive aerobes and anaerobes. While it possesses activity against staphylococci and enterococci, it is used primarily for its bactericidal activity against <u>Clostridium difficile</u>. Because of the unique target site, cross-resistance with other antibiotic classes has not been documented. Following oral administration, *fidaxomicin* has minimal systemic absorption and primarily remains within the gastrointestinal tract. This is ideal for the treatment of <u>C. difficile</u> infection, which occurs in the gut. The most common adverse effects include nausea, vomiting, and abdominal pain. Anemia and neutropenia have been observed infrequently. Hypersensitivity reactions including angioedema, dyspnea, and pruritus have occurred. *Fidaxomicin* should be used with caution in patients with a macrolide allergy, as they may be at increased risk for hypersensitivity.

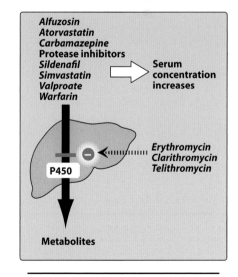

Figure 30.14
Inhibition of the cytochrome P450 system by *erythromycin*, *clarithromycin*, and *telithromycin*.

VII. CHLORAMPHENICOL

The use of *chloramphenicol* [klor-am-FEN-i-kole], a broad-spectrum antibiotic, is restricted to life-threatening infections for which no alternatives exist.

A. Mechanism of action

Chloramphenicol binds reversibly to the bacterial 50S ribosomal subunit and inhibits protein synthesis at the peptidyl transferase reaction (Figure 30.2). Because of some similarity of mammalian mitochondrial ribosomes to those of bacteria, protein and ATP synthesis in these organelles may be inhibited at high circulating *chloramphenicol* concentrations, producing bone marrow toxicity. [Note: The oral formulation of *chloramphenicol* was removed from the US market due to this toxicity.]

B. Antibacterial spectrum

Chloramphenicol is active against many types of microorganisms including chlamydiae, rickettsiae, spirochetes, and anaerobes. The drug is primarily bacteriostatic, but it may exert bactericidal activity depending on the dose and organism.

C. Resistance

Resistance is conferred by the presence of enzymes that inactivate *chloramphenicol*. Other mechanisms include decreased ability to penetrate the organism and ribosomal binding site alterations.

D. Pharmacokinetics

Chloramphenicol is administered intravenously and is widely distributed throughout the body. It reaches therapeutic concentrations in the CSF. *Chloramphenicol* primarily undergoes hepatic metabolism to an inactive glucuronide, which is secreted by the renal tubule and eliminated in the urine. Dose reductions are necessary in patients with liver dysfunction or cirrhosis. *Chloramphenicol* is also secreted into breast milk and should be avoided in breastfeeding mothers.

E. Adverse effects

1. **Anemias:** Patients may experience dose-related anemia, hemolytic anemia (observed in patients with glucose-6-phosphate dehydrogenase deficiency), and aplastic anemia. [Note: Aplastic anemia is independent of dose and may occur after therapy has ceased.]

2. **Gray baby syndrome:** Neonates have a low capacity to glucuronidate the antibiotic, and they have underdeveloped renal function, which decreases their ability to excrete the drug. This leads to drug accumulation to concentrations that interfere with the function of mitochondrial ribosomes, causing poor feeding, depressed breathing, cardiovascular collapse, cyanosis (hence the term "gray baby"), and death. Adults who have received very high doses of *chloramphenicol* may also exhibit this toxicity.

3. **Drug interactions:** *Chloramphenicol* inhibits some of the hepatic mixed-function oxidases, preventing the metabolism of drugs such as *warfarin* and *phenytoin*, which may potentiate their effects.

VIII. CLINDAMYCIN

Clindamycin [klin-da-MYE-sin] has a mechanism of action that is similar to that of the macrolides. *Clindamycin* is used primarily in the treatment of infections caused by gram-positive organisms, including MRSA and streptococcus, and anaerobic bacteria. Resistance mechanisms are the same as those for *erythromycin,* and cross-resistance has been described. C. difficile is resistant to *clindamycin*, and the utility of *clindamycin* for gram-negative anaerobes (for example, Bacteroides sp.) is decreasing due to increasing resistance. *Clindamycin* is available in both IV and oral formulations, but use of oral *clindamycin* is limited by gastrointestinal intolerance. It distributes well into all body fluids but exhibits poor entry into the CSF. *Clindamycin* undergoes extensive oxidative metabolism to active and inactive products and is excreted into bile and urine. Low urinary excretion of active drug limits its clinical utility for urinary tract infections (Figure 30.15). Accumulation has been reported in patients with either severe renal impairment or hepatic failure. In addition to skin rash, the most common adverse effect is diarrhea, which may represent a serious pseudomembranous colitis caused by overgrowth of C. difficile. Oral administration of either *metronidazole* or *vancomycin* is usually effective in the treatment of C. difficile infection.

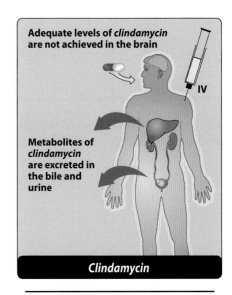

Figure 30.15
Administration and fate of *clindamycin.*

IX. QUINUPRISTIN/DALFOPRISTIN

Quinupristin/dalfopristin [KWIN-yoo-pris-tin/DAL-foh-pris-tin] is a mixture of two streptogramins in a ratio of 30 to 70, respectively. Due to significant adverse effects, this combination drug is normally reserved for the treatment of severe infections caused by *vancomycin*-resistant Enterococcus faecium (VRE) in the absence of other therapeutic options.

A. Mechanism of action

Each component of this combination drug binds to a separate site on the 50S bacterial ribosome. *Dalfopristin* disrupts elongation by interfering with the addition of new amino acids to the peptide chain. *Quinupristin* prevents elongation similar to the macrolides and causes release of incomplete peptide chains. Thus, they synergistically interrupt protein synthesis. The combination drug has bactericidal activity against most susceptible organisms and has a long PAE.

B. Antibacterial spectrum

Quinupristin/dalfopristin is active primarily against gram-positive cocci, including those resistant to other antibiotics. Its primary use is for the treatment of E. faecium infections, including VRE strains, against which it is bacteriostatic. The drug is not effective against E. faecalis.

C. Resistance

Enzymatic processes commonly account for resistance to these agents. For example, the presence of a ribosomal enzyme that methylates the target bacterial 23S ribosomal RNA site can interfere in *quinupristin* binding. In some cases, the enzymatic modification can change the action from bactericidal to bacteriostatic. Plasmid-associated acetyltransferase inactivates *dalfopristin.* An active efflux pump can also decrease levels of the antibiotics in bacteria.

D. Pharmacokinetics

Quinupristin/dalfopristin is available intravenously. It does not achieve therapeutic concentrations in CSF. Both compounds undergo hepatic metabolism, with excretion mainly in the feces.

E. Adverse effects

Venous irritation commonly occurs when *quinupristin/dalfopristin* is administered through a peripheral rather than a central line. Hyperbilirubinemia occurs in about 25% of patients, resulting from a competition with the antibiotic for excretion. Arthralgia and myalgia have been reported when higher doses are administered. *Quinupristin/dalfopristin* inhibits the cytochrome P450 CYP3A4 isoenzyme, and concomitant administration with drugs that are metabolized by this pathway may lead to toxicities.

X. OXAZOLIDINONES

Linezolid [lih-NEH-zo-lid] and *tedizolid* [ted-eye-ZOE-lid] are synthetic oxazolidinones developed to combat gram-positive organisms, including resistant isolates such as *methicillin*-resistant <u>Staphylococcus aureus</u>, VRE, and *penicillin*-resistant streptococci.

A. Mechanism of action

Linezolid and *tedizolid* bind to the bacterial 23S ribosomal RNA of the 50S subunit, thereby inhibiting the formation of the 70S initiation complex (Figure 30.2) and translation of bacterial proteins.

B. Antibacterial spectrum

The antibacterial action of the oxazolidinones is directed primarily against gram-positive organisms such as staphylococci, streptococci, and enterococci, <u>Corynebacterium</u> species and <u>Listeria monocytogenes</u>. It is also moderately active against <u>Mycobacterium tuberculosis</u> (Figure 30.16). The main clinical use of *linezolid* and *tedizolid* is to treat infections caused by drug-resistant gram-positive organisms. Like other agents that interfere with bacterial protein synthesis, *linezolid* and *tedizolid* are bacteriostatic; however, *linezolid* has bactericidal activity against streptococci. *Linezolid* is an alternative to *daptomycin* for infections caused by VRE. Because they are bacteriostatic, the oxazolidinones are not recommended as first-line treatment for MRSA bacteremia.

C. Resistance

Resistance primarily occurs via reduced binding at the target site. Reduced susceptibility and resistance have been reported in <u>S. aureus</u> and <u>Enterococcus</u> sp. Cross-resistance with other protein synthesis inhibitors does not occur.

D. Pharmacokinetics

Linezolid and *tedizolid* are well absorbed after oral administration. IV formulations are also available. These drugs distribute widely

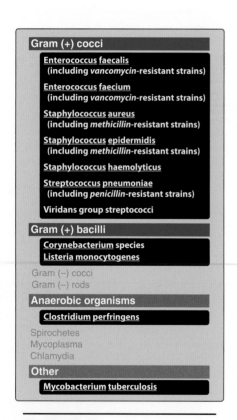

Gram (+) cocci

<u>Enterococcus faecalis</u>
(including *vancomycin*-resistant strains)

<u>Enterococcus faecium</u>
(including *vancomycin*-resistant strains)

<u>Staphylococcus aureus</u>
(including *methicillin*-resistant strains)

<u>Staphylococcus epidermidis</u>
(including *methicillin*-resistant strains)

<u>Staphylococcus haemolyticus</u>

<u>Streptococcus pneumoniae</u>
(including *penicillin*-resistant strains)

Viridans group streptococci

Gram (+) bacilli

<u>Corynebacterium</u> species
<u>Listeria monocytogenes</u>

Gram (–) cocci
Gram (–) rods

Anaerobic organisms

<u>Clostridium perfringens</u>

Spirochetes
Mycoplasma
Chlamydia

Other

<u>Mycobacterium tuberculosis</u>

Figure 30.16
Antimicrobial spectrum of oxazolidinones.

throughout the body. Although the metabolic pathway of *linezolid* has not been fully determined, it is known that it is metabolized via oxidation to two inactive metabolites. The drug is excreted both by renal and nonrenal routes. *Tedizolid* is metabolized by sulfation, and the majority of elimination occurs via the liver, and drug is mainly excreted in the feces. No dose adjustments are required for either agent for renal or hepatic dysfunction.

E. Adverse effects

The most common adverse effects are gastrointestinal upset, nausea, diarrhea, headache, and rash. Thrombocytopenia has been reported, usually in patients taking the drug for longer than 10 days. *Linezolid* and *tedizolid* possess nonselective monoamine oxidase activity and may lead to serotonin syndrome if given concomitantly with large quantities of tyramine-containing foods, selective serotonin reuptake inhibitors, or monoamine oxidase inhibitors. The condition is reversible when the drug is discontinued. Irreversible peripheral neuropathies and optic neuritis causing blindness have been associated with greater than 28 days of use, limiting utility for extended-duration treatments.

Study Questions

Choose the ONE best answer.

30.1 Which of the following adverse effects is often employed as a therapeutic use for erythromycin?

A. QTc prolongation
B. Increased gastrointestinal motility
C. Photosensitivity
D. Deposition in bone

Correct answer = B. Macrolides, but especially erythromycin, cause GI distress and increase motility of the GI tract, which is often used to treat gastroparesis and/or postoperative ileus. QTc prolongation is an adverse effect of erythromycin but not one employed therapeutically. Photosensitivity and deposition in bone are adverse effects of tetracyclines.

30.2 Which of the following describes the mechanism of action of tetracycline antibiotics?

A. Bind the 30S subunit of the bacterial ribosome, preventing binding of tRNA to the mRNA–ribosome complex.
B. Bind the 30S ribosomal subunit, interfering with assembly of the functional ribosomal apparatus.
C. Bind irreversibly to a site on the 50S subunit of the bacterial ribosome, inhibiting translocation steps of protein synthesis.
D. Bind the bacterial 23S ribosomal RNA of the 50S subunit, inhibiting the formation of the 70S initiation complex.

Correct answer = A. Tetracyclines enter susceptible organisms via passive diffusion and also by an energy-dependent transport protein mechanism unique to the bacterial inner cytoplasmic membrane. The drugs bind reversibly to the 30S subunit of the bacterial ribosome. This action prevents binding of tRNA to the mRNA–ribosome complex, thereby inhibiting bacterial protein synthesis. B is the mechanism for aminoglycosides, C is the mechanism for macrolides, and D is the mechanism for oxazolidinones.

30.3 Linezolid would be a good choice for antibiotic treatment in which of the following patient scenarios?

A. Bacteremia caused by Staphylococcus aureus
B. Urinary tract infection caused by Escherichia coli
C. Pneumonia caused by drug-resistant Streptococcus pneumoniae
D. Diabetic foot infection caused by Pseudomonas aeruginosa

Correct answer = C. Linezolid does have coverage against resistant S. pneumoniae. It is not an optimal choice for treatment of bacteremia. Linezolid also does not have gram-negative coverage against E. coli and P. aeruginosa.

30.4 After 5 days of clindamycin treatment for a skin infection, a patient develops diarrhea (10 watery stools/day), severe abdominal pain, and fever. Which of the following organisms would you be concerned about as the causative pathogen of diarrhea?

A. Escherichia coli
B. Bacteroides fragilis
C. Staphylococcus aureus
D. Clostridium difficile

Correct answer = D. Clindamycin use has been associated with Clostridium difficile–associated diarrhea. This infection should be considered in a patient who presents with diarrhea while on clindamycin.

30.5 Which of the following statements accurately describes the difference in spectrum of activity between erythromycin and azithromycin?

A. Azithromycin has better activity against respiratory pathogens such as Haemophilus influenzae and Moraxella catarrhalis but less potent activity against staphylococci and streptococci.
B. Erythromycin has the same activity as azithromycin against gram-positives and gram-negatives.
C. Azithromycin has better activity against staphylococci and streptococci compared to erythromycin.
D. Erythromycin has better activity against gram-negatives such as H. influenza.

Correct answer = A. Erythromycin has better activity against gram-positive organisms, so B and C are incorrect. D is incorrect as azithromycin has better activity against H. influenza.

30.6 Which of the following antibiotic agents should not be given to children less than 8 years of age due to its deposition in bone and teeth?

A. Azithromycin
B. Doxycycline
C. Linezolid
D. Quinupristin/dalfopristin

Correct answer = B. Tetracyclines are contraindicated in this age group because they are deposited in tissues undergoing calcification, such as teeth and bone, and can stunt growth.

30.7 A 77-year-old woman was started on antibiotics for pneumonia treatment. After 3 days of antibiotic therapy, the serum creatinine doubled. Which of the following antibiotics is most likely responsible for this increase in serum creatinine?

A. Doxycycline
B. Clarithromycin
C. Tobramycin
D. Linezolid

Correct answer = C. Aminoglycosides such as tobramycin accumulate in the proximal tubular cells of the kidney and disrupt calcium-mediated transport processes. This results in kidney damage ranging from mild, reversible renal impairment to severe, potentially irreversible acute tubular necrosis. Nephrotoxicity is not commonly associated with tetracyclines, macrolides or oxazolidinones.

30.8 A 24-year-old pregnant woman was diagnosed with community-acquired pneumonia and will be managed in the outpatient setting. Which antibiotic is a safe option for this patient to treat her pneumonia?

A. Azithromycin
B. Doxycycline
C. Fidaxomicin
D. Gentamicin

Correct answer = A. Azithromycin is available orally and considered safe in pregnancy. Doxycycline should not be used in pregnancy due to its ability to cross the placenta and affect bone and skeletal development in the fetus. Fidaxomicin does not reach therapeutic concentrations in serum or at this site of infection. It concentrates in the gut. Gentamicin crosses the placental barrier and may accumulate in fetal plasma and amniotic fluid. It would also not be used clinically in this outpatient scenario.

30.9 Parents of a 1-month-old baby are told their child has developed "gray baby syndrome." Which of the following antibiotics did the baby likely receive?

A. Tobramycin
B. Linezolid
C. Erythromycin
D. Chloramphenicol

Correct answer = D. Gray baby syndrome is an adverse effect caused by chloramphenicol in neonates due to their underdeveloped renal function and low capacity to glucuronidate the antibiotic. The other agents do not undergo this glucuronidation.

30.10 Aminoglycosides are commonly used for their concentration-dependent bactericidal activity against which group of organisms?

    A. Gram-positive aerobes

    B. Gram-negative aerobes

    C. Gram-positive anaerobes

    D. Gram-negative anaerobes

Correct answer = B. Although aminoglycosides (such as gentamicin) are sometimes used synergistically against gram-positive aerobes, this is not their most common use. They are typically used for their activity against gram-negative aerobes. Aminoglycosides do not have good anaerobic activity.

Quinolones, Folic Acid Antagonists, and Urinary Tract Antiseptics

Kenneth P. Klinker and Joseph Pardo

31

I. FLUOROQUINOLONES

Discovery of quinolone antimicrobials led to the development of numerous compounds utilized in clinical practice. Following synthesis of *nalidixic acid* in the early 1960s, continued modification of the quinolone nucleus expanded the spectrum of activity, improved pharmacokinetics, and stabilized compounds against common mechanisms of resistance. Due to these enhancements, quinolone antimicrobials were rapidly integrated into human and agricultural medicine. Unfortunately, overuse resulted in rising rates of resistance in gram-negative and gram-positive organisms, increased frequency of <u>Clostridium difficile</u> infections, and identification of numerous untoward adverse effects. Consequently, these agents have been relegated to second-line options for various indications. This chapter reviews key characteristics of fluoroquinolones and their role in therapy. The fluoroquinolones and other antibiotics discussed in this chapter are listed in Figure 31.1.

A. Mechanism of action

Most bacterial species maintain two distinct type II topoisomerases that assist with deoxyribonucleic acid (DNA) replication, DNA gyrase, and topoisomerase IV. DNA gyrase is responsible for reducing torsional stress ahead of replicating forks by breaking double-strand DNA and introducing negative supercoils. Topoisomerase IV assists in separating daughter chromosomes once replication is completed. Following cell wall entry through porin channels, fluoroquinolones bind to these enzymes and interfere with DNA ligation. This interference increases the number of permanent chromosomal breaks, triggering cell lysis. In general, fluoroquinolones have different targets for gram-negative (DNA gyrase) and gram-positive organisms (topoisomerase IV), resulting in rapid cell death.

FLUOROQUINOLONES
Ciprofloxacin CIPRO
Delafloxacin BAXDELA
Gemifloxacin FACTIVE
Levofloxacin LEVAQUIN
Moxifloxacin AVELOX, MOXEZA, VIGAMOX
Ofloxacin GENERIC ONLY
INHIBITORS OF FOLATE SYNTHESIS
Mafenide SULFAMYLON
Silver sulfadiazine SILVADENE, SSD, THERMAZENE
Sulfadiazine GENERIC ONLY
Sulfasalazine AZULFIDINE
INHIBITORS OF FOLATE REDUCTION
Pyrimethamine DARAPRIM
Trimethoprim PRIMSOL, TRIMPEX
COMBINATION OF INHIBITORS OF FOLATE SYNTHESIS AND REDUCTION
Cotrimoxazole (trimethoprim + sulfamethoxazole) BACTRIM, SEPTRA
URINARY TRACT ANTISEPTICS
Methenamine HIPREX, UREX
Nitrofurantoin MACROBID, MACRODANTIN

Figure 31.1
Summary of drugs described in this chapter.

B. Antimicrobial spectrum

Fluoroquinolones are bactericidal and exhibit area-under-the-curve/minimum inhibitory concentration (AUC/MIC)-dependent killing. A major facet of their development centered on improving microbiologic coverage. Modifications to the quinolone nucleus steadily improved topoisomerase inhibitory activity and facilitated bacterial cell wall penetration. These changes enhanced activity against a variety of pathogens including aerobic gram-negative and gram-positive organisms, atypical organisms (for example, Chlamydia, Legionella, and Mycoplasma spp.), and anaerobes. Based on the impact of these structural changes, fluoroquinolones are often classified according to spectrum of activity.

First-generation compounds (for example, *nalidixic acid*) were narrow spectrum agents with activity against aerobic gram-negative bacilli, mostly Enterobacteriaceae. Second-generation compounds (for example, *ciprofloxacin*) exhibit improved intracellular penetration and broadened coverage, which includes Enterobacteriaceae, Pseudomonas aeruginosa, Haemophilus influenzae, Neisseria spp., Chlamydia spp., and Legionella spp. Third-generation compounds (for example, *levofloxacin*) maintain the bacterial spectrum of second-generation agents, with improved activity against Streptococcus spp., including S. pneumoniae, *methicillin*-susceptible Staphylococcus aureus, Stenotrophomonas maltophilia, and Mycobacterium spp. Fourth-generation compounds (*moxifloxacin*, *gemifloxacin*, and *delafloxacin*) have enhanced gram-positive activity, including Staphylococcus and Streptococcus spp. *Delafloxacin* has activity against *methicillin*-resistant Staphylococcus aureus (MRSA) and Enterococcus faecalis. Further, *delafloxacin* and *moxifloxacin* have activity against Bacteroides fragilis and Prevotella spp., while maintaining activity against Enterobacteriaceae and Haemophilus influenzae. From this group, only *delafloxacin* has activity against Pseudomonas aeruginosa. Lastly, these agents maintain atypical coverage, with *moxifloxacin* and *delafloxacin* showing activity against Mycobacteria spp. Common therapeutic applications of fluoroquinolones are shown in Figure 31.2.

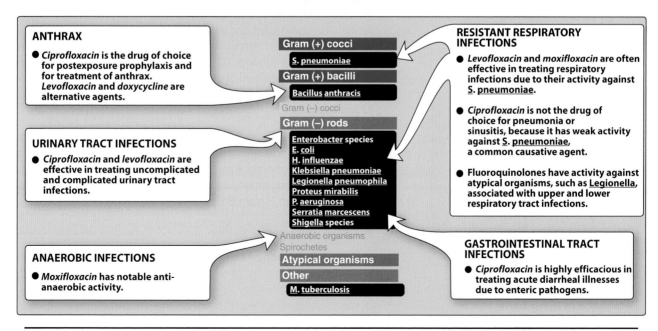

Figure 31.2
Typical therapeutic applications of fluoroquinolones.

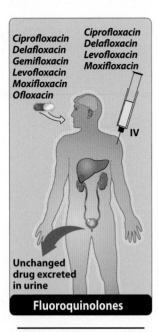

Figure 31.3
Administration and fate
of the fluoroquinolones.

C. Resistance

Numerous mechanisms of fluoroquinolone resistance exist in clinical pathogens. High-level fluoroquinolone resistance is primarily driven by chromosomal mutations within topoisomerases, although decreased entry, efflux systems, and modifying enzymes play a role. Mechanisms responsible for resistance include the following:

1. **Altered target binding:** Mutations in bacterial genes encoding DNA gyrase or topoisomerase IV (for example, gyrA or parC) alter target site structure and reduce binding efficiency of fluoroquinolones.

2. **Decreased accumulation:** Reduced intracellular concentration is linked to 1) a reduction in membrane permeability or 2) efflux pumps. Alterations in membrane permeability are mediated through a reduction in outer membrane porin proteins, thus limiting drug access to topoisomerases. Efflux pumps actively remove fluoroquinolones from the cell.

3. **Fluoroquinolone degradation:** An aminoglycoside acetyltransferase variant can acetylate fluoroquinolones, rendering them inactive.

D. Pharmacokinetics

1. **Absorption:** Fluoroquinolones are well absorbed after oral administration, with *levofloxacin* and *moxifloxacin* having a bioavailability that exceeds 90% (Figure 31.3). Ingestion of fluoroquinolones with *sucralfate*, aluminum- or magnesium-containing antacids, or dietary supplements containing iron or zinc can reduce the absorption. Calcium and other divalent cations also interfere with the absorption of these agents (Figure 31.4).

2. **Distribution:** Binding to plasma proteins ranges from 20% to 84%. Fluoroquinolones distribute well into all tissues and body fluids. Concentrations are high in bone, urine (except *moxifloxacin*), kidney, prostatic tissue (but not prostatic fluid), and lungs as compared to serum. Penetration into cerebrospinal fluid is good, and these agents may be considered in certain central nervous system (CNS) infections. Accumulation in macrophages and polymorphonuclear leukocytes results in activity against intracellular organisms such as <u>Listeria</u>, <u>Chlamydia</u>, and <u>Mycobacterium</u>.

3. **Elimination:** Most fluoroquinolones are excreted renally. Therefore, dosage adjustments are needed in renal dysfunction. *Moxifloxacin* is metabolized primarily by the liver, and while there is some renal excretion, no dose adjustment is required for renal impairment (see Figure 31.3).

E. Adverse reactions

In general, fluoroquinolones are well tolerated (Figure 31.5). Common adverse effects leading to discontinuation are nausea, vomiting, headache, and dizziness. These agents carry boxed warnings for tendinitis, tendon rupture, peripheral neuropathy, and CNS effects

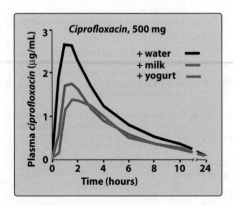

Figure 31.4
Effect of dietary calcium on the
absorption of *ciprofloxacin*.

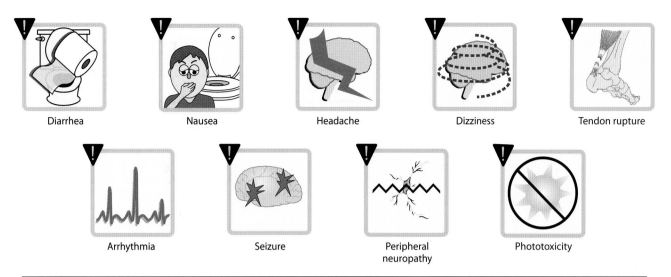

Figure 31.5
Some adverse reactions to fluoroquinolones.

(hallucinations, anxiety, insomnia, confusion, and seizures). Patients taking fluoroquinolones are at risk for phototoxicity resulting in exaggerated sunburn reactions. Patients should use sunscreen and avoid excessive exposure to ultraviolet (UV) light. Arthropathy is uncommon, but arthralgia and arthritis are reported with fluoroquinolone use in pediatric patients. Use in the pediatric population should be limited to distinct clinical scenarios (for example, cystic fibrosis exacerbation). Hepatotoxicity or blood glucose disturbances (usually in diabetic patients receiving oral hypoglycemic agents or insulin) have been observed. Identification of any of these events should result in prompt removal of the agent. Fluoroquinolones may prolong the QT_c interval, and these agents should be avoided in patients predisposed to arrhythmias or taking medication associated with QT prolongation. *Ciprofloxacin* inhibits P450 1A2- and 3A4-mediated metabolism. Serum concentrations of medications such as *theophylline, tizanidine, warfarin, ropinirole, duloxetine, caffeine, sildenafil,* and *zolpidem* may be increased (Figure 31.6).

F. Examples of clinically useful fluoroquinolones

Due to increasing resistance and boxed warnings, fluoroquinolones should be used with caution in select circumstances. They may be considered in patients who do not tolerate other agents (for example, severe beta-lactam allergies) or as definitive therapy once susceptibilities are available. Listed below are potential indications for these agents.

1. **Ciprofloxacin:** *Ciprofloxacin* [SIP-roe-FLOX-a-sin] has good activity against gram-negative bacilli, including P. aeruginosa. *Ciprofloxacin* is used in the treatment of traveler's diarrhea, typhoid fever, and anthrax. It is a second-line agent for infections arising from intra-abdominal, lung, skin, or urine sources. Of note, high-dose therapy should be employed when treating Pseudomonas infections.

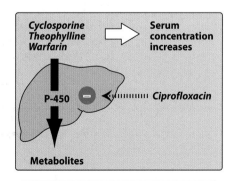

Figure 31.6
Drug interactions with *ciprofloxacin.*

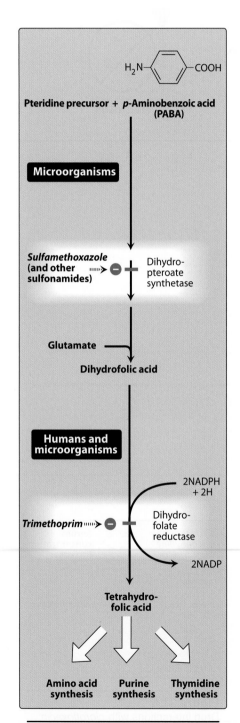

Figure 31.7
Inhibition of tetrahydrofolate synthesis by sulfonamides and *trimethoprim*.

2. **Levofloxacin:** *Levofloxacin* [leev-oh-FLOX-a-sin] has similar activity to *ciprofloxacin* and they are often interchanged when managing gram-negative bacilli, including P. aeruginosa. *Levofloxacin* has enhanced activity against S. pneumoniae and is first-line therapy for community-acquired pneumonia (CAP). It is a second-line agent for the treatment of S. maltophilia.

3. **Moxifloxacin:** *Moxifloxacin* [mox-ee-FLOX-a-sin] has enhanced activity against gram-positive organisms (for example, S. pneumoniae), gram-negative anaerobes, and Mycobacterium spp. The drug may be used for CAP, but not hospital-acquired pneumonia due to poor coverage of P. aeruginosa. It may be considered for mild-to-moderate intra-abdominal infections, but should be avoided if patients have fluoroquinolone exposure within previous three months, due to increasing B. fragilis resistance. *Moxifloxacin* may be considered as a second-line agent for management of drug-susceptible tuberculosis.

4. **Gemifloxacin:** *Gemifloxacin* [gem-ee-FLOX-a-sin] is indicated for management of community-acquired respiratory infections. Unlike the other compounds, it is only available as an oral formulation.

5. **Delafloxacin:** *Delafloxacin* [del-a-FLOX-a-sin] has improved activity against gram-positive cocci, including MRSA and Enterococcus spp. Due to its spectrum of activity, it is an option for managing acute bacterial skin and skin structure infections. It is available as an intravenous and oral formulation.

II. FOLATE ANTAGONISTS

Folic acid is a coenzyme essential in the synthesis of ribonucleic acid (RNA), DNA, and certain amino acids. In the absence of folate, cells cannot grow or divide. Humans use dietary folate to synthesize the critical folate derivative, tetrahydrofolic acid. By contrast, many bacteria are impermeable to folate derivatives, and rely on their ability to synthesize folate de novo (Figure 31.7). Sulfonamides (sulfa drugs) are a family of antibiotics that inhibit de novo synthesis of folate. A second type of folate antagonist, *trimethoprim*, prevents microorganisms from converting dihydrofolic acid to tetrahydrofolic acid. Thus, both sulfonamides and *trimethoprim* interfere with the ability of an infecting bacterium to perform DNA synthesis and other essential cellular functions. The combination of the sulfonamide *sulfamethoxazole* with *trimethoprim* (the generic name for the combination is *cotrimoxazole*) provides a synergistic effect.

III. SULFONAMIDES

Sulfa drugs were among the first antibiotics used in clinical practice. Today, they are seldom prescribed alone except in developing countries, where they are employed because of low cost and efficacy.

A. Mechanism of action

Microorganisms use the enzyme dihydropteroate synthetase to create dihydrofolic acid from the precursor molecule *p*-aminobenzoic acid (PABA). Sulfonamides are synthetic analogs of PABA. Because of their structural similarity, sulfonamides compete with PABA to inhibit dihydropteroate synthetase and the genesis of bacterial dihydrofolic acid (see Figure 31.7). These agents, including *cotrimoxazole*, are bacteriostatic.

B. Antibacterial spectrum

Sulfa drugs have in vitro activity against gram-negative and gram-positive organisms. Common organisms include Enterobacteriaceae, Haemophilus influenzae, Streptococcus spp., Staphylococcus spp., and Nocardia. Additionally, *sulfadiazine* [sul-fa-DYE-a-zeen] in combination with the dihydrofolate reductase inhibitor *pyrimethamine* [py-ri-METH-a-meen] is the preferred treatment for toxoplasmosis.

C. Resistance

Bacteria that obtain folate from their environment are naturally resistant to sulfa drugs. Acquired bacterial resistance to the sulfa drugs can arise from plasmid transfers or random mutations. Resistance may be due to 1) altered dihydropteroate synthetase, 2) decreased cellular permeability to sulfa drugs, or 3) enhanced production of the natural substrate, PABA. [Note: Organisms resistant to one member of this drug family are resistant to all.]

D. Pharmacokinetics

1. **Absorption:** Most sulfa drugs are well absorbed following oral administration (Figure 31.8). An exception is *sulfasalazine* [sul-fa-SAL-a-zeen]. It is not absorbed when administered orally or as a suppository and, therefore, is reserved for treatment of chronic inflammatory bowel diseases. [Note: Intestinal flora split *sulfasalazine* into sulfapyridine and 5-aminosalicylate, with the latter exerting the anti-inflammatory effect. Absorption of sulfapyridine can lead to toxicity in patients who are slow acetylators.] Intravenous sulfonamides are generally reserved for patients who are unable to take oral preparations or have severe infections. Because of the risk of sensitization, sulfa drugs are not usually applied topically. However, in burn units, *silver sulfadiazine* [sul-fa-DYE-ah-zeen] or *mafenide* [mah-FEN-ide] *acetate* (α-amino-p-toluenesulfonamide) creams have been effective in reducing burn-associated sepsis because they prevent colonization of bacteria. [Note: *Silver sulfadiazine* is preferred because *mafenide* produces pain on application and its absorption may contribute to acid–base disturbances.]

2. **Distribution:** Sulfa drugs are bound to serum albumin in circulation and widely distribute throughout body tissues. Sulfa drugs penetrate well into cerebrospinal fluid (even in the absence of inflammation) and cross the placental barrier to enter fetal tissues.

3. **Metabolism:** Sulfa drugs are acetylated and conjugated primarily in the liver. The acetylated product is devoid of antimicrobial activity but retains the toxic potential to precipitate at neutral or acidic pH. This causes crystalluria ("stone formation"; see below) and potential damage to the kidney.

4. **Excretion:** Unchanged sulfa drug and metabolites are eliminated via glomerular filtration and secretion, requiring dose adjustments with renal impairment. Sulfonamides may be eliminated in breast milk.

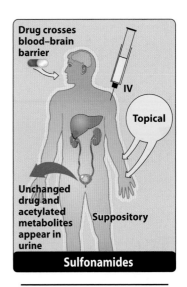

Figure 31.8
Administration and fate of the sulfonamides.

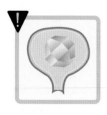

Crystalluria

Hypersensitivity

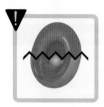

Hemolytic anemia

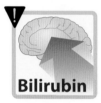

Kernicterus

Bilirubin

Figure 31.9
Some adverse reactions to sulfonamides.

E. Adverse effects

1. **Crystalluria:** Nephrotoxicity may develop as a result of crystalluria (Figure 31.9). Adequate hydration and alkalinization of urine can prevent the problem by reducing the concentration of drug and promoting its ionization.

2. **Hypersensitivity:** Hypersensitivity reactions, such as rashes, angioedema, or Stevens-Johnson syndrome, may occur. When patients report previous sulfa allergies, it is paramount to acquire a description of the reaction to direct appropriate therapy.

3. **Hematopoietic disturbances:** Hemolytic anemia is encountered in patients with glucose-6-phosphate dehydrogenase (G6PD) deficiency. Granulocytopenia and thrombocytopenia can also occur. Fatal reactions have been reported from associated agranulocytosis, aplastic anemia, and other blood dyscrasias.

4. **Kernicterus:** Bilirubin-associated brain damage (kernicterus) may occur in newborns, because sulfa drugs displace bilirubin from binding sites on serum albumin. The bilirubin is then free to pass into the CNS, because the blood–brain barrier is not fully developed.

5. **Drug potentiation:** *Sulfamethoxazole* potentiates the anticoagulant effect of *warfarin* due to inhibition of CYP2C9, resulting in reduced clearance of *warfarin*. Sulfonamides may also displace *warfarin* from binding sites on serum albumin. Serum *methotrexate* levels may rise through protein binding displacement. Other CYP2C9 substrates, such as *phenytoin*, may have increased concentrations when given with sulfonamides.

6. **Contraindications:** Due to the danger of kernicterus, sulfa drugs should be avoided in newborns and infants less than 2 months of age, as well as in pregnant women at term. Sulfonamides should not be given to patients receiving *methenamine*, since they can crystallize in the presence of formaldehyde produced by this agent.

IV. TRIMETHOPRIM

Trimethoprim [try-METH-oh-prim], a potent inhibitor of bacterial dihydrofolate reductase, was initially available in combination with the sulfonamide *sulfamethoxazole* [sul-fa-meth-OX-a-zole], and later approved for use as a single agent. Today, *trimethoprim* is most commonly used in combination with *sulfamethoxazole*.

A. Mechanism of action

Trimethoprim is a potent inhibitor of bacterial dihydrofolate reductase (see Figure 31.7). Inhibition of this enzyme prevents the formation of the metabolically active form of folic acid, tetrahydrofolic acid, and thus, interferes with normal bacterial cell functions. *Trimethoprim* binds to bacterial dihydrofolate reductase more readily than it does to human dihydrofolate reductase, which accounts for the selective toxicity of the drug.

B. Antibacterial spectrum

The antibacterial spectrum of *trimethoprim* is similar to that of *sulfamethoxazole*. However, *trimethoprim* is 20- to 50-fold more potent than the sulfonamides. *Trimethoprim* may be used alone in the treatment of urinary tract infections (UTIs) and in the treatment of bacterial prostatitis (although fluoroquinolones and *cotrimoxazole* are preferred).

C. Resistance

Resistance in gram-negative bacteria is due to the presence of an altered dihydrofolate reductase that has a lower affinity for *trimethoprim*. Efflux pumps and decreased permeability to the drug may play a role.

D. Pharmacokinetics

Trimethoprim is rapidly absorbed following oral administration. Because the drug is a weak base, higher concentrations of *trimethoprim* are achieved in the relatively acidic prostatic and vaginal fluids. The drug is widely distributed into body tissues and fluids, including penetration into the cerebrospinal fluid. *Trimethoprim* undergoes some O-demethylation, but 60% to 80% is renally excreted unchanged.

E. Adverse effects

Trimethoprim can produce the effects of folic acid deficiency. These effects include megaloblastic anemia, leukopenia, and granulocytopenia, especially in pregnant patients and those with nutrient-poor diets. These blood disorders may be reversed by simultaneous administration of *folinic acid* (also known as *leucovorin*), which does not enter bacteria. *Trimethoprim* has a potassium-sparing effect and may cause hyperkalemia, especially at higher doses and when administered with other medication that causes hyperkalemia (for example, angiotensin converting enzyme inhibitors).

V. COTRIMOXAZOLE

The combination of *trimethoprim* with *sulfamethoxazole*, called *cotrimoxazole* [co-try-MOX-a-zole], shows greater antimicrobial activity than equivalent quantities of either drug used alone (Figure 31.10). The combination was selected because of the synergistic activity and the similarity in the half-lives of the two drugs.

A. Mechanism of action

The synergistic antimicrobial activity of *cotrimoxazole* results from its inhibition of two sequential steps in the synthesis of tetrahydrofolic acid. *Sulfamethoxazole* inhibits the incorporation of PABA into dihydrofolic acid precursors, and *trimethoprim* prevents reduction of dihydrofolate to tetrahydrofolate (Figure 31.7).

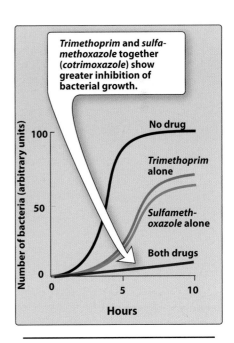

Trimethoprim and *sulfamethoxazole* together (*cotrimoxazole*) show greater inhibition of bacterial growth.

Figure 31.10
Synergism between *trimethoprim* and *sulfamethoxazole* inhibits growth of E. coli.

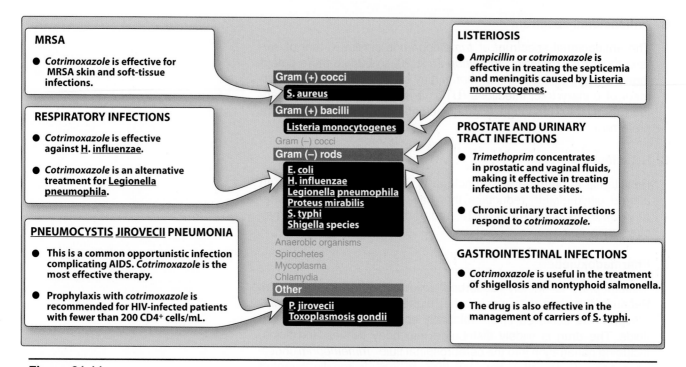

Figure 31.11
Typical therapeutic applications of *cotrimoxazole* (*sulfamethoxazole* plus *trimethoprim*).

B. Antibacterial spectrum

Cotrimoxazole has a broader spectrum of antibacterial action than the sulfa drugs alone (Figure 31.11). It is effective in treating UTIs and respiratory tract infections, as well as Pneumocystis jirovecii, toxoplasmosis, Listeria monocytogenes, and Salmonella infections. It has activity against *methicillin*-resistant S. aureus and can be particularly useful for skin and soft tissue infections caused by this organism. It is the drug of choice for infections caused by susceptible Nocardia spp. and Stenotrophomonas maltophilia.

C. Resistance

Resistance to the *trimethoprim–sulfamethoxazole* combination is encountered less frequently than resistance to either of the drugs alone, because it requires bacterium to maintain simultaneous resistance to both drugs. Significant resistance has been documented in a number of clinically relevant organisms, including E. coli.

D. Pharmacokinetics

Cotrimoxazole is generally administered orally (Figure 31.12). Intravenous administration may be utilized in patients with severe pneumonia caused by Pneumocystis jirovecii. Both agents distribute throughout the body. *Trimethoprim* concentrates in the relatively acidic milieu of prostatic fluids, and this accounts for the use of *trimethoprim–sulfamethoxazole* in the treatment of prostatitis. *Cotrimoxazole* readily crosses the blood–brain barrier. Both parent drugs and their metabolites are excreted in the urine.

E. Adverse effects

Adverse reactions and drug interactions related to *cotrimoxazole* are similar to those expected with each of the individual components, *sulfamethoxazole* and *trimethoprim* (Figure 31.13). The most common adverse reactions are nausea and vomiting, skin rash, hematologic toxicity, and hyperkalemia.

VI. URINARY TRACT ANTISEPTICS/ANTIMICROBIALS

UTIs are one of the most common bacterial infections in the world, primarily impacting women and the elderly. Historically, fluoroquinolones and *cotrimoxazole* have been first-line therapy for the treatment of UTIs. Unfortunately, resistance has increased among common pathogens (for example, E. coli). As a result, *methenamine*, *nitrofurantoin*, and *fosfomycin* (see Chapter 29) can be considered for treatment or suppression of recurrence, due to their efficacy against common pathogens and high concentrations in the urine.

A. Methenamine

1. **Mechanism of action:** *Methenamine* [meth-EN-a-meen] salts are hydrolyzed to ammonia and formaldehyde in acidic urine (pH ≤ 5.5). Formaldehyde denatures proteins and nucleic acids, resulting in bacterial cell death. *Methenamine* is combined with a weak acid (for example, hippuric acid) to maintain urine acidity and promote production of formaldehyde (Figure 31.14).

2. **Antibacterial spectrum:** *Methenamine* is primarily used for chronic suppressive therapy to reduce the frequency of UTIs. *Methenamine* is active against E. coli, Enterococcus spp., and Staphylococcus spp. It has some activity against Proteus spp. and Pseudomonas aeruginosa, but urine pH must be kept acidic to achieve bactericidal activity. The main benefit of *methenamine* is the lack of selection for resistant organisms.

3. **Pharmacokinetics:** *Methenamine* is orally absorbed, with up to 30% decomposing in gastric juices, unless protected by enteric coating. It reaches the urine through tubular secretion and glomerular filtration. Concentrations are sufficient to treat susceptible organisms. Due to ammonia formation, use should be avoided in hepatic insufficiency.

4. **Adverse effects:** The major adverse effect of *methenamine* is gastrointestinal distress, although at higher doses, albuminuria, hematuria, and rashes may develop. *Methenamine mandelate* is contraindicated in patients with renal insufficiency, because mandelic acid may precipitate. The *methenamine hippurate* formulation should be used instead. [Note: Sulfonamides, such as *cotrimoxazole*, react with formaldehyde and must not be used concomitantly with *methenamine*. The combination increases the risk of crystalluria and mutual antagonism.]

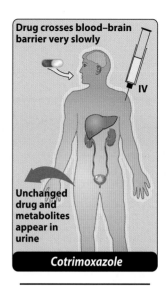

Figure 31.12
Administration and fate of *cotrimoxazole*.

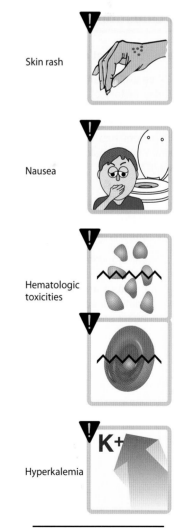

Figure 31.13
Some adverse reactions to *cotrimoxazole*.

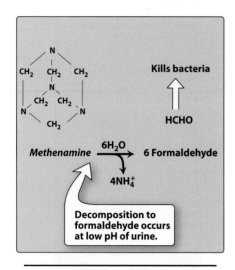

Figure 31.14
Formation of formaldehyde from
methenamine at acid pH.

B. Nitrofurantoin

Nitrofurantoin [NYE-troe-fue-RAN-toin] was introduced into clinical practice for the management of cystitis in the early 1950s. For decades, it was rarely used, but was resurrected due to increasing antibiotic resistance among Enterobacteriaceae and is considered first-line therapy for uncomplicated cystitis. *Nitrofurantoin* works by inhibiting DNA and RNA synthesis. Susceptible organisms include E. coli, Klebsiella spp., Enterococcus spp., and Staphylococcus spp. Following oral administration, it is rapidly absorbed, with nearly 40% excreted unchanged in the urine. Overall, *nitrofurantoin* is well tolerated. Common adverse events include nausea, vomiting, and diarrhea. Use of the microcrystalline formulation decreases the incidence of gastrointestinal toxicity. Rare complications of therapy include pulmonary fibrosis, neuropathy, and autoimmune hepatitis. These events are observed with prolonged exposure greater than 1 month. Additionally, patients with impaired renal function should not receive *nitrofurantoin* due to an increased risk of adverse events.

Study Questions

Choose the ONE best answer.

31.1 A 32-year-old man presents to an outpatient clinic with a 5-day history of productive cough, purulent sputum, and shortness of breath. He is diagnosed with community-acquired pneumonia (CAP). It is noted that this patient has a severe ampicillin allergy (anaphylaxis). Which would be an acceptable treatment for this patient?

A. Levofloxacin
B. Ciprofloxacin
C. Penicillin VK
D. Nitrofurantoin

Correct answer = A. Streptococcus pneumoniae is a common cause of CAP, and the respiratory fluoroquinolones levofloxacin and moxifloxacin provide good coverage. Ciprofloxacin does not cover S. pneumoniae well and is a poor choice for treatment of CAP. Penicillin would be a poor choice due to allergy. Nitrofurantoin has no clinical utility for respiratory tract infections.

31.2 A 22-year-old woman presents with a 2-day history of dysuria with increased urinary frequency and urgency. A urine culture and urinalysis are done. She is diagnosed with a urinary tract infection caused by E. coli. Which agent should be avoided in the treatment of her UTI?

A. Levofloxacin
B. Cotrimoxazole
C. Moxifloxacin
D. Nitrofurantoin

Correct answer = C. Moxifloxacin does not concentrate in the urine and would be ineffective for treatment of a UTI. All other answers are viable alternatives, and the resistance profile for the E. coli can be utilized to direct therapy.

31.3 Which drug is correctly matched with the appropriate adverse effect?

A. Levofloxacin—hyperkalemia
B. Nitrofurantoin—pulmonary fibrosis
C. Cotrimoxazole—hepatic encephalopathy
D. Methenamine—nystagmus

Correct answer = B. Hyperkalemia may be caused by cotrimoxazole, not fluoroquinolones. Hepatic encephalopathy may be related to therapy with methenamine in patients with hepatic insufficiency. Nystagmus is not associated with methenamine therapy.

31.4 Cotrimoxazole provides activity against which organism?

    A. MRSA

    B. Pseudomonas aeruginosa

    C. Anaerobes

    D. Mycoplasma

> Correct answer = A. Cotrimoxazole is effective against MRSA. It does not have activity against Pseudomonas, anaerobes, or Mycoplasma.

31.5 A 55-year-old man presents to primary care clinic with an erythematous and tender abscess on his left thigh. He has a history of MRSA skin infections. Which is an appropriate antibiotic for empiric treatment?

    A. Ciprofloxacin

    B. Cotrimoxazole

    C. Pyrimethamine

    D. Cephalexin

> Correct answer = B. Cotrimoxazole is the only agent with reliable activity against MRSA. Ciprofloxacin does have some minor activity, but resistance has readily increased and it is no longer a valid recommendation. The other agents do not have activity against MRSA.

31.6 Which is a common adverse effect of cotrimoxazole?

    A. Hyperkalemia

    B. Pulmonary fibrosis

    C. Tendon rupture

    D. Blood glucose disturbances

> Correct answer = A. Trimethoprim acts as a potassium-sparing agent, resulting in an increase in serum potassium concentrations. Pulmonary fibrosis is an adverse effect of nitrofurantoin. Tendon rupture and blood glucose disturbances are adverse effects of fluoroquinolones.

31.7 A 21-year-old marathon runner reports to the clinic with acute Achilles tendon rupture. The nurse noted that the patient recently took an antibiotic for community-acquired pneumonia. Which antibiotic may have contributed to tendon rupture?

    A. Amoxicillin/clavulanate

    B. Cefdinir

    C. Levofloxacin

    D. Minocycline

> Correct answer = C. Levofloxacin is associated with tendon ruptures and tendinopathy. The other agents are not associated with this adverse effect.

31.8 A 70-year-old woman with acute cystitis presents to the Family Medicine clinic for assessment. She has a past medical history of hypertension and chronic kidney disease. The team recommends initiation of nitrofurantoin for cystitis. After reviewing her antimicrobial therapy, which actions should be taken prior to clinic discharge?

    A. Continue current therapy and counsel on gastrointestinal effects of nitrofurantoin.

    B. Change nitrofurantoin to alternative agent due to chronic kidney disease.

    C. Reduce nitrofurantoin dose due to impaired renal function.

    D. Counsel patient regarding neuropathy associated with short-term therapy.

> Correct answer = B. The key issue with the antibiotic recommendation is that nitrofurantoin should not be administered in patients with poor kidney function. Adjusting the dose and continuing the current regimen are not acceptable modifications. Neuropathy is more common with therapy greater than 1 month.

31.9 Which recommendation should be provided to avoid phototoxicity associated with fluoroquinolone therapy?

    A. Use sunscreen and avoid excessive exposure to UV light.

    B. Take the medication at night to avoid high drug concentrations during the day.

    C. Take with food.

    D. Drink with 1 L of water per day to minimize drug buildup in skin tissue.

Correct answer = A. Patients taking a fluoroquinolone should apply sunscreen and take precautions to minimize risk of phototoxicity. Adjusting the timing of the dose or taking with food or additional water does not change the risk of an event.

31.10 What is the main benefit for prescribing methenamine for treatment of a urinary tract infection?

    A. Safe to use in patients with hepatic failure.

    B. Available in intravenous and oral formulations.

    C. Broad spectrum of activity.

    D. Minimal development of resistance.

Correct answer = D. Methenamine does not select for resistance. Due to its conversion to formaldehyde, this compound is the least likely compound to select for resistant isolates. Methenamine should be avoided in patients with hepatic failure. This agent is only available as an oral formulation, and it has a narrow spectrum of activity.

Antimycobacterial Drugs

32

Charles A. Peloquin and Eric F. Egelund

I. OVERVIEW

Mycobacteria are rod-shaped aerobic bacilli that multiply slowly, every 18 to 24 hours in vitro. Their cell walls contain mycolic acids, which give the genus its name. Mycolic acids are long-chain, β-hydroxylated fatty acids. Mycobacteria produce highly lipophilic cell walls that stain poorly with Gram stain. Once stained, the bacilli are not decolorized easily by acidified organic solvents. Hence, the organisms are called "acid-fast bacilli." Mycobacterial infections classically result in the formation of slow-growing, granulomatous lesions that cause tissue destruction anywhere in the body.

Mycobacterium tuberculosis can cause latent tuberculosis infection (LTBI) and the disease known as tuberculosis (TB). [Note: In LTBI, the patient is infected with M. tuberculosis without signs or symptoms of active TB disease.] TB is the leading infectious cause of death worldwide, and a quarter of the world's population is infected with TB. Increasing in frequency are diseases caused by nontuberculous mycobacteria (NTM). These species include M. avium-intracellulare, M. chelonae, M. abscessus, M. kansasii, and M. fortuitum. Finally, M. leprae causes leprosy.

TB treatment generally includes four first-line drugs (Figure 32.1). Second-line drugs are typically less effective, more toxic, and less extensively studied. They are used for patients who cannot tolerate the first-line drugs or who are infected with resistant TB. No drugs are specifically developed for NTM infections. Macrolides, rifamycins, and aminoglycosides are frequently included, but NTM regimens vary widely by organism.

II. CHEMOTHERAPY FOR TUBERCULOSIS

M. tuberculosis is slow growing and requires treatment for months to years. LTBI can be treated for 9 months with *isoniazid (INH)* monotherapy or with 12 once-weekly higher doses of *INH* and *rifapentine*. In contrast, active TB disease must be treated with several drugs. Treatment for drug-susceptible TB lasts for at least 6 months, while treatment of multidrug-resistant TB (MDR-TB) typically lasts for about 2 years.

DRUGS USED TO TREAT TUBERCULOSIS
Ethambutol MYAMBUTOL
Isoniazid GENERIC ONLY
Pyrazinamide GENERIC ONLY
Rifabutin MYCOBUTIN
Rifampin RIFADIN
Rifapentine PRIFTIN
DRUGS USED TO TREAT TUBERCULOSIS (2ND LINE)
Aminoglycosides
Aminosalicylic acid PASER
Bedaquiline SIRTURO
Capreomycin CAPASTAT
Cycloserine SEROMYCIN
Ethionamide TRECATOR
Fluoroquinolones
Macrolides
DRUGS USED TO TREAT LEPROSY
Clofazimine LAMPRENE
Dapsone GENERIC ONLY
Rifampin (Rifampicin) RIFADIN

Figure 32.1
Summary of drugs used to treat mycobacterial infections.

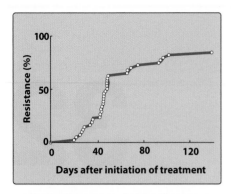

Figure 32.2
Cumulative percentage of strains of
Mycobacterium tuberculosis showing
resistance to *streptomycin*.

A. Strategies for addressing drug resistance

Populations of M. tuberculosis contain small numbers of organisms that are naturally resistant to a particular drug. Under selective pressure from inadequate treatment, especially from monotherapy, these resistant organisms can emerge as the dominant population. Figure 32.2 shows that resistance develops rapidly in TB patients given only *streptomycin*. Multidrug therapy is employed to suppress these resistant organisms. The first-line drugs *isoniazid*, *rifampin*, *ethambutol*, and *pyrazinamide* are preferred because of their high efficacy and acceptable incidence of toxicity. *Rifabutin* or *rifapentine* may replace *rifampin* under certain circumstances. Active disease always requires treatment with multidrug regimens, and preferably three or more drugs with proven in vitro activity against the isolate. Although clinical improvement can occur in the first several weeks of treatment, therapy is continued much longer to eradicate persistent organisms and to prevent relapse.

Standard short-course chemotherapy for tuberculosis includes *isoniazid*, *rifampin*, *ethambutol*, and *pyrazinamide* for 2 months (the intensive phase), followed by *isoniazid* and *rifampin* for 4 months (the continuation phase; Figure 32.3). Once susceptibility data are available, the drug regimen can be individually tailored. Second-line regimens for MDR-TB (TB resistant to at least *isoniazid* and *rifampin*) normally include an aminoglycoside (*streptomycin*, *kanamycin*, or *amikacin*) or *capreomycin* (all injectable agents), a fluoroquinolone (typically *levofloxacin* or *moxifloxacin*), any first-line drugs that remain active, and one or more of the following: *cycloserine*, *ethionamide*, or *p-aminosalicylic acid*. For extensively drug-resistant TB (XDR-TB), other drugs such as *clofazimine* and *linezolid* may be employed empirically.

Patient adherence can be low when multidrug regimens last for 6 months or longer. One successful strategy for achieving better treatment completion rates is directly observed therapy (DOT). Patients take the medications under observation of a member of the health care team. DOT decreases drug resistance and improves cure rates. Most public health departments offer DOT services.

B. Isoniazid

Isoniazid [eye-so-NYE-a-zid], along with *rifampin*, is one of the two most important TB drugs.

1. **Mechanism of action:** *Isoniazid* is a prodrug activated by a mycobacterial catalase–peroxidase (KatG). *Isoniazid* targets the enzymes acyl carrier protein reductase (InhA) and β-ketoacyl-ACP synthase (KasA), which are essential for the synthesis of mycolic acid. Inhibiting mycolic acid leads to a disruption in the bacterial cell wall.

2. **Antibacterial spectrum:** *Isoniazid* is specific for treatment of M. tuberculosis, although M. kansasii may be susceptible at higher drug concentrations. Most NTM are resistant to *INH*. The drug is particularly effective against rapidly growing bacilli and is also active against intracellular organisms.

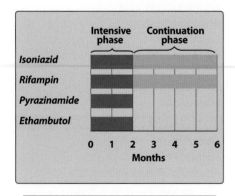

Figure 32.3
One of several recommended
multidrug schedules for the treatment
of tuberculosis.

3. **Resistance:** Resistance follows chromosomal mutations, including 1) mutation or deletion of KatG (producing mutants incapable of prodrug activation), 2) varying mutations of the acyl carrier proteins, or 3) overexpression of the target enzyme InhA. Cross-resistance may occur between *isoniazid* and *ethionamide*.

4. **Pharmacokinetics:** *Isoniazid* is readily absorbed after oral administration. Absorption is impaired if *isoniazid* is taken with food, particularly high-fat meals. The drug diffuses into all body fluids, cells, and caseous material (necrotic tissue resembling cheese that is produced in tuberculous lesions). Drug concentrations in the cerebrospinal fluid (CSF) are similar to those in the serum. *Isoniazid* undergoes *N*-acetylation and hydrolysis, resulting in inactive products. *Isoniazid* acetylation is genetically regulated, with fast acetylators exhibiting a 90-minute serum half-life, as compared with 3 to 4 hours for slow acetylators (Figure 32.4). Excretion is through glomerular filtration and secretion, predominantly as metabolites (Figure 32.5). Slow acetylators excrete more of the parent compound.

5. **Adverse effects:** Hepatitis is the most serious adverse effect associated with *isoniazid*. If hepatitis goes unrecognized, and if *isoniazid* is continued, it can be fatal. The incidence increases with age (greater than 35 years old), among patients who also take *rifampin*, or among those who drink alcohol daily. Peripheral neuropathy, manifesting as paresthesia of the hands and feet, appears to be due to a relative pyridoxine deficiency caused by *isoniazid*. This can be avoided by daily supplementation of pyridoxine (vitamin B_6). Central nervous system (CNS) adverse effects can occur, including convulsions in patients prone to seizures. Hypersensitivity reactions with *isoniazid* include rashes and fever. Because *isoniazid* inhibits the metabolism of *carbamazepine* and *phenytoin* (Figure 32.6), *isoniazid* can potentiate the adverse effects of these drugs (for example, nystagmus and ataxia).

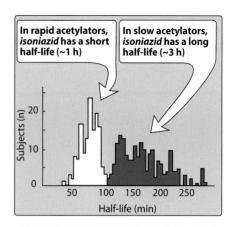

Figure 32.4
Bimodal distribution of *isoniazid* half-lives caused by rapid and slow acetylation of the drug.

C. Rifamycins: rifampin, rifabutin, and rifapentine

Rifampin, *rifabutin*, and *rifapentine* are all considered rifamycins, a group of structurally similar macrocyclic antibiotics, which are first-line oral agents for tuberculosis.

1. **Rifampin:** *Rifampin* [ri-FAM-pin] has broader antimicrobial activity than *isoniazid* and can be used as part of treatment for several different bacterial infections. Because resistant strains rapidly emerge during monotherapy, it is never given as a single agent in the treatment of active tuberculosis.

   a. **Mechanism of action:** *Rifampin* blocks RNA transcription by interacting with the β subunit of mycobacterial DNA-dependent RNA polymerase.

   b. **Antimicrobial spectrum:** *Rifampin* is bactericidal for both intracellular and extracellular mycobacteria, including M. tuberculosis, and NTM, such as M. kansasii and Mycobacterium avium complex (MAC). It is effective against many gram-positive and gram-negative organisms and is used

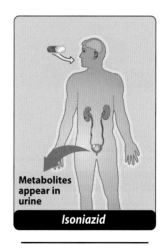

Figure 32.5
Administration and fate of *isoniazid*.

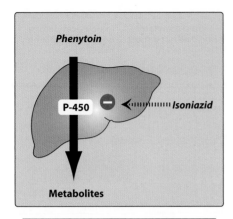

Figure 32.6
Isoniazid potentiates the adverse effects of *phenytoin*.

prophylactically for individuals exposed to meningitis caused by meningococci or Haemophilus influenzae. *Rifampin* also is highly active against M. leprae.

c. **Resistance:** Resistance to *rifampin* is caused by mutations in the affinity of the bacterial DNA-dependent RNA polymerase gene for the drug.

d. **Pharmacokinetics:** Absorption is adequate after oral administration. Distribution of *rifampin* occurs to all body fluids and organs. Concentrations attained in the CSF are variable, often 10% to 20% of blood concentrations. The drug is taken up by the liver and undergoes enterohepatic recycling. *Rifampin* can induce hepatic cytochrome P450 enzymes and transporters (see Chapter 1), leading to numerous drug interactions. Unrelated to its effects on cytochrome P450 enzymes, *rifampin* undergoes autoinduction, leading to a shortened elimination half-life over the first 1 to 2 weeks of dosing. Elimination of *rifampin* and its metabolites is primarily through the bile and into the feces; a small percentage is cleared in the urine (Figure 32.7). [Note: Urine, feces, and other secretions have an orange-red color, so patients should be forewarned. Tears may even stain soft contact lenses orange-red.]

e. **Adverse effects:** *Rifampin* is generally well tolerated. The most common adverse reactions include nausea, vomiting, and rash. Hepatitis and death due to liver failure are rare. However, the drug should be used judiciously in older patients, alcoholics, or those with chronic liver disease. There is a modest increase in the incidence of hepatic dysfunction when *rifampin* is coadministered with *isoniazid* and *pyrazinamide*. When *rifampin* is dosed intermittently, especially with higher doses, a flu-like syndrome can occur, with fever, chills, and myalgia, sometimes extending to acute renal failure, hemolytic anemia, and shock.

f. **Drug interactions:** Because *rifampin* induces a number of phase I cytochrome P450 enzymes and phase II enzymes (see Chapter 1), it can decrease the half-lives of coadministered drugs that are metabolized by these enzymes (Figure 32.8). This may necessitate higher dosages for coadministered drugs, a switch to drugs less affected by *rifampin*, or replacement of *rifampin* with *rifabutin*.

2. **Rifabutin:** *Rifabutin* [rif-a-BYOO-tin], a derivative of *rifampin*, is preferred for TB patients coinfected with the human immunodeficiency virus (HIV) who are receiving protease inhibitors or several of the nonnucleoside reverse transcriptase inhibitors. *Rifabutin* is a less potent inducer (approximately 40% less) of cytochrome P450 enzymes, thus lessening drug interactions. *Rifabutin* has adverse effects similar to those of *rifampin* but can also cause uveitis, skin hyperpigmentation, and neutropenia.

3. **Rifapentine:** *Rifapentine* [rih-fa-PEN-teen] has a longer half-life than that of *rifampin*. In combination with *isoniazid*, *rifapentine*

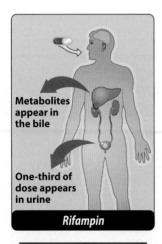

Figure 32.7
Administration and fate of *rifampin*. [Note: Patient should be warned that urine and tears may turn orange-red in color.]

may be used once weekly in patients with LTBI and in select HIV-negative patients with minimal pulmonary TB.

D. Pyrazinamide

Pyrazinamide [peer-a-ZIN-a-mide] is a synthetic, orally effective short-course agent used in combination with *isoniazid*, *rifampin*, and *ethambutol*. The precise mechanism of action is unclear. *Pyrazinamide* must be enzymatically hydrolyzed by pyrazinamidase to pyrazinoic acid, which is the active form of the drug. Some resistant strains lack the pyrazinamidase enzyme. *Pyrazinamide* is active against tuberculosis bacilli in acidic lesions and in macrophages. The drug distributes throughout the body, penetrating the CSF. *Pyrazinamide* may contribute to liver toxicity. Uric acid retention is common, but rarely precipitates a gouty attack. Most of the clinical benefit from *pyrazinamide* occurs early in treatment. Therefore, this drug is usually discontinued after 2 months of a 6-month regimen.

E. Ethambutol

Ethambutol [e-THAM-byoo-tole] is bacteriostatic and specific for mycobacteria. *Ethambutol* inhibits arabinosyl transferase—an enzyme important for the synthesis of the mycobacterial cell wall. *Ethambutol* is used in combination with *pyrazinamide*, *isoniazid*, and *rifampin* pending culture and susceptibility data. [Note: *Ethambutol* may be discontinued if the isolate is determined to be susceptible to *isoniazid*, *rifampin*, and *pyrazinamide*.] *Ethambutol* distributes well throughout the body. Penetration into the CNS is variable, and it is questionably adequate for tuberculous meningitis. Both the parent drug and its hepatic metabolites are primarily excreted in the urine. The most important adverse effect is optic neuritis, which results in diminished visual acuity and loss of ability to discriminate between red and green. The risk of optic neuritis increases with higher doses and in patients with renal impairment. Visual acuity and color discrimination should be tested prior to initiating therapy and periodically thereafter. Uric acid excretion is decreased by *ethambutol*, and caution should be exercised in patients with gout.

Figure 32.9 summarizes some of the characteristics of first-line drugs.

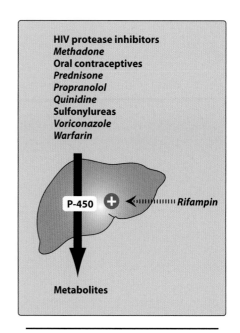

Figure 32.8
Induces cytochrome P450, which can decrease the half-lives of coadministered drugs that are metabolized by this system.

DRUG	ADVERSE EFFECTS	COMMENTS
Ethambutol	Optic neuritis with blurred vision, red-green color blindness	Establish baseline visual acuity and color vision; test monthly.
Isoniazid	Hepatic enzyme elevation, hepatitis, peripheral neuropathy	Take baseline hepatic enzyme measurements; repeat if abnormal or patient is at risk or symptomatic. Clinically significant interaction with *phenytoin* and *carbamazepine*.
Pyrazinamide	Nausea, hepatitis, hyperuricemia, rash, joint ache, gout (rare)	Take baseline hepatic enzymes and uric acid measurements; repeat if abnormal or patient is at risk or symptomatic.
Rifampin	Hepatitis, GI upset, rash, flu-like syndrome, significant interaction with several drugs	Take baseline hepatic enzyme measurements and CBC; repeat if abnormal or patient is at risk or symptomatic. Warn patient that urine and tears may turn red-orange in color.

Figure 32.9
Some characteristics of first-line drugs used in treating tuberculosis. CBC = complete blood count; GI = gastrointestinal.

F. Alternate second-line drugs

Streptomycin [strep-toe-MY-sin], *para-aminosalicylic* [a-mee-noe-sal-i-SIL-ik] *acid*, *capreomycin* [kap-ree-oh-MYE-sin], *cycloserine* [sye-kloe-SER-een], *ethionamide* [e-thye-ON-am-ide], *bedaquiline* [bed-AK-wi-leen], fluoroquinolones, and macrolides are second-line TB drugs. In general, these agents are less effective and more toxic than the first-line agents. Figure 32.10 summarizes some of the characteristics of second-line drugs.

1. **Streptomycin:** *Streptomycin*, an aminoglycoside antibiotic (see Chapter 30), was one of the first effective agents for TB. Its action appears to be greater against extracellular organisms. Infections due to *streptomycin*-resistant organisms may be treated with *kanamycin* or *amikacin*, to which these bacilli usually remain susceptible.

2. **Para-aminosalicylic acid:** *Para-aminosalicylic acid* (*PAS*) works via folic acid inhibition. While largely replaced by *ethambutol* for drug-susceptible TB, *PAS* remains an important component of many regimens for MDR-TB.

3. **Capreomycin:** This is a parenterally administered polypeptide that inhibits protein synthesis similar to aminoglycosides. *Capreomycin* is primarily reserved for the treatment of MDR-TB. Careful monitoring of renal function and hearing is necessary to minimize nephrotoxicity and ototoxicity, respectively.

4. **Cycloserine:** *Cycloserine* is an orally effective, tuberculostatic drug that disrupts D-alanine incorporation into the bacterial cell

DRUG	ADVERSE EFFECTS	COMMENTS
Fluoroquinolones	GI intolerance, tendonitis, CNS toxicity including caffeine-like effects	Monitor LFTs, serum creatinine/BUN, QT interval prolongation. Avoid concomitant ingestion with antacids, multivitamins or drugs containing di- or trivalent cations.
Aminoglycosides, *Capreomycin*	Nephrotoxicity, ototoxicity	Not available orally. Monitor for vestibular, auditory and renal toxicity.
Macrolides	GI intolerance, tinnitus	Monitor LFTs, serum creatinine/BUN, QT interval prolongation. Monitor for drug interactions due to CYP inhibition (except *azithromycin*).
Ethionamide	GI intolerance, hepatotoxicity, hypothyroidism	Monitor LFTs, TSH. A majority of patients experience GI intolerance. Cross-resistance with *isoniazid* is possible.
Para-aminosalicylic acid (PAS)	GI intolerance, hepatotoxicity, hypothyroidism	Monitor LFTs, TSH. Patients with G6PD deficiency are at increased risk of hemolytic anemia.
Cycloserine	CNS toxicity	Close monitoring is needed for depression, anxiety, confusion, etc. Seizures may be exacerbated in patients with epilepsy. Monitor serum creatinine.

Figure 32.10
Some characteristics of second-line drugs used in treating tuberculosis. BUN = blood urea nitrogen; CNS = central nervous system; CYP = cytochrome; G6PD = glucose-6-phosphate dehydrogenase; GI = gastrointestinal; LFTs = liver function tests; TSH = thyroid-stimulating hormone.

wall. It distributes well throughout body fluids, including the CSF. *Cycloserine* is primarily excreted unchanged in urine. Accumulation occurs with renal insufficiency. Adverse effects involve CNS disturbances (for example, lethargy, difficulty concentrating, anxiety, and suicidal tendency), and seizures may occur.

5. **Ethionamide:** *Ethionamide* is a structural analog of *isoniazid* that also disrupts mycolic acid synthesis. The mechanism of action is not identical to *isoniazid*, but there is some overlap in the resistance patterns. *Ethionamide* is widely distributed throughout the body, including the CSF. Metabolism is extensive, most likely in the liver, to active and inactive metabolites. Adverse effects that limit its use include nausea, vomiting, and hepatotoxicity. Hypothyroidism, gynecomastia, alopecia, impotence, and CNS effects also have been reported.

6. **Fluoroquinolones:** The fluoroquinolones (see Chapter 31), specifically *moxifloxacin* and *levofloxacin*, have an important place in the treatment of multidrug-resistant tuberculosis. Some NTM also are susceptible.

7. **Macrolides:** The macrolides (see Chapter 30) *azithromycin* and *clarithromycin* are included in regimens for several NTM infections, including MAC. *Azithromycin* may be preferred for patients at greater risk for drug interactions, since *clarithromycin* is both a substrate and inhibitor of cytochrome P450 enzymes.

8. **Bedaquiline:** *Bedaquiline,* a diarylquinoline, is an ATP synthase inhibitor. It is approved for the treatment of MDR-TB. *Bedaquiline* is administered orally, and it is active against many types of mycobacteria. *Bedaquiline* has a boxed warning for QT prolongation, and monitoring of the electrocardiogram is recommended. Elevations in liver enzymes have also been reported and liver function should be monitored during therapy. This agent is metabolized via CYP3A4, and administration with strong CYP3A4 inducers (for example, *rifampin*) should be avoided.

III. DRUGS FOR LEPROSY

Leprosy (or Hansen disease) is uncommon in the United States; however, worldwide, it is a much larger problem (Figure 32.11). Leprosy can be treated effectively with *dapsone* and *rifampin* (Figure 32.12).

A. Dapsone

Dapsone [DAP-sone] is structurally related to the sulfonamides and similarly inhibits dihydropteroate synthase in the folate synthesis pathway. It is bacteriostatic for <u>M. leprae</u>, and resistant strains may be encountered. *Dapsone* also is used in the treatment of pneumonia caused by <u>Pneumocystis jirovecii</u> in immunosuppressed patients. The drug is well absorbed from the gastrointestinal tract and is distributed throughout the body, with high concentrations in the skin. The parent drug undergoes hepatic acetylation. Both parent drug and metabolites are eliminated in the urine. Adverse reactions include hemolysis

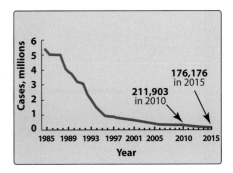

Figure 32.11
Reported prevalence of leprosy worldwide.

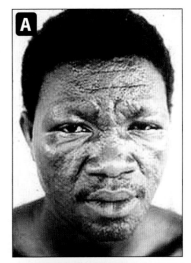

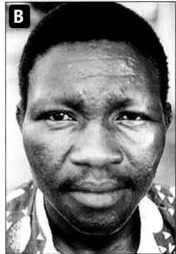

Figure 32.12
Patient with leprosy.

(especially in patients with glucose-6-phosphate dehydrogenase deficiency), methemoglobinemia, and peripheral neuropathy.

B. Clofazimine

Clofazimine [kloe-FAZ-i-meen] is a phenazine dye. Its mechanism of action may involve binding to DNA, although alternative mechanisms have been proposed. Its redox properties may lead to the generation of cytotoxic oxygen radicals that are toxic to the bacteria. *Clofazimine* is bactericidal to M. leprae, and it has potentially useful activity against M. tuberculosis and NTM. The drug is recommended by the World Health Organization as part of a shorter regimen (9 to 12 months) for MDR-TB. Following oral absorption, *clofazimine* accumulates in tissues, allowing intermittent therapy but does not enter the CNS. Patients typically develop a pink to brownish-black discoloration of the skin and should be informed of this in advance. Eosinophilic and other forms of enteritis, sometimes requiring surgery, have been reported. *Clofazimine* has some anti-inflammatory and anti-immune activities. Thus, erythema nodosum leprosum may not develop in patients treated with this drug.

Study Questions

Choose the ONE best answer.

32.1 A 22-year-old female intravenous drug user was admitted to the hospital with a 4-week history of cough and fever. A chest radiograph showed left upper lobe cavitary infiltrate. Cultures of sputum yielded M. tuberculosis susceptible to all antimycobacterial drugs. The patient received self-administered isoniazid, rifampin, pyrazinamide, and ethambutol. Two weeks following initiation of therapy, the patient is concerned that her urine is a "funny-looking reddish color." Which drug is the most likely cause?

A. Isoniazid
B. Rifampin
C. Pyrazinamide
D. Ethambutol

Correct answer = B. Rifampin (as well as rifabutin and rifapentine) and its metabolites may color urine, feces, saliva, sputum, sweat, and tears a bright red-orange. Patients should be counseled that this is an adverse effect which is not harmful, but can stain clothes and contact lenses.

32.2 A 32-year-old man has been on standard four-drug therapy for active pulmonary tuberculosis for the past 2 months. He has no other comorbid conditions. At his regular clinic visit, he complains of a "pins and needles" sensation in his feet. Which drug is most likely causing this?

A. Isoniazid
B. Rifampin
C. Pyrazinamide
D. Ethambutol

Correct answer = A. Standard four-drug therapy for active pulmonary tuberculosis includes isoniazid. Isoniazid can cause peripheral neuropathy with symptoms including paresthesias, such as "pins and needles" and numbness.

32.3 A 32-year-old man who takes standard four-drug therapy for active pulmonary tuberculosis complains about a "pins and needles" feeling in his feet. He is diagnosed with peripheral neuropathy. Which vitamin should have been included in the regimen for this patient to reduce the risk of neuropathy?

A. Niacin
B. Pyridoxine
C. Thiamine
D. Ascorbic acid

Correct answer = B. Concurrent administration of pyridoxine (vitamin B_6) prevents the neuropathic actions of isoniazid. The relative deficiency of pyridoxine appears to be due to the interference of isoniazid with its activation and enhancement of the excretion of pyridoxine.

32.4 A 23-year-old man was started on standard four-drug antimycobacterial therapy for treatment of active TB. He has epilepsy, which is controlled with carbamazepine. He has had no seizures in 5 years; however, upon return to clinic at 1 month, he reports having two seizures since his last visit. Which drug may be the reason his carbamazepine is less effective?

A. Isoniazid
B. Rifampin
C. Pyrazinamide
D. Ethambutol

Correct answer = B. Rifampin is a potent inducer of cytochrome P450–dependent drug-metabolizing enzymes and may reduce the concentration of carbamazepine. None of the other drugs listed induce cytochrome P450 enzymes.

32.5 A 26-year-old female HIV patient was recently diagnosed with active tuberculosis. Currently, she is on a stable HIV regimen consisting of two protease inhibitors and two nucleoside reverse transcriptase inhibitors. Which is the most appropriate regimen for treatment of her tuberculosis?

A. Rifampin + isoniazid + pyrazinamide + ethambutol
B. Rifabutin + isoniazid + pyrazinamide + ethambutol
C. Rifapentine + isoniazid + pyrazinamide + ethambutol
D. Rifampin + moxifloxacin + pyrazinamide + ethambutol

Correct answer = B. Rifabutin is recommended in place of rifampin in patients coinfected with HIV, since it is a less potent inducer of CYP enzymes than rifampin. However, rifabutin is a CYP3A4 substrate and "bidirectional" interactions may result. That is, other medications, such as the protease inhibitors, may affect the concentration of rifabutin, requiring dose adjustment of rifabutin or use of alternative HIV agents.

32.6 A 28-year-old man with MDR-TB is receiving the following medications for treatment: pyrazinamide, ethionamide, moxifloxacin, streptomycin, and para-aminosalicylic acid. Which drug in his regimen requires monitoring for QT prolongation?

A. Pyrazinamide
B. Ethionamide
C. Moxifloxacin
D. Streptomycin

Correct answer = C. While rare, prolongation of the QT interval is associated with the fluoroquinolones. QT interval prolongation is due to the blocking of voltage-gated potassium channels. Of the available quinolones, moxifloxacin has the greatest risk. The risk may be minimized by avoiding coadministration of other medications, which may prolong the QT interval. The other agents are not associated with QT prolongation.

32.7 A 46-year-old male patient with active tuberculosis is to be initiated on the four-drug regimen of isoniazid, rifampin, pyrazinamide, and ethambutol. The patient reports no other conditions except gout. Which pair of antituberculosis drugs has the potential to worsen his gout?

A. Rifampin and isoniazid
B. Ethambutol and pyrazinamide
C. Rifampin and ethambutol
D. Isoniazid and ethambutol

Correct answer = B. Ethambutol and especially pyrazinamide both may increase uric acid concentrations and have the potential to precipitate gouty attacks. Pyrazinamide- and ethambutol-induced hyperuricemia may be controlled by use of antigout medications, such as xanthine oxidase inhibitors. Symptoms of gout must be monitored closely.

32.8 A 24-year-old man returns to the clinic 1 month after starting treatment for tuberculosis. He is receiving isoniazid, rifampin, pyrazinamide, and ethambutol. He states that he feels fine, but now is having difficulty reading and feels he may need to get glasses. Which drug may be causing his decline in vision?

A. Isoniazid
B. Rifampin
C. Pyrazinamide
D. Ethambutol

Correct answer = D. Optic neuritis, exhibited as a decrease in visual acuity or loss of color discrimination, is the most important side effect associated with ethambutol. Visual disturbances generally are dose related and more common in patients with reduced renal function. They are reversible (weeks to months) if ethambutol is discontinued promptly.

32.9 A 36-year-old woman with multidrug-resistant tuberculosis is being treated with the following agents: streptomycin, cycloserine, pyrazinamide, ethionamide, and p-aminosalicylic acid. Her physician recently noticed that she appears confused and anxious, and has a slight tremor. Which drug is most likely contributing to her current state?

A. Streptomycin
B. Cycloserine
C. Pyrazinamide
D. Ethionamide

Correct answer = B. Cycloserine easily penetrates the CNS and may cause adverse effects involving the nervous system, including psychoses, drowsiness, tremor, paresthesia, aggression, and suicidal ideation, among others. Patients should be monitored continually for these signs and symptoms.

32.10 Which is correct regarding clofazimine in the treatment of leprosy?

A. Clofazimine should not be used in patients with a deficiency in glucose-6-phosphate dehydrogenase (G6PD).
B. Peripheral neuropathy is one of the most common adverse effects seen with the drug.
C. Clofazimine may cause skin discoloration over time.
D. The risk of erythema nodosum leprosum is increased in patients given clofazimine.

Correct answer = C. Clofazimine is a phenazine dye and causes bronzing (the skin pigment color will change color, from pink to brownish-black), especially in fair-skinned patients. This occurs in a majority of patients, and generally is not considered harmful but may take several months to years to fade after discontinuing the medication.

Antifungal Drugs

33

Lindsey Childs-Kean

I. OVERVIEW

Infectious diseases caused by fungi are called mycoses, and they are often chronic in nature. Mycotic infections may involve only the skin (cutaneous mycoses extending into the epidermis), or may cause subcutaneous or systemic infections. Unlike bacteria, fungi are eukaryotic, with rigid cell walls composed largely of chitin rather than peptidoglycan (a characteristic component of most bacterial cell walls). In addition, the fungal cell membrane contains ergosterol rather than the cholesterol found in mammalian membranes. These structural characteristics are useful targets for chemotherapeutic agents against mycoses. Fungi are generally resistant to antibiotics; conversely, bacteria are resistant to antifungal agents. The incidence of mycoses such as candidemia has been on the rise for the last few decades. This is attributed to an increased number of patients with chronic immune suppression due to organ transplantation, cancer chemotherapy, or human immunodeficiency virus (HIV) infection. Simultaneously, new therapeutic options have become available for the treatment of mycoses. Figure 33.1 summarizes clinically useful agents for cutaneous and systemic mycoses. Figure 33.2 lists the common pathogenic organisms of the Kingdom Fungi, and Figure 33.3 provides an overview of the mechanism of action of the various antifungal agents.

II. DRUGS FOR SUBCUTANEOUS AND SYSTEMIC MYCOTIC INFECTIONS

A. Amphotericin B

Amphotericin [am-foe-TER-i-sin] *B* is a naturally occurring polyene antifungal produced by <u>Streptomyces</u> <u>nodosus</u>. In spite of its toxic potential, *amphotericin B* remains the drug of choice for the treatment of several life-threatening mycoses.

1. **Mechanism of action:** *Amphotericin B* binds to ergosterol in the plasma membranes of fungal cells. There, it forms pores (channels) that require hydrophobic interactions between the lipophilic

DRUGS FOR SUBCUTANEOUS AND SYSTEMIC MYCOSES
Amphotericin B VARIOUS
Anidulafungin ERAXIS
Caspofungin CANCIDAS
Fluconazole DIFLUCAN
Flucytosine ANCOBON
Isavuconazole CRESEMBA
Itraconazole ONMEL, SPORANOX
Ketoconazole EXTINA, NIZORAL, XOLEGEL
Micafungin MYCAMINE
Posaconazole NOXAFIL
Voriconazole VFEND

DRUGS FOR CUTANEOUS MYCOSES
Butenafine LOTRIMIN ULTRA, MENTAX
Butoconazole GYNAZOLE
Clotrimazole CRUEX, DESENEX, LOTRIMIN AF, VARIOUS
Ciclopirox LOPROX, PENLAC
Econazole ECOZA, SPECTAZOLE
Efinaconazole JUBLIA
Griseofulvin GRIS-PEG
Miconazole VARIOUS
Naftifine NAFTIN
Nystatin VARIOUS
Oxiconazole OXISTAT
Sertaconazole ERTACZO
Sulconazole EXELDERM
Tavaborole KERYDIN
Terbinafine LAMISIL
Terconazole TERAZOL
Tioconazole MONISTAT-1, VAGISTAT-1
Tolnaftate LAMISIL AF, TINACTIN

Figure 33.1
Summary of antifungal drugs.

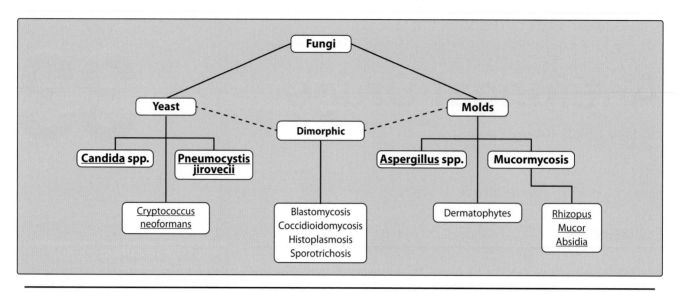

Figure 33.2
Common pathogenic organisms of Kingdom Fungi.

segment of the polyene antifungal and the sterol (Figure 33.4). The pores disrupt membrane function, allowing electrolytes (particularly potassium) and small molecules to leak from the cell, resulting in cell death.

2. **Antifungal spectrum:** *Amphotericin B* is either fungicidal or fungistatic, depending on the organism and the concentration of the drug. It is effective against a wide range of fungi, including <u>Candida albicans</u>, <u>Histoplasma capsulatum</u>, <u>Cryptococcus neoformans</u>,

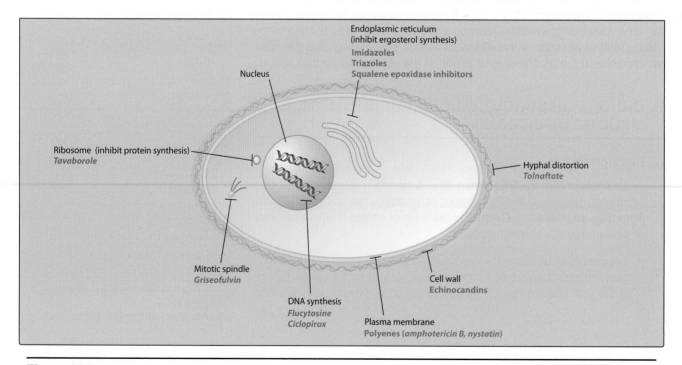

Figure 33.3
Cellular targets of antifungal drugs.

<u>Coccidioides</u> <u>immitis</u>, <u>Blastomyces</u> <u>dermatitidis</u>, and many strains of <u>Aspergillus</u>. [Note: *Amphotericin B* is also used in the treatment of the protozoal infection leishmaniasis.]

3. **Resistance:** Fungal resistance to *amphotericin B*, although infrequent, is associated with decreased ergosterol content of the fungal membrane.

4. **Pharmacokinetics:** *Amphotericin B* is administered by slow intravenous (IV) infusion (Figure 33.5). *Amphotericin B* is insoluble in water and must be coformulated with sodium deoxycholate (conventional) or artificial lipids to form liposomes. The liposomal preparations are associated with reduced renal and infusion toxicity but are more costly. *Amphotericin B* is extensively bound to plasma proteins and is distributed throughout the body. Inflammation favors penetration into various body fluids, but little of the drug is found in the cerebral spinal fluid (CSF), vitreous humor, peritoneal fluid, or synovial fluid. Low levels of the drug and its metabolites are excreted primarily in the urine over a long period of time.

5. **Adverse effects:** *Amphotericin B* has a low therapeutic index. Toxic manifestations are outlined below (Figure 33.6).

a. **Fever and chills:** These occur most commonly 1 to 3 hours after starting the IV administration but usually subside with repeated administration of the drug. Premedication with a corticosteroid or an antipyretic helps to prevent this problem.

b. **Renal impairment:** Despite the low levels of the drug excreted in the urine, patients may exhibit a decrease in glomerular filtration rate and renal tubular function. Serum creatinine may increase, creatinine clearance can decrease, and potassium and magnesium are lost. Renal function usually returns with discontinuation of the drug, but residual damage is likely at high doses. Azotemia is exacerbated by other nephrotoxic drugs, such as aminoglycosides, *cyclosporine*, and *vancomycin*, although adequate hydration can decrease its severity. Sodium loading with infusions of normal saline prior to administration of the conventional formulation or use of the liposomal *amphotericin B* products minimizes the risk of nephrotoxicity.

c. **Hypotension:** A shock-like fall in blood pressure accompanied by hypokalemia may occur, requiring potassium supplementation. Care must be exercised in patients taking *digoxin* and other drugs that can cause potassium fluctuations.

d. **Thrombophlebitis:** Adding *heparin* to the infusion can alleviate this problem.

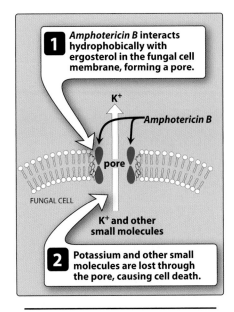

Figure 33.4
Model of a pore formed by *amphotericin B* in the lipid bilayer membrane.

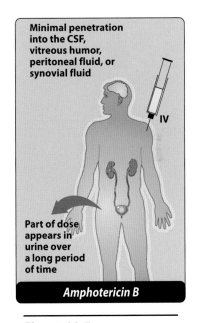

Figure 33.5
Administration and fate of *amphotericin B*. CSF = cerebrospinal fluid.

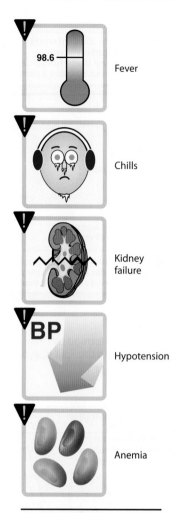

Figure 33.6
Adverse effects of *amphotericin B*.

B. Antimetabolite antifungals

Flucytosine [floo-SYE-toe-seen] *(5-FC)* is a synthetic pyrimidine antimetabolite that is often used in combination with other antifungal agents.

1. **Mechanism of action:** *5-FC* enters the fungal cell via a cytosine-specific permease, an enzyme not found in mammalian cells. It is subsequently converted to a series of compounds, including *5-fluorouracil (5-FU)* and 5-fluorodeoxyuridine 5′-monophosphate, which disrupt nucleic acid and protein synthesis (Figure 33.7). [Note: *Amphotericin B* increases cell permeability, allowing more *5-FC* to penetrate the cell leading to synergistic effects.]

2. **Antifungal spectrum:** *5-FC* is fungistatic. It is effective in combination with *itraconazole* for treating chromoblastomycosis. It is also used in combination with *amphotericin B* for the treatment of systemic mycoses and for meningitis caused by C. neoformans and C. albicans. *Flucytosine* can also be used for Candida urinary tract infections when *fluconazole* is not appropriate; however, resistance can occur with repeated use.

3. **Resistance:** Resistance may occur due to decreased levels of any of the enzymes in the conversion of *5-FC* to *5-FU* and other metabolites. The emergence of resistant fungal cells is lower with a combination of *5-FC* plus a second antifungal agent. Thus, *5-FC* is not used as a single antimycotic drug.

4. **Pharmacokinetics:** *5-FC* is well absorbed after oral administration. It distributes throughout the body water and penetrates well into the CSF. *5-FU* is detectable in patients and is probably the result of metabolism of *5-FC* by intestinal bacteria. Excretion of both the parent drug and metabolites is via glomerular filtration, and the dose must be adjusted in patients with compromised renal function.

5. **Adverse effects:** *5-FC* causes reversible neutropenia, thrombocytopenia, and dose-related bone marrow depression. Reversible hepatic dysfunction with elevation of serum transaminases has been observed. Nausea, vomiting, and diarrhea are common, and severe enterocolitis may occur.

C. Azole antifungals

Azole antifungals are made up of two different classes of drugs—imidazoles and triazoles. Although these drugs have similar mechanisms of action and spectra of activity, their pharmacokinetics and therapeutic uses vary significantly. In general, imidazoles are applied topically for cutaneous infections, whereas triazoles are administered systemically for the treatment or prophylaxis of cutaneous and systemic mycoses. [Note: Imidazole antifungals are discussed in the section on agents for cutaneous mycotic infections.] The systemic triazole antifungals include *fluconazole*, *itraconazole*, *posaconazole*, *voriconazole*, and *isavuconazole*.

1. **Mechanism of action:** Azoles are predominantly fungistatic. They inhibit 14-α demethylase (a cytochrome P450 [CYP450] enzyme), thereby blocking the demethylation of lanosterol to ergosterol (Figure 33.8). The inhibition of ergosterol biosynthesis disrupts fungal membrane structure and function, which, in turn, inhibits fungal cell growth.

2. **Resistance:** Resistance to azole antifungals is becoming a significant clinical problem, particularly with protracted therapy required in immunocompromised patients, such as those who have advanced HIV infection or bone marrow transplant. Mechanisms of resistance include mutations in the 14-α demethylase gene that lead to decreased azole binding and efficacy. Additionally, some strains of fungi develop efflux pumps that pump the drug out of the cell or have reduced ergosterol in the cell wall.

3. **Drug interactions:** All azoles inhibit the hepatic CYP450 3A4 isoenzyme to varying degrees. Patients on concomitant medications that are substrates for this isoenzyme may have increased concentrations and risk for toxicity. Several azoles, including *itraconazole* and *voriconazole*, are metabolized by CYP450 3A4 and other CYP450 isoenzymes. Therefore, concomitant use of potent CYP450 inhibitors (for example, *ritonavir*) and inducers (for example, *rifampin*, *phenytoin*) can lead to increased adverse effects or clinical failure of these azoles, respectively.

4. **Contraindications:** Azoles are considered teratogenic, and they should be avoided in pregnancy unless the potential benefit outweighs the risk to the fetus.

D. Fluconazole

Fluconazole [floo-KON-a-zole] was the first triazole antifungal agent. It is the least active of all triazoles, with most of its spectrum limited to yeasts and some dimorphic fungi. It has no role in the treatment of aspergillosis or zygomycosis. It is highly active against <u>Cryptococcus neoformans</u> and certain species of <u>Candida</u>, including <u>C. albicans</u> and <u>C. parapsilosis</u>. Resistance is a concern, however, with other species, including <u>C. krusei</u> and <u>C. glabrata</u>. *Fluconazole* is used for prophylaxis against invasive fungal infections in recipients of bone marrow transplants. It is the drug of choice for <u>Cryptococcus neoformans</u> after induction therapy with *amphotericin B* and *flucytosine* and is used for the treatment of candidemia and coccidioidomycosis. *Fluconazole* is effective against most forms of mucocutaneous candidiasis. It is commonly used as a single-dose oral treatment for vulvovaginal candidiasis. *Fluconazole* is available in oral and IV dosage formulations. It is well absorbed after oral administration and distributes widely to body fluids and tissues. The majority of the drug is excreted unchanged via the urine, and doses must be reduced in patients with renal dysfunction. The most common adverse effects with *fluconazole* are nausea, vomiting, headache, and skin rashes.

E. Itraconazole

Itraconazole [it-ra-KON-a-zole] is a synthetic triazole that has a broad antifungal spectrum compared to *fluconazole*. *Itraconazole* is a drug of choice for the treatment of blastomycosis, sporotrichosis, paracoccidioidomycosis, and histoplasmosis. It is rarely used for treatment

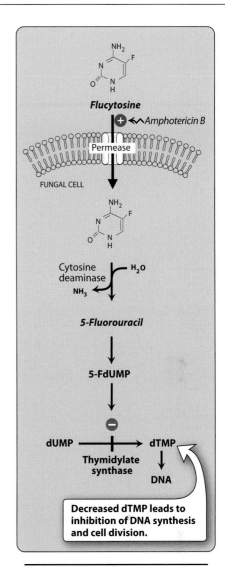

Figure 33.7
Mode of action of *flucytosine*.
5-FdUMP = 5-fluorodeoxyuridine 5′-monophosphate; dTMP = deoxythymidine 5′-monophosphate.

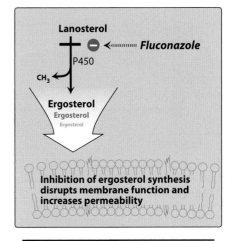

Figure 33.8
Mode of action of azole antifungals.

of infections due to <u>Candida</u> and <u>Aspergillus</u> species because of the availability of more effective agents. *Itraconazole* is available as a capsule, tablet, or oral solution. The capsule and tablet should be taken with food, and ideally an acidic beverage, to increase absorption. By contrast, the solution should be taken on an empty stomach, as food decreases the absorption. The drug distributes well in most tissues, including bone and adipose tissues. *Itraconazole* is extensively metabolized by the liver, and the drug and inactive metabolites are excreted in the urine and feces. Adverse effects include nausea, vomiting, rash (especially in immunocompromised patients), hypokalemia, hypertension, edema, and headache. Liver toxicity can also occur, especially when given with other hepatotoxic drugs. *Itraconazole* has a negative inotropic effect and should be avoided in patients with evidence of ventricular dysfunction, such as heart failure.

F. Posaconazole

Posaconazole [poe-sa-KONE-a-zole], a synthetic triazole, is a broad-spectrum antifungal structurally similar to *itraconazole*. It is available as an oral suspension, oral tablet, or IV formulation. *Posaconazole* is commonly used for the treatment and prophylaxis of invasive <u>Candida</u> and <u>Aspergillus</u> infections in severely immunocompromised patients. Because of its broad spectrum of activity, *posaconazole* is used in the treatment of invasive fungal infections caused by <u>Scedosporium</u> and <u>Zygomycetes</u>. The drug has low oral bioavailability and should be given with food. Unlike other azoles, *posaconazole* is not metabolized by CYP450, but is eliminated via glucuronidation. Drugs that increase gastric pH (for example, proton pump inhibitors) may decrease the absorption of oral *posaconazole* and should be avoided if possible. Due to its potent inhibition of CYP450 3A4, concomitant use of *posaconazole* with a number of agents (for example, ergot alkaloids, *atorvastatin*, *citalopram*, and *risperidone*) is contraindicated.

G. Voriconazole

Voriconazole [vor-i-KON-a-zole], a synthetic triazole related to *fluconazole*, is a broad-spectrum antifungal agent that is available in both IV and oral dosage forms. *Voriconazole* has replaced *amphotericin B* as the drug of choice for invasive aspergillosis. It is also approved for treatment of invasive candidiasis, as well as serious infections caused by <u>Scedosporium</u> and <u>Fusarium</u> species. *Voriconazole* has high oral bioavailability and penetrates into tissues well. It is extensively metabolized by CYP450 2C19, 2C9, and 3A4 isoenzymes, and the metabolites are primarily excreted via the urine. Inhibitors and inducers of these isoenzymes may impact levels of *voriconazole*, leading to toxicity or clinical failure, respectively. *Voriconazole* displays nonlinear kinetics, which can be affected by drug interactions and pharmacogenetic variability, particularly CYP450 2C19 polymorphisms. High trough concentrations have been associated with visual and auditory hallucinations and an increased incidence of hepatotoxicity. *Voriconazole* is also an inhibitor of CYP2C19, 2C9, and 3A4 isoenzymes. Drugs that are substrates of these isoenzymes are impacted by *voriconazole* (Figure 33.9). Because of significant interactions, use of *voriconazole* is contraindicated with many drugs (for example, *rifampin*, *rifabutin*, *carbamazepine*, and *St. John's wort*).

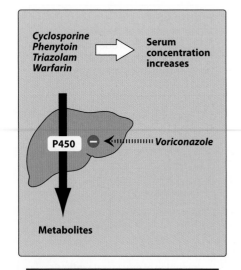

Figure 33.9
By inhibiting cytochrome P450, *voriconazole* can potentiate the toxicities of other drugs.

H. Isavuconazole

Isavuconazole [eye-sa-voo-KON-a-zole] is a broad-spectrum anti-fungal agent, which is supplied as the prodrug *isavuconazonium* in IV and oral dosage forms. *Isavuconazonium* is rapidly hydrolyzed by esterases in the blood to *isavuconazole*. *Isavuconazole* has a spectrum of activity similar to *voriconazole* and is approved for invasive aspergillosis and invasive mucormycosis. *Isavuconazonium* has high bioavailability after oral administration and distributes well into tissues. The drug is metabolized by CYP450 3A4/5 and uridine diphosphate-glucuronosyltransferases. Coadministration of *isavuconazole* with potent CYP450 3A4 inhibitors and inducers is contraindicated. *Isavuconazole* is also an inhibitor of the CYP450 3A4 isoenzyme, thereby increasing the concentrations of drugs that are substrates of CYP450 3A4. Nausea, vomiting, diarrhea, and hypokalemia are common adverse effects.

Figures 33.10 and 33.11 summarize the azole antifungal agents.

I. Echinocandins

Echinocandins interfere with the synthesis of the fungal cell wall by inhibiting the synthesis of $\beta(1,3)$-D-glucan, leading to lysis and cell death. *Caspofungin*, *micafungin*, and *anidulafungin* are available for IV administration once daily. *Micafungin* is the only echinocandin that does not require a loading dose. The echinocandins have potent activity against Aspergillus and most Candida species, including those species resistant to azoles. However, they have minimal activity against other fungi. The most common adverse effects are

	FLUCONAZOLE	ITRACONAZOLE	ISAVUCONAZOLE	VORICONAZOLE	POSACONAZOLE
SPECTRUM OF ACTIVITY	+	++	+++	+++	++++
ROUTE(S) OF ADMINISTRATION	Oral, IV	Oral	Oral, IV	Oral, IV	Oral, IV
ORAL BIOAVAILABILITY (%)	95	55 (solution)	98	96	Variable
DRUG LEVELS AFFECTED BY FOOD OR GASTRIC pH	No	Yes	No	No	Yes
PROTEIN BINDING (%)	10	99	99	58	99
PRIMARY ROUTE OF ELIMINATION	Renal	Hepatic CYP3A4	Hepatic CYP3A4, UGT	Hepatic CYP2C19, 2C9, 3A4	Hepatic glucuronidation
CYTOCHROME P450 ENZYMES INHIBITED	CYP3A4, 2C9, 2C19	CYP3A4, 2C9	CYP3A4	CYP2C19, 2C9, 3A4	CYP3A4
HALF-LIFE ($t_{1/2}$)	25 h	30–40 h	130 h	Dose dependent	20–66 h
CSF PENETRATION	Yes	No	Yes	Yes	Yes
RENAL EXCRETION OF ACTIVE DRUG (%)	>90	<2	45	<2	<2
TDM RECOMMENDED (RATIONALE)	No	Yes (efficacy)	Unknown (therapeutic levels not yet determined)	Yes (efficacy and safety)	Yes (efficacy)

Figure 33.10
Summary of triazole antifungals. CSF = cerebrospinal fluid; TDM = therapeutic drug monitoring.

INTERACTING DRUG	AZOLE DRUG	EFFECT ON DRUG EXPOSURE	MAIN CLINICAL CONSEQUENCE OF INTERACTION
Amiodarone, dronedarone, citalopram, pimozide, quinidine	*Isavuconazole, itraconazole, fluconazole, voriconazole, posaconazole**	↑ Exposure to interacting drugs	QT interval prolongation with risk of torsades de pointes
Carbamazepine	*Isavuconazole, voriconazole*	↓ Exposure to *voriconazole*	Treatment failure of *voriconazole*
Efavirenz	*Isavuconazole, voriconazole*	↓ Exposure to *voriconazole*	Treatment failure of *voriconazole*
		↑ Exposure to *efavirenz*	Risk of *efavirenz* toxicity
Ergot alkaloids	*Isavuconazole, itraconazole, fluconazole, voriconazole, posaconazole**	↑ Exposure to ergot alkaloid	Ergotism
Lovastatin, simvastatin	*Itraconazole, voriconazole, posaconazole*	↑ Exposure to HMG-CoA reductase inhibitor	Risk of rhabdomyolysis
Midazolam, triazolam	*Isavuconazole, itraconazole, voriconazole, posaconazole*	↑ Exposure to benzodiazepine	Sleepiness
Phenytoin	*Isavuconazole, voriconazole, posaconazole*	↓ Exposure to *voriconazole, posaconazole*	Treatment failure
		↑ Exposure to *phenytoin*	Nystagmus, ataxia
Rifabutin	*Isavuconazole, voriconazole, posaconazole*	↓ Exposure to *voriconazole*	Treatment failure of *voriconazole*
		↑ Exposure to *rifabutin*	Uveitis
Rifampicin (rifampin)	*Isavuconazole, voriconazole, posaconazole*	↓ Exposure to *voriconazole*	Treatment failure of *voriconazole*
High-dose *ritonavir* (400 mg twice daily)	*Isavuconazole, voriconazole*	↓ Exposure to *voriconazole*	Treatment failure of *voriconazole*
Vincristine, vinblastine	*Isavuconazole, itraconazole, voriconazole, posaconazole*	↑ Exposure to vinca alkaloids	Neurotoxicity
Sirolimus	*Isavuconazole, voriconazole, posaconazole*	↑ Exposure to *sirolimus*	Risk of *sirolimus* toxicity

Figure 33.11
Major or life-threatening drug interactions of azole drugs. ↑ indicates increased; ↓ indicates decreased. *Where an interaction has been reported for one triazole, the contraindication has been extended to all others.

fever, rash, nausea, and phlebitis at the infusion site. They should be administered via a slow IV infusion, as they can cause a histamine-like reaction (flushing) when infused rapidly.

1. **Caspofungin:** *Caspofungin* [kas-poh-FUN-jin] is a first-line option for patients with invasive candidiasis, including candidemia, and a second-line option for invasive aspergillosis in patients who have failed or cannot tolerate *amphotericin B* or an azole. The dose of *caspofungin* should be adjusted with moderate hepatic dysfunction. Concomitant administration of *caspofungin* with CYP450 enzyme inducers (for example, *rifampin*) may require an increase in *caspofungin* dose. *Caspofungin* should not be coadministered with *cyclosporine* due to a high incidence of elevated hepatic transaminases with concurrent use.

2. Micafungin and anidulafungin: *Micafungin* [mi-ka-FUN-jin] and *anidulafungin* [ay-nid-yoo-la-FUN-jin] are first-line options for the treatment of invasive candidiasis, including candidemia. *Micafungin* is also indicated for the prophylaxis of invasive Candida infections in patients who are undergoing hematopoietic stem cell transplantation. These agents are not substrates for CYP450 enzymes and do not have any associated drug interactions.

III. DRUGS FOR CUTANEOUS MYCOTIC INFECTIONS

Mold-like fungi that cause cutaneous infections are called dermatophytes or tinea. Tinea infections are classified by the affected site (for example, tinea pedis, which refers to an infection of the feet). Common dermatomycoses, such as tinea infections that appear as rings or round red patches with clear centers, are often referred to as "ringworm." This is a misnomer because fungi rather than worms cause the disease. The three different fungi that cause the majority of cutaneous infections are Trichophyton, Microsporum, and Epidermophyton. The drugs used in the treatment of cutaneous mycoses are listed in Figure 33.1.

A. Squalene epoxidase inhibitors

These agents act by inhibiting squalene epoxidase, thereby blocking the biosynthesis of ergosterol, an essential component of the fungal cell membrane (Figure 33.12). Accumulation of toxic amounts of squalene results in increased membrane permeability and death of the fungal cell.

1. Terbinafine: Oral *terbinafine* [TER-bin-a-feen] is the drug of choice for treating dermatophyte onychomycoses (fungal infections of nails). It is better tolerated, requires a shorter duration of therapy, and is more effective than either *itraconazole* or *griseofulvin* for Trichophyton. Therapy is prolonged (usually about 3 months) but considerably shorter than that with *griseofulvin*. Oral *terbinafine* may also be used for tinea capitis (infection of the scalp). [Note: Oral antifungal therapy (*griseofulvin, terbinafine, itraconazole*) is needed for tinea capitis. Topical antifungals are ineffective.] Topical *terbinafine* (1% cream, gel or solution) is used to treat tinea pedis, tinea corporis (ringworm), tinea cruris (infection of the groin or "jock itch"), and tinea versicolor due to Malassezia furfur. Duration of treatment is usually 1 week.

a. Antifungal spectrum: *Terbinafine* is active against Trichophyton. It may also be effective against Candida, Epidermophyton, and Scopulariopsis, but the efficacy in treating clinical infections due to these pathogens has not been established.

b. Pharmacokinetics: *Terbinafine* is available for oral and topical administration. The bioavailability after oral administration is only 40% due to first-pass metabolism. *Terbinafine* is highly protein bound and is deposited in the skin, nails, and adipose tissue. A prolonged terminal half-life of 200 to 400 hours may reflect the slow release from these tissues. Oral *terbinafine* is extensively metabolized by several CYP450 isoenzymes

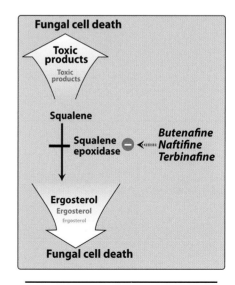

Figure 33.12
Mode of action of squalene epoxidase inhibitors.

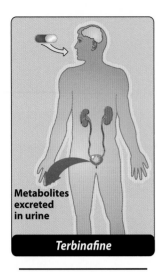

Figure 33.13
Administration and fate
of *terbinafine*.

and is excreted mainly via the urine (Figure 33.13). The drug should be avoided in patients with moderate to severe renal impairment or hepatic dysfunction. *Terbinafine* is an inhibitor of the CYP450 2D6 isoenzyme, and concomitant use with substrates of CYP450 2D6 may result in an increased risk of adverse effects with those agents.

    c. Adverse effects: Common adverse effects include diarrhea, dyspepsia, nausea, headache, and rash. Taste and visual disturbances have been reported, as well as elevations in serum hepatic transaminases.

2. Naftifine: *Naftifine* [NAF-ti-feen] is active against <u>Trichophyton</u>, <u>Microsporum</u>, and <u>Epidermophyton</u>. *Naftifine* cream and gel are used for topical treatment of tinea corporis, tinea cruris, and tinea pedis. Duration of treatment is usually 2 to 4 weeks.

3. Butenafine: *Butenafine* [byoo-TEN-a-feen] is active against <u>Trichophyton</u> <u>rubrum</u>, <u>Epidermophyton</u>, and <u>Malassezia</u>. Like *naftifine*, *butenafine* cream is used for topical treatment of tinea infections.

B. Griseofulvin

Griseofulvin [gris-ee-oh-FUL-vin] causes disruption of the mitotic spindle and inhibition of fungal mitosis (Figure 33.14). It has been largely replaced by oral *terbinafine* for the treatment of onychomycosis, although it is still used for dermatophytosis of the scalp and hair. *Griseofulvin* is fungistatic and requires a long duration of treatment (for example, 6 to 12 months for onychomycosis). Duration of therapy is dependent on the rate of replacement of healthy skin and nails. Ultrafine crystalline preparations are absorbed adequately from the gastrointestinal tract, and absorption is enhanced by high-fat meals. The drug concentrates in skin, hair, nails, and adipose tissue. *Griseofulvin* induces hepatic CYP450 activity, which increases the rate of metabolism of a number of drugs, including anticoagulants. The use of *griseofulvin* is contraindicated in pregnancy and patients with porphyria.

C. Nystatin

Nystatin [nye-STAT-in] is a polyene antifungal, and its structure, chemistry, mechanism of action, and resistance profile resemble those of *amphotericin B.* It is used for the treatment of cutaneous and oral <u>Candida</u> infections. The drug is negligibly absorbed from the gastrointestinal tract, and it is not used parenterally due to systemic toxicity (acute infusion-related adverse effects and nephrotoxicity). It is administered as an oral agent ("swish and swallow" or "swish and spit") for the treatment of oropharyngeal candidiasis (thrush), intravaginally for vulvovaginal candidiasis, or topically for cutaneous candidiasis.

D. Imidazoles

Imidazoles are azole derivatives, which currently include *butoconazole* [byoo-toe-KON-a-zole], *clotrimazole* [kloe-TRIM-a-zole], *econazole* [ee-KON-a-zole], *ketoconazole* [kee-toe-KON-a-zole], *miconazole*

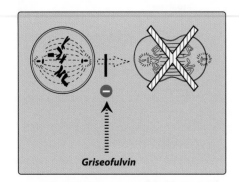

Figure 33.14
Inhibition of mitosis by *griseofulvin*.

[my-KON-a-zole], *oxiconazole* [oks-i-KON-a-zole], *sertaconazole* [serta-KON-a-zole], *sulconazole* [sul-KON-a-zole], *terconazole* [ter-KON-a-zole], and *tioconazole* [tee-oh-KON-a-zole]. As a class of topical agents, they have a wide range of activity against <u>Epidermophyton</u>, <u>Microsporum</u>, <u>Trichophyton</u>, <u>Candida</u>, and <u>Malassezia</u>, depending on the agent. The topical imidazoles have a variety of uses, including tinea corporis, tinea cruris, tinea pedis, and oropharyngeal and vulvovaginal candidiasis. Topical use is associated with contact dermatitis, vulvar irritation, and edema. *Clotrimazole* is also available as a troche (lozenge), and *miconazole* is available as a buccal tablet for the treatment of thrush. Oral *ketoconazole* is rarely used today due to the risk of severe liver injury, adrenal insufficiency, and adverse drug interactions.

E. Efinaconazole

Efinaconazole [eff-in-a-KON-a-zole] is a topical triazole antifungal agent approved for the treatment of toenail onychomycosis caused by <u>Trichophyton</u> <u>rubrum</u> and <u>Trichophyton</u> <u>mentagrophytes</u>. Duration of treatment is 48 weeks. It has also shown activity against <u>Candida</u> <u>albicans</u>.

F. Ciclopirox

Ciclopirox [sye-kloe-PEER-oks], a pyridine antimycotic, inhibits the transport of essential elements in the fungal cell, disrupting the synthesis of DNA, RNA, and proteins. *Ciclopirox* is active against <u>Trichophyton</u>, <u>Epidermophyton</u>, <u>Microsporum</u>, <u>Candida</u>, and <u>Malassezia</u>. It is available in a number of formulations. *Ciclopirox* shampoo is used for treatment of seborrheic dermatitis. Tinea pedis, tinea corporis, tinea cruris, cutaneous candidiasis, and tinea versicolor may be treated with the cream, gel, or suspension. Onychomycosis can be treated with the nail lacquer formulation.

G. Tavaborole

Tavaborole [tav-a-BOOR-ole] inhibits an aminoacyl-transfer ribonucleic acid synthetase, preventing fungal protein synthesis. *Tavaborole* is active against <u>Trichophyton</u> <u>rubrum</u>, <u>Trichophyton</u> <u>mentagrophytes</u>, and <u>Candida</u> <u>albicans</u>. A topical solution is approved for the treatment of toenail onychomycosis, requiring 48 weeks of treatment.

H. Tolnaftate

Tolnaftate [tole-NAF-tate], a topical thiocarbamate, distorts the hyphae and stunts mycelial growth in susceptible fungi. *Tolnaftate* is active against <u>Epidermophyton</u>, <u>Microsporum</u>, and <u>Malassezia</u> <u>furfur</u>. [Note: *Tolnaftate* is not effective against <u>Candida</u>.] *Tolnaftate* is used to treat tinea pedis, tinea cruris, and tinea corporis. It is available as a solution, cream, and powder.

Study Questions

Choose the ONE best answer.

33.1 Which antifungal agent is MOST likely to cause renal insufficiency?

A. Fluconazole
B. Amphotericin B
C. Itraconazole
D. Posaconazole

Correct answer = B. Amphotericin B is the best choice since nephrotoxicity is commonly associated with this medication. Although the dose of fluconazole must be adjusted for renal insufficiency, it is not associated with causing nephrotoxicity. Itraconazole and posaconazole are metabolized by the liver and are not associated with nephrotoxicity.

33.2 A 55-year-old woman presents to the hospital with shortness of breath, fever, and malaise. She has a history of breast cancer and is receiving chemotherapy. Her chest x-ray shows pneumonia, and respiratory cultures are positive for Aspergillus fumigatus. Which is the MOST appropriate choice for treatment?

A. Voriconazole
B. Fluconazole
C. Flucytosine
D. Ketoconazole

Correct answer = A. Voriconazole is the drug of choice for aspergillosis. Studies have found it to be superior to other regimens including amphotericin B. Fluconazole, flucytosine, and ketoconazole do not have reliable in vitro activity and are therefore not recommended.

33.3 Which antifungal agent should be avoided in patients with evidence of ventricular dysfunction?

A. Micafungin
B. Itraconazole
C. Terbinafine
D. Posaconazole

Correct answer = B. There is a black box warning that warns against the use of itraconazole in patients with evidence of ventricular dysfunction, including patients with heart failure.

33.4 A 56-year-old woman with diabetes complains of thickening of the nail of the right big toe and a change in color (yellow). The podiatrist diagnoses the patient with onychomycosis of the toenails. Which is the most appropriate choice for treating this infection?

A. Terbinafine
B. Micafungin
C. Itraconazole
D. Griseofulvin

Correct answer = A. Terbinafine is better tolerated, requires a shorter duration of therapy, and is more effective than either itraconazole or griseofulvin. Micafungin is not active for this type of infection.

33.5 A 44-year-old man presents to clinic with fevers and chills, headaches, and shortness of breath. He reports that he was exploring caves about 5 weeks ago. He is diagnosed with mild/moderate acute pulmonary histoplasmosis. Which is the most appropriate choice for treating this infection?

A. Micafungin
B. Itraconazole
C. Terbinafine
D. Griseofulvin

Correct answer = B. Itraconazole is the treatment of choice in patients with mild/moderate acute pulmonary histoplasmosis who have had symptoms for more than 1 month. Micafungin, terbinafine, and griseofulvin are not active for this type of infection.

33.6 A 32-year-old HIV-positive woman is admitted to the hospital with severe confusion and dizziness. She has been nonadherent with her HIV medications for several months. She is diagnosed with meningitis caused by <u>Cryptococcus neoformans</u>. Which is the most appropriate choice for treating the infection in this patient?

    A. Anidulafungin alone

    B. Amphotericin B plus flucytosine

    C. Flucytosine alone

    D. Isavuconazole plus anidulafungin

> Correct answer = B. The treatment of choice for initial therapy for cryptococcal meningitis is the combination of amphotericin B and flucytosine. Flucytosine should not be given alone because of the rapid development of resistance. Anidulafungin is not active against this type of infection. Isavuconazole has not been studied for the treatment of cryptococcal meningitis.

33.7 A 22-year-old woman reports a cottage cheese–like vaginal discharge and slight dysuria for 1 week. The patient is diagnosed with vulvovaginal candidiasis. She requests as short a course of treatment as possible due to her busy schedule. Which antifungal is the best choice?

    A. Oral fluconazole

    B. Topical miconazole

    C. Oral terbinafine

    D. Topical efinaconazole

> Correct answer = A. Oral fluconazole can be given as a one-time dose for vulvovaginal candidiasis. Topical miconazole requires multiple days of therapy. Terbinafine and efinaconazole are not used clinically for vulvovaginal candidiasis.

33.8 Which drug is relatively free of drug–drug interactions?

    A. Voriconazole

    B. Itraconazole

    C. Micafungin

    D. Terbinafine

> Correct answer = C. The echinocandins (including micafungin) are not metabolized by the CYP450 enzyme system, so they have very few drug–drug interactions. Voriconazole, itraconazole, and terbinafine are all metabolized by the CYP450 enzyme system, so they have significant drug–drug interactions.

33.9 Which drug works by creating pores/channels in the fungal cell membrane?

    A. Fluconazole

    B. Anidulafungin

    C. Amphotericin B

    D. Flucytosine

> Correct answer = C. Amphotericin B creates pores/channels in the fungal cell membrane. Fluconazole works by inhibiting the conversion of lanosterol to ergosterol. Anidulafungin inhibits the synthesis of β-D-glucan. Flucytosine disrupts nucleic acid and protein synthesis.

33.10 Which drug requires a loading dose?

    A. Caspofungin

    B. Micafungin

    C. Liposomal amphotericin B

    D. Tavaborole

> Correct answer = A. Caspofungin is the only drug listed that requires a loading dose before starting the maintenance dosing.

Antiviral Drugs

Elizabeth Sherman

34

I. OVERVIEW

Viruses are obligate intracellular parasites. They lack both a cell wall and a cell membrane, and they do not carry out metabolic processes. Viruses use much of the metabolic machinery of the host, and few drugs are selective enough to prevent viral replication without injury to the infected host cells. Therapy for viral diseases is further complicated by the fact that clinical symptoms appear late in the course of the disease, at a time when most of the virus particles have replicated. At this stage of viral infection, administration of drugs that block viral replication has limited effectiveness in many cases. However, a few virus groups respond to available antiviral drugs, and some antiviral agents are useful as prophylactic agents. These agents are discussed in this chapter. To assist in the review of these drugs, they are grouped according to the type of viral infection they target (Figure 34.1).

II. TREATMENT OF RESPIRATORY VIRAL INFECTIONS

Viral respiratory tract infections for which treatments exist include influenza A and B and respiratory syncytial virus (RSV). [Note: Immunization against influenza is the preferred approach. However, antiviral agents are used when patients are allergic to the vaccine or outbreaks occur.]

A. Neuraminidase inhibitors

The neuraminidase inhibitors *oseltamivir* [os-el-TAM-i-veer] and *zanamivir* [za-NA-mi-veer] are effective against both type A and type B influenza viruses. They do not interfere with the immune response to influenza vaccine. Administered prior to exposure, neuraminidase inhibitors prevent infection and, when administered within 24 to 48 hours after the onset of symptoms, they modestly decrease the intensity and duration of symptoms.

FOR RESPIRATORY VIRUS INFECTIONS
Amantadine GENERIC ONLY
Oseltamivir TAMIFLU
Ribavirin VIRAZOLE
Rimantadine FLUMADINE
Zanamivir RELENZA

FOR HEPATIC VIRAL INFECTIONS: HEPATITIS B
Adefovir HEPSERA
Entecavir BARACLUDE
Lamivudine EPIVIR-HBV
Peginterferon alfa-2a PEGASYS
Tenofovir alafenamide VEMLIDY
Tenofovir disoproxil fumarate VIREAD

FOR HEPATIC VIRAL INFECTIONS: HEPATITIS C
Daclatasvir DAKLINZA
Elbasvir/grazoprevir ZEPATIER
Glecaprevir/pibrentasvir MAVYRET
Ledipasvir/sofosbuvir HARVONI
Paritaprevir/ritonavir/ombitasvir TECHNIVIE
Paritaprevir/ritonavir/ombitasvir + dasabuvir VIEKIRA
Ribavirin MODERIBA, REBETOL
Sofosbuvir SOVALDI
Sofosbuvir/velpatasvir EPCLUSA
Sofosbuvir/velpatasvir/ voxilaprevir VOSEVI

FOR HERPESVIRUS AND CYTOMEGALOVIRUS INFECTIONS
Acyclovir ZOVIRAX
Cidofovir GENERIC ONLY
Famciclovir GENERIC ONLY
Foscarnet FOSCAVIR
Ganciclovir CYTOVENE
Penciclovir DENAVIR
Trifluridine VIROPTIC
Valacyclovir VALTREX
Valganciclovir VALCYTE

FOR HIV: NUCLEOSIDE AND NUCLEOTIDE REVERSE TRANSCRIPTASE INHIBITORS
Abacavir ZIAGEN
Didanosine VIDEX
Emtricitabine EMTRIVA
Lamivudine EPIVIR
Stavudine ZERIT
Tenofovir disoproxil fumarate VIREAD
Zidovudine RETROVIR

Figure 34.1
Summary of antiviral drugs. HIV = human immunodeficiency virus. *Part of a fixed-dose combination. (Figure continues on next page)

1. **Mechanism of action:** Influenza viruses employ a specific neuraminidase that is inserted into the host cell membrane for the purpose of releasing newly formed virions. This enzyme is essential for the virus life cycle. *Oseltamivir* and *zanamivir* selectively inhibit neuraminidase, thereby preventing the release of new virions and their spread from cell to cell.

2. **Pharmacokinetics:** *Oseltamivir* is an orally active prodrug that is rapidly hydrolyzed by the liver to its active form. *Zanamivir* is not active orally and is administered via inhalation. Both drugs are eliminated unchanged in the urine (Figure 34.2).

3. **Adverse effects:** The most common adverse effects of *oseltamivir* are gastrointestinal (GI) discomfort and nausea, which can be alleviated by taking the drug with food. Irritation of the respiratory tract occurs with *zanamivir*. It should be used with caution in individuals with asthma or chronic obstructive pulmonary disease, because bronchospasm may occur.

4. **Resistance:** Mutations of the neuraminidase enzyme have been identified in adults treated with either of the neuraminidase inhibitors. These mutants, however, are often less infective and virulent than the wild type.

B. Adamantane antivirals

The therapeutic spectrum of the adamantane derivatives, *amantadine* [a-MAN-ta-deen] and *rimantadine* [ri-MAN-ta-deen], is limited to influenza A infections. Due to widespread resistance, the adamantanes are not recommended in the United States for the treatment or prophylaxis of influenza A.

C. Ribavirin

Ribavirin [rye-ba-VYE-rin], a synthetic guanosine analog, is effective against a broad spectrum of RNA and DNA viruses. For example, *ribavirin* is used in the treatment of immunosuppressed infants and young children with severe RSV infections. *Ribavirin* is also effective in chronic hepatitis C infections when used in combination with other direct-acting antivirals (DAAs).

1. **Mechanism of action:** *Ribavirin* inhibits replication of RNA and DNA viruses. The drug is first phosphorylated to the 5′-phosphate derivatives. The major product *ribavirin* triphosphate exerts its antiviral action by inhibiting guanosine triphosphate formation, preventing viral messenger RNA (mRNA) capping, and blocking RNA-dependent RNA polymerase.

2. **Pharmacokinetics:** *Ribavirin* is effective orally and by inhalation. An aerosol is used in the treatment of RSV infection. Absorption is increased if the oral drug is taken with a fatty meal. The drug and its metabolites are eliminated in urine (Figure 34.3).

FOR HIV: NONNUCLEOSIDE REVERSE TRANSCRIPTASE INHIBITORS
Delavirdine RESCRIPTOR
Efavirenz SUSTIVA
Etravirine INTELENCE
Nevirapine VIRAMUNE
Rilpivirine EDURANT

FOR HIV: PROTEASE INHIBITORS
Atazanavir REYATAZ
Darunavir PREZISTA
Fosamprenavir LEXIVA
Indinavir CRIXIVAN
Lopinavir/ritonavir KALETRA
Nelfinavir VIRACEPT
Saquinavir INVIRASE
Tipranavir APTIVUS

FOR HIV: ENTRY INHIBITORS
Enfuvirtide FUZEON
Maraviroc SELZENTRY

FOR HIV: INTEGRASE INHIBITORS
Bictegravir*
Dolutegravir TIVICAY
Elvitegravir*
Raltegravir ISENTRESS

FOR HIV: PHARMACOKINETIC ENHANCERS
Cobicistat TYBOST
Ritonavir NORVIR

FOR HIV: FIXED-DOSE COMBINATIONS
Abacavir + lamivudine EPZICOM
Abacavir + lamivudine + dolutegravir TRIUMEQ
Abacavir + zidovudine + lamivudine TRIZIVIR
Bictegravir + tenofovir alafenamide + emtricitabine BIKTARVY
Efavirenz + emtricitabine + tenofovir disoproxil fumarate ATRIPLA
Elvitegravir + cobicistat + tenofovir alafenamide + emtricitabine GENVOYA
Elvitegravir + cobicistat + tenofovir disoproxil fumarate + emtricitabine STRIBILD
Emtricitabine + tenofovir alafenamide DESCOVY
Emtricitabine + tenofovir disoproxil fumarate TRUVADA
Rilpivirine + tenofovir alafenamide + emtricitabine ODEFSEY
Rilpivirine + tenofovir disoproxil fumarate + emtricitabine COMPLERA
Zidovudine + lamivudine COMBIVIR

Figure 34.1 (continued)
Summary of antiviral drugs.
HIV = human immunodeficiency virus.

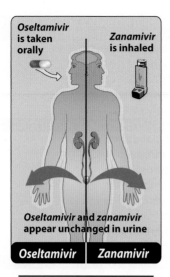

Figure 34.2
Administration and fate of
oseltamivir and *zanamivir*.

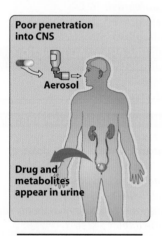

Figure 34.3
Administration and fate
of *ribavirin*.

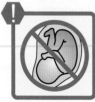

Figure 34.4
Ribavirin
causes
teratogenic
effects.

3. **Adverse effects:** Adverse effects of *ribavirin* include dose-dependent transient anemia. Elevated bilirubin has also been reported. The aerosol may be safer, although respiratory function in infants can deteriorate quickly after initiation of aerosol treatment. Therefore, monitoring is essential. *Ribavirin* is contraindicated in pregnancy (Figure 34.4).

III. TREATMENT OF HEPATIC VIRAL INFECTIONS

The hepatitis viruses currently identified (A, B, C, D, and E) each have a pathogenesis, which specifically involves replication in and destruction of hepatocytes. Of this group, hepatitis B (a DNA virus) and hepatitis C (an RNA virus) are the most common causes of chronic hepatitis, cirrhosis, and hepatocellular carcinoma (Figure 34.5) and are the only hepatic viral infections for which therapy is currently available. [Note: Hepatitis A is a commonly encountered infection caused by oral ingestion of the virus, but it is not a chronic disease.] Chronic hepatitis B may be treated with *peginterferon-α-2a* [peg-in-ter-FEER-on AL-fa], which is injected subcutaneously once weekly. Oral therapy for chronic hepatitis B virus (HBV) includes *lamivudine* [la-MIV-yoo-deen], *adefovir* [a-DEF-o-veer], *entecavir* [en-TEK-a-vir], and *tenofovir* [ten-OF-oh-vir] (see Section VIII for *tenofovir*). The preferred treatment for chronic hepatitis C virus (HCV) is a combination of DAAs, the selection of which is based on the hepatitis C genotype. In certain cases, *ribavirin* is added to a DAA regimen to enhance virologic response. With the introduction of new DAAs, *pegylated interferon-α* is no longer commonly used in HCV, and it is not recommended in current guidelines due to inferior efficacy and poor tolerability.

IV. TREATMENT OF HEPATITIS B

A. Interferons

Interferons are a family of naturally occurring, inducible glycoproteins that interfere with the ability of viruses to infect cells. The interferons are synthesized by recombinant DNA technology. At least three types of interferons exist—α, β, and γ (Figure 34.6). In "pegylated" formulations, bis-monomethoxy polyethylene glycol has been covalently attached to *interferon-α* to increase the size of the molecule. The larger molecular size delays absorption from the injection site, lengthens the duration of action of the drug, and also decreases its clearance.

1. **Mechanism of action:** The antiviral mechanism is incompletely understood. It appears to involve the induction of host cell enzymes that inhibit viral RNA translation, ultimately leading to the degradation of viral mRNA and tRNA.

2. **Therapeutic uses:** *Peginterferon alfa-2a* is approved for the treatment of chronic HBV infection. It is also indicated for the treatment of HCV in combination with other agents, although use is uncommon due to availability of more effective agents.

3. **Adverse effects:** These include flu-like symptoms, such as fever, chills, myalgias, arthralgias, and GI disturbances. Fatigue and mental depression are common. The principal dose-limiting toxicities are bone marrow suppression, severe fatigue and weight loss, neurotoxicity characterized by somnolence and behavioral disturbances, autoimmune disorders such as thyroiditis and, rarely, cardiovascular problems such as heart failure.

B. Lamivudine

This cytosine analog is an inhibitor of both hepatitis B virus (HBV) and human immunodeficiency virus (HIV) reverse transcriptases (RTs). *Lamivudine* must be phosphorylated by host cellular enzymes to the triphosphate (active) form. This compound competitively inhibits HBV RNA-dependent DNA polymerase. As with many nucleotide analogs, the intracellular half-life of the triphosphate is many hours longer than its plasma half-life. The rate of HBV resistance is high following long-term therapy with *lamivudine* and, therefore, *lamivudine* is no longer recommended in current hepatitis B guidelines.

C. Adefovir

Adefovir is a nucleotide analog that is phosphorylated by cellular kinases to adefovir diphosphate, which is then incorporated into viral DNA. This leads to termination of chain elongation and prevents replication of HBV. *Adefovir* is administered once daily and is renally excreted via glomerular filtration and tubular secretion. As with other agents, discontinuation of *adefovir* may result in severe exacerbation of hepatitis. Nephrotoxicity may occur with chronic use, and the drug should be used cautiously in patients with existing renal dysfunction. *Adefovir* is no longer recommended in current hepatitis B guidelines due to lower efficacy compared to other agents.

D. Entecavir

Entecavir is a guanosine nucleoside analog for the treatment of HBV infection. Following intracellular phosphorylation to the triphosphate, it competes with the natural substrate, deoxyguanosine triphosphate, for viral RT. *Entecavir* is effective against *lamivudine*-resistant strains of HBV and is dosed once daily. The drug is primarily excreted unchanged in the urine and dosage adjustments are needed in renal dysfunction. Concomitant use of drugs with renal toxicity should be avoided.

V. TREATMENT OF HEPATITIS C

Hepatitis C virus (HCV) enters the hepatocyte following interaction with cellular entry factors. Once inside the cell, a viral genome is released from the nucleocapsid and an HCV polyprotein is translated using the internal ribosome entry site. The polyprotein is then cleaved by cellular and viral proteases to yield structural and nonstructural proteins. The core NS3

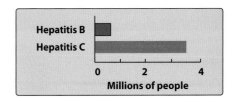

Figure 34.5
The prevalence of chronic hepatitis B and C in the United States.

Interferon-α	*Interferon-β*	*Interferon-γ*
Chronic hepatitis B and C	Relapsing-remitting multiple sclerosis	Chronic granulomatous disease
Genital warts caused by papilloma-virus		
Hairy cell leukemia,		
Chronic myelogenous leukemia		
Kaposi sarcoma		

Figure 34.6
Some approved indications for *interferon*.

GENERIC NAME(S)	BRAND NAME(S)	APPROVED HCV GENOTYPES
Elbasvir/grazoprevir	Zepatier	1, 4
Glecaprevir/pibrentasvir	Mavyret	1, 2, 3, 4, 5, 6
Paritaprevir/ritonavir/ombitasvir	Technivie	4
Paritaprevir/ritonavir/ombitasvir + dasabuvir	Viekira Pak, Viekira XR	1
Sofosbuvir + daclatasvir	Sovaldi + Daklinza	1, 3
Sofosbuvir/ledipasvir	Harvoni	1, 4, 5, 6
Sofosbuvir/velpatasvir	Epclusa	1, 2, 3, 4, 5, 6
Sofosbuvir/velpatasvir/voxilaprevir	Vosevi	1, 2, 3, 4, 5, 6

Figure 34.7
Combinations of direct-acting antiviral agents for treatment of hepatitis C virus. HCV = hepatitis C virus.

and NS5A proteins form the replication complex on lipid droplets and serve as a scaffold for RNA polymerase to replicate the viral genome, which is then packaged in envelope glycoproteins before noncytolytic secretion of mature virions. Several direct-acting antiviral agents targeting the NS3/NS4A protease, NS5B polymerase, and NS5A involved in HCV replication and assembly are available.

Combination therapy with DAAs is necessary to optimize HCV treatment response rates. Current combinations employ multiple DAAs that target different stages of the HCV life cycle simultaneously (Figure 34.7). With combination therapy, the agents are collectively able to suppress both wild-type and drug-resistant viral populations. Certain combinations may have different efficacy based on the genotype of HCV. It is anticipated that additional agents will be available in the near future. For a summary of current guidelines and regimens recommended in specific scenarios, see www.hcvguidelines.org.

A. NS3/NS4A protease inhibitors

The viral NS3/NS4A serine protease is crucial for processing the single polyprotein encoded by HCV RNA into individually active proteins, NS4A, NS4B, NS5A, and NS5B. Without these serine proteins, RNA replication does not occur and the HCV life cycle is effectively disrupted. *Paritaprevir* [PAR-i-TAP-re-vir] (which requires *ritonavir* [rit-OH-na-vir] boosting), *grazoprevir* [graz-OH-pre-vir], *voxilaprevir* [VOX-i-LA-pre-vir], and *glecaprevir* [glec-A-pre-vir] are DAAs that inhibit the NS3/NS4A serine protease as their primary mechanism of action. [Note: HCV protease inhibitors often have the ending "-previr."] These drugs have a lower barrier to resistance than other agents, such as *sofosbuvir*. Use of HCV protease inhibitors presents significant potential for drug–drug interactions due to their metabolism by CYP3A enzymes. Adverse effects of NS3/NS4A protease inhibitors include rash, pruritus, nausea, fatigue, and anemia.

B. NS5B polymerase inhibitors

NS5B is the sole RNA polymerase responsible for HCV replication and is processed with other HCV proteins into an individual polypeptide by the viral NS3/NS4A serine protease. There are two types of NS5B RNA polymerase inhibitors—nucleoside/nucleotide analogues that compete for the enzyme active site and nonnucleoside analogues that target allosteric sites. *Sofosbuvir* [soe-FOS-bue-vir] is currently the only NS5B nucleotide polymerase inhibitor for the treatment of HCV infection, and *dasabuvir* [da-SAB-ue-vir] is the only nonnucleoside analogue. [Note: NS5B inhibitors often end in "-buvir."] NS5B polymerase inhibitors are well tolerated with few adverse effects.

C. NS5A replication complex inhibitors

NS5A is a viral protein that is essential for HCV RNA replication and assembly. Its role in replication appears to be the formation of a membranous web along with viral protein NS4B, and this web provides a platform for replication. The currently available NS5A inhibitors include *ledipasvir* [le-DIP-as-vir], *ombitasvir* [om-BIT-as-vir], *elbasvir* [ELB-as-vir], *velpatasvir* [vel-PAT-as-vir], *pibrentasvir* [pi-BRENT-as-vir], and *daclatasvir* [dak-LAT-as-vir]. [Note: NS5A inhibitors often in "-asvir."] With the exception of *daclatasvir*, these agents are all coformulated with other direct-acting antivirals (see Figure 34.7). NS5A inhibitors have a number of clinically significant drug interactions due to their metabolism by hepatic CYP450 isoenzymes and inhibition of P-glycoprotein (P-gp). For example, *daclatasvir* is extensively metabolized via hepatic CYP3A4 enzymes, and the drug is contraindicated in combination with strong CYP3A4 inducers because of the potential for reduced efficacy. In addition, the dose of *daclatasvir* should be decreased when coadministered with strong CYP3A4 inhibitors and increased when coadministered with moderate CYP3A4 inducers. Absorption of *ledipasvir* is reduced when gastric pH is increased. Patients receiving proton pump inhibitors should either stop these agents during HCV therapy with *ledipasvir* or take the proton pump inhibitor with *ledipasvir*-containing regimens under fasted conditions to ensure that gastric pH is at its lowest point at the time of drug administration.

D. Ribavirin

Ribavirin is approved for the treatment of chronic HCV when used in combination with standard or *pegylated interferon* or with DAAs. *Ribavirin*, a guanosine analogue, improves viral clearance, decreases relapse rates, and improves rates of sustained virologic response when used in combination with other agents. The addition of *ribavirin* to DAA-based regimens is based on HCV genotype/subtype, cirrhosis status, mutational status, and treatment history. Despite its use in patients with HCV for more than 20 years, the precise mechanism(s) by which *ribavirin* improves outcomes is unknown. *Ribavirin* remains an important component of HCV therapy, even in the age of DAA therapy. Whether use of *ribavirin* will

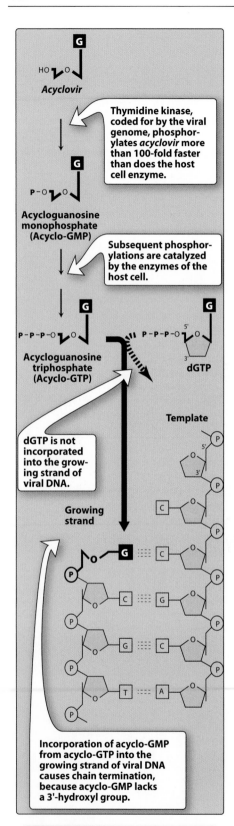

Figure 34.8
Incorporation of *acyclovir* into
replicating viral DNA, causing chain
termination. dGTP = deoxyguanosine
triphosphate.

be necessary with future DAAs is not known. The dose of *ribavirin* is always weight-based, and it is administered in two daily divided doses with food.

VI. TREATMENT OF HERPES VIRUS INFECTIONS

Herpes viruses are associated with a broad spectrum of diseases, for example, cold sores, viral encephalitis, and genital infections. The drugs that are effective against these viruses exert their actions during the acute phase of viral infections and are without effect during the latent phase.

A. Acyclovir

Acyclovir [ay-SYE-kloe-veer] is the prototypic antiherpetic therapeutic agent. Herpes simplex virus (HSV) types 1 and 2, varicella-zoster virus (VZV), and some Epstein-Barr virus–mediated infections are sensitive to *acyclovir*. It is the treatment of choice in HSV encephalitis. The most common use of *acyclovir* is in therapy for genital herpes infections. It is also given prophylactically to seropositive patients before bone marrow transplant and post-heart transplant to protect such individuals from herpetic infections.

1. **Mechanism of action:** *Acyclovir*, a guanosine analog, is monophosphorylated in the cell by the herpesvirus-encoded enzyme thymidine kinase (Figure 34.8). Therefore, virus-infected cells are most susceptible. The monophosphate analog is converted to the di- and triphosphate forms by the host cell kinases. Acyclovir triphosphate competes with deoxyguanosine triphosphate as a substrate for viral DNA polymerase and is itself incorporated into the viral DNA, causing premature DNA chain termination.

2. **Pharmacokinetics:** *Acyclovir* is administered by intravenous (IV), oral, or topical routes. [Note: The efficacy of topical applications is questionable.] The drug distributes well throughout the body, including the cerebrospinal fluid (CSF). *Acyclovir* is partially metabolized to an inactive product. Excretion into the urine occurs both by glomerular filtration and tubular secretion (Figure 34.9). *Acyclovir* accumulates in patients with renal failure. The valyl ester, *valacyclovir* [val-a-SYE-kloe-veer], has greater oral bioavailability than *acyclovir*. This ester is rapidly hydrolyzed to *acyclovir* and achieves levels of the latter comparable to those of *acyclovir* following IV administration.

3. **Adverse effects:** Adverse effects of *acyclovir* treatment depend on the route of administration. For example, local irritation may occur from topical application; headache, diarrhea, nausea, and vomiting may result after oral administration. Transient renal dysfunction may occur at high doses or in a dehydrated patient receiving the drug intravenously.

4. Resistance: Altered or deficient thymidine kinase and DNA polymerases have been found in some resistant viral strains and are most commonly isolated from immunocompromised patients. Cross-resistance to the other agents in this family occurs.

B. Cidofovir

Cidofovir [si-DOE-foe-veer] is indicated for the treatment of cytomegalovirus (CMV) retinitis in patients with AIDS. [Note: CMV is a member of the herpesvirus family.] *Cidofovir* is a nucleotide analog of cytosine, the phosphorylation of which is not dependent on viral or cellular enzymes. It inhibits viral DNA synthesis. Slow elimination of the active intracellular metabolite permits prolonged dosage intervals and eliminates the permanent venous access needed for *ganciclovir* therapy. *Cidofovir* is administered intravenously. *Cidofovir* produces significant renal toxicity (Figure 34.10), and it is contraindicated in patients with preexisting renal impairment and in those taking nephrotoxic drugs. Neutropenia and metabolic acidosis also occur. Oral *probenecid* and IV normal saline are coadministered with *cidofovir* to reduce the risk of nephrotoxicity. Since the introduction of highly active antiretroviral therapy, the prevalence of CMV infections in immunocompromised hosts has markedly declined, as has the importance of *cidofovir* in the treatment of these patients.

C. Foscarnet

Unlike most antiviral agents, *foscarnet* [fos-KAR-net] is not a purine or pyrimidine analog. Instead, it is a pyrophosphate derivative and does not require activation by viral (or cellular) kinases. *Foscarnet* is approved for CMV retinitis in immunocompromised hosts and for *acyclovir*-resistant HSV infections. *Foscarnet* works by reversibly inhibiting viral DNA and RNA polymerases, thereby interfering with viral DNA and RNA synthesis. Mutation of the polymerase structure is responsible for resistant viruses. *Foscarnet* is poorly absorbed orally and must be injected intravenously. It must also be given frequently to avoid relapse when plasma levels fall. It is dispersed throughout the body, and greater than 10% enters the bone matrix, from which it slowly disperses. The parent drug is eliminated by glomerular filtration and tubular secretion (Figure 34.11). Adverse effects include nephrotoxicity, anemia, nausea, and fever. Due to chelation with divalent cations, hypocalcemia and hypomagnesemia are also seen. In addition, hypokalemia, hypo- and hyperphosphatemia, seizures, and arrhythmias have been reported.

D. Ganciclovir

Ganciclovir [gan-SYE-kloe-veer] is an analog of *acyclovir* that has greater activity against CMV. It is used for the treatment of CMV retinitis in immunocompromised patients and for CMV prophylaxis in transplant patients.

1. Mechanism of action: Like *acyclovir*, *ganciclovir* is activated through conversion to the nucleoside triphosphate by viral

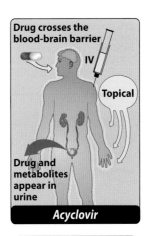

Figure 34.9
Administration and fate of *acyclovir*. IV = intravenous.

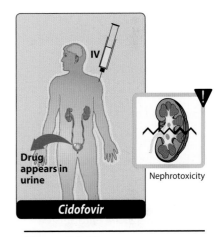

Figure 34.10
Administration, fate, and toxicity of *cidofovir*. IV = intravenous.

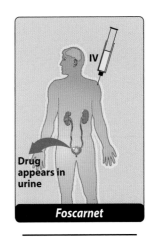

Figure 34.11
Administration and fate of *foscarnet*.

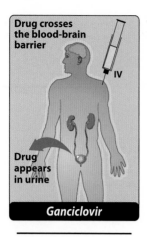

Figure 34.12
Administration and
fate of *ganciclovir*.

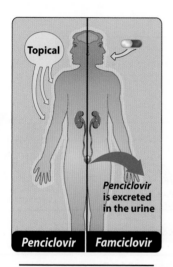

Figure 34.13
Administration and
fate of *penciclovir* and
famciclovir.

and cellular enzymes. The nucleotide inhibits viral DNA polymerase and can be incorporated into the DNA resulting in chain termination.

2. **Pharmacokinetics:** *Ganciclovir* is administered IV and distributes throughout the body, including the CSF. Excretion into the urine occurs through glomerular filtration and tubular secretion (Figure 34.12). Like *acyclovir*, *ganciclovir* accumulates in patients with renal failure. *Valganciclovir* [val-gan-SYE-kloe-veer], an oral drug, is the valyl ester of *ganciclovir*. Like *valacyclovir*, *valganciclovir* has high oral bioavailability, because rapid hydrolysis in the intestine and liver after oral administration leads to high levels of *ganciclovir*.

3. **Adverse effects:** Adverse effects include severe, dose-dependent neutropenia. *Ganciclovir* is carcinogenic as well as teratogenic and carries a boxed warning for use in pregnancy.

4. **Resistance:** Resistant CMV strains have been detected that have lower levels of ganciclovir triphosphate.

E. Penciclovir and famciclovir

Penciclovir [pen-SYE-kloe-veer] is an acyclic guanosine nucleoside derivative that is active against HSV-1, HSV-2, and VZV. *Penciclovir* is administered topically (Figure 34.13). It is monophosphorylated by viral thymidine kinase, and cellular enzymes form the nucleoside triphosphate, which inhibits HSV DNA polymerase. Penciclovir triphosphate has an intracellular half-life much longer than acyclovir triphosphate. *Penciclovir* is negligibly absorbed upon topical application and is well tolerated. *Famciclovir* [fam-SYE-kloe-veer], another acyclic analog of 2′-deoxyguanosine, is a prodrug that is metabolized to the active *penciclovir*. The antiviral spectrum is similar to that of *ganciclovir*, and it is approved for treatment of acute herpes zoster, genital HSV infection, and recurrent herpes labialis. The drug is effective orally (Figure 34.13). Adverse effects include headache and nausea.

F. Trifluridine

Trifluridine [trye-FLURE-i-deen] is a fluorinated pyrimidine nucleoside analog that is structurally similar to thymidine. Once converted to the triphosphate, the agent is believed to inhibit the incorporation of thymidine triphosphate into viral DNA and, to a lesser extent, lead to the synthesis of defective DNA that renders the virus unable to replicate. *Trifluridine* is active against HSV-1, HSV-2, and vaccinia virus. It is indicated for treatment of HSV keratoconjunctivitis and recurrent epithelial keratitis. Because the triphosphate form of *trifluridine* can also incorporate to some degree into cellular DNA, the drug is too toxic for systemic use. Therefore, the use of *trifluridine* is restricted to a topical ophthalmic preparation. A short half-life necessitates that the drug be applied frequently. Adverse effects include a transient irritation of the eye and palpebral (eyelid) edema.

Figure 34.14 summarizes selected antiviral agents.

Antiviral drug	Mechanism of action	Viruses or diseases affected
Acyclovir	Metabolized to acyclovir triphosphate, which inhibits viral DNA polymerase	Herpes simplex, varicella-zoster, cytomegalovirus
Amantadine	Blockage of the M2 protein ion channel and its ability to modulate intracellular pH	Influenza A
Cidofovir	Inhibition of viral DNA polymerase	Cytomegalovirus; indicated only for virus-induced retinitis
Famciclovir	Same as *penciclovir*	Herpes simplex, varicella-zoster
Foscarnet	Inhibition of viral DNA polymerase and reverse transcriptase at the pyrophosphate-binding site	Cytomegalovirus, *acyclovir*-resistant herpes simplex, *acyclovir*-resistant varicella-zoster
Ganciclovir	Inhibits viral DNA polymerase	Cytomegalovirus
Interferon-α	Induction of cellular enzymes that interfere with viral protein synthesis	Hepatitis B and C, human herpesvirus 8, papilloma virus, Kaposi sarcoma, hairy cell leukemia, chronic myelogenous leukemia
Lamivudine	Inhibition of viral DNA polymerase and reverse transcriptase	Hepatitis B (chronic cases), human immunodeficiency virus type 1
Oseltamivir	Inhibition of viral neuraminidase	Influenza A and B
Penciclovir	Metabolized to penciclovir triphosphate, which inhibits viral DNA polymerase	Herpes simplex
Ribavirin	Interference with viral messenger RNA	Lassa fever, hantavirus (hemorrhagic fever renal syndrome), hepatitis C (in combination with direct-acting antiviral agents), RSV in children and infants
Rimantadine	Blockage of the M2 protein ion channel and its ability to modulate intracellular pH	Influenza A
Valacyclovir	Same as *acyclovir*	Herpes simplex, varicella-zoster, cytomegalovirus
Zanamivir	Inhibition of viral neuraminidase	Influenza A and B

Figure 34.14
Summary of selected antiviral agents. RSV = respiratory syncytial virus.

VII. TREATMENT OF HIV INFECTION

Prior to approval of *zidovudine* [zye-DOE-vyoo-deen] in 1987, treatment of HIV infections focused on decreasing the occurrence of opportunistic infections that caused a high degree of morbidity and mortality in AIDS patients. Today, the viral life cycle is understood (Figure 34.15), and a combination of drugs is used to suppress replication of HIV and restore the number of CD4 cells and immunocompetence to the host. This multidrug regimen is commonly referred to as antiretroviral therapy, or ART (Figure 34.16). There are five classes of antiretroviral drugs, each of which targets one of the four viral processes. These classes of drugs are nucleoside and nucleotide reverse transcriptase inhibitors (NRTIs), nonnucleoside reverse transcriptase inhibitors (NNRTIs), protease

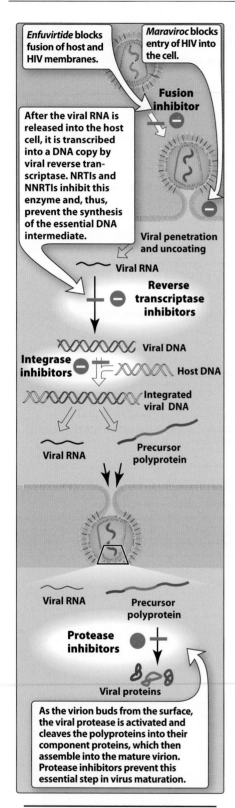

Figure 34.15
Drugs used to prevent HIV from replicating. NRTI = nucleoside and nucleotide reverse transcriptase inhibitor; NNRTI = nonnucleoside reverse transcriptase inhibitor.

inhibitors (PIs), entry inhibitors, and the integrase inhibitors. There are also two pharmacokinetic enhancers, also known as "boosters," which lack anti-HIV activity themselves, but rather serve to increase drug levels of concomitantly administered antiretroviral agents and allow for less frequent dosing and less variation in drug levels. Initial therapy for HIV consists of a combination of two NRTIs with an integrase inhibitor, an NNRTI, or a boosted PI. Selection of the appropriate combination is based on 1) avoidance of the use of two agents of the same nucleoside analog; 2) avoidance of overlapping toxicities and genotypic and phenotypic characteristics of the virus; 3) patient factors, such as disease symptoms and concurrent illnesses; 4) impact of drug interactions; and 5) ease of adherence to the regimen. The goals of therapy are to maximally and durably suppress HIV RNA replication, to restore and preserve immunologic function, to reduce HIV-related morbidity and mortality, and to improve quality of life.

VIII. NRTIS USED TO TREAT HIV INFECTION

A. Overview of NRTIs

NRTIs were the first agents available to treat HIV infection, and currently, the use of two NRTIs is a mainstay of most initial antiretroviral regimens. Available NRTIs include *zidovudine, lamivudine, emtricitabine* [em-trye-SYE-ta-been], *tenofovir, didanosine* [dye-DAN-oh-seen], *stavudine* [STA-vue-deen], and *abacavir* [a-BAK-a-veer]. The most commonly used NRTIs are *tenofovir, abacavir, emtricitabine,* and *lamivudine,* and these NRTIs are recommended parts of initial regimens for most patients with HIV. *Tenofovir disoproxil fumarate* in combination with *emtricitabine* can also be used for preexposure prophylaxis in individuals at high risk for HIV acquisition.

1. **Mechanism of action:** These agents are inhibitors of HIV reverse transcriptase. NRTIs are analogs of native ribosides (nucleosides or nucleotides containing ribose), which all lack a 3′-hydroxyl group. Once they enter cells, they are phosphorylated by cellular enzymes to the corresponding triphosphate analog, which is preferentially incorporated into the viral DNA by RT. Because the 3′-hydroxyl group is not present, a 3′,5′-phosphodiester bond between an incoming nucleoside triphosphate and the growing DNA chain cannot be formed, and DNA chain elongation is terminated. Affinities of the drugs for many host cell DNA polymerases are lower than they are for HIV RT, although mitochondrial DNA polymerase γ appears to be susceptible at therapeutic concentrations.

2. **Pharmacokinetics:** All of the NRTIs are administered orally. [Note: *Zidovudine* is also available as an intravenous formulation.] *Tenofovir* is available in two different salt forms as *tenofovir disoproxil fumarate* (TDF) and *tenofovir alafenamide* (TAF); both prodrugs of *tenofovir.* The *tenofovir* prodrug is converted by lymphoid cellular enzymes to tenofovir diphosphate, which is the active form of the drug and an inhibitor of HIV RT. TAF achieves improved anti-HIV activity at lower doses than TDF, resulting in a five- to

sevenfold increase in intracellular diphosphate in the lymphoid cell and in lower circulating plasma *tenofovir* levels. Because of this, TAF has fewer adverse effects (renal insufficiency and loss of bone mineral density) than TDF. The NRTIs are primarily renally excreted, and all require dosage adjustment in renal insufficiency except *abacavir*, which is metabolized by alcohol dehydrogenase and glucuronyl transferase.

3. **Adverse effects:** Many toxicities of the NRTIs are believed to be due to inhibition of the mitochondrial DNA polymerase in certain tissues. As a general rule, the dideoxynucleosides, such as *didanosine* and *stavudine*, have a greater affinity for the mitochondrial DNA polymerase, leading to toxicities such as peripheral neuropathy, pancreatitis, and lipoatrophy. Because of these mitochondrial toxicities, *didanosine* and *stavudine* are rarely used in current antiretroviral regimens. When more than one NRTI is given, care is taken to avoid overlapping toxicities. All NRTIs have been associated with potentially fatal liver toxicity characterized by lactic acidosis and hepatomegaly with steatosis. *Abacavir* is associated with a hypersensitivity reaction, which affects approximately 5% of patients and is usually characterized by drug fever, plus a rash, GI symptoms, malaise, or respiratory distress (Figure 34.17). Sensitized individuals should *never* be rechallenged with *abacavir* because of rapidly appearing, severe reactions that may lead to death. A genetic test (HLA-B*5701) is available to screen patients for the potential of this reaction. Figure 34.18 shows some adverse reactions commonly seen with nucleoside analogs.

4. **Drug interactions:** Due to the renal excretion of the NRTIs, there are not many drug interactions encountered with these agents except for *zidovudine* and *tenofovir*.

5. **Resistance:** NRTI resistance is well characterized, and the most common resistance pattern is a mutation at viral RT codon 184, which confers a high degree of resistance to *lamivudine* and *emtricitabine* but, more importantly, restores sensitivity to *zidovudine* and *tenofovir*. Because cross-resistance and antagonism occur between agents of the same analog class (thymidine, cytosine, guanosine, and adenosine), concomitant use of agents with the same analog target is contraindicated (for example, *zidovudine* and *stavudine* are both analogs of thymidine and should not be used together).

IX. NNRTIS USED TO TREAT HIV INFECTION

NNRTIs are highly selective, noncompetitive inhibitors of HIV RT. They bind to HIV RT at an allosteric hydrophobic site adjacent to the active site, inducing a conformational change that results in enzyme inhibition. They do not require activation by cellular enzymes. These drugs have common characteristics that include cross-resistance with other NNRTIs, drug interactions, and a high incidence of hypersensitivity reactions,

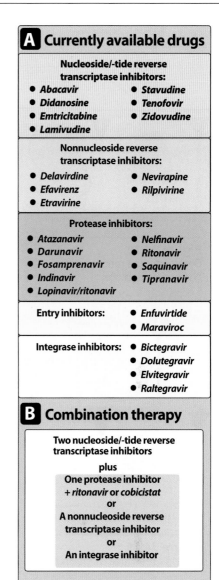

A Currently available drugs

Nucleoside/-tide reverse transcriptase inhibitors:
- *Abacavir*
- *Didanosine*
- *Emtricitabine*
- *Lamivudine*
- *Stavudine*
- *Tenofovir*
- *Zidovudine*

Nonnucleoside reverse transcriptase inhibitors:
- *Delavirdine*
- *Efavirenz*
- *Etravirine*
- *Nevirapine*
- *Rilpivirine*

Protease inhibitors:
- *Atazanavir*
- *Darunavir*
- *Fosamprenavir*
- *Indinavir*
- *Lopinavir/ritonavir*
- *Nelfinavir*
- *Ritonavir*
- *Saquinavir*
- *Tipranavir*

Entry inhibitors:
- *Enfuvirtide*
- *Maraviroc*

Integrase inhibitors:
- *Bictegravir*
- *Dolutegravir*
- *Elvitegravir*
- *Raltegravir*

B Combination therapy

Two nucleoside/-tide reverse transcriptase inhibitors

plus

One protease inhibitor
+ *ritonavir* or *cobicistat*
or
A nonnucleoside reverse transcriptase inhibitor
or
An integrase inhibitor

Figure 34.16
Antiretroviral therapy for treatment of HIV. [Note: *Elvitegravir* is coformulated with *cobicistat*. *Cobicistat* inhibits the metabolism of *elvitegravir*, thereby increasing its concentration in the plasma.]

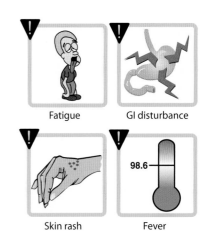

Fatigue   GI disturbance

Skin rash   Fever

Figure 34.17
Hypersensitivity reactions to *abacavir*.

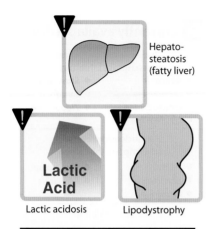

Figure 34.18
Some adverse reactions of nucleoside analogs.

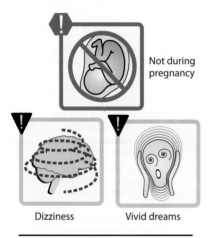

Figure 34.19
Adverse reactions of *efavirenz*.

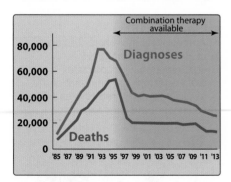

Figure 34.20
Estimated number of AIDS cases and deaths due to AIDS in the United States. *Green* background indicates years in which combination antiretroviral therapy came into common usage.

including rash. The NNRTIs include *nevirapine* [ne-VYE-ra-peen], *delavirdine* [de-LA-vir-deen], *efavirenz* [e-FA-veer-enz], *etravirine* [et-ra-VYE-rine], and *rilpivirine* [ril-pi-VIR-een]. *Efavirenz* (Figure 34.19) and *rilpivirine* are recommended in initial antiretroviral regimens in certain clinical situations. For example, *efavirenz* is safe to use in patients co-infected with tuberculosis because of its lower potential for drug interactions with rifamycins, and *rilpivirine* has the smallest tablet size, making it ideal for patients with difficulty swallowing. *Etravirine* is a second-generation NNRTI active against many HIV strains that are resistant to the first-generation NNRTIs; its use is limited to HIV treatment–experienced, multidrug-resistant patients who have evidence of ongoing viral replication. *Delavirdine* and *nevirapine* are rarely used due to toxicities and/or inferior antiviral efficacy.

X. PROTEASE INHIBITORS USED TO TREAT HIV INFECTION

Inhibitors of HIV protease have significantly altered the course of this devastating viral disease. Shortly after their introduction, the number of deaths in the United States due to AIDS decreased and continues to remain on the decline (Figure 34.20). Available PIs include *atazanavir* (ATV), *darunavir* (DRV) [da-ROON-a-veer], *fosamprenavir* (FPV) [FOS-am-PREN-a-veer], *indinavir* (IDV) [in-DIN-a-veer], *lopinavir* (LPV) [loe-PIN-a-vir], *nelfinavir* (NFV) [nel-FIN-a-veer], *saquinavir* (SQV) [sa-KWIN-a-veer], and *tipranavir* (TPV) [tip-RA-na-veer]. However, current HIV guidelines only list a select few (for example, *atazanavir* or *darunavir*) due to improved adverse effect profile, virologic efficacy, and ease of dosing. Due to their high genetic barrier to resistance, protease inhibitors are recommended in initial regimens in certain clinical situations (for example, patients with uncertain adherence or when resistance testing results are not yet available).

A. Overview

These potent agents have several common features that characterize their pharmacology.

1. **Mechanism of action:** Drugs in this group are reversible inhibitors of the HIV aspartyl protease (retropepsin), which is the viral enzyme responsible for cleavage of the viral polyprotein into a number of essential enzymes (RT, protease, and integrase) and several structural proteins. The inhibition prevents maturation of the viral particles and results in the production of noninfectious virions.

2. **Pharmacokinetics:** High-fat meals substantially increase the bioavailability of some PIs, such as *nelfinavir* and *saquinavir*, whereas the bioavailability of *indinavir* is decreased, and others are essentially unaffected. The HIV PIs are all substantially bound to plasma proteins. These agents are substrates for the CYP3A4 isoenzyme, and individual PIs are also metabolized by other CYP450 isoenzymes. Metabolism is extensive, and very little drug is excreted unchanged in urine.

3. **Adverse effects:** PIs commonly cause nausea, vomiting, and diarrhea (Figure 34.21). Disturbances in glucose and lipid metabolism also occur, including diabetes, hypertriglyceridemia, and hypercholesterolemia. Chronic administration results in fat redistribution, including loss of fat from the extremities, fat accumulation in the abdomen and the base of the neck ("buffalo hump"; Figure 34.22), and breast enlargement. These physical changes may indicate to others that an individual is HIV infected.

4. **Drug interactions:** Drug interactions are a common problem for PIs, because they are substrates and also potent inhibitors of CYP450 isoenzymes. Drugs that rely on metabolism for their termination of action may accumulate to toxic levels. Examples of potentially dangerous interactions with PIs include rhabdomyolysis from *simvastatin* or *lovastatin*, excessive sedation from *midazolam* or *triazolam*, and respiratory depression from *fentanyl* (Figure 34.23). Other drug interactions that require dosage modification and cautious use include *warfarin, sildenafil,* and *phenytoin* (Figure 34.24). In addition, inducers of CYP450 isoenzymes may decrease PI plasma concentrations to suboptimal levels, contributing to treatment failures. Thus, drugs such as *rifampin* and *St. John's wort* are also contraindicated with PIs.

5. **Resistance:** Resistance occurs as an accumulation of stepwise mutations of the protease gene. Initial mutations result in decreased ability of the virus to replicate, but as the mutations accumulate, virions with high levels of resistance to the protease inhibitors emerge. Suboptimal concentrations of PI result in the more rapid appearance of resistant strains.

B. Atazanavir

Atazanavir is well absorbed after oral administration. It must be taken with food to increase absorption and bioavailability. *Atazanavir* requires an acidic environment for absorption. Thus, unboosted *atazanavir* is contraindicated with concurrent use of proton pump inhibitors, and administration must be spaced apart from H_2-blockers and antacids. *Atazanavir* can be boosted by *ritonavir* or *cobicistat*. The drug is highly protein bound and undergoes extensive metabolism by CYP3A4 isoenzymes. It is excreted primarily in bile. It has a half-life of about 7 hours, but it may be administered once daily. *Atazanavir* is a competitive inhibitor of glucuronyl transferase, and benign hyperbilirubinemia and jaundice are known adverse effects. In addition, the drug may prolong the PR interval. *Atazanavir* exhibits a decreased risk of hyperlipidemia compared with other PIs.

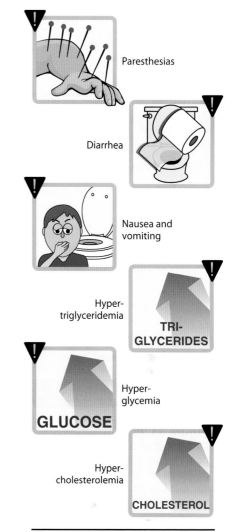

Figure 34.21
Some adverse effects of the HIV protease inhibitors.

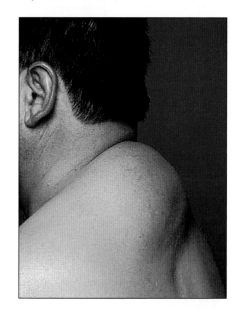

Figure 34.22
Accumulation of fat at the base of the neck in a patient receiving a protease inhibitor.

DRUG CLASS	EXAMPLE
ANTIARRHYTHMICS	*Amiodarone*
ERGOT DERIVATIVES	*Ergotamine*
ANTIMYCOBACTERIAL DRUGS	*Rifampin*
BENZODIAZEPINES	*Triazolam*
INHALED STEROIDS	*Fluticasone*
HERBAL SUPPLEMENTS	*St. John's wort*
HMG CoA REDUCTASE INHIBITORS	*Lovastatin Simvastatin*
NARCOTICS	*Fentanyl*
β-2 AGONIST	*Salmeterol*

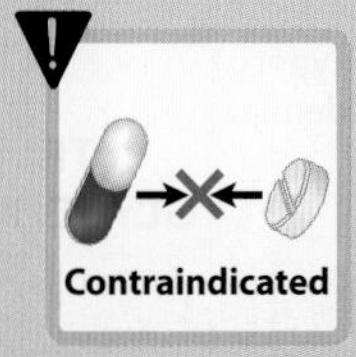

Contraindicated

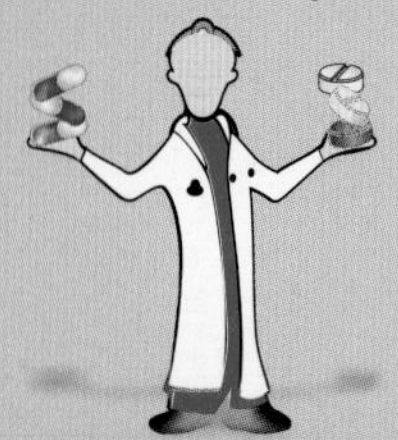

PROTEASE INHIBITORS

Figure 34.23
Drugs that should not be coadministered with any protease inhibitor.

DRUG CLASS	EXAMPLE
ANTICOAGULANTS	*Warfarin*
ANTICONVULSANTS	*Phenytoin*
ANTIFUNGALS	*Voriconazole*
ANTIMYCOBACTERIALS	*Rifabutin*
ERECTILE DYSFUNCTION AGENTS	*Sildenafil Tadalafil Vardenafil*
LIPID-LOWERING AGENTS	*Atorvastatin*
NARCOTICS	*Methadone*

PROTEASE INHIBITORS

C. Darunavir

Darunavir [da-RU-na-veer] is coadministered with *cobicistat* or a low dose of *ritonavir*. *Darunavir* is approved for initial therapy in treatment-naive HIV-infected patients, as well as for treatment-experienced patients with HIV resistant to other PIs. *Darunavir* must be taken with food to increase absorption. The elimination half-life is 15 hours when combined with *ritonavir*. *Darunavir* is extensively metabolized by the CYP3A enzymes and is also an inhibitor of the CYP3A4 isoenzyme. Adverse effects are similar to those of the other PIs. In addition, *darunavir* therapy has been associated with a rash.

A summary of PIs is presented in Figure 34.25.

XI. ENTRY INHIBITORS

A. Enfuvirtide

Enfuvirtide [en-FYOO-vir-tide] is a fusion inhibitor. For HIV to gain entry into the host cell, it must fuse its membrane with that of the host cell. This is accomplished by changes in the conformation of the viral transmembrane glycoprotein gp41, which occurs when HIV binds to the host cell surface. *Enfuvirtide* is a polypeptide that binds to gp41, preventing the conformational change. *Enfuvirtide*, in combination with other antiretroviral agents, is indicated for therapy of treatment-experienced patients with evidence of viral replication despite ongoing antiretroviral drug therapy. As a peptide, it must be given subcutaneously. Most of the adverse effects are related to the injection, including pain, erythema, induration, and nodules, which occur in almost all patients. *Enfuvirtide* must be reconstituted prior to administration.

B. Maraviroc

Maraviroc [ma-RAV-i-rok] is an entry inhibitor that blocks the CCR5 coreceptor that works with gp41 to facilitate HIV entry through the membrane into the cell. HIV may express preference for either the CCR5 coreceptor or the CXCR4 coreceptor, or both (dual-tropic). Prior to use of *maraviroc*, a test to determine viral tropism is required to distinguish whether the strain of HIV virus uses the CCR5 coreceptor, the CXCR4 coreceptor, or is dual-tropic. Only strains of HIV that use CCR5 to gain access to the cell can be successfully treated with *maraviroc*. The drug is well absorbed after oral administration. *Maraviroc* is metabolized mainly by the hepatic CYP3A isoenzyme, and the dose must be reduced when given with most PIs or strong CYP450 inhibitors. Conversely, it should be increased in patients receiving *efavirenz*, *etravirine*, or strong CYP450 inducers. *Maraviroc* is generally well tolerated. The drug has been associated with severe hepatotoxicity, which may be preceded by a fever or rash. Monitoring of liver function is recommended.

Figure 34.24
Drugs that require dose modifications or cautious use with any protease inhibitor.

XII. INTEGRASE INHIBITORS

Raltegravir [ral-TEG-ra-veer], elvitegravir [el-vi-TEG-ra-vir], dolutegravir [doe-loo-TEG-ra-vir], and bictegravir [bik-TEG-ra-vir] are integrase strand transfer inhibitors (INSTIs), often called integrase inhibitors. These agents work by inhibiting the insertion of proviral DNA into the host cell genome. The active site of the integrase enzyme binds to the host cell DNA and includes two divalent metal cations that serve as chelation targets for the INSTIs. As a result, when an INSTI is present, the active site of the enzyme is occupied and the integration process is halted. The half-life of elvitegravir is 3 hours when administered alone, but increases to approximately 9 hours when boosted by cobicistat. Pharmacokinetic boosting of elvitegravir allows once-daily dosing with food. The INSTIs are generally well tolerated, with nausea and diarrhea being the most commonly reported adverse effects. Importantly, INSTIs are subject to chelation interactions with antacids, resulting in significant reductions in bioavailability. Therefore, INSTI doses should be separated from antacids and other polyvalent cations by several hours. Resistance to INSTIs occurs with single-point mutations within the integrase gene. Cross-resistance between raltegravir and elvitegravir can occur, although dolutegravir has limited cross-resistance to other INSTIs.

XIII. PHARMACOKINETIC ENHANCERS

A. Ritonavir

Ritonavir [ri-TOE-na-veer] is no longer used as a single PI but, instead, is used as a pharmacokinetic enhancer or "booster" of other PIs. Ritonavir is a potent inhibitor of CYP3A, and concomitant ritonavir administration at low doses increases the bioavailability of the second PI, often allowing for longer dosing intervals. The resulting higher C_{min} levels of the "boosted" PI also help to prevent the development of HIV resistance. Therefore, "boosted" PIs are recommended for use in initial HIV regimens in certain clinical situations. Metabolism by CYP3A4 and CYP2D6 and biliary excretion are the primary methods of elimination. Ritonavir has a half-life of 3 to 5 hours. Although ritonavir is primarily an inhibitor of CYP450 isoenzymes, it may also induce several CYP450 isoenzymes, and numerous drug interactions have been identified.

B. Cobicistat

Cobicistat [koe-BIK-i-stat] is a pharmacokinetic enhancer or booster drug used in combination treatments for HIV. This agent inhibits CYP3A isoenzymes and is used to enhance the bioavailability of the protease inhibitors atazanavir and darunavir, and the integrase inhibitor elvitegravir. Because cobicistat inhibits CYP3A, CYP2D6, and the transporter P-gp, numerous drug interactions exist. Cobicistat may also cause elevations in serum creatinine due to inhibition of tubular creatinine secretion.

DRUGS	MAJOR TOXICITIES AND CONCERNS
Atazanavir	Nausea, abdominal discomfort, skin rash, hyperbilirubinemia
Darunavir	Nausea, abdominal discomfort, headache, skin rash
Fosamprenavir	Nausea, diarrhea, vomiting, oral and perioral paresthesia, and rash
Indinavir	Benign hyperbilirubinemia, nephrolithiasis; take 1 hour before or 2 hours after food; may take with skim milk or a low-fat meal; drink >1.5 L of liquid daily
Lopinavir	Gastrointestinal, hyperlipidemia, insulin resistance
Nelfinavir	Diarrhea, nausea, flatulence, rash
Ritonavir	Diarrhea, nausea, taste perversion, vomiting, anemia, increased hepatic enzymes, increased triglycerides. Capsules require refrigeration, tablets do not. Take with meals; chocolate milk improves the taste
Saquinavir	Diarrhea, nausea, abdominal discomfort, elevated transaminase levels. Take with high-fat meal or within 2 hours of a full meal
Tipranavir	Nausea, vomiting, diarrhea, rash, severe hepatotoxicity, intracranial hemorrhage

Figure 34.25
Summary of protease inhibitors. [Note: Lopinavir is coformulated with ritonavir. Ritonavir inhibits the metabolism of lopinavir, thereby increasing its level in the plasma.]

Study Questions

Choose the ONE best answer.

34.1 A 30-year-old man with human immunodeficiency virus infection is being treated with an antiretroviral regimen. Four weeks after initiating therapy, he presents to the emergency department complaining of fever, rash, and gastrointestinal upset. His HLA-B*5701 test is positive. Which drug is most likely the cause of his symptoms?

A. Zidovudine
B. Abacavir
C. Efavirenz
D. Darunavir

Correct answer = B. The abacavir hypersensitivity reaction is characterized by fever, rash, and gastrointestinal upset. The patient must stop therapy and should not be rechallenged with abacavir.

34.2 A 75-year-old man with chronic obstructive pulmonary disease is diagnosed with suspected influenza based on complaints of flu-like symptoms that began 24 hours ago. Which agent is most appropriate to initiate for the treatment of influenza?

A. Oseltamivir
B. Zanamivir
C. Rimantadine
D. Amantadine

Correct answer = A. Oseltamivir is the best choice since it is administered orally and not associated with resistance. Zanamivir is administered via inhalation and is not recommended for patients with underlying COPD. High rates of resistance have developed to adamantanes (amantadine, rimantadine), and these drugs are infrequently indicated.

34.3 A 24-year-old woman is diagnosed with genital herpes simplex virus infection. Which agent is indicated for use in this diagnosis?

A. Valacyclovir
B. Cidofovir
C. Ganciclovir
D. Zanamivir

Correct answer = A. Valacyclovir, famciclovir, penciclovir, and acyclovir are all indicated for herpes simplex virus infection. Cidofovir and ganciclovir are used for CMV retinitis. Zanamivir is indicated for influenza.

34.4 A woman who is being treated for chronic hepatitis B develops nephrotoxicity while on treatment. Which medication is most likely to be included in her HBV treatment?

A. Entecavir
B. Ribavirin
C. Lamivudine
D. Adefovir

Correct answer = D. Nephrotoxicity is the most commonly seen with adefovir in the treatment of HBV. This adverse effect is uncommon with lamivudine and entecavir. Ribavirin is used for the treatment of hepatitis C infection (not HBV).

34.5 Which class of direct-acting antivirals for hepatitis C works by inhibiting formation of the membranous web that provides a platform for viral replication?

A. NS3/NS4A protease inhibitors
B. NS5B polymerase inhibitors
C. NS5A replication complex inhibitors
D. Interferons

Correct answer = C. NS5A inhibitors work to inhibit the formation of proteins that form a membranous web, which serves as a platform for viral replication. NS3/NS4A protease inhibitors prevent processing of the single polyprotein encoded by HCV RNA into individually active proteins. NS5B polymerase inhibitors act on the RNA polymerase responsible for HCV replication. The mechanism of interferons has not been fully defined.

34.6 Which antiretroviral drug class chelates with polyvalent cations and, as such, their administration must be separated from antacids by several hours?

A. Integrase inhibitors
B. Nonnucleoside reverse transcriptase inhibitors
C. Protease inhibitors
D. Entry inhibitors

Correct answer = A. Integrase inhibitors bind to other positively charged ions, rendering them ineffective. As such, separation of doses of these agents from aluminum-, magnesium-, and calcium-containing antacids is recommended.

34.7 A 62-year-old man with human immunodeficiency virus infection is being treated with an antiretroviral regimen containing elvitegravir/cobicistat/emtricitabine/tenofovir disoproxil fumarate and has achieved a sustained undetectable level of HIV RNA. His prescriber would like to change his therapy to elvitegravir/cobicistat/emtricitabine/tenofovir alafenamide. Which information should the prescriber provide to the patient that best summarizes the advantage of tenofovir alafenamide over tenofovir disoproxil fumarate?

A. Removal of food restrictions
B. Fewer drug interactions
C. Twice daily dosing
D. Improved renal and bone safety profile

Correct answer = D. Tenofovir alafenamide delivers the same active drug as tenofovir disoproxil fumarate, but with a lower incidence of renal and bone adverse effects. Both tenofovir-containing combinations are dosed once daily and should be taken with food. No change in drug interactions is expected, since tenofovir alafenamide is a prodrug which, like TDF, is metabolized to tenofovir.

34.8 A 37-year-old woman with GERD and chronic hepatitis C genotype 1a infection is preparing to begin treatment with ledipasvir/sofosbuvir. Which is the most appropriate information for the patient regarding use of a proton pump inhibitor during treatment with ledipasvir/sofosbuvir?

A. Absorption of ledipasvir is increased with increasing pH.
B. A proton pump inhibitor can be safely administered with ledipasvir/sofosbuvir without regard to timing of the dose or food intake.
C. The patient should either stop using the proton pump inhibitor or take it with ledipasvir/sofosbuvir under fasted conditions.
D. Absorption of ledipasvir is not affected by gastric pH.

Answer = C. Absorption of ledipasvir is reduced when gastric pH is increased. Patients receiving proton pump inhibitors should stop these agents during HCV therapy with ledipasvir or take the proton pump inhibitor with ledipasvir/sofosbuvir under fasted conditions to ensure that gastric pH is at its lowest point of the day at the time of drug administration.

34.9 Which HIV antiretroviral is an orally administered entry inhibitor?

A. Maraviroc
B. Enfuvirtide
C. Rilpivirine
D. Raltegravir

Answer = A. Maraviroc is the only orally administered entry inhibitor for HIV infection. Enfuvirtide is an entry inhibitor (fusion inhibitor), but it is injected. Rilpivirine is an NNRTI, and raltegravir is an INSTI for HIV infection.

34.10 Which drug is a pharmacokinetic enhancer used to boost levels of some HIV protease inhibitors and elvitegravir?

A. Cobicistat
B. Dolutegravir
C. Entecavir
D. Tenofovir

Answer = A. Cobicistat is a pharmacokinetic enhancer used to boost serum levels of HIV protease inhibitors atazanavir, darunavir, and the integrase inhibitor elvitegravir. Like elvitegravir, dolutegravir is an INSTI. Entecavir is a guanosine nucleoside analog for the treatment of HBV infection. Tenofovir is a nucleoside reverse transcriptase inhibitor used in the treatment of HIV and HBV.

Anticancer Drugs

Kourtney LaPlant and Paige May

35

I. OVERVIEW

It is estimated that over 25% of the population of the United States will face a diagnosis of cancer during their lifetime, with more than 1.6 million new cancer patients diagnosed each year. Less than a quarter of these patients will be cured solely by surgery and/or local radiation. Most of the remainder will receive systemic chemotherapy at some time during their illness. In a small fraction (approximately 10%) of patients with cancer representing selected neoplasms, the chemotherapy will result in a cure or a prolonged remission. However, in most cases, drug therapy will produce only a regression of the disease, and complications and/or relapse may eventually lead to death. Thus, the overall 5-year survival rate for cancer patients is about 68%, ranking cancer second only to cardiovascular disease as a cause of mortality. Figure 35.1 provides a list of the anticancer agents discussed in this chapter.

II. PRINCIPLES OF CANCER CHEMOTHERAPY

Cancer chemotherapy strives to cause a lethal cytotoxic event or apoptosis in the cancer cells that can arrest the progression of tumor growth. The attack is generally directed toward DNA or against metabolic sites essential to cell replication, for example, the availability of purines and pyrimidines, which are the building blocks for DNA or RNA synthesis (Figure 35.2). Ideally, anticancer drugs should interfere only with cellular processes that are unique to malignant cells. Unfortunately, most traditional anticancer drugs do not specifically recognize neoplastic cells but, rather, affect all kinds of proliferating cells, both normal and abnormal. Therefore, almost all antitumor agents have a steep dose–response curve for both therapeutic and toxic effects. Newer agents are being developed that take a different approach to cancer treatment by blocking checkpoints and allowing the patient's own immune system to attack cancer cells. While this strategy is showing great promise, adverse effects are also a concern and present as autoimmune toxicity, as compared to the myelosuppressive profile with traditional chemotherapy agents.

A. Treatment strategies

1. **Goals of treatment:** The ultimate goal of chemotherapy is a cure (that is, long-term, disease-free survival). A true cure requires the eradication of every neoplastic cell. If a cure is not attainable, then

ANTIMETABOLITES	
Azacitidine	VIDAZA
Capecitabine	XELODA
Cladribine	GENERIC ONLY
Cytarabine	DEPOCYT
Fludarabine	GENERIC ONLY
5-Fluorouracil	ADRUCIL
Gemcitabine	GEMZAR
6-Mercaptopurine	PURINETHOL
Methotrexate **(MTX)**	TREXALL
Pemetrexed	ALIMTA
Pralatrexate	FOLOTYN

ANTIBIOTICS	
Bleomycin	GENERIC ONLY
Daunorubicin	CERUBIDINE
Doxorubicin	ADRIAMYCIN, DOXIL
Epirubicin	ELLENCE
Idarubicin	IDAMYCIN
Mitoxantrone	GENERIC ONLY

ALKYLATING AGENTS	
Busulfan	MYLERAN
Carmustine	BICNU
Chlorambucil	LEUKERAN
Cyclophosphamide	CYTOXAN
Dacarbazine	GENERIC ONLY
Ifosfamide	IFEX
Lomustine	GLEOSTINE
Melphalan	ALKERAN
Temozolomide	TEMODAR

MICROTUBULE INHIBITORS	
Docetaxel	TAXOTERE
Paclitaxel	TAXOL
Vinblastine	GENERIC ONLY
Vincristine	VINCASAR PFS
Vinorelbine	NAVELBINE

Figure 35.1
Summary of chemotherapeutic agents.

the goal becomes control of the disease (prevent the cancer from enlarging and spreading) to extend survival and maintain quality of life. Thus, the individual maintains a "near-normal" existence, with the cancer treated as a chronic disease. In either case, the neoplastic cell burden is initially reduced (debulked), either by surgery and/or by radiation, followed by chemotherapy, immunotherapy, therapy using biological modifiers, or a combination of these treatment modalities (Figure 35.3). In advanced stages of cancer, the likelihood of controlling the cancer is low, and the goal is palliation (alleviation of symptoms and avoidance of life-threatening toxicity). This means that chemotherapeutic drugs may be used to relieve symptoms caused by the cancer and improve the quality of life, even though the drugs may not extend survival. The goal of treatment should always be kept in mind, as it often influences treatment decisions. Figure 35.4 illustrates how treatment goals can be dynamic.

2. **Indications for treatment:** Chemotherapy is sometimes used when neoplasms are disseminated and are not amenable to surgery. Chemotherapy may also be used as a supplemental treatment to attack micrometastases following surgery and radiation treatment, in which case it is called adjuvant chemotherapy. Chemotherapy given prior to the surgical procedure in an attempt to shrink the cancer is referred to as neoadjuvant chemotherapy, and chemotherapy given in lower doses to assist in prolonging remission is known as maintenance chemotherapy.

3. **Tumor susceptibility and the growth cycle:** The fraction of tumor cells that are in the replicative cycle ("growth fraction") influences susceptibility to most cancer chemotherapeutic agents. Rapidly dividing cells are generally more sensitive to chemotherapy, whereas slowly proliferating cells are less sensitive to chemotherapy. In general, nondividing cells (those in the G_0 phase; Figure 35.5) usually survive the toxic effects of many chemotherapeutic agents.

   a. **Cell cycle specificity of drugs:** Both normal cells and tumor cells go through growth cycles (Figure 35.5). However, the number of cells that are in various stages of the cycle may differ in normal and neoplastic tissues. Chemotherapeutic agents that are effective only against replicating cells (that is, those cells that are dividing) are said to be cell cycle specific (Figure 35.5), whereas other agents are cell cycle nonspecific. Although the nonspecific drugs generally have greater toxicity in cycling cells, they are also useful against tumors that have a low percentage of replicating cells.

   b. **Tumor growth rate:** The growth rate of most solid tumors is initially rapid, but growth rate usually decreases as the tumor size increases (see Figure 35.3). This is due to a deficiency of nutrients and oxygen caused by inadequate vascularization and lack of blood circulation. Tumor burden can be reduced through surgery, radiation, or use of cell cycle–nonspecific drugs that promote the remaining cells into active proliferation, thus increasing susceptibility to cell cycle–specific chemotherapeutic agents.

STEROID HORMONES AND THEIR ANTAGONISTS
Anastrozole ARIMIDEX
Bicalutamide CASODEX
Enzalutamide XTANDI
Exemestane AROMASIN
Flutamide GENERIC ONLY
Fulvestrant FASLODEX
Goserelin ZOLADEX
Letrozole FEMARA
Leuprolide LUPRON
Nilutamide NILANDRON
Raloxifene EVISTA
Tamoxifen GENERIC ONLY
Triptorelin TRELSTAR

MONOCLONAL ANTIBODIES
Bevacizumab AVASTIN
Cetuximab ERBITUX
Daratumumab DARZALEX
Panitumumab VECTIBIX
Ramucirumab CYRAMZA
Rituximab RITUXAN
Trastuzumab HERCEPTIN

TYROSINE KINASE INHIBITORS
Afatinib GILOTRIF
Dabrafenib TAFINLAR
Dasatinib SPRYCEL
Erlotinib TARCEVA
Ibrutinib IMBRUVICA
Idelalisib ZYDELIG
Imatinib GLEEVEC
Nilotinib TASIGNA
Osimertinib TAGRISSO
Pazopanib VOTRIENT
Sorafenib NEXAVAR
Sunitinib SUTENT
Trametinib MEKINIST
Vemurafenib ZELBORAF

OTHERS
Abiraterone ZYTIGA
Bortezomib VELCADE
Carboplatin GENERIC ONLY
Carfilzomib KYPROLIS
Cisplatin PLATINOL
Etoposide TOPOSAR
Ixazomib NINLARO
Lenalidomide REVLIMID
Nivolumab OPDIVO
Oxaliplatin ELOXATIN
Pembrolizumab KEYTRUDA
Pomalidomide POMALYST
Thalidomide THALOMID
Topotecan HYCAMTIN

Figure 35.1 (continued)

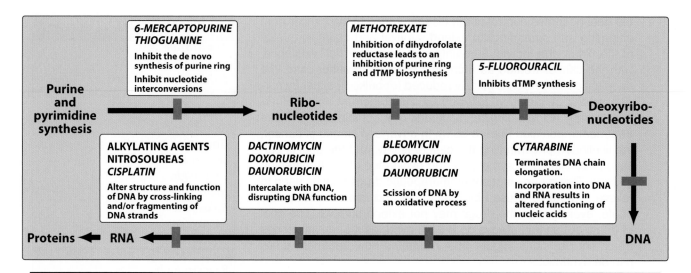

Figure 35.2
Examples of chemotherapeutic agents affecting RNA and DNA. dTMP = deoxythymidine monophosphate.

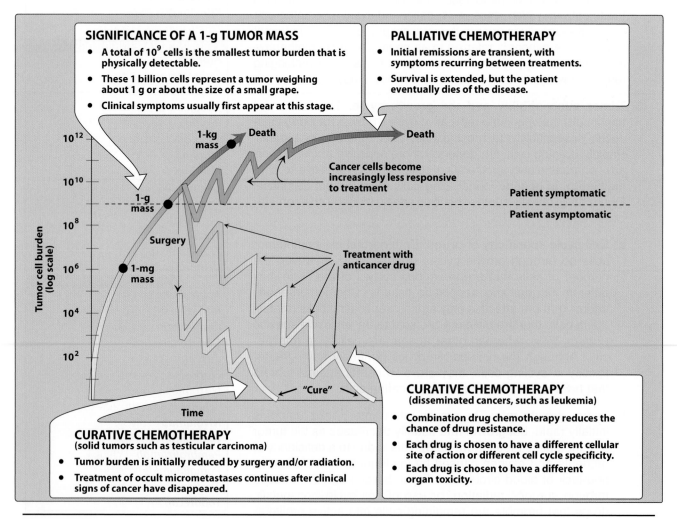

Figure 35.3
Effects of various treatments on the cancer cell burden in a hypothetical patient.

B. Treatment regimens and scheduling

Drug dosages are usually calculated on the basis of body surface area, in an effort to tailor the dosage to each patient.

1. **Log kill phenomenon:** Destruction of cancer cells by chemotherapeutic agents follows first-order kinetics (that is, a given dose of drug destroys a constant fraction of cells). The term "log kill" is used to describe this phenomenon. For example, a diagnosis of leukemia is generally made when there are about 10^9 (total) leukemic cells. Consequently, if treatment leads to a 99.999% kill, then 0.001% of 10^9 cells (or 10^4 cells) remain. This is defined as a 5-log kill (reduction of 10^5 cells). At this point, the patient becomes asymptomatic, and the patient is in remission (see Figure 35.3). For most bacterial infections, a 5-log (100,000-fold) reduction in the number of microorganisms results in a cure, because the immune system can destroy the remaining bacterial cells. However, tumor cells are not as readily eliminated, and additional treatment is required to totally eradicate the leukemic cell population.

2. **Pharmacologic sanctuaries:** Leukemic or other tumor cells find sanctuary in tissues such as the central nervous system (CNS), where transport constraints prevent certain chemotherapeutic agents from entrance. Therefore, a patient may require irradiation of the craniospinal axis or intrathecal administration of drugs to eliminate leukemic cells at that site. Similarly, drugs may be unable to penetrate certain areas of solid tumors.

3. **Treatment protocols:** Combination chemotherapy is more successful than single-drug treatment in most cancers for which chemotherapy is effective.

   a. **Combination chemotherapy:** Cytotoxic agents with different toxicities, and with different molecular sites and mechanisms of action, are usually combined at full doses. This results in higher response rates, due to additive and/or potentiated cytotoxic effects, and nonoverlapping host toxicities. In contrast, agents with similar dose-limiting toxicities, such as myelosuppression, nephrotoxicity, or cardiotoxicity, can be combined safely only by reducing the doses of each.

   b. **Advantages of combinations:** The advantages of combination chemotherapy are that it 1) provides maximal cell killing within the range of tolerated toxicity, 2) is effective against a broader range of cell lines in the heterogeneous tumor population, and 3) may delay or prevent the development of resistant cell lines.

   c. **Treatment protocols:** Many cancer treatment protocols have been developed, and each is applicable to a particular neoplastic state. They are usually identified by an acronym. For example, a common regimen called R-CHOP, used for the treatment of non-Hodgkin lymphoma, consists of *rituximab, cyclophosphamide, hydroxydaunorubicin (doxorubicin), Oncovin (vincristine),* and *prednisone.* Therapy is scheduled

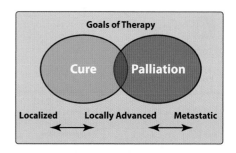

Figure 35.4
Goals of treatment with chemotherapeutic agents.

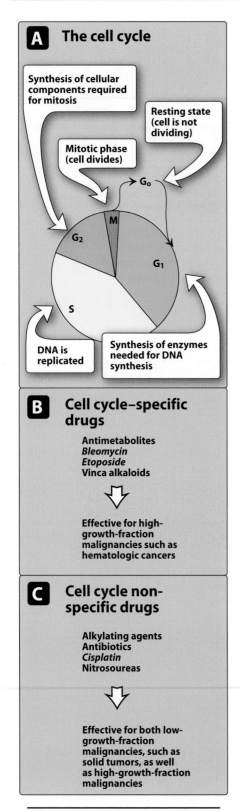

Figure 35.5
Effects of chemotherapeutic agents on the growth cycle of mammalian cells.

intermittently to allow recovery or rescue of the immune system, which is also affected by the chemotherapeutic agents, thus reducing the risk of serious infection.

C. Resistance and toxicity with chemotherapy

Cancer drugs are toxins that present a lethal threat to the cells. It is, therefore, not surprising that cells have evolved elaborate defense mechanisms to protect themselves from chemical toxins, including chemotherapeutic agents.

1. **Resistance:** Some neoplastic cells (for example, melanoma) are inherently resistant to most anticancer drugs. Other tumor types may acquire resistance to the cytotoxic effects of a drug by mutating, particularly after prolonged administration of suboptimal doses. The development of drug resistance is minimized by short-term, intensive, intermittent therapy with combinations of drugs. Drug combinations are also effective against a broader range of resistant cells in the tumor population.

2. **Multidrug resistance:** Stepwise selection of an amplified gene that codes for a transmembrane protein (P-glycoprotein for "permeability" glycoprotein; Figure 35.6) is responsible for multidrug resistance. This resistance is due to adenosine triphosphate–dependent pumping of drugs out of the cell in the presence of P-glycoprotein. Cross-resistance following the use of structurally unrelated agents also occurs. For example, cells that are resistant to the cytotoxic effects of the Vinca alkaloids are also resistant to *dactinomycin* and to the anthracycline antibiotics, as well as to *colchicine*, and vice versa. These drugs are all naturally occurring substances, each of which has a hydrophobic aromatic ring and a positive charge at neutral pH. [Note: P-glycoprotein is normally expressed at low levels in most cell types, but higher levels are found in the kidney, liver, pancreas, small intestine, colon, and adrenal gland. It has been suggested that the presence of P-glycoprotein may account for the intrinsic resistance to chemotherapy observed with adenocarcinomas.] Certain drugs at high concentrations (for example, *verapamil*) can inhibit the pump and, thus, interfere with the efflux of the anticancer agent. However, these drugs are undesirable because of adverse pharmacologic actions of their own. Pharmacologically inert pump blockers are being sought.

3. **Toxicity:** Therapy aimed at killing rapidly dividing cancer cells also affects normal cells undergoing rapid proliferation (for example, cells of the buccal mucosa, bone marrow, gastrointestinal [GI] mucosa, and hair follicles), contributing to the toxic manifestations of chemotherapy.

   a. **Common adverse effects:** Most chemotherapeutic agents have a narrow therapeutic index. Severe vomiting, stomatitis, bone marrow suppression, and alopecia occur to varying extents during therapy with most antineoplastic agents. Vomiting is often controlled by administration of antiemetic drugs. Some toxicities, such as myelosuppression that predisposes to infection, are common to many chemotherapeutic agents (Figure 35.7), whereas other adverse reactions are confined to specific agents, such as bladder toxicity with *cyclophosphamide,* cardiotoxicity with *doxorubicin*, and pulmonary fibrosis with *bleomycin*. The duration of the adverse effects varies widely. For example, alopecia is transient, but the cardiac, pulmonary, and bladder toxicities can be irreversible.

b. Minimizing adverse effects: Some toxic reactions may be ameliorated by interventions, such as the use of cytoprotectant drugs, local perfusion of the tumor (for example, a sarcoma of the arm), removal of some marrow of the patient prior to intensive treatment and then reimplantation afterward, or intensive hydration and diuresis to prevent bladder toxicities. The megaloblastic anemia that occurs with *methotrexate* can be effectively counteracted by administering *folinic acid* (*leucovorin*). With the availability of human granulocyte colony-stimulating factors, the neutropenia associated with treatment of cancer by many drugs can be partially reversed.

4. Treatment-induced tumors: Because most antineoplastic agents are mutagens, neoplasms (for example, acute nonlymphocytic leukemia) may arise 10 or more years after the original cancer was cured. [Note: Treatment-induced neoplasms are especially a problem after therapy with alkylating agents.] Most tumors that develop from cancer chemotherapeutic agents respond well to treatment strategies.

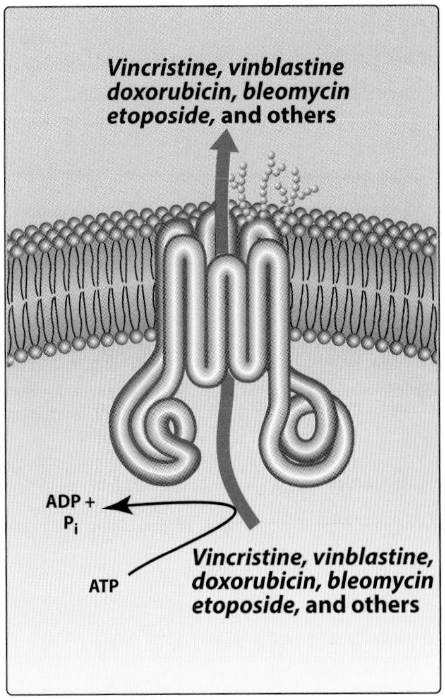

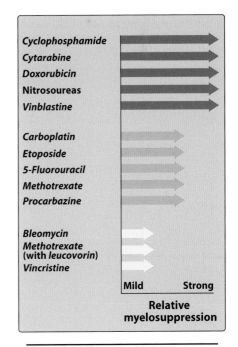

Figure 35.6
The six membrane-spanning loops of the P-glycoprotein form a central channel for the ATP-dependent pumping of drugs from the cell.

III. ANTIMETABOLITES

Antimetabolites are structurally related to normal compounds that exist within the cell (Figure 35.8). They generally interfere with the availability of normal purine or pyrimidine nucleotide precursors, either by inhibiting their synthesis or by competing with them in DNA or RNA synthesis. Their maximal cytotoxic effects are in S phase and are, therefore, cell cycle specific.

A. Methotrexate, pemetrexed, and pralatrexate

The vitamin folic acid plays a central role in a variety of metabolic reactions involving the transfer of one-carbon units and is essential for cell replication. Folic acid is obtained mainly from dietary sources and from that produced by intestinal flora. *Methotrexate* [meth-oh-TREK-sate] (*MTX*), *pemetrexed* [pem-e-TREX-ed], and *pralatrexate* [pral-a-TREX-ate] are antifolate agents.

1. Mechanism of action: *MTX* is structurally related to folic acid and acts as an antagonist of the vitamin by inhibiting mammalian dihydrofolate reductase (DHFR), the enzyme that converts folic acid to its active, coenzyme form, tetrahydrofolic acid (FH$_4$) (Figure 35.9). The inhibition of DHFR can only be reversed by a 1000-fold excess of the natural substrate, dihydrofolate (FH$_2$), or by administration of *leucovorin,* which bypasses the blocked enzyme and replenishes the folate pool (Figure 35.9). [Note: *Leucovorin*, or *folinic acid*, is the N^5-formyl group–carrying form of FH$_4$.] *MTX* is

Figure 35.7
Comparison of myelosuppressive potential of chemotherapeutic drugs.

DRUG	ROUTE	ADVERSE EFFECTS	NOTABLE DRUG INTERACTIONS	MONITORING PARAMETERS	NOTES
Methotrexate	IV/PO/ IM/IT	N/V/D, stomatitis, rash, alopecia, myelosuppression, high-dose: renal damage IT: neurologic toxicities	*Omeprazole, folic acid, warfarin,* NSAIDs, penicillins, cephalosporins	CBC; renal, hepatic function; *methotrexate* levels (after high-dose infusion)	Some adverse effects can be prevented or reversed by administering *leucovorin*. Adjust dose in renal impairment.
6-Mercaptopurine (6-MP)	PO	N/V/D, myelosuppression, anorexia, hepatotoxicity (jaundice)	*Warfarin, allopurinol, SMZ/TMP*	CBC; renal, hepatic function	Reduce dose of *6-MP* by 50%–75% when used with *allopurinol* to prevent toxicity
Fludarabine	IV	N/V/D, myelosuppression, rash, immunosuppression, fever, edema, neurologic toxicity	*Cytarabine, cyclophosphamide, cisplatin, mitoxantrone, pentostatin*	CBC; renal, hepatic function; tumor lysis syndrome	Immunosuppression increases risk of opportunistic infections. Adjust dose in renal impairment.
Cladribine	IV/SC	Neutropenia, immunosuppression, fever, N/V, teratogenic, peripheral neuropathy		CBC; renal function; tumor lysis syndrome	Immunosuppression increases risk of opportunistic infections.
5-Fluorouracil (5-FU)	IV	D, alopecia, severe mucositis, myelosuppression (bolus), "hand-foot syndrome" (continuous infusion), coronary vasospasm	*Methotrexate* (antifolate analogs)	CBC; renal, hepatic function; D	"Hand-foot syndrome"/palmar-plantar erythrodysesthesia is an erythematous desquamation of the palms and soles.
Capecitabine	PO	D, mucositis, myelosuppression, "hand-foot syndrome," chest pain	*Warfarin, phenytoin*	CBC; renal, hepatic function; D	Should be taken within 30 min of a meal; keep skin well moisturized.
Cytarabine	IV/IT	N/V/D, myelosuppression, hepatotoxicity; neurologic toxicity, conjunctivitis (high dose)	*Digoxin, alkylating agents, methotrexate*	CBC; renal, hepatic function; CNS toxicity	Administer steroid eye drops with high dose to prevent conjunctivitis.
Azacitidine	IV/SC	Myelosuppression (neutropenia, thrombocytopenia), N/V, constipation, hypokalemia, renal toxicity		CBC; renal, hepatic function	Stability of prepared drug (IV) is only 60 min.
Gemcitabine	IV	Myelosuppression, (thrombocytopenia), N/V, alopecia, rash, flu-like syndrome	Potent radiosensitizer	CBC; hepatic function, rash	

Figure 35.8
Summary of antimetabolites. CBC = complete blood count; CNS = central nervous system; D = diarrhea; IM = intramuscular; IT = intrathecal; IV = intravenous; N = nausea; NSAID = nonsteroidal anti-inflammatory drug; PO = oral; SC = subcutaneous; SMZ/TMP = sulfamethoxazole/trimethoprim; V = vomiting.

specific for the S phase of the cell cycle. *Pemetrexed* is an antimetabolite similar in mechanism to *methotrexate*. However, in addition to inhibiting DHFR, it also inhibits thymidylate synthase and other enzymes involved in folate metabolism and DNA synthesis. *Pralatrexate* is an antimetabolite that also inhibits DHFR.

2. **Therapeutic uses:** *MTX*, usually in combination with other drugs, is effective against acute lymphocytic leukemia, Burkitt lymphoma in children, breast cancer, bladder cancer, and head and neck carcinomas. In addition, low-dose *MTX* is effective as a single agent against certain inflammatory diseases, such as severe psoriasis and rheumatoid arthritis, as well as Crohn disease. All patients receiving *MTX* require close monitoring for possible toxic effects. *Pemetrexed* is primarily used in non–small cell lung cancer. *Pralatrexate* is used in relapsed or refractory T-cell lymphoma.

3. **Pharmacokinetics:** *MTX* is variably absorbed at low doses from the GI tract, but it can also be administered by intramuscular, intravenous (IV), and intrathecal routes (Figure 35.10). Because *MTX* does not easily penetrate the blood–brain barrier, it can be

administered intrathecally to destroy neoplastic cells that thrive in the sanctuary of the CNS. High concentrations of the drug are found in the intestinal epithelium, liver, and kidney, as well as in ascites and pleural effusions. *MTX is* also distributed to the skin. Small amounts of *MTX* undergo hydroxylation at the 7th position to form 7-hydroxymethotrexate. This derivative is less water soluble than *MTX* and may lead to crystalluria. Therefore, it is important to keep the urine alkaline and the patient well hydrated to avoid renal toxicity. Excretion of the parent drug and the 7-OH metabolite occurs primarily via urine.

4. **Adverse effects:** Adverse effects of *MTX* are outlined in Figure 35.8. *Pemetrexed* and *pralatrexate* should be given with folic acid and vitamin B_{12} supplements to reduce hematologic and GI toxicities. Pretreatment with corticosteroids to prevent cutaneous reactions is recommended with *pemetrexed*.

B. 6-Mercaptopurine

6-Mercaptopurine [mer-kap-toe-PYOOR-een] (*6-MP*), a purine antimetabolite, is the thiol analog of hypoxanthine. *6-MP* and *6-thioguanine* were the first purine analogs to prove beneficial for treating neoplastic disease. [Note: *Azathioprine*, an immunosuppressant, exerts its cytotoxic effects after conversion to *6-MP*.] *6-MP* is used principally in the maintenance of remission in acute lymphoblastic leukemia. *6-MP* and its analog, *azathioprine*, are also beneficial in the treatment of Crohn disease. Adverse effects are noted in Figure 35.8.

C. Fludarabine

Fludarabine [floo-DARE-a-been] is the 5'-phosphate of 2-fluoroadenine arabinoside, a purine nucleotide analog. It is useful in the treatment of chronic lymphocytic leukemia, hairy cell leukemia, and indolent non-Hodgkin lymphoma. *Fludarabine* is a prodrug, and the phosphate is removed in the plasma to form 2-F-araA, which is taken up into cells and again phosphorylated (initially by deoxycytidine kinase). Although the exact cytotoxic mechanism is uncertain, the triphosphate is incorporated into both DNA and RNA. This decreases their synthesis in the S phase and affects their function. Resistance is associated with reduced uptake into cells, lack of deoxycytidine kinase, and decreased affinity for DNA polymerase, as well as other mechanisms. *Fludarabine* is administered IV rather than orally, because intestinal bacteria split off the sugar to yield the very toxic metabolite, fluoroadenine.

D. 5-Fluorouracil

5-Fluorouracil [flure-oh-YOOR-ah-sil] (*5-FU*), a pyrimidine analog, has a stable fluorine atom in place of a hydrogen atom at position 5 of the uracil ring. The fluorine interferes with the conversion of deoxyuridylic acid to thymidylic acid, thus depriving the cell of thymidine, one of the essential precursors for DNA synthesis. *5-FU* is employed primarily in the treatment of slow-growing solid tumors (for example, colorectal, breast, ovarian, pancreatic, and gastric carcinomas). When applied topically, *5-FU* is also effective for the treatment of superficial basal cell carcinomas.

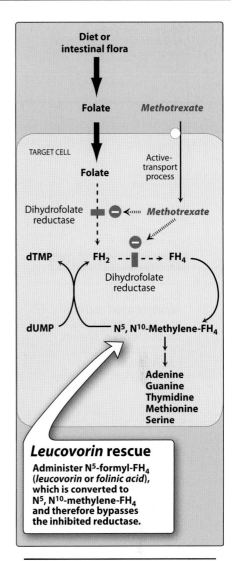

Figure 35.9
Mechanism of action of *methotrexate* and the effect of administration of *leucovorin*. FH_2 = dihydrofolate; FH_4 = tetrahydrofolate; dTMP = deoxythymidine monophosphate; dUMP = deoxyuridine monophosphate.

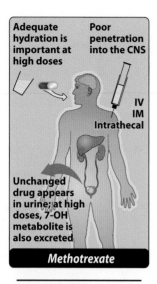

| Adequate hydration is important at high doses | Poor penetration into the CNS |

IV
IM
Intrathecal

Unchanged drug appears in urine; at high doses, 7-OH metabolite is also excreted

Methotrexate

Figure 35.10
Administration and fate of *methotrexate*. CNS = central nervous system; IV = intravenous; IM = intramuscular.

1. **Mechanism of action:** *5-FU* itself is devoid of antineoplastic activity. It enters the cell through a carrier-mediated transport system and is converted to the corresponding deoxynucleotide (5-fluoro-deoxyuridine monophosphate [5-FdUMP]; Figure 35.11), which competes with deoxyuridine monophosphate for thymidylate synthase, thus inhibiting its action. DNA synthesis decreases due to lack of thymidine, leading to imbalanced cell growth and "thymidine-less death" of rapidly dividing cells. [Note: *Leucovorin* is administered with *5-FU*, because the reduced folate coenzyme is required in the thymidylate synthase inhibition. For example, a standard regimen for advanced colorectal cancer is *irinotecan* plus *5-FU/leucovorin*.] *5-FU* is also incorporated into RNA, and low levels have been detected in DNA. In the latter case, a glyco-sylase excises the *5-FU*, damaging the DNA. *5-FU* produces the anticancer effect in the S phase of the cell cycle.

2. **Pharmacokinetics:** Because of severe toxicity to the GI tract, *5-FU* is administered IV or, in the case of skin cancer, topically. The drug penetrates well into all tissues, including the CNS. *5-FU* is rapidly metabolized in the liver, lung, and kidney. It is eventually converted to fluoro-β-alanine, which is removed in the urine. Elevated levels of dihydropyrimidine dehydrogenase (DPD) can increase the rate of *5-FU* catabolism and decrease its bioavailability. The level of DPD varies from individual to individual and may differ by as much as six-fold in the general population. Patients with DPD deficiency may experience severe toxicity manifested by pancytopenia, mucositis, and life-threatening diarrhea. Knowledge of DPD activity in an individual should allow more appropriate dosing of *5-FU*.

E. Capecitabine

Capecitabine [KAP-e-SYE-ta-been] is a fluoropyrimidine carbamate. It is used in the treatment of colorectal and metastatic breast cancer. *Capecitabine* is well absorbed following oral administration. After being absorbed, *capecitabine,* which is itself nontoxic, undergoes a series of enzymatic reactions, the last of which is hydrolysis to *5-FU*. This step is catalyzed by thymidine phosphorylase, an enzyme that is concentrated primarily in tumors (Figure 35.12). Thus, the cyto-toxic activity of *capecitabine* is the same as that of *5-FU* and is tumor specific. The most important enzyme inhibited by *5-FU* (and, thus, *capecitabine*) is thymidylate synthase.

F. Cytarabine

Cytarabine [sye-TARE-ah-been] (*cytosine arabinoside or ara-C*) is an analog of 2′-deoxycytidine in which the natural ribose residue is replaced by D-arabinose. *Cytarabine* acts as a pyrimidine antagonist. The major clinical use of *cytarabine* is in acute nonlymphocytic (myelogenous) leukemia (AML). *Cytarabine* enters the cell by a carrier-mediated process and, like the other purine and pyrimidine antagonists, must be sequentially phosphorylated by deoxycytidine kinase and other nucleotide kinases to the nucleotide form (cytosine arabinoside triphosphate or ara-CTP) to be cytotoxic. Ara-CTP is an effective inhibitor of DNA polymerase. The nucleotide is also incorporated into nuclear DNA and can terminate chain elongation. It is, therefore, S phase (and, hence, cell cycle) specific.

1. **Pharmacokinetics:** *Cytarabine* is not effective when given orally, because of deamination to the noncytotoxic ara-U by cytidine deaminase in the intestinal mucosa and liver. Given IV, it distributes throughout the body but does not penetrate the CNS in sufficient amounts. Therefore, it may also be injected intrathecally. *Cytarabine* undergoes extensive oxidative deamination in the body to ara-U, a pharmacologically inactive metabolite. Both *cytarabine* and ara-U are excreted in urine.

G. Azacitidine

Azacitidine [A-zuh-SITE-i-dine] is a pyrimidine nucleoside analog of cytidine. It is used for the treatment of myelodysplastic syndromes and AML. *Azacitidine* undergoes activation to the nucleotide metabolite azacitidine triphosphate and gets incorporated into RNA to inhibit RNA processing and function. It is S-phase cell cycle specific.

H. Gemcitabine

Gemcitabine [jem-SITE-ah-been] is an analog of the nucleoside deoxycytidine. It is used most commonly for pancreatic cancer and non–small cell lung cancer. *Gemcitabine* is a substrate for deoxycytidine kinase, which phosphorylates the drug to 2′,2′-difluorodeoxycytidine triphosphate (Figure 35.13). *Gemcitabine* is administered by IV infusion. It is deaminated to difluorodeoxyuridine, which is not cytotoxic, and is excreted in urine.

IV. ANTIBIOTICS

The antitumor antibiotics (Figure 35.14) owe their cytotoxic action primarily to their interactions with DNA, leading to disruption of DNA function. In addition to intercalation, their abilities to inhibit topoisomerases (I and II) and produce free radicals also play a major role in their cytotoxic effect. They are cell cycle nonspecific, with *bleomycin* as an exception.

A. Anthracyclines: Doxorubicin, daunorubicin, idarubicin, epirubicin, and mitoxantrone

Doxorubicin [dox-oh-ROO-bi-sin] and *daunorubicin* [daw-noe-ROO-bi-sin] are classified as anthracycline antibiotics. *Doxorubicin* is the hydroxylated analog of *daunorubicin*. *Idarubicin* [eye-da-ROO-bi-sin], the 4-demethoxy analog of *daunorubicin, epirubicin* [eh-pee-ROO-bih-sin], and *mitoxantrone* [mye-toe-ZAN-trone] are also available. Therapeutic uses for these agents differ despite their structural similarity and apparently similar mechanisms of action. *Doxorubicin* is one of the most important and widely used anticancer drugs. It is used in combination with other agents for treatment of sarcomas and a variety of carcinomas, including breast cancer, as well as for treatment of acute lymphocytic leukemia and lymphomas. *Daunorubicin* and *idarubicin* are used in the treatment of acute leukemias, and *mitoxantrone* is used in prostate cancer.

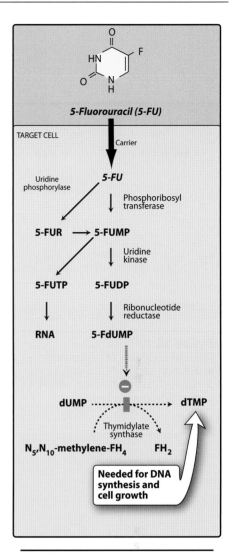

Figure 35.11
Mechanism of the cytotoxic action of *5-FU*. *5-FU* is converted to 5-fluorodeoxyuridine monophosphate (5-FdUMP), which competes with deoxyuridine monophosphate (dUMP) for the enzyme thymidylate synthase. *5-FU = 5-fluorouracil*; 5-FUR = 5-fluorouridine; 5-FUMP = 5-fluorouridine monophosphate; 5-FUDP = 5-fluorouridine diphosphate; 5-FUTP = 5-fluorouridine triphosphate; dUMP = deoxyuridine monophosphate; dTMP = deoxythymidine monophosphate.

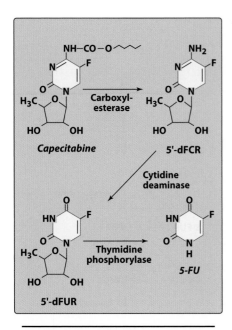

Figure 35.12
Metabolic pathway of *capecitabine*
to *5-fluorouracil* (*5-FU*). 5′-dFCR =
5′-deoxy-5-fluorocytidine; 5′-dFUR =
5′-deoxy-5-fluorouridine.

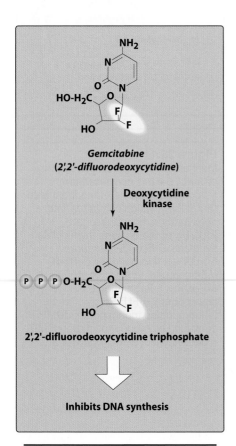

Figure 35.13
Mechanism of action of *gemcitabine*.

1. **Mechanism of action:** *Doxorubicin* and other anthracyclines induce cytotoxicity through several different mechanisms. For example, *doxorubicin*-derived free radicals can induce membrane lipid peroxidation, DNA strand scission, and direct oxidation of purine or pyrimidine bases, thiols, and amines (Figure 35.15).

2. **Pharmacokinetics:** These agents must be administered intravenously, because they are inactivated in the GI tract. Extravasation is a serious problem that can lead to tissue necrosis. The anthracycline antibiotics bind to plasma proteins as well as to other tissue components, where they are widely distributed. They do not penetrate the blood–brain barrier or the testes. These agents undergo extensive hepatic metabolism, and dosage adjustments are needed in patients with impaired hepatic function. Biliary excretion is the major route of elimination. Because of the dark red color of the anthracycline drugs, the veins may become visible surrounding the site of infusion, and red discoloration of urine may occur.

3. **Adverse effects:** Irreversible, dose-dependent cardiotoxicity is the most serious adverse reaction and is more common with *daunorubicin* and *doxorubicin* than with *idarubicin* and *epirubicin*. Cardiotoxicity apparently results from the generation of free radicals and lipid peroxidation. Addition of *trastuzumab* to protocols with *doxorubicin* or *epirubicin* increases the risk of congestive heart failure. There has been some success with the iron chelator *dexrazoxane* in protecting against the cardiotoxicity of *doxorubicin*. The liposomal-encapsulated *doxorubicin* is reported to be less cardiotoxic than the standard formulation.

B. Bleomycin

Bleomycin [blee-oh-MYE-sin] is a mixture of different copper-chelating glycopeptides that, like the anthracycline antibiotics, cause scission of DNA by an oxidative process. *Bleomycin* is cell cycle specific and causes cells to accumulate in the G$_2$ phase. It is primarily used in the treatment of testicular cancers and Hodgkin lymphoma.

1. **Mechanism of action:** A DNA–*bleomycin*–Fe^{2+} complex appears to undergo oxidation to *bleomycin*–Fe^{3+}. The liberated electrons react with oxygen to form superoxide or hydroxyl radicals, which, in turn, attack the phosphodiester bonds of DNA, resulting in strand breakage and chromosomal aberrations (Figure 35.16).

2. **Pharmacokinetics:** *Bleomycin* is administered by a number of routes. The *bleomycin*-inactivating enzyme (a hydrolase) is high in a number of tissues (for example, liver and spleen) but is low in the lung and absent in the skin, accounting for toxicity in those tissues. Most of the parent drug is excreted unchanged in the urine, necessitating dose adjustment in patients with renal failure.

3. **Adverse effects:** Pulmonary toxicity is the most serious adverse effect, progressing from rales, cough, and infiltrate to potentially fatal fibrosis. The pulmonary fibrosis that is caused by *bleomycin* is often referred as "*bleomycin* lung." Hypertrophic skin changes and hyperpigmentation of the hands are prevalent. *Bleomycin* is unusual in that myelosuppression is rare.

DRUG	ROUTE	ADVERSE EFFECTS	NOTABLE DRUG INTERACTIONS	MONITORING PARAMETERS	NOTES
Doxorubicin	IV	Myelosuppression, N/V/D, mucositis, cardiac toxicity, alopecia, red coloration of urine. Strong vesicants	*Phenytoin, trastuzumab* (cardiotoxicity), *digoxin*	CBC; renal, hepatic function; cardiac function (ECHO or MUGA); adjust in hepatic dysfunction	Cumulative doses >450 mg/m² increase risk of cardiotoxicity. Vesicant!
Daunorubicin	IV				Cumulative doses >550 mg/m² increase risk of cardiotoxicity. Vesicant!
Liposomal Doxorubicin	IV				Not a substitute for *doxorubicin*, less cardiotoxicity
Epirubicin	IV		*Cimetidine*		Cumulative doses >900 mg/m² increase risk of cardiotoxicity. Vesicant! Less N/V
Idarubicin	IV			As with other anthracyclines plus tumor lysis syndrome	Cumulative doses >150 mg/m² increase risk of cardiotoxicity. Vesicant!
Bleomycin	IV/SC/IM	Pulmonary fibrosis, alopecia, skin reactions, hyperpigmentation of hands, fever, chills, anaphylaxis	Phenothiazines, *cisplatin* (renal), radiation (pulmonary)	Pulmonary function tests; adjust in renal dysfunction; anaphylaxis	"Bleomycin lung" pulmonary fibrosis can be fatal. Discontinue if any signs of lung dysfunction.

Figure 35.14
Summary of antitumor antibiotics. CBC = complete blood count; D = diarrhea; IM = intramuscular; IV = intravenous; N = nausea; SC = subcutaneous; V = vomiting.

V. ALKYLATING AGENTS

Alkylating agents (Figure 35.17) exert their cytotoxic effects by covalently binding to nucleophilic groups on various cell constituents. Alkylation of DNA is probably the crucial cytotoxic reaction that is lethal to the tumor cells. Alkylating agents do not discriminate between cycling and resting cells, even though they are most toxic for rapidly dividing cells. They are used in combination with other agents to treat a wide variety of lymphatic and solid cancers. In addition to being cytotoxic, all are mutagenic and carcinogenic and can lead to secondary malignancies such as acute leukemia.

A. Cyclophosphamide and ifosfamide

These drugs are very closely related mustard agents that share most of the same primary mechanisms and toxicities. They are cytotoxic only after generation of their alkylating species, which are produced through hydroxylation by cytochrome P450 (CYP450). These agents have a broad clinical spectrum and are used as single agents or in combinations in the treatment of a wide variety of neoplastic diseases, such as non-Hodgkin lymphoma, sarcoma, and breast cancer.

1. **Mechanism of action:** *Cyclophosphamide* [sye-kloe-FOSS-fah-mide] is the most commonly used alkylating agent. Both *cyclophosphamide* and *ifosfamide* [eye-FOSS-fah-mide] are first biotransformed to hydroxylated intermediates primarily in the liver by the CYP450 system (Figure 35.18). The hydroxylated intermediates then undergo metabolism to form the active compounds, phosphoramide mustard and acrolein. Reaction of the phosphoramide mustard with DNA is considered to be the cytotoxic step.

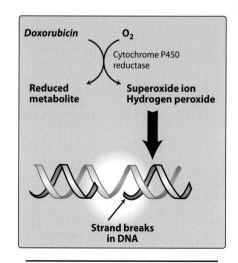

Figure 35.15
Doxorubicin interacts with molecular oxygen, producing superoxide ions and hydrogen peroxide, which cause single-strand breaks in DNA.

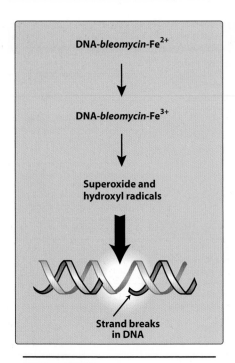

DNA-*bleomycin*-Fe^{2+}

↓

DNA-*bleomycin*-Fe^{3+}

↓

Superoxide and hydroxyl radicals

Strand breaks in DNA

Figure 35.16
Bleomycin causes breaks in DNA by an oxidative process.

2. **Pharmacokinetics:** *Cyclophosphamide* is available in oral and IV preparations, whereas *ifosfamide* is IV only. *Cyclophosphamide* is metabolized in the liver to active and inactive metabolites, and minimal amounts are excreted in the urine as unchanged drug. *Ifosfamide* is metabolized primarily by CYP450 3A4 and 2B6 isoenzymes. It is mainly renally excreted.

3. **Adverse effects:** A unique toxicity of both drugs is hemorrhagic cystitis, which can lead to fibrosis of the bladder. Bladder toxicity has been attributed to acrolein in the urine in the case of *cyclophosphamide* and to toxic metabolites of *ifosfamide*. Adequate hydration as well as IV injection of *mesna* (sodium 2-mercaptoethane sulfonate), which neutralizes the toxic metabolites, can minimize this problem. Neurotoxicity has been reported in patients on high-dose *ifosfamide*, probably due to the metabolite, chloroacetaldehyde.

B. Nitrosoureas

Carmustine [KAR-mus-teen, BCNU] and *lomustine* [LOE-mus-teen, CCNU] are closely related nitrosoureas. Because of their ability to penetrate the CNS, the nitrosoureas are primarily employed in the treatment of brain tumors.

1. **Mechanism of action:** The nitrosoureas exert cytotoxic effects by an alkylation that inhibits replication and, eventually, RNA and

DRUG	ROUTE	ADVERSE EFFECTS	NOTABLE DRUG INTERACTIONS	MONITORING PARAMETERS	NOTES
Cyclophosphamide	IV/PO	Myelosuppression, hemorrhagic cystitis, N/V/D, alopecia, amenorrhea, secondary malignancies	*Phenobarbital, phenytoin* (P450); *digoxin,* anticoagulants	Urinalysis; CBC; renal, hepatic function	Good hydration to prevent bladder toxicity (*mesna* with high doses)
Ifosfamide	IV	Myelosuppression, hemorrhagic cystitis, N/V, neurotoxicity, alopecia, amenorrhea	*Phenobarbital, phenytoin* (P450); *cimetidine, allopurinol, warfarin*	Urinalysis; neurotoxicity	Use *mesna* and hydration to prevent bladder toxicity
Carmustine (BCNU)	IV	Myelosuppression, N/V, facial flushing, hepatotoxicity, pulmonary toxicity, impotence, infertility	*Cimetidine, amphotericin B, digoxin, phenytoin*	CBC; PFTs; renal, hepatic function	Also available as an implantable wafer (brain)
Lomustine (CCNU)	PO	Myelosuppression, N/V, pulmonary toxicity, impotence, infertility, neurotoxicity	*Cimetidine,* alcohol	CBC; PFTs; renal function	Administer on an empty stomach
Dacarbazine	IV	Myelosuppression, N/V, flu-like syndrome, CNS toxicity, hepatotoxicity, photosensitivity	*Phenytoin, phenobarbital* (P450)	CBC; renal, hepatic function	Vesicant
Temozolomide	PO	N/V, myelosuppression, headache, fatigue, photosensitivity		CBC; renal, hepatic function	Requires <u>Pneumocystis</u> pneumonia prophylaxis
Melphalan	IV/PO	Myelosuppression, N/V/D, mucositis, hypersensitivity (IV)	*Cimetidine,* steroids, *cyclosporine*	CBC; renal, hepatic function	Take on an empty stomach
Chlorambucil	PO	Myelosuppression, skin rash, pulmonary fibrosis (rare), hyperuricemia, seizures	*Phenobarbital, phenytoin* (P450)	CBC; renal, hepatic function; uric acid	Take with food
Busulfan	IV/PO	Myelosuppression, N/V/D, mucositis, skin rash, pulmonary fibrosis, hepatotoxicity	*Acetaminophen, itraconazole, phenytoin*	CBC; pulmonary symptoms; renal, hepatic function	"Busulfan lung"

Figure 35.17
Summary of alkylating agents. CBC = complete blood count; CNS = central nervous system; D = diarrhea; IV = intravenous; N = nausea; PFT = pulmonary function test; PO = by mouth; V = vomiting.

protein synthesis. Although they alkylate DNA in resting cells, cytotoxicity is expressed primarily in cells that are actively dividing. Therefore, nondividing cells can escape death if DNA repair occurs. Nitrosoureas also inhibit several key enzymatic processes by carbamoylation of amino acids in proteins in the targeted cells.

2. **Pharmacokinetics:** *Carmustine* is administered IV and as chemotherapy wafer implants, whereas *lomustine* is given orally. Because of their lipophilicity, these agents distribute widely in the body and readily penetrate the CNS. The drugs undergo extensive metabolism. *Lomustine* is metabolized to active products. The kidney is the major excretory route for the nitrosoureas (Figure 35.19).

C. Dacarbazine and temozolomide

Dacarbazine [dah-KAR-bah-zeen] is an alkylating agent that must undergo biotransformation to an active metabolite, methyltriazeno-imidazole carboxamide (MTIC). The metabolite is responsible for the alkylating activity of this agent by forming methyl carbonium ions that attack the nucleophilic groups in the DNA molecule. The cytotoxic action of *dacarbazine* has been attributed to the ability of its metabolite to methylate DNA on the O-6 position of guanine. *Dacarbazine* has found use in the treatment of melanoma and Hodgkin lymphoma. *Temozolomide* [te-moe-ZOE-loe-mide] is related to *dacarbazine*, because both must undergo biotransformation to an active metabolite, MTIC, which is likely responsible for the methylation of DNA on the O-6 and N-7 position of guanine. Unlike *dacarbazine*, *temozolomide* does not require the CYP450 system for metabolic transformation, and it undergoes chemical transformation at normal physiological pH. *Temozolomide* also inhibits the repair enzyme, O-6-guanine-DNA alkyltransferase. *Temozolomide* differs from *dacarbazine* in that it crosses the blood–brain barrier and, therefore, is used in the treatment of brain tumors such as glioblastomas and astrocytomas. It is also used in metastatic melanoma. *Temozolomide* is administered intravenously or orally and has excellent bioavailability after oral administration. The parent drug and metabolites are excreted in urine (Figure 35.20).

D. Other alkylating agents

Mechlorethamine [mek-lor-ETH-ah-meen] was developed as a vesicant (nitrogen mustard) during World War I. Its ability to cause lymphocytopenia led to its use in lymphatic cancers. *Melphalan* [MEL-fah-lan], a phenylalanine derivative of nitrogen mustard, is used in the treatment of multiple myeloma. This is a bifunctional alkylating agent that can be given orally, although the plasma concentration differs from patient to patient due to variation in intestinal absorption and metabolism. The dose of *melphalan* is carefully adjusted by monitoring the platelet and white blood cell counts. *Chlorambucil* [clor-AM-byoo-sil] is another bifunctional alkylating agent that is used in the treatment of chronic lymphocytic leukemia. *Busulfan* [byoo-SUL-fan] is an alkylating agent that is effective against chronic myelogenous leukemia. This agent can cause pulmonary fibrosis ("*busulfan* lung"). Like other alkylating agents, all of these agents are leukemogenic.

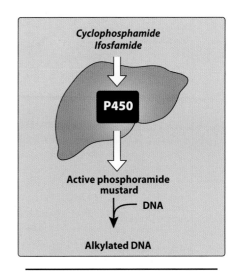

Figure 35.18
Activation of *cyclophosphamide* and *ifosfamide* by hepatic cytochrome P450.

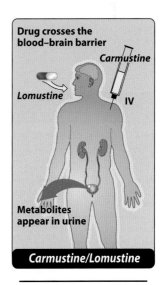

Figure 35.19
Administration and fate of *carmustine/lomustine*. IV = intravenous.

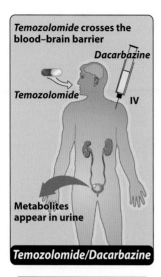

Figure 35.20
Administration and fate of *temozolomide* and *dacarbazine*. IV = intravenous.

VI. MICROTUBULE INHIBITORS

The mitotic spindle is part of a larger, intracellular skeleton (cytoskeleton) that is essential for the movements of structures occurring in the cytoplasm of all eukaryotic cells. The mitotic spindle consists of chromatin plus a system of microtubules composed of the protein tubulin. The mitotic spindle is essential for the equal partitioning of DNA into the two daughter cells that are formed when a eukaryotic cell divides. Several plant-derived substances used as anticancer drugs disrupt this process by affecting the equilibrium between the polymerized and depolymerized forms of the microtubules, thereby causing cytotoxicity. The microtubule inhibitors are summarized in Figure 35.21.

A. Vincristine and vinblastine

Vincristine [vin-KRIS-teen] (*VX*) and *vinblastine* [vin-BLAS-teen] (*VBL*) are structurally related compounds derived from the periwinkle plant, Vinca rosea. They are, therefore, referred to as the Vinca alkaloids. A less neurotoxic agent is *vinorelbine* [vye-NOR-el-been] (*VRB*). Although the Vinca alkaloids are structurally similar, their therapeutic indications are different. They are generally administered in combination with other drugs. *VX* is used in the treatment of acute lymphoblastic leukemia in children, Wilms tumor, Ewing soft tissue sarcoma, and Hodgkin and non-Hodgkin lymphomas, as well as some other rapidly proliferating neoplasms. [Note: *VX* (former trade name, *Oncovin*) is the "O" in the R-CHOP regimen for lymphoma. Due to relatively mild myelosuppressive activity, *VX* is used in a number of other protocols.] *VBL* is administered with *bleomycin* and *cisplatin* for the treatment of metastatic testicular carcinoma. It is also used in the treatment of systemic Hodgkin and non-Hodgkin lymphomas. *VRB* is beneficial in the treatment of advanced non–small cell lung cancer, either as a single agent or with *cisplatin*.

1. **Mechanism of action:** These agents are cell cycle specific and phase specific, because they block mitosis in metaphase (M phase). Their binding to the microtubular protein, tubulin, blocks

DRUG	ROUTE	ADVERSE EFFECTS	NOTABLE DRUG INTERACTIONS	MONITORING PARAMETERS	NOTES
Vincristine	IV	Neurotoxicity, constipation	*Phenytoin, phenobarbital, carbamazepine*, azole antifungal drugs	CBC, hepatic function, peripheral neuropathy	Vesicants; IT administration may result in death
Vinblastine	IV	Myelosuppression, neurotoxicity		CBC, hepatic function	
Vinorelbine	IV	Granulocytopenia			
Paclitaxel	IV	Neutropenia, neurotoxicity, alopecia, N, V	*Repaglinide, gemfibrozil, rifampin* (CYP2C8)	CBC, hepatic function, peripheral neuropathy	Hypersensitivity reactions (dyspnea, urticaria, hypotension); require premedications
Docetaxel	IV	Neutropenia, neurotoxicity, fluid retention, alopecia, N, V, D	*Ketoconazole, ritonavir* (CYP3A4)		

Figure 35.21
Summary of microtubule inhibitors. CBC = complete blood count; D = diarrhea; IT = intrathecal; IV = intravenous; N = nausea; V = vomiting.

the ability of tubulin to polymerize to form microtubules. Instead, paracrystalline aggregates consisting of tubulin dimers and the alkaloid drug are formed. The resulting dysfunctional spindle apparatus, frozen in metaphase, prevents chromosomal segregation and cell proliferation (Figure 35.22).

2. **Pharmacokinetics:** IV injection of these agents leads to rapid cytotoxic effects and cell destruction. This, in turn, can cause hyperuricemia due to the oxidation of purines that are released from fragmenting DNA molecules. The Vinca alkaloids are concentrated and metabolized in the liver by the CYP450 pathway and eliminated in bile and feces. Dosage adjustment is required in patients with impaired hepatic function or biliary obstruction.

3. **Adverse effects:** *VX* and *VBL* are both associated with phlebitis or cellulitis if extravasation occurs during injection, as well as nausea, vomiting, diarrhea, and alopecia. *VBL* is a potent myelosuppressant, whereas peripheral neuropathy (paresthesias, loss of reflexes, foot drop, and ataxia) and constipation are more common with *VX*. These agents should not be administered intrathecally. This potential drug error can result in death, and special precautions should be in place for administration.

B. Paclitaxel and docetaxel

Paclitaxel [PAK-li-tax-el] was the first member of the taxane family to be used in cancer chemotherapy. Semisynthetic *paclitaxel* is available through chemical modification of a precursor found in the needles of Pacific yew species. An albumin-bound form is also available. Substitution of a side chain resulted in *docetaxel* [doe-see-TAX-el], which is the more potent of the two drugs. *Paclitaxel* has good activity against advanced ovarian cancer and metastatic breast cancer, as well as non–small cell lung cancer when administered with *cisplatin*. *Docetaxel* is commonly used in prostate, breast, GI, and non–small cell lung cancers.

1. **Mechanism of action:** Both drugs are active in the G$_2$/M phase of the cell cycle, but unlike the Vinca alkaloids, they promote polymerization and stabilization of the polymer rather than disassembly, leading to the accumulation of microtubules (Figure 35.23). The microtubules formed are overly stable and nonfunctional, and chromosome desegregation does not occur. This results in cell death.

2. **Pharmacokinetics:** These agents undergo hepatic metabolism by the CYP450 system and are excreted via the biliary system. Dosages should be reduced in patients with hepatic dysfunction.

3. **Adverse effects:** The dose-limiting toxicities of *paclitaxel* and *docetaxel* are neutropenia and leukopenia. Peripheral neuropathy is also a common adverse effect with the taxanes. [Note: Because of serious hypersensitivity reactions (including dyspnea, urticaria, and hypotension), patients who are treated with *paclitaxel* should be premedicated with *dexamethasone* and *diphenhydramine*, as well as with an H$_2$ receptor antagonist.]

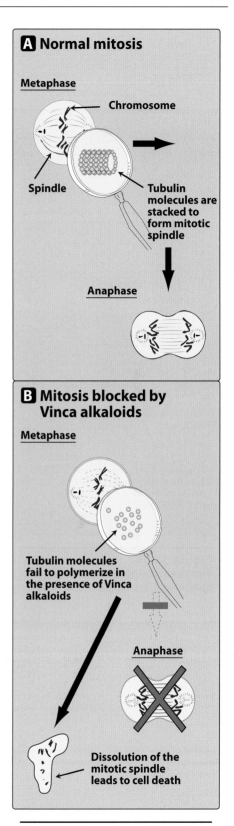

Figure 35.22
Mechanism of action of the microtubule inhibitors.

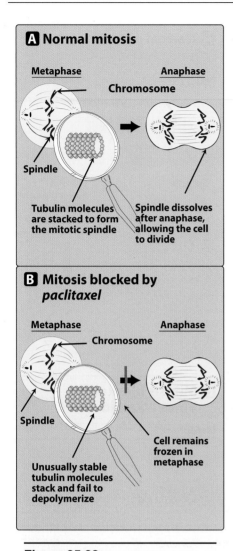

A Normal mitosis

Metaphase									Anaphase

Chromosome

Spindle

Tubulin molecules			Spindle dissolves
are stacked to form			after anaphase,
the mitotic spindle			allowing the cell
									to divide

B Mitosis blocked by *paclitaxel*

Metaphase									Anaphase

Chromosome

Spindle

Cell remains
frozen in
metaphase

Unusually stable
tubulin molecules
stack and fail to
depolymerize

Figure 35.23
Paclitaxel stabilizes microtubules, rendering them nonfunctional.

VII. STEROID HORMONES AND THEIR ANTAGONISTS

Tumors that are sensitive to steroid hormones may be either 1) hormone responsive, in which the tumor regresses following treatment with a specific hormone; or 2) hormone dependent, in which removal of a hormonal stimulus causes tumor regression; or 3) both. Removal of hormonal stimuli from hormone-dependent tumors can be accomplished by surgery (for example, in the case of orchiectomy—surgical removal of one or both testes—for patients with advanced prostate cancer) or by drugs (for example, in breast cancer treatment with the antiestrogen *tamoxifen* prevents estrogen stimulation of breast cancer cells; Figure 35.24). For a steroid hormone to influence a cell, that cell must have intracellular (cytosolic) receptors that are specific for that hormone (Figure 35.25A).

A. Tamoxifen

Tamoxifen [tah-MOX-ih-fen] is a selective estrogen modulator (SERM). It is an estrogen antagonist in breast tissue and an agonist in other tissues, such as bone and the endometrium. *Tamoxifen* is used for first-line therapy in the treatment of estrogen receptor–positive breast cancer. It is also used for prevention of breast cancer in high-risk women.

1. **Mechanism of action:** *Tamoxifen* competes with estrogen for binding to estrogen receptors in the breast tissue, and inhibits estrogen-induced growth of breast cancer (Figure 35.25B). The result is a depletion (down-regulation) of estrogen receptors, and the growth-promoting effects of the natural hormone and other growth factors are suppressed.

2. **Pharmacokinetics:** *Tamoxifen* is effective after oral administration. It is partially metabolized by the liver. Some metabolites possess estrogen antagonist activity, whereas others have agonist activity. Unchanged drug and metabolites are excreted predominantly through the bile into the feces. *Tamoxifen* is an inhibitor of CYP3A4 and P-glycoprotein.

DRUG	ROUTE	ADVERSE EFFECTS	NOTABLE DRUG INTERACTIONS	MONITORING PARAMETERS	NOTES
Tamoxifen	PO	Hot flashes, N, V, vaginal bleeding, hypercalcemia, thromboembolism	*Warfarin, rifampin*	Vaginal bleeding, new breast lumps	May cause endometrial cancer
Anastrozole, Letrozole	PO	Hot flashes, N, joint pain, ischemic cardiovascular events, osteoporosis	Estrogen-containing products	Hepatic function, bone mineral density monitoring, cholesterol monitoring	Contraindicated in premenopausal or pregnant women
Leuprolide, Goserelin, Triptorelin	Depot, SC IM	Tumor flare, hot flashes, asthenia, gynecomastia		Bone mineral density monitoring, serum testosterone, PSA	
Flutamide, Nilutamide, Bicalutamide	PO	Hot flashes, N, gynecomastia, pain, constipation	*Warfarin*	Hepatic function, PSA	Combined with LHRH agonists or surgical castration

Figure 35.24
Summary of steroid hormones and their antagonists. IM = intramuscular; LHRH = luteinizing hormone–releasing hormone; N = nausea; PO = oral administration; PSA = prostate-specific antigen; SC = subcutaneous; V = vomiting.

3. **Adverse effects:** Adverse effects caused by *tamoxifen* include hot flashes, nausea, vomiting, skin rash, and vaginal bleeding and discharge (due to estrogenic activity of the drug and some of its metabolites in the endometrial tissue). *Tamoxifen* has the potential to cause endometrial cancer. Other toxicities include thromboembolism and effects on vision.

B. Fulvestrant and raloxifene

Fulvestrant [fool-VES-trant] is an estrogen receptor antagonist that is given via intramuscular injection to patients with hormone receptor–positive metastatic breast cancer. This agent binds to and causes estrogen receptor down-regulation on tumors and other targets. *Raloxifene* [ral-OKS-i-feen] is an oral SERM that blocks estrogen effects in the uterine and breast tissues, while promoting effects in the bone to inhibit resorption. This agent reduces the risk of estrogen receptor–positive invasive breast cancer in postmenopausal women. Both drugs are known to cause hot flashes, arthralgias, and myalgias.

C. Aromatase inhibitors

The aromatase reaction is responsible for extra-adrenal synthesis of estrogen from androstenedione, which takes place in liver, fat, muscle, skin, and breast tissues, including breast malignancies. Peripheral aromatization is an important source of estrogen in postmenopausal women. Aromatase inhibitors decrease the production of estrogen in these women.

1. **Anastrozole and letrozole:** *Anastrozole* [an-AS-troe-zole] and *letrozole* [LE-troe-zole] are nonsteroidal aromatase inhibitors. These agents are considered first-line drugs for the treatment of breast cancer in postmenopausal women. They are orally active and cause almost a total suppression of estrogen synthesis. *Anastrozole* and *letrozole* do not predispose patients to endometrial cancer. Both drugs are extensively metabolized in the liver, and metabolites and parent drug are excreted primarily in the urine.

2. **Exemestane:** A steroidal, irreversible inhibitor of aromatase, *exemestane* [ex-uh-MES-tane], is well absorbed after oral administration and widely distributed. Hepatic metabolism occurs via the CYP3A4 isoenzyme. Because the metabolites are excreted in urine, doses of the drug must be adjusted in patients with renal failure. Major toxicities are nausea, fatigue, and hot flashes. Alopecia and dermatitis have also been noted.

D. Leuprolide, goserelin, and triptorelin

Gonadotropin-releasing hormone (GnRH) is normally secreted by the hypothalamus and stimulates the anterior pituitary to secrete the gonadotropic hormones: 1) luteinizing hormone (LH), the primary stimulus for the secretion of testosterone by the testes, and 2) follicle-stimulating hormone (FSH), which stimulates the secretion of estrogen. *Leuprolide* [loo-PROE-lide], *goserelin* [GOE-se-rel-in], and *triptorelin* [TRIP-to-rel-in] are synthetic analogs of GnRH. As GnRH analogs, they occupy the GnRH receptor in the pituitary, which leads

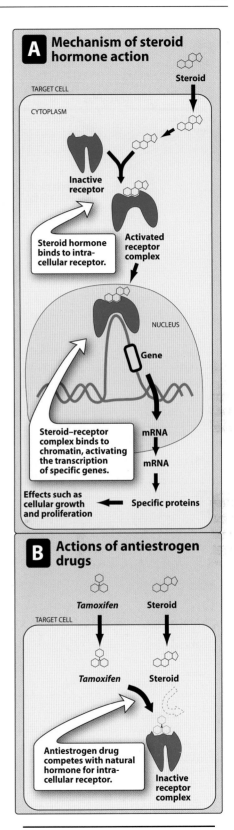

Figure 35.25
Action of steroid hormones and antiestrogen agents. mRNA = messenger RNA.

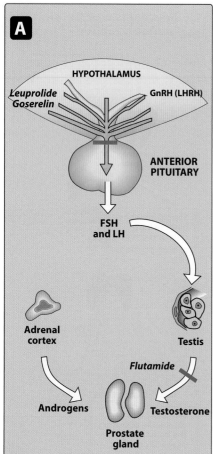

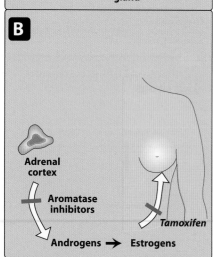

Figure 35.26
Effects of some anticancer drugs on the endocrine system. **A.** In therapy for prostatic cancer. **B.** In therapy of postmenopausal breast cancer. FSH = follicle-stimulating hormone; GnRH = gonadotropin-releasing hormone; LH = luteinizing hormone; LHRH = luteinizing hormone–releasing hormone.

to its desensitization and, consequently, inhibition of release of FSH and LH. Thus, both androgen and estrogen synthesis are reduced (Figure 35.26). Response to *leuprolide* in prostatic cancer is equivalent to that of orchiectomy with regression of tumor and relief of bone pain. These drugs have some benefit in premenopausal women with advanced breast cancer and have largely replaced estrogens in therapy for prostate cancer. *Leuprolide* is available as 1) a subcutaneous daily injection, 2) a subcutaneous depot injection, or 3) an intramuscular depot injection to treat metastatic carcinoma of the prostate. *Goserelin acetate* is a subcutaneous implant, and *triptorelin pamoate* is injected intramuscularly. Levels of androgen in prostate cancer patients may initially rise, but then fall to castration levels. The adverse effects of these drugs, including impotence, hot flashes, and tumor flare, are minimal compared to those experienced with estrogen treatment.

E. Antiandrogens

Flutamide [FLOO-ta-mide], *nilutamide* [nye-LOO-ta-mide], *bicalutamide* [bye-ka-LOO-ta-mide], and *enzalutamide* [enz-a-LOO-ta-mide] are oral antiandrogens used in the treatment of prostate cancer. They compete with the natural hormone for binding to the androgen receptor and prevent its action in the prostate (see Figure 35.26). Adverse effects include gynecomastia, constipation, nausea, and abdominal pain. Rarely, liver failure has occurred with *flutamide*. *Nilutamide* can cause visual problems.

VIII. PLATINUM COORDINATION COMPLEXES

A. Cisplatin, carboplatin, and oxaliplatin

Cisplatin [SIS-pla-tin] was the first member of the platinum coordination complex class of anticancer drugs, but because of severe toxicity, *carboplatin* [KAR-boe-pla-tin] was developed. The potency, pharmacokinetics, patterns of distribution, and dose-limiting toxicities differ significantly (Figure 35.27) between the two drugs. *Cisplatin* has synergistic cytotoxicity with radiation and other chemotherapeutic agents. It has found wide application in the treatment of solid tumors, such as metastatic testicular carcinoma in combination with *VBL* and *bleomycin*, ovarian carcinoma in combination with *cyclophosphamide*, or alone for bladder carcinoma. *Carboplatin* is used when patients cannot be vigorously hydrated, as is required for *cisplatin* treatment, or if they suffer from kidney dysfunction or are prone to neuro- or ototoxicity. *Oxaliplatin* [ox-AL-ih-pla-tin] is a closely related analog of *carboplatin* used in the setting of colorectal cancer.

1. **Mechanism of action:** The mechanism of action for these agents is similar to that of the alkylating agents. In the high-chloride milieu of the plasma, *cisplatin* persists as the neutral species, which enters the cell and loses chloride in the low-chloride milieu. It then binds to guanine in DNA, forming inter- and intrastrand cross-links. The resulting cytotoxic lesion inhibits both polymerases for DNA replication and RNA synthesis. Cytotoxicity can occur at any stage of the cell cycle, but cells are most vulnerable to the actions of these drugs in the G_1 and S phases.

DRUG	ROUTE	ADVERSE EFFECTS	NOTABLE DRUG INTERACTIONS	MONITORING PARAMETERS	NOTES
Cisplatin	IV, IP, IA	Neurotoxicity, myelosuppression, ototoxicity, N, V, electrolyte wasting, infusion reaction, nephrotoxicity	Anticonvulsants	CBC, CMP, electrolytes, hearing	Aggressive pre- and posthydration required, high incidence of N/V
Carboplatin	IV, IP, IA	Myelosuppression, N, V, infusion reaction	Aminoglycosides	CBC	Dose calculated using AUC
Oxaliplatin	IV	Neurotoxicity, N, V, infusion reaction, hepatotoxicity, myelosuppression	*Warfarin*	CBC, neurologic function, hepatic function	Cold-related and cumulative peripheral neuropathy

Figure 35.27
Summary of platinum coordination complexes. AUC = area under the curve; CBC = complete blood count; CMP = complete metabolic panel; IA = intra-arterially; IP = intraperitoneally; IV = intravenous; N = nausea; V = vomiting.

2. **Pharmacokinetics:** These agents are administered via IV infusion. *Cisplatin* and *carboplatin* can also be given intraperitoneally for ovarian cancer and intra-arterially to perfuse other organs. The highest concentrations of the drugs are found in the liver, kidney, and intestinal, testicular, and ovarian cells, but little penetrates into the cerebrospinal fluid (CSF). The renal route is the main pathway of excretion.

3. **Adverse effects:** Severe nausea and vomiting occurs in most patients after administration of *cisplatin* and may continue for as long as 5 days. Premedication with antiemetic agents is required. The major limiting toxicity is dose-related nephrotoxicity, involving the distal convoluted tubule and collecting ducts. This can be prevented by aggressive hydration. Other toxicities include ototoxicity with high-frequency hearing loss and tinnitus. Unlike *cisplatin*, *carboplatin* causes only mild nausea and vomiting, and it is rarely nephro-, neuro-, or ototoxic. The dose-limiting toxicity is myelosuppression. *Oxaliplatin* has a distinct adverse effect of cold-induced peripheral neuropathy that usually resolves within 72 hours of administration. It also causes myelosuppression and cumulative peripheral neuropathy. Hepatotoxicity has also been reported. These agents may cause hypersensitivity reactions ranging from skin rashes to anaphylaxis.

IX. TOPOISOMERASE INHIBITORS

These agents exert their mechanism of action via inhibition of topoisomerase enzymes, a class of enzymes that reduce supercoiling of DNA (Figure 35.28).

DRUG	ROUTE	ADVERSE EFFECTS	NOTABLE DRUG INTERACTIONS	MONITORING PARAMETERS	NOTES
Irinotecan	IV	Diarrhea, myelosuppression, N, V	CYP3A4 substrates	CBC, electrolytes	Acute and delayed (life-threatening) diarrhea
Topotecan	IV, PO	Myelosuppression, N, V	P-glycoprotein inhibitors (PO)	CBC	Diarrhea common with PO
Etoposide	IV, PO	Myelosuppression, hypotension, alopecia, N, V		CBC	May cause secondary malignancies (leukemias)

Figure 35.28
Summary of topoisomerase inhibitors. CBC = complete blood count; IV = intravenous; N = nausea; PO = oral administration; V = vomiting.

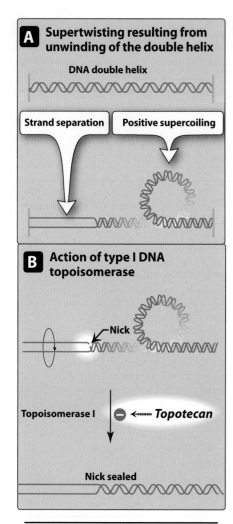

Figure 35.29
Action of type I DNA topoisomerases.

A. Camptothecins

Camptothecins are plant alkaloids originally isolated from the Chinese tree Camptotheca. *Irinotecan* [eye-rin-oh-TEE-kan] and *topotecan* [toe-poe-TEE-kan] are semisynthetic derivatives of *camptothecin* [camp-toe-THEE-sin]. *Topotecan* is used in metastatic ovarian cancer when primary therapy has failed and also in the treatment of small cell lung cancer. *Irinotecan* is used with *5-FU* and *leucovorin* for the treatment of colorectal carcinoma.

1. **Mechanism of action:** These drugs are S-phase specific and inhibit topoisomerase I, which is essential for the replication of DNA in human cells (Figure 35.29). SN-38 (the active metabolite of *irinotecan*) is approximately 1000 times as potent as *irinotecan* as an inhibitor of topoisomerase I. The topoisomerases relieve torsional strain in DNA by causing reversible, single-strand breaks.

2. **Adverse effects:** Bone marrow suppression, particularly neutropenia, is the dose-limiting toxicity for *topotecan*. Frequent blood counts should be performed in patients receiving this drug. Myelosuppression is also seen with *irinotecan*. Acute and delayed diarrhea with *irinotecan* may be severe and require treatment with *atropine* during the infusion or high doses of *loperamide* in the days following the infusion.

B. Etoposide

Etoposide [e-toe-POE-side] is a semisynthetic derivative of the plant alkaloid, podophyllotoxin. This agent blocks cells in the late S to G$_2$ phase of the cell cycle, and the major target is topoisomerase II. Binding of the drug to the enzyme–DNA complex results in persistence of the transient, cleavable form of the complex and, thus, renders it susceptible to irreversible double-strand breaks (Figure 35.30). *Etoposide* finds its major clinical use in the treatment of lung cancer and in combination with *bleomycin* and *cisplatin* for testicular carcinoma. *Etoposide* may be administered either IV or orally. Dose-limiting myelosuppression (primarily leukopenia) is the major toxicity.

X. ANTIBODIES

Monoclonal antibodies (Figure 35.31) are an active area of drug development for anticancer therapy and other nonneoplastic diseases, because they are directed at specific targets and often have different adverse effect profiles as compared to traditional chemotherapy agents. [Note: Monoclonal antibodies also find application in a number of other disorders, such as inflammatory bowel disease, psoriasis, and rheumatoid arthritis.] All of these agents are administered intravenously, and infusion-related reactions are common.

XI. TYROSINE KINASE INHIBITORS

The tyrosine kinases are a family of enzymes that are involved in several important processes within a cell, including signal transduction and cell division. [Note: At least 50 tyrosine kinases mediate cell growth or division by phosphorylation of signaling proteins. They have been implicated in the development of many neoplasms.] The tyrosine kinase inhibitors are administered orally, and these agents have a wide variety of applications in the treatment of cancer (Figure 35.32).

XII. IMMUNOTHERAPY

Immunotherapy with intravenous immune checkpoint inhibitors is a rapidly evolving option for cancer treatment. The goal of immune checkpoint inhibitors is to block the checkpoint molecules, such as the programmed death (PD-1) receptor, that normally help to keep the immune system in check. By blocking these molecules, the immune system is better able to attack the tumor and cause destruction. The two most commonly used checkpoint inhibitors are *pembrolizumab* [PEM-broe-LIZ-ue-mab] and *nivolumab* [nye-VOL-ue-mab]. The adverse reaction profiles of these agents consist of potentially severe and even fatal immune-mediated adverse events. This is because turning off the immune checkpoints allows attack of the tumor, but can also lead to unchecked autoimmune response to normal tissues. Adverse events include diarrhea, colitis, pneumonitis, hepatitis, nephritis, neurotoxicity, dermatologic toxicity in the form of severe skin rashes, and endocrinopathies such as hypo- or hyperthyroidism. Patients should be closely monitored for the potential development of signs and symptoms of toxicity and promptly treated with corticosteroids if necessary.

XIII. MISCELLANEOUS AGENTS

A. Abiraterone acetate

Abiraterone [ab-er-AT-er-own] *acetate* is an oral agent used in the treatment of metastatic castration–resistant prostate cancer. *Abiraterone acetate* is used in conjunction with *prednisone* to inhibit the CYP17 enzyme (an enzyme required for androgen synthesis), resulting in reduced testosterone production. Coadministration with *prednisone* is required to help lessen the effects of mineralocorticoid excess resulting from CYP17 inhibition. Hepatotoxicity may occur, and patients should be closely monitored for hypertension, hypokalemia, and fluid retention. Joint and muscle discomfort, hot flushes, and diarrhea are common adverse effects with this agent.

B. Immunomodulating agents

Thalidomide [tha-LID-oh-mide], *lenalidomide* [LEN-a-LID-oh-mide], and *pomalidomide* [pom-a-LID-oh-mide] are oral agents used in the treatment of multiple myeloma. Their exact mechanism of action is not clear, but they possess antimyeloma properties including antiangiogenic, immune-modulation, anti-inflammatory and antiproliferative effects. These agents are often combined with *dexamethasone* or other chemotherapeutic agents. Adverse effects include thromboembolism, myelosuppression, fatigue, rash, and constipation. *Thalidomide* was previously given to pregnant women to prevent

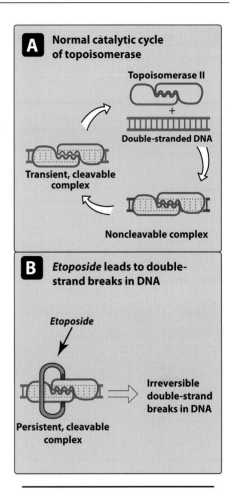

Figure 35.30
Mechanism of action of *etoposide*.

DRUG	MECHANISM OF ACTION	ADVERSE EFFECTS	MONITORING PARAMETERS	NOTES
Bevacizumab	Binds VEGF and prevents binding of VEGF to its receptors on endothelial cells Inhibits vascularization of the tumor	Hypertension, GI perforation, proteinuria, wound healing problems, bleeding	BP, urine protein, signs and symptoms of bleeding	Hold for recent or upcoming surgical procedures
Cetuximab	Binds to EGFR and competitively inhibits the binding of epidermal growth factor and other ligands Inhibits tumor cell growth and increases apoptosis	Skin rash, electrolyte wasting, infusion reaction, diarrhea	Electrolytes, vital signs during infusion	Premedication with antihistamine required before infusion; rash equated with increased response
Daratumumab	Binds to the transmembrane protein CD38 on multiple myeloma cells and causes cell lysis	Infusion reactions, diarrhea, fatigue, pyrexia	CBC with differential, vital signs during infusion	Can bind CD38 on red blood cells Type and screen patients before starting therapy Premedication with antihistamines, antipyretics, and corticosteroids required
Ramucirumab	Binds VEGF receptor 2 and blocks binding of VEGF receptor ligands	Proteinuria, hypertension, wound healing problems, bleeding	BP, urine protein, signs and symptoms of bleeding	Hold for recent or upcoming surgical procedures
Rituximab	Targets the CD20 antigen expressed on the surface of pre-B lymphocytes and mature B lymphocytes	Fatal infusion reaction, TLS, mucocutaneous reactions, PML	Vital signs during infusion, TLS labs	Fatal reactivation of hepatitis B Premedication with antihistamine and acetaminophen required Increased risk of nephrotoxicity when given with *cisplatin*
Trastuzumab	Inhibits the proliferation of human tumor cells that overexpress HER2	Cardiomyopathy, infusion-related fever and chills, pulmonary toxicity, headache, nausea/vomiting	LVEF, CBC, pulmonary toxicity due to infusion reaction	Embryo-fetal toxicity Neutropenia in combination with chemotherapy Premedication with antihistamine and *acetaminophen* required

Figure 35.31
Summary of monoclonal antibodies. BP = blood pressure; CBC = complete blood count; EGFR = epidermal growth factor receptor; HER2 = human epidermal growth factor receptor protein 2; GI = gastrointestinal; LVEF = left ventricular ejection fraction; PML = progressive multifocal leukoencephalopathy; TLS = tumor lysis syndrome; VEGF = vascular endothelial growth factor.

morning sickness. However, severe birth defects were prevalent in children born to mothers who used *thalidomide*. Because of their structurally similarities to *thalidomide*, *lenalidomide* and *pomalidomide* are contraindicated in pregnancy.

C. Proteasome inhibitors

Bortezomib [bore-TEZ-o-mib], *ixazomib* [ix-az-O-mib], and *carfilzomib* [kar-FIL-zo-mib] are proteasome inhibitors commonly used as the backbone therapy in the treatment of multiple myeloma. These agents work by inhibiting proteasomes, which in turn prevents the degradation of proapoptotic factors, thus leading to a promotion in programmed cell death (apoptosis). Malignant cells readily depend on suppression of the apoptotic pathway; therefore, proteasome inhibition works well in multiple myeloma. *Bortezomib* can be administered IV, but the subcutaneous route is preferred because it is associated with less neuropathy. Other adverse effects include myelosuppression, diarrhea, nausea, fatigue, and herpes zoster reactivation. Patients should receive antiviral prophylaxis if they are receiving therapy with *bortezomib*. *Ixazomib* is an oral agent with an adverse effect profile similar to *bortezomib*.

DRUG	MECHANISM OF ACTION	ADVERSE EFFECTS	NOTABLE DRUG INTERACTIONS	MONITORING PARAMETERS	NOTES
Afatinib	Inhibits EGFR tyrosine kinase	Diarrhea, rash, stomatitis, paronychia, nausea, vomiting, pruritus	P-gp inhibitors and inducers	CBC, CMP	Administer on an empty stomach. Reduce dose for significant diarrhea. Use effective contraception for female patients
Dabrafenib	Inhibits mutated BRAF kinases	Pyrexia, rash, arthralgia, cough, embryo-fetal toxicity	CYP3A4 inhibitors and substrates; CYP2C8 inhibitors and substrates; substrates of CYP2C9, CYP2C19, or CYP2B6	Glucose, symptoms of heart failure or bleeding, CBC, BMP, INR (if *warfarin*)	Use effective contraception for female patients. Administer on empty stomach. May cause new primary malignancies
Dasatinib	Inhibits BCR-ABL tyrosine kinase	Myelosuppression, fluid retention, diarrhea	CYP3A4 substrates, acid-reducing agents	CBC, BCR-ABL, electrolytes	QT prolongation
Erlotinib	Inhibits EGFR tyrosine kinase	Rash, ILD, hepatoxicity	CYP3A4 substrates, acid-reducing agents, *warfarin*	CMP	Rash equated with increased response
Ibrutinib	Inhibits Bruton tyrosine kinase	Neutropenia, thombocytopenia, diarrhea, anemia, pain, rash, nausea, bruising, fatigue, hemorrhage, pyrexia	CYP3A inhibitors and inducers	CBC, CMP, atrial fibrillation, BP, tumor lysis syndrome	Avoid grapefruit juice and Seville oranges. Can cause hepatitis B reactivation. Use effective contraceptive
Idelalisib	Inhibits phosphatidylinositol 3-kinase	Diarrhea, fatigue, nausea, cough, pyrexia, abdominal pain, pneumonia, rash, neutropenia, infection	CYP3A inducers and substrates	CBC, LFTs, pulmonary symptoms, infection	Use effective contraception for female patients
Imatinib	Inhibits BCR-ABL tyrosine kinase	Myelosuppression, fluid retention, CHF	CYP3A4 substrates, *warfarin*	CBC, BCR-ABL	Monitor for development of heart failure
Nilotinib	Inhibits BCR-ABL tyrosine kinase	Myelosuppression, QT prolongation, hepatotoxicity	CYP3A4 substrates, acid-reducing agents	CBC, BCR-ABL, electrolytes	QT prolongation. Administer on empty stomach
Osimertinib	Inhibits EGFR tyrosine kinase	Diarrhea, rash, dry skin, nail toxicity, fatigue	Strong CYP3A inducers	CBC, ECG, electrolytes	Use effective contraceptive for female patients
Pazopanib	Multi–tyrosine kinase inhibitor	Diarrhea, hypertension, hair color changes, nausea, anorexia, vomiting	CYP3A4 inhibitors, inducers, and substrates; CYP2D6 or CYP2C8 substrates; *simvastatin*; drugs that reduce gastric pH	ECG, electrolytes, thyroid function tests, LFTs, UA, CBC, BP	Use effective contraceptive for female patients
Sorafenib	Inhibits multiple intracellular and cell surface kinases	Hypertension, hand-foot syndrome, rash, diarrhea, fatigue	CYP3A4 inducers, *warfarin*	BP, CMP	Wound healing complications, cardiac events
Sunitinib	Multi–tyrosine kinase inhibitor	Hypertension, hand-foot syndrome, rash, diarrhea, fatigue, hepatotoxicity, hypothyroidism	CYP3A4 substrates	BP, CMP, TSH	Monitor for development of heart failure
Trametinib	Reversible inhibitor of mitogen-activated extracellular kinases	Pyrexia, rash, diarrhea, vomiting, lymphedema	CYP2C8 substrates, P-gp	Fever, new cutaneous malignancies, serum glucose, LVEF, CBC, CMP	Used in combination with *dabrafenib*. Administer on empty stomach
Vemurafenib	Inhibits mutated BRAF serine-threonine kinase	Arthralgia, rash, alopecia, fatigue, photosensitivity, pruritus, skin papilloma	CYP3A4 inhibitors and inducers, CYP1A2 substrates	ECG, electrolytes, CMP, uveitis	May cause new primary cutaneous malignancies. Use effective contraception in female patients

Figure 35.32
Summary of tyrosine kinase inhibitors. BMP = basic metabolic panel; BP = blood pressure; CBC = complete blood count; CHF = congestive heart failure; CMP = complete metabolic panel; ECG = electrocardiogram; EGFR = epidermal growth factor receptor; ILD = interstitial lung disease; INR = international normalized ratio; LFT = liver function test; LVEF = left ventricular ejection fraction; P-gp = P-glycoprotein; TSH = thyroid-stimulating hormone; UA = urinalysis.

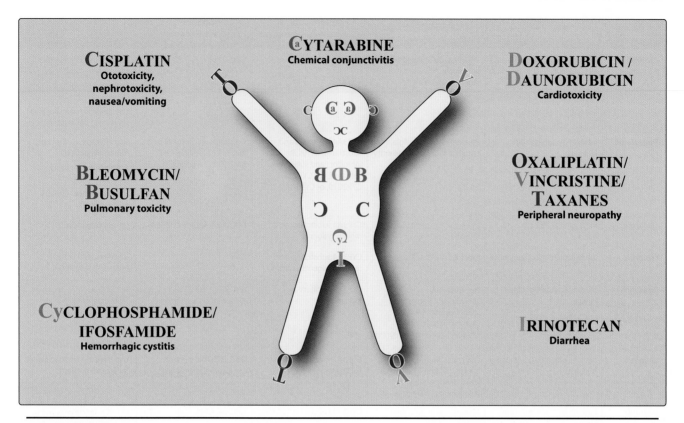

Figure 35.33
Chemo Man—a summary of toxicity of chemotherapeutic agents.

Carfilzomib is administered intravenously, and common adverse effects include myelosuppression, fatigue, nausea, diarrhea, and fever.

"Chemo Man" is a useful tool to help remember the most common toxicities of these drugs (Figure 35.33).

Study Questions

Choose the ONE best answer.

35.1   A patient is about to undergo three cycles of chemotherapy prior to surgery for bladder cancer. Which best describes chemotherapy in this setting?

   A. Adjuvant
   B. Neoadjuvant
   C. Palliative
   D. Maintenance

Correct answer = B. Chemotherapy given *before* the surgical procedure in an attempt to shrink the cancer is referred to as neoadjuvant chemotherapy. Chemotherapy is indicated when neoplasms are disseminated and are not amenable to surgery (palliative). Chemotherapy is also used as a supplemental treatment to attack micrometastases following surgery and radiation treatment, in which case it is called adjuvant chemotherapy. Chemotherapy given in lower doses to assist in prolonging a remission is known as maintenance chemotherapy.

35.2 A 45-year-old man is being treated with ABVD chemotherapy for Hodgkin lymphoma. He presents for cycle 4 of a planned 6 cycles with a new-onset cough. He states it started a week ago and he also feels like he has a little trouble catching his breath. Which drug in the ABVD regimen is the most likely cause of his pulmonary toxicity?

A. Doxorubicin (Adriamycin)
B. Bleomycin
C. Vinblastine
D. Dacarbazine

Correct answer = B. Pulmonary toxicity is the most serious adverse effect of bleomycin, progressing from rales, cough, and infiltrate to potentially fatal fibrosis. The pulmonary fibrosis that is caused by bleomycin is often referred as "bleomycin lung."

35.3 A patient is about to begin therapy with doxorubicin and cyclophosphamide. Which test should be ordered for baseline assessment before treatment?

A. Baseline PFTs
B. Baseline stress test
C. Baseline echocardiogram
D. Baseline urinalysis

Correct answer = C. Irreversible, dose-dependent cardiotoxicity, apparently a result of the generation of free radicals and lipid peroxidation, is the most serious adverse reaction of anthracyclines, such as doxorubicin. Cardiac function should be assessed prior to therapy, and then periodically throughout therapy.

35.4 A 64-year-old man is scheduled to undergo chemotherapy for rhabdomyosarcoma, and the regimen includes ifosfamide. Which is most appropriate to include in chemotherapy orders for this patient?

A. IV hydration, mesna, and frequent urinalyses
B. Leucovorin and frequent urinalyses
C. Allopurinol and frequent urinalyses
D. IV hydration, prophylactic antibiotics, and frequent urinalyses

Correct answer = A. A unique toxicity of ifosfamide is hemorrhagic cystitis. This bladder toxicity has been attributed to toxic metabolites of ifosfamide. Adequate hydration as well as IV injection of mesna (sodium 2-mercaptoethane sulfonate), which neutralizes the toxic metabolites, can minimize this problem. Frequent urinalyses to monitor for red blood cells should be ordered. Leucovorin is used with methotrexate or *5-FU* (not ifosfamide). Allopurinol has a drug interaction with ifosfamide and is not an agent that prevents hemorrhagic cystitis. IV fluids are correct; however, mesna is also needed.

35.5 Development of signs of which condition should be monitored in patients receiving chemotherapy with ifosfamide?

A. Hand-foot syndrome
B. Rash
C. Cardiotoxicity
D. Neurotoxicity

Correct answer = D. A fairly high incidence of neurotoxicity has been reported in patients on high-dose ifosfamide, probably due to the metabolite, chloroacetaldehyde. Hand-foot syndrome is an adverse effect of *5-FU* and derivatives. Rash is possible with many drugs, but is not the most appropriate answer here. Cardiotoxicity is an adverse effect of the anthracyclines.

35.6 Which chemotherapy drug can cause nephrotoxicity, neurotoxicity, ototoxicity, electrolyte abnormalities, and severe nausea and vomiting?

A. Cyclophosphamide
B. Oxaliplatin
C. Etoposide
D. Cisplatin

Correct answer = D. Cisplatin can cause renal failure, neuropathy, hearing loss, electrolyte wasting, and significant nausea and vomiting. Oxaliplatin rarely causes ototoxicity or nephrotoxicity. Cyclophosphamide and etoposide have myelosuppression as the dose-limiting toxicity.

35.7 A patient was mistakenly administered vincristine instead of cytarabine intrathecally. What is the likely outcome of this drug error?

A. Neuropathy
B. Death
C. Renal failure
D. Hearing loss

Correct answer = B. Death. Vincristine is fatal if given intrathecally.

35.8 The appearance of a facial rash with cetuximab is associated with a(n)

A. Negative response to therapy.
B. Positive response to therapy.
C. Drug allergy.
D. Infusion reaction.

Correct answer = B. Patients undergoing therapy with an epidermal growth factor receptor (EGFR) inhibitor such as cetuximab often develop an acneiform-like rash on the face, chest, upper back, and arms. The appearance of such a rash has been correlated with an increased response as compared to patients who do not experience a rash during therapy.

35.9 Which of the following should be administered prior to an infusion of the monoclonal antibody rituximab?

A. Allopurinol and acetaminophen.
B. Folic acid and H_2 receptor antagonist.
C. Antihistamine and acetaminophen.
D. Hepatitis B vaccine and vitamin B_{12}.

Correct answer = C. Patients receiving rituximab may experience an infusion reaction, usually on the first cycle. Hypotension, bronchospasm, and angioedema may occur. Chills and fever may occur, especially in patients with high circulating levels of neoplastic cells, because of rapid activation of complement, which results in the release of tumor necrosis factor-α and interleukins. Pretreatment with diphenhydramine, acetaminophen, and corticosteroids and a slower infusion rate can lessen the chance of this reaction.

35.10 Patients should receive antiviral prophylaxis for herpes zoster while undergoing treatment with which agent for multiple myeloma?

A. Dabrafenib
B. Ipilimumab
C. Cisplatin
D. Bortezomib

Correct answer = D. Bortezomib is known to cause herpes zoster reactivation in patients receiving treatment for multiple myeloma. Patients should receive antiviral prophylaxis while on bortezomib therapy.

Immunosuppressants

36

Jennifer Jebrock and Jane Revollo

I. OVERVIEW

The importance of the immune system in protecting the body against harmful foreign molecules is well recognized. The immune system is one of the most complex organ systems in the body, which can make it difficult to manipulate. Immunosuppressants are drugs that reduce the activation or efficacy of the immune system to treat certain conditions, such as autoimmune diseases, or to lower the body's ability to reject a transplanted organ. Autoimmune diseases can arise when the immune system mistakenly identifies an individual's own tissues as foreign and directs a destructive response against them. The goal of treatment for these diseases is to use drug therapy to stop this inappropriate and harmful process. In the case of organ transplantation, foreign tissue is purposely implanted into the recipient, but the goal remains the same—to use drug therapy to limit the damage inflicted by the immune system and potential rejection of the transplanted organ. Transplantation of organs and tissues (for example, kidney, heart, or bone marrow) has become routine due to improved surgical techniques and better tissue typing. Available drugs now more selectively inhibit rejection of transplanted tissues while preventing the patient from immunological compromise and prolonging the life of transplanted organs (Figure 36.1). Earlier drugs were nonselective, and patients frequently succumbed to infection due to suppression of both the antibody-mediated (humoral) and cell-mediated arms of the immune system. Today, the principal approach to immunosuppressive therapy is to alter lymphocyte function using drugs or antibodies against immune proteins. Because of their severe toxicities when used as monotherapy, a combination of immunosuppressive agents, usually at lower doses, is generally employed. Immunosuppressive drug regimens typically consist of two to four agents with different mechanisms of action that disrupt various levels of T-cell activation. [Note: Although this chapter focuses on immunosuppressive agents in the context of organ transplantation, these agents may be used in the treatment of other disorders. For example, *cyclosporine* may be useful in the treatment of psoriasis, and various monoclonal antibodies have applications in a number of disorders, including rheumatoid arthritis, multiple sclerosis, Crohn disease, and ulcerative colitis.]

ANTIBODIES
Alemtuzumab CAMPATH
Antithymocyte globulins ATGAM, THYMOGLOBULIN
Basiliximab SIMULECT
Rituximab RITUXAN
CALCINEURIN INHIBITORS
Cyclosporine NEORAL, SANDIMMUNE
Tacrolimus ASTAGRAF XL, ENVARSUS XR, PROGRAF
COSTIMULATION BLOCKER
Belatacept NULOJIX
mTOR INHIBITORS
Everolimus ZORTRESS
Sirolimus RAPAMUNE
ANTI-PROLIFERATIVES
Azathioprine IMURAN
Mycophenolate mofetil CELLCEPT
Mycophenolate sodium MYFORTIC
ADRENOCORTICOIDS
Methylprednisolone MEDROL, SOLU-MEDROL
Prednisolone ORAPRED, PRELONE
Prednisone GENERIC ONLY
OTHER
Bortezomib VELCADE
Intravenous immunoglobulin VARIOUS

Figure 36.1
Immunosuppressant drugs. mTOR = mammalian target of *rapamycin*.

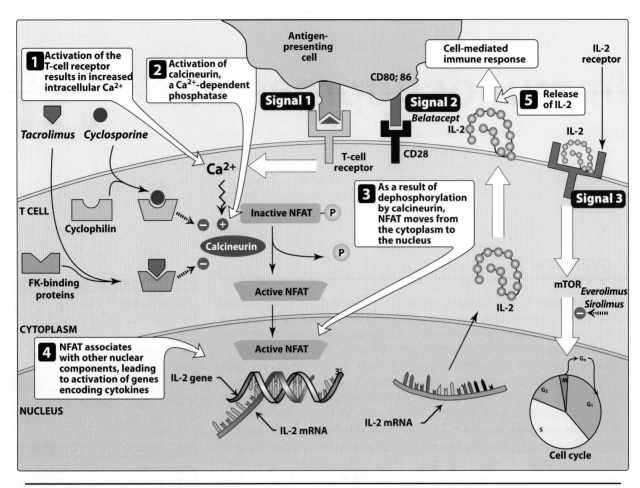

Figure 36.2
Mechanism of action of immunosuppressive agents. IL-2 = interleukin 2; mRNA = messenger RNA; mTOR = mammalian target of *rapamycin*; NFAT = nuclear factor of activated T cells; mRNA = messenger RNA cells.

The immune activation cascade can be described as a three-signal model (Figure 36.2). Signal 1 constitutes T-cell triggering at the CD3 receptor complex by an antigen on the surface of an antigen-presenting cell (APC). Signal 1 alone is insufficient for T-cell activation and requires signal 2. Signal 2, also referred to as costimulation, occurs when CD80 and CD86 (also known as B7.1 and B7.2) on the surface of APCs engage CD28 on T cells. Both signals 1 and 2 activate several intracellular signal transduction pathways, one of which is the calcium–calcineurin pathway. These pathways trigger the production of cytokines such as interleukin (IL)-2. IL-2 then binds to the IL-2 receptor (also known as CD25) on the surface of other T cells, thereby providing signal 3, activating the cell cycle via mammalian target of *rapamycin* (mTOR), and leading to T-cell proliferation.

Immunosuppressants can be broadly categorized by their place in therapy and their mechanism of action. More potent immunosuppressant drugs, such as monoclonal and polyclonal antibodies, are often used in induction therapy, which powerfully suppresses the immune system at the time of transplant, allowing the new organ to start functioning in the recipient and preventing early graft rejection. Maintenance immunosuppressant drugs, on the other hand, are less potent and provide long-term immunological protection for the transplanted organs, with lower risk of infection than with the induction drugs. As noted above, maintenance immunosuppressant medications are frequently combined in regimens to maintain adequate immunosuppression while minimizing adverse effects.

II. INDUCTION AND REJECTION IMMUNOSUPPRESSANT MEDICATIONS

The use of antibodies plays a central role in prolonging allograft survival. [Note: An allograft is a transplant of an organ or tissue from one person to another who is not genetically identical.] Antibodies are prepared by immunization of either rabbits or horses with human lymphoid cells (producing a mixture of polyclonal antibodies or monoclonal antibodies) or by hybridoma technology (producing antigen-specific monoclonal antibodies). Hybridomas are produced by fusing mouse antibody-producing cells with tumor cells. Hybrid cells are selected and cloned, and the antibody specificity of the clones is determined. Clones of interest can be cultured in large quantities to produce clinically useful amounts of the desired antibody. Recombinant deoxyribonucleic acid (DNA) technology can also be used to replace part of the mouse gene sequence with human genetic material, thus "humanizing" the antibodies and making them less antigenic. The names of monoclonal antibodies conventionally contain "xi" or "zu" if they are chimerized or humanized, respectively. The suffix "-mab" (monoclonal antibody) identifies the category of drug. The polyclonal antibodies, although relatively inexpensive to produce, are variable and less specific, which is in contrast to monoclonal antibodies, which are homogeneous and specific (Figure 36.3).

DRUG	CLASS	MECHANISM OF ACTION	INDICATIONS	ADVERSE EFFECTS
Alemtuzumab	Humanized monoclonal antibody	Binds to CD52 on B and T lymphocytes, causing T- and B-cell depletion	Induction, treatment of rejection	Infusion-related effects (chills, fever), severe and prolonged leukopenia, neutropenia, thrombocytopenia, infections (CMV, HSV, and other viruses/fungi)
Antithymocyte globulins	Polyclonal antibodies	T-cell depletion	Induction, treatment of rejection	Infusion-related effects (chills, fever), leukopenia, thrombocytopenia, pulmonary edema, infections due to CMV or other viruses, skin rash
Basiliximab	Chimeric monoclonal antibody	Binds to CD25 (IL-2R) and inhibits IL-2 mediated T-cell proliferation (nondepleting)	Induction	Generally well tolerated vs. placebo
Bortezomib	Proteasome inhibitor	Proteasome inhibition leads to plasma cell depletion	Treatment of antibody-mediated rejection	Leukopenia, anemia, thrombocytopenia, nausea/vomiting, diarrhea, peripheral neuropathy, hypotension, hepatotoxicity (less common)
Intravenous Immunoglobulin (IVIg)	Immune globulin	Antibodies, B cells	Induction for highly sensitized patients, treatment of rejection	Infusion-related reactions, headache, hypotension, hemolytic anemia, pulmonary edema, thromboembolic events, aseptic meningitis, acute renal failure
Methylprednisolone	Corticosteroid	Nonspecific interleukin and TNF inhibition	Induction, treatment of rejection, maintenance	HTN, HLD, hyperglycemia, peripheral edema, mood disturbance, osteoporosis, weight gain
Rituximab	Chimeric monoclonal antibody	CD20$^+$ B-cell depletion	Induction, treatment of rejection	Infusion-related effects (chills, fever), infections (reactivation of hepatitis B virus, CMV, and other viruses/fungi), PML, leukopenia, thrombocytopenia, mucocutaneous reactions

Figure 36.3
Medications used for induction and/or rejection immunosuppressant therapy. CMV = cytomegalovirus; HLD = hyperlipidemia; HSV = herpes simplex virus; HTN = hypertension; IL = interleukin; PML = progressive multifocal leukoencephalopathy; TNF = tumor necrosis factor.

A. Antithymocyte globulins

Antithymocyte globulins are polyclonal antibodies produced by isolating gamma-globulin fractions of serum obtained from rabbits or horses after immunization with human thymocytes. They cause depletion of circulating T cells and apoptosis of activated T cells. Rabbit preparations are preferred over horse preparations because of greater potency and less toxicity.

Antithymocyte globulin (rabbit) is primarily used at the time of transplantation to prevent early allograft rejection, along with other immunosuppressive agents. It may also be used to treat severe rejection episodes or corticosteroid-resistant acute rejection. It is usually used for 3 to 10 days to produce profound lymphopenia that may last beyond 1 year.

The antibodies are slowly infused intravenously and their half-life extends from 3 to 9 days. Premedication with corticosteroids, *acetaminophen*, and antihistamines may help reduce infusion-related reactions. Prolonged use may be associated with profound immunosuppression and an increased risk of opportunistic infections and/or posttransplant lymphoproliferative disease (PTLD).

B. Basiliximab

Basiliximab [bass-il-IX-im-ab] is a chimeric murine/human monoclonal antibody that binds to the α chain of the IL-2 receptor (CD25) on activated T cells and, thus, interferes with the proliferation of these cells. Blockade of this receptor foils the ability of any antigenic stimulus to activate the T-cell response system.

Basiliximab is approved for prophylaxis of acute rejection in renal transplantation in combination with *cyclosporine* and corticosteroids. This may allow for reduced doses or delayed introduction of calcineurin inhibitors. The drug may be beneficial in those with delayed graft function and may reduce the risk of calcineurin inhibitor–associated renal toxicity. *Basiliximab* is not T-cell depleting and, therefore, is mainly used in induction protocols as opposed to the treatment of rejection. *Basiliximab* is given as an IV infusion. The serum half-life of *basiliximab* is about 7 days. Usually, two doses of this drug are administered—the first at 2 hours prior to transplantation and the second at 4 days after the surgery. The drug is generally well tolerated.

C. Alemtuzumab

Alemtuzumab [AL-em-TOOZ-ue-mab] is a humanized monoclonal antibody that binds to CD52 on both T and B cells, resulting in depletion of both lymphoid cell lines. Depletion of T and B cells is observed soon after infusion and recovery of these cells is gradual. T cells recover over 6 to 12 months, and B cells recover in 6 months or less. It is approved for the treatment of chronic lymphocytic leukemia, but has been used in transplantation as an induction and antirejection agent for both acute cellular rejection and antibody-mediated rejection (AMR) due to its activity against both T and B cells. Because of the potent and prolonged immunosuppressive effect, it is recommended to initiate or continue prophylaxis for <u>Pneumocystis</u> pneumonia and herpes viruses after administration of *alemtuzumab*.

Alemtuzumab was removed from the US market by the manufacturer in 2012 in preparation for relabeling for use in multiple sclerosis, but it can still be obtained through the Campath Distribution Program for use in transplant patients.

D. Rituximab

Rituximab [ri-TUX-i-mab] is a chimeric monoclonal antibody against the antigen CD20 on pre-B cells, mature B cells, and memory B cells. *Rituximab* causes B-cell depletion by inducing B-cell lysis and blocking B-cell activation and eventual maturation to antibody-forming plasma cells. Existing plasma cells do not express the CD20 antigen and, therefore, are unaffected by *rituximab*. The drug is approved for use in the treatment of B-cell lymphomas, PTLD, and rheumatoid arthritis. The benefit of using *rituximab* in transplantation is for antibody removal, which has been utilized in ABO (blood type) incompatible transplants, desensitization protocols, and treatment of AMR.

Intravenous administration of *rituximab* leads to rapid and sustained depletion of B lymphocytes, with B-cell counts returning to normal within 9 to 12 months. *Rituximab* has a boxed warning for reactivation of JC virus leading to progressive multifocal leukoencephalopathy (PML), which has been reported in the nontransplant population. Activation of hepatitis B infection has also been reported following treatment, and hepatitis serologies should be monitored.

E. Bortezomib

AMR involves the production of high levels of antibodies by plasma cells, either newly made from B cells or from those that existed prior to transplant. One mechanism to control AMR is to target antibody production by plasma cells. *Bortezomib* [bor-TEZ-oh-mib] is a proteasome inhibitor that leads to cell cycle arrest and apoptosis of normal plasma cells, thereby decreasing antibody production in sensitized patients.

Bortezomib is approved for the treatment of multiple myeloma, but it has been adapted for use in the treatment of AMR in transplant patients. It can be administered via intravenous bolus or subcutaneous injection, so it has a low potential for infusion-related reactions. *Bortezomib* is metabolized primarily by cytochrome P450 enzymes and hepatic dysfunction has rarely been reported when multiple cycles are given.

F. Intravenous immunoglobulin

Intravenous immunoglobulin (*IVIG*) contains immunoglobulins prepared by human plasma pooled from many donors. It has an immunomodulatory effect and is often used for autoimmune diseases, pretransplant desensitization protocols, and treatment of AMR. The immunomodulatory effects on T and B cells occur at high doses, and it is also used at lower doses to prevent infection by replacing immunoglobulins removed during plasmapheresis. The mechanism of action is not well defined, but high doses of *IVIG* appear to induce B-cell apoptosis and modulate B-cell signaling. It also inhibits binding of antibodies to the transplanted graft and activation of the complement system. The serum half-life of *IVIG* is about 3 to 4 weeks.

Adverse effects of IVIG include headache, fever, chills, myalgias, and hypotension/hypertension, which can be reduced by slowing the infusion rate. Serious adverse effects are rare and can include aseptic meningitis, acute renal failure, and thrombotic events.

III. MAINTENANCE IMMUNOSUPPRESSANT MEDICATIONS

Maintenance immunosuppressants are intended to provide adequate immunosuppression to prevent allograft rejection, while minimizing infection, malignancy, and drug-induced adverse effects. Often they are combined in regimens of two to four drugs, using medications with different mechanisms of action to minimize drug toxicity. These drugs can be further divided into four main classes: 1) calcineurin inhibitors (*cyclosporine* and *tacrolimus*), 2) costimulation blockers (*belatacept*), 3) mTOR inhibitors (*sirolimus* and *everolimus*), and 4) antiproliferatives (*mycophenolate* and *azathioprine*) (Figure 36.4).

DRUG	CLASS	INDICATIONS	PHARMACOKINETICS	ADVERSE EFFECTS
Azathioprine	Antiproliferative	SOT (renal), RA	Activated by glutathione S-transferase DDIs (*allopurinol, warfarin*)	Myelosuppression, nausea, vomiting, diarrhea, pancreatitis, hepatotoxicity
Belatacept	Costimulation blockade	SOT (renal)	Elimination half-life ~10 days	Anemia, leukopenia
Cyclosporine	Calcineurin inhibitor	SOT (renal, liver, heart), psoriasis, RA, acute GVHD	Metabolism by CYP3A4 Numerous DDIs	HTN, HLD, hyperglycemia, hyperkalemia, hirsutism, gingival hyperplasia, neurotoxicity, nephrotoxicity
Everolimus	mTOR inhibitor	SOT (renal, liver), oncology	Metabolism by CYP3A4 Numerous DDIs	HTN, HLD (particularly TG, TC), stomatitis, proteinuria, impaired wound healing, rash, myelosuppression
Methylprednisolone, prednisolone, prednisone	Corticosteroid	Numerous indications	Activated to *prednisolone*	HTN, HLD, hyperglycemia, peripheral edema, mood disturbance, osteoporosis, weight gain
Mycophenolate	Antiproliferative	SOT (renal, liver, heart)	Metabolism by glucuronidation DDI (bile acid sequestrants)	Leukopenia, thrombocytopenia, nausea, vomiting, diarrhea
Sirolimus	mTOR inhibitor	SOT (renal), lymphangio-leiomyomatosis	Metabolism by CYP3A4 Numerous DDIs	HTN, HLD (particularly TG, TC), stomatitis, proteinuria, impaired wound healing, rash, myelosuppression, pneumonitis
Tacrolimus	Calcineurin inhibitor	SOT (renal, liver, heart)	Metabolism by CYP3A4 Numerous DDIs	HTN, HLD, hyperglycemia, hyperkalemia, alopecia, neurotoxicity (hand tremor, headache, seizure), nephrotoxicity

Figure 36.4
Medications used for maintenance immunosuppressant therapy. DDI = drug–drug interaction; GVHD = graft versus host disease; HLD = hyperlipidemia; HTN = hypertension; mTOR = mammalian target of *rapamycin*; RA = rheumatoid arthritis; SOT = solid organ transplant; TC = total cholesterol; TG = triglycerides.

A. Calcineurin inhibitors

Calcineurin inhibitors *cyclosporine* [sye-kloe-SPOR-een] and *tacrolimus* [tac-RO-li-mus] block signal transduction through the calcium–calcineurin pathway, activated downstream of signal 1, to impair T-cell activation. Calcineurin, a calcium-dependent protein phosphatase, dephosphorylates nuclear factor of activated T cells (NFAT), allowing NFAT to enter the T-cell nucleus and bind to DNA, leading to transcription and production of cytokines, including IL-2. *Cyclosporine* binds to cyclophilin, whereas *tacrolimus* binds a protein called FK-binding protein (FKBP). These drug–protein complexes inhibit the activity of calcineurin, thereby preventing T-cell activation (see Figure 36.2). *Tacrolimus* is the preferred calcineurin inhibitor due to its decreased rate of allograft rejection as compared to *cyclosporine*. Although it is approved for renal, liver, and heart transplant, *tacrolimus* is the mainstay of maintenance immunosuppressants for all solid organ transplants.

Enzymes CYP3A4, CYP3A5, and P-glycoprotein (P-gp) expressed in the gastrointestinal tract and liver are responsible for the interindividual variability in oral absorption and metabolism of *cyclosporine* and *tacrolimus*. Dosing titration is based on 12-hour trough levels, with goal trough levels varying between different organs, time from transplant, and transplant center-specific protocols.

One of the primary limitations to the use of calcineurin inhibitors is nephrotoxicity, which has led to the development of regimens using these agents in combination with other immunosuppressant drugs. As with all immunosuppressants, infections are possible with use of calcineurin inhibitors, and recipients are often given prophylactic medications posttransplant. Hirsutism, or excessive hair growth, is a common adverse effect of *cyclosporine*.

B. Costimulation blocker

Belatacept [bel-a-TA-sept], a second-generation costimulation blocker, is a recombinant fusion protein of CTLA-4, which like CD28, binds to CD80 and CD86 on APCs. Binding of *belatacept* to CD80 and CD86 prevents CD28 from binding to those molecules and, thus, inhibits signal 2 of the T-cell activation pathway. *Belatacept* is approved for kidney transplantation in combination with *basiliximab*, *mycophenolate mofetil*, and corticosteroids. This drug can substitute for calcineurin inhibitors to avoid the detrimental long-term nephrotoxic, cardiovascular, and metabolic complications seen with *cyclosporine* and *tacrolimus*. [Note: The first-generation costimulation blocker *abatacept* is approved for rheumatoid arthritis.]

Belatacept is the first IV maintenance immunosuppressant and is dosed in two phases. Initially, it is administered four times in the first month at a higher dose to build up drug levels and then decreased to once-monthly dosing. After 4 months, the dose is also decreased. Monthly dosing may be beneficial in patients for whom medication compliance is an issue. Clearance of *belatacept* is not affected by age, sex, race, renal, or hepatic function. *Belatacept* increases the risk of PTLD, particularly of the central nervous system. Therefore, it is contraindicated in patients who are seronegative to Epstein-Barr virus (EBV), a common cause of PTLD. Serological titers to EBV are typically obtained to confirm exposure.

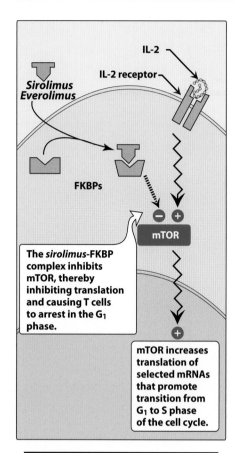

Figure 36.5
Mechanism of action of *sirolimus* and *everolimus*. FKBP = FK-binding protein; IL = interleukin; mRNA = messenger RNA; mTOR = mammalian target of *rapamycin*.

C. mTOR inhibitors

Sirolimus [sih-RO-lih-mus] (also known as *rapamycin*) and *everolimus* [e-ve-RO-lih-mus] inhibit the protein mTOR, blocking the signal transduction pathway activated by signal 3. Progression into the cell cycle and T-cell proliferation is subsequently prevented (Figure 36.5). The mTOR inhibitors are commonly used in multidrug regimens, frequently to minimize the dose of calcineurin inhibitors and spare their nephrotoxic adverse effects.

Like the calcineurin inhibitors, both *sirolimus* and *everolimus* are metabolized by CYP3A4, are substrates for P-gp, and are subject to numerous drug–drug interactions. Both agents require drug monitoring of trough concentrations to optimize therapy. *Sirolimus* has a longer half-life than the calcineurin inhibitors or *everolimus*, and is dosed only once daily, which may improve medication compliance. The antiproliferative action of *sirolimus* is also valuable in cardiology where *sirolimus*-coated stents are used to inhibit restenosis of the blood vessels by reducing proliferation of the endothelial cells. *Everolimus* is also used in oncology to treat many different types of cancer, including breast, renal cell, and neuroendocrine tumors. However, the doses for tumor treatment are higher than those used in transplantation.

D. Antiproliferatives

The antiproliferatives *azathioprine* [ay-za-THYE-oh-preen] and *mycophenolate* [mye-koe-FEN-oh-late] block lymphocyte proliferation by inhibiting nucleic acid synthesis. *Azathioprine*, which was one of the first agents to achieve widespread use in organ transplantation, is a prodrug that is converted first to *6-mercaptopurine* (*6-MP*) and then to the corresponding nucleotide analog, thioinosinic acid. The analog is incorporated into nucleic acid chains and blocks further elongation of the DNA. *Mycophenolate* is a potent, reversible, noncompetitive inhibitor of inosine monophosphate dehydrogenase, which blocks the de novo formation of guanosine monophosphate (Figure 36.6). Because lymphocytes are unable to

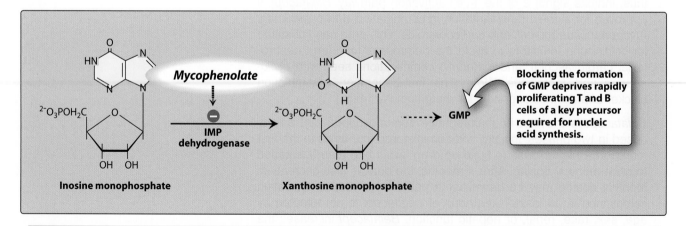

Figure 36.6
Mechanism of action of *mycophenolate*. IMP = inosine-5′-monophosphate; GMP = guanosine monophosphate.

utilize the salvage pathway of nucleotide synthesis, *mycophenolate* effectively blocks T- and B-cell proliferation by eliminating de novo production of guanosine monophosphate.

These medications are used as adjunctive immunosuppressant agents, primarily with calcineurin inhibitors with or without corticosteroids. However, *mycophenolate* has largely replaced *azathioprine* in this role due to its improved safety and efficacy profile. The main dose-limiting adverse effect of *azathioprine* is bone marrow suppression. *Allopurinol* inhibits the metabolism of *azathioprine*, thereby enhancing the adverse effects of *azathioprine*. Thus, concomitant use of *allopurinol* requires a significant reduction in *azathioprine* dose.

Mycophenolate is available in two formulations—as a prodrug *mycophenolate mofetil* and as an active drug *mycophenolic acid*. *Mycophenolate mofetil* is rapidly hydrolyzed in the gastrointestinal tract to *mycophenolic acid*. Glucuronidation of *mycophenolic acid* in the liver produces an inactive metabolite, but enterohepatic recirculation occurs, prolonging the effect of the drug. *Mycophenolic acid* is an enteric-coated tablet designed to theoretically reduce the gastrointestinal upset commonly experienced with *mycophenolate mofetil*.

E. Corticosteroids

The corticosteroids (see Chapter 26) were the first pharmacologic agents to be used as immunosuppressives, both in transplantation and in various autoimmune disorders. They are still one of the mainstays for attenuating rejection episodes. For transplantation, the most common agents are *prednisone* and *methylprednisolone,* whereas *prednisone* and *prednisolone* are used for autoimmune conditions. [Note: In transplantation, they are used in combination with agents described previously in this chapter.] The steroids are used to suppress acute rejection of solid organ allografts and in chronic graft versus host disease. In addition, they are effective against a wide variety of autoimmune conditions, including refractory rheumatoid arthritis, systemic lupus erythematosus, temporal arteritis, and asthma. The exact mechanism responsible for the immunosuppressive action of the corticosteroids is unclear. The T lymphocytes are most affected. The steroids are able to rapidly reduce lymphocyte populations by lysis or redistribution. On entering cells, they bind to the glucocorticoid receptor. The complex passes into the nucleus and regulates the transcription of DNA. Among the genes affected are those involved in inflammatory responses. The use of these agents is associated with numerous adverse effects. For example, they are diabetogenic and can cause hypercholesterolemia, cataracts, osteoporosis, and hypertension with prolonged use. Consequently, efforts are being directed toward reducing or eliminating the use of steroids in the maintenance of allografts.

Study Questions

Choose the ONE best answer.

36.1 A 45-year-old man who received a renal transplant 3 months ago and is being maintained on tacrolimus, prednisone, and mycophenolate mofetil is found to have increased creatinine levels and a kidney biopsy indicates severe rejection. Which course of therapy would be appropriate?

A. Increased dose of prednisone.
B. Treatment with rabbit antithymocyte globulin.
C. Treatment with sirolimus.
D. Treatment with azathioprine.

Correct answer = B. This patient is apparently undergoing an acute rejection of the kidney. The most effective treatment would be administration of an antibody. Increasing the dose of prednisone may have some effect but would not be enough to treat the rejection. Sirolimus is used prophylactically with cyclosporine to prevent renal rejection but is less effective when an episode is occurring. Azathioprine has no benefit over mycophenolate.

36.2 Which combination of immunosuppressive drugs should be avoided?

A. Basiliximab, belatacept, mycophenolate mofetil, and prednisone.
B. Tacrolimus, mycophenolate mofetil, and prednisone.
C. Tacrolimus, cyclosporine, and prednisone.
D. Tacrolimus, sirolimus, and prednisone.

Correct answer = C. Tacrolimus and cyclosporine are both calcineurin inhibitors and have the same mechanism of action. Immunosuppressive drug regimens should work synergistically at different places in the T-cell activation cascade. Additionally, cyclosporine and tacrolimus are both extremely nephrotoxic and when used together would cause harm to patients. All of the other combinations are reasonable.

36.3 Which drug used to prevent allograft rejection can cause hyperlipidemia?

A. Basiliximab
B. Belatacept
C. Mycophenolate mofetil
D. Sirolimus

Correct answer = D. Patients who are receiving sirolimus can develop elevated cholesterol and triglyceride levels, which can be controlled by statin therapy. None of the other agents have this adverse effect.

36.4 Which drug specifically inhibits calcineurin in the activated T lymphocytes?

A. Basiliximab
B. Tacrolimus
C. Sirolimus
D. Mycophenolate mofetil

Correct answer = B. Tacrolimus binds to FKBP-12, which, in turn, inhibits calcineurin and interferes in the cascade of reactions that synthesize interleukin-2 (IL-2) and lead to T-lymphocyte proliferation. Although basiliximab also interferes with T-lymphocyte proliferation, it does so by binding to the CD25 site on the IL-2 receptor. Sirolimus, while also binding to FKBP-12, does not inhibit calcineurin. Mycophenolate mofetil exerts its immunosuppressive action by inhibiting inosine monophosphate dehydrogenase, thus depriving the cells of guanosine monophosphate, a key precursor of nucleic acids.

36.5 An 18-year-old woman who received a kidney transplant 6 months ago comes in to clinic complaining of facial hair growth and does not want to take an immunosuppressant anymore. Which treatment option would be the most appropriate to address her concerns?

A. Switch cyclosporine to tacrolimus.
B. Switch mycophenolate mofetil to sirolimus.
C. Stop prednisone and add methylprednisolone.
D. Switch mycophenolate mofetil to mycophenolic acid.

Correct answer = A. Hirsutism, or excessive hair growth, is a well-known adverse effect of cyclosporine. Many patients experience dark, coarse facial or body hair growth while taking cyclosporine. Switching cyclosporine to tacrolimus would eliminate this adverse effect and keep the patient on a calcineurin inhibitor that is effective in preventing rejection. Mycophenolate and prednisone are not known to cause hirsutism.

36.6 Which immunosuppressant medication avoids the need for therapeutic drug monitoring?

   A. Cyclosporine
   B. Tacrolimus
   C. Mycophenolate mofetil
   D. Sirolimus

Correct answer = C. Calcineurin inhibitors (cyclosporine and tacrolimus) and mTOR inhibitors (sirolimus and everolimus) require therapeutic drug monitoring in order to maximize efficacy (prevent rejection episodes) and minimize toxicity (adverse effects). Mycophenolate mofetil is the correct answer since there is no role for routine monitoring with this medication.

36.7 Which clinical situation is least appropriate for immunosuppression with sirolimus?

   A. A patient with primary renal failure.
   B. A patient who has failed calcineurin inhibitors due to neurotoxicity.
   C. A patient who is 6 months postliver transplant and the incision site is fully healed.
   D. A patient with an abnormal lipid profile.

Correct answer = D. A patient with an abnormal lipid profile is a poor candidate for immunosuppression with sirolimus, since this medication is known to cause or exacerbate hyperlipidemia, particularly triglycerides and total cholesterol. A patient with primary renal failure would be a candidate for sirolimus, since it does not cause nephrotoxicity as calcineurin inhibitors do. It would be appropriate to switch a patient who has failed calcineurin inhibitors due to neurotoxicity to sirolimus for immunosuppression since it is not associated with that adverse effect. Sirolimus is known to impair wound healing, but a patient with a fully healed incision site could appropriately be placed on sirolimus.

36.8 Which statement is correct regarding the difference between induction immunosuppression (IS) and maintenance IS?

   A. Maintenance IS is less important than induction IS for long-term graft survival.
   B. Induction IS is more intense than maintenance IS.
   C. Maintenance IS includes lymphocyte-depleting antibodies, while induction IS does not.
   D. Induction IS increases the risk of infection, while maintenance IS does not.

Correct answer = B. Induction IS is more intense than maintenance IS, as it provides IS during the intraoperative and early postoperative period to combat the body's initial immune response to the transplanted graft. Both maintenance and induction IS are important for the long-term survival of the graft. Lymphocyte-depleting antibodies are used as induction IS and not as maintenance. Although induction IS is more potent, all IS (both induction and maintenance) can increase the risk of infection.

36.9 A 39-year-old man is admitted 3 months after liver transplant with increased liver function tests. A liver biopsy is performed and the results show acute rejection, severe. The team decides to start treatment with antithymocyte globulin, rabbit. What additional drug therapy is required for appropriate administration of this medication?

   A. No additional medications are required.
   B. Diphenhydramine, acetaminophen.
   C. Diphenhydramine, ketorolac, corticosteroids.
   D. Diphenhydramine, acetaminophen, corticosteroids.

Correct answer = D. Infusion-related reactions are common with the administration of antithymocyte globulins due to cytokine release. Common symptoms include chills, fever, hypotension, and pulmonary edema. Premedication with acetaminophen, diphenhydramine, and corticosteroids should be administered 30 minutes prior to the start of the infusion to prevent this syndrome. Although diphenhydramine and acetaminophen are correct, corticosteroids are also needed as premedication. Ketorolac is not the most appropriate for use as premedication for antithymocyte globulin.

36.10 A 21-year-old woman is admitted to receive a kidney transplant from her father. Since she has a low-to-moderate risk of rejection, she will receive induction with the antibody basiliximab. Which statement indicates the uniqueness of the therapy she is receiving compared with other antibody agents?

   A. Basiliximab is generally well tolerated and does not require premedications prior to administration.
   B. Basiliximab binds to CD52 and targets B and T lymphocytes.
   C. Basiliximab is used only in combination with antithymocyte globulin.
   D. Basiliximab targets B cells, not T cells.

Correct answer = A. Basiliximab does not require premedication since it is a nondepleting agent and would not be expected to cause cytokine release or infusion reactions. It can be used in combination with antithymocyte globulin, but most commonly it is used alone. Basiliximab binds to CD25 (not CD52) and affects T cells. It does not have any effect on B cells.

Histamine and Serotonin

Nancy Borja-Hart and Carol Motycka

37

I. OVERVIEW

Histamine and serotonin, along with prostaglandins, belong to a group of endogenous compounds called autacoids. These heterogeneous substances have widely differing structures and pharmacologic activities. They all have the common feature of being formed by the tissues on which they act and, therefore, function as local hormones. [Note: The word "autacoid" comes from the Greek: *autos* (self) and *akos* (medicinal agent, or remedy).] The autacoids also differ from circulating hormones in that they are produced by many tissues rather than in specific endocrine glands. The drugs described in this chapter are either autacoids or autacoid antagonists (compounds that inhibit the synthesis of certain autacoids or that interfere with their interactions with receptors).

II. HISTAMINE

Histamine is a chemical messenger mostly generated in mast cells. Histamine, via multiple receptor systems, mediates a wide range of cellular responses, including allergic and inflammatory reactions, gastric acid secretion, and neurotransmission in parts of the brain. Histamine has no clinical applications, but agents that inhibit the action of histamine (antihistamines or histamine receptor blockers) have important therapeutic applications. Figure 37.1 provides a summary of the antihistamines.

A. Location, synthesis, and release of histamine

1. **Location:** Histamine is present in practically all tissues, with significant amounts in the lungs, skin, blood vessels, and gastrointestinal (GI) tract. It is found in high concentrations in mast cells and basophils. Histamine functions as a neurotransmitter in the brain. It also occurs as a component of venoms and in secretions from insect stings.

H1 ANTIHISTAMINES
Alcaftadine LASTACAFT
Azelastine ASTEPRO
Bepotastine BEPREVE
Brompheniramine BROMAX, LO-HIST
Cetirizine ZYRTEC
Chlorpheniramine CHLOR-TRIMETON
Clemastine TAVIST
Cyclizine MAREZINE
Cyproheptadine GENERIC ONLY
Desloratadine CLARINEX
Dimenhydrinate DRAMAMINE
Diphenhydramine BENADRYL
Doxylamine UNISOM SLEEPTABS
Emedastine EMADINE
Fexofenadine ALLEGRA
Hydroxyzine VISTARIL
Ketotifen ALAWAY, ZADITOR
Levocetirizine XYZAL
Loratadine ALAVERT, CLARITIN
Meclizine BONINE, ANTIVERT
Olopatadine PATADAY, PATANASE, PATANOL
Promethazine PHENERGAN
Triprolidine HISTEX

Figure 37.1
Summary of antihistamines.

493

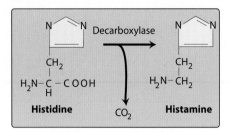

Figure 37.2
Biosynthesis of histamine.

H₁ Receptors

EXOCRINE EXCRETION

Increased production of nasal and bronchial mucus, resulting in respiratory symptoms.

BRONCHIAL SMOOTH MUSCLE

Constriction of bronchioles results in symptoms of asthma and decreased lung capacity.

INTESTINAL SMOOTH MUSCLE

Constriction results in intestinal cramps and diarrhea.

SENSORY NERVE ENDINGS

Causes itching and pain.

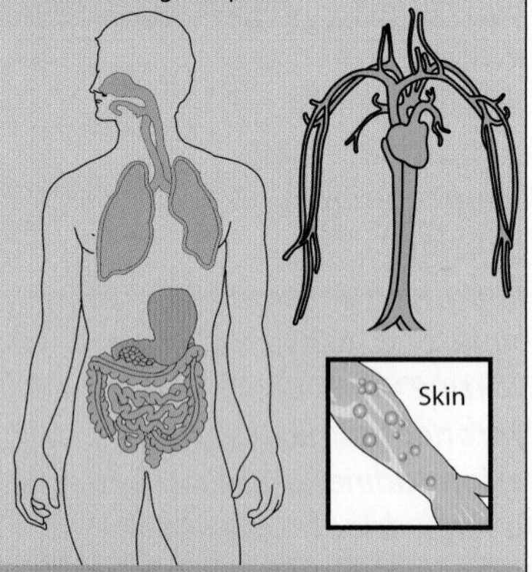

Skin

H₁ and H₂ Receptors

CARDIOVASCULAR SYSTEM

Lowers systemic blood pressure by reducing peripheral resistance. Causes positive chronotropism (mediated by H₂ receptors) and a positive inotropism (mediated by both H₁ and H₂ receptors).

SKIN

Dilation and increased permeability of the capillaries results in leakage of proteins and fluid into the tissues. In the skin, this results in the classic "triple response": wheal formation, reddening due to local vasodilation, and flare ("halo").

H₂ Receptors

STOMACH

Stimulation of gastric hydrochloric acid secretion.

2. **Synthesis:** Histamine is an amine formed by the decarboxylation of the amino acid histidine by the enzyme histidine decarboxylase, which is expressed in cells throughout the body, including neurons, gastric parietal cells, mast cells, and basophils (Figure 37.2). In mast cells, histamine is stored in granules. If histamine is not stored, it is rapidly inactivated by the enzyme amine oxidase.

3. **Release of histamine:** Most often, histamine is just one of several chemical mediators released in response to stimuli. The stimuli for release of histamine from tissues may include destruction of cells as a result of cold, toxins from organisms, venoms from insects and spiders, and trauma. Allergies and anaphylaxis can also trigger significant release of histamine.

B. Mechanism of action

Histamine released in response to certain stimuli exerts its effects by binding to various types of histamine receptors (H₁, H₂, H₃, and H₄). H₁ and H₂ receptors are widely expressed and are the targets of clinically useful drugs. Histamine has a wide range of pharmacologic effects that are mediated by both H₁ and H₂ receptors. For example, the H₁ receptors are important in producing smooth muscle contraction and increasing capillary permeability (Figure 37.3). Histamine promotes vasodilation of small blood vessels by causing the vascular endothelium to release nitric oxide. In addition, histamine can enhance the secretion of proinflammatory cytokines in several cell types and in local tissues. Histamine H₁ receptors mediate many pathological processes, including allergic rhinitis, atopic dermatitis, conjunctivitis, urticaria, bronchoconstriction, asthma, and anaphylaxis. Moreover, histamine stimulates the parietal cells in the stomach, causing an increase in acid secretion via the activation of H₂ receptors.

C. Role in allergy and anaphylaxis

The symptoms resulting from intravenous injection of histamine are similar to those associated with anaphylactic shock and allergic reactions. These include contraction of airway smooth muscle, stimulation of secretions, dilation and increased permeability of the capillaries, and stimulation of sensory nerve endings. Symptoms associated with allergy and anaphylactic shock result from the release of certain mediators from their storage sites. Such mediators include histamine, serotonin, leukotrienes, and the eosinophil chemotactic factor of anaphylaxis. In some cases, these mediators cause a localized allergic reaction, producing, for example, actions on the skin or respiratory tract. Under other conditions, these mediators may cause a full-blown anaphylactic response. It is thought that the difference between these two situations results from differences in the sites from which mediators are released and in their rates of release. For example, if the release of histamine is slow enough to permit its inactivation before it enters the bloodstream, a local allergic reaction results. However, if histamine release is too fast for efficient inactivation, a full-blown anaphylactic reaction occurs.

Figure 37.3
Actions of histamine.

III. H₁ ANTIHISTAMINES

The term antihistamine refers primarily to the classic H₁-receptor blockers. The H₁-receptor blockers can be divided into first- and second-generation drugs (Figure 37.4). The older first-generation drugs are still widely used because they are effective and inexpensive. However, most of these drugs penetrate the central nervous system (CNS) and cause sedation. Furthermore, they tend to interact with other receptors, producing a variety of unwanted adverse effects. By contrast, the second-generation agents are specific for peripheral H₁ receptors. The second-generation antihistamines are made polar, mainly by adding carboxyl groups (for example, *cetirizine* is the carboxylated derivative of *hydroxyzine*), and, therefore, these agents do not penetrate the blood–brain barrier and cause less CNS depression than do the first-generation drugs. Among the second-generation agents, *desloratadine* [des-lor-AH-tah-deen], *fexofenadine* [fex-oh-FEN-a-deen], and *loratadine* [lor-AT-a-deen] show the least sedation (Figure 37.5). *Cetirizine* [seh-TEER-ih-zeen] and *levocetirizine* [lee-voe-seh-TEER-ih-zeen] are partially sedating second-generation agents.

A. Actions

The action of all H₁-receptor blockers is qualitatively similar. Most of these compounds do not influence the formation or release of histamine. Rather, they block the receptor-mediated response of a target tissue. They are much more effective in preventing symptoms than reversing them once they have occurred. However, most of these agents have additional effects unrelated to their ability to block H₁ receptors. These effects reflect binding of the H₁-receptor antagonists to cholinergic, adrenergic, or serotonin receptors (Figure 37.6). For example, *cyproheptadine* [SYE-proe-HEP-ta-deen] also acts as a serotonin antagonist on the appetite center, resulting in appetite stimulation. Antihistamines such as *azelastine* [a-ZEL-uh-steen] and *ketotifen* [kee-toe-TYE-fen] also have mast cell–stabilizing effects in addition to their histamine receptor–blocking effects.

B. Therapeutic uses

1. **Allergic and inflammatory conditions:** H₁-receptor blockers are useful in treating and preventing allergic reactions caused by antigens acting on immunoglobulin E antibody. For example, oral antihistamines are the drugs of choice in controlling the symptoms of allergic rhinitis and urticaria because histamine is the principal mediator released by mast cells. Ophthalmic antihistamines, such as *azelastine*, *olopatadine* [oh-loe-PAT-a-deen], *ketotifen*, and others, are useful for the treatment of allergic conjunctivitis. However, the H₁-receptor blockers are not indicated in treating bronchial asthma, because histamine is only one of several mediators that are responsible for causing bronchial reactions. [Note: *Epinephrine* has actions on smooth muscle that are opposite to those of histamine. It acts via β₂ receptors on smooth muscle,

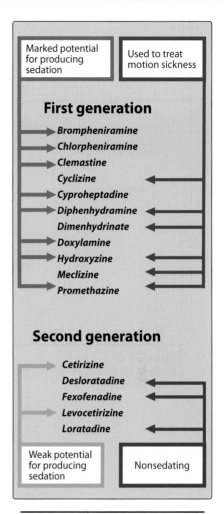

Figure 37.4
Summary of therapeutic advantages and disadvantages of some H₁ histamine receptor–blocking agents.

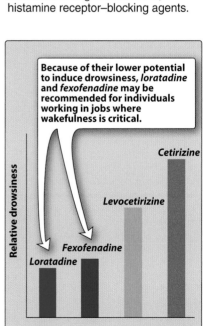

Figure 37.5
Relative potential for causing drowsiness in patients receiving second-generation H₁ antihistamines.

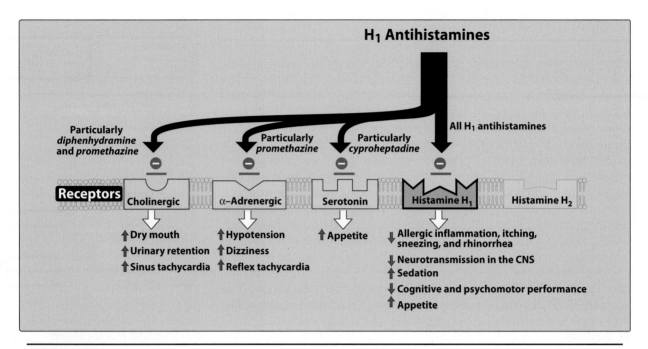

Figure 37.6
Effects of H$_1$ antihistamines at histamine, adrenergic, cholinergic, and serotonin-binding receptors. CNS = central nervous system.

causing cAMP-mediated relaxation. Therefore, *epinephrine* is the drug of choice in treating systemic anaphylaxis and other conditions that involve massive release of histamine.]

2. **Motion sickness and nausea:** Along with the antimuscarinic agent *scopolamine*, certain H$_1$-receptor blockers, such as *diphenhydramine* [dye-fen-HYE-dra-meen], *dimenhydrinate* [dye-men-HYE-dri-nate] (a chemical combination of *diphenhydramine* and a chlorinated theophylline derivative), *cyclizine* [SYE-kli-zeen], *meclizine* [MEK-li-zeen], and *promethazine* [proe-METH-a-zeen], are the most effective agents for prevention of the symptoms of motion sickness. They are usually not effective if symptoms are already present and, thus, should be taken prior to expected travel. The antihistamines prevent or diminish nausea and vomiting mediated by both the chemoreceptor and vestibular pathways. The antiemetic action of these medications seems to be due to their blockade of central H$_1$ and M$_1$ muscarinic receptors. *Meclizine* is also useful for the treatment of vertigo associated with vestibular disorders.

3. **Insomnia:** Although they are not the medications of choice, many first-generation antihistamines, such as *diphenhydramine* and *doxylamine* [dox-IL-a-meen], have strong sedative properties and are used in the treatment of insomnia. The use of first-generation H$_1$ antihistamines is contraindicated in the treatment of individuals working in jobs in which wakefulness is critical. The second-generation antihistamines have no value as somnifacients.

C. **Pharmacokinetics**

H$_1$-receptor blockers are well absorbed after oral administration, with maximum serum levels occurring at 1 to 2 hours. The average plasma half-life is 4 to 6 hours, except for that of *meclizine* and the second-generation agents, which is 12 to 24 hours, allowing for once-daily dosing. First-generation H₁-receptor blockers are distributed in all tissues, including the CNS. All first-generation H₁ antihistamines and some second-generation H₁ antihistamines, such as *desloratadine* and *loratadine*, are metabolized by the hepatic cytochrome P450 system. *Levocetirizine* is the active enantiomer of *cetirizine*. *Cetirizine* and *levocetirizine* are excreted largely unchanged in urine, and *fexofenadine* is excreted largely unchanged in feces. After a single oral dose, the onset of action occurs within 1 to 3 hours. *Azelastine*, *olopatadine*, *ketotifen*, *alcaftadine* [al-KAF-ta-deen], *bepotastine* [bep-oh-TAS-teen], and *emedastine* [em-e-DAS-teen] are available in ophthalmic formulations that allow for more targeted tissue delivery. *Azelastine* and *olopatadine* have intranasal formulations, as well.

D. Adverse effects

First-generation H₁-receptor blockers have a low specificity, interacting not only with histamine receptors but also with muscarinic cholinergic receptors, α-adrenergic receptors, and serotonin receptors (Figure 37.6). The extent of interaction with these receptors and, as a result, the nature of the side effects varies with the structure of the drug. Some side effects may be undesirable, and others may be of therapeutic value. Furthermore, the incidence and severity of adverse reactions for a given drug varies between individual subjects.

1. **Sedation:** First-generation H₁ antihistamines, such as *chlorpheniramine* [klor-fen-IR-a-meen], *diphenhydramine*, *hydroxyzine* [hye-DROX-ee-zeen], and *promethazine*, bind to H₁ receptors and block the neurotransmitter effect of histamine in the CNS. The most frequently observed adverse reaction is sedation (Figure 37.7); however, *diphenhydramine* may cause paradoxical hyperactivity in young children. Other central actions include fatigue, dizziness, lack of coordination, and tremors. Elderly patients are more sensitive to these effects. Sedation is less common with the second-generation drugs, since they do not readily enter the CNS. Second-generation H₁ antihistamines are specific for peripheral H₁ receptors.

2. **Other effects:** First-generation antihistamines exert anticholinergic effects, leading to dryness in the nasal passage and oral cavity. They also may cause blurred vision and retention of urine. The most common adverse reaction associated with second-generation antihistamines is headache. Topical formulations of *diphenhydramine* can cause local hypersensitivity reactions such as contact dermatitis.

3. **Drug interactions:** Interaction of H₁-receptor blockers with other drugs can cause serious consequences, such as potentiation of effects of other CNS depressants, including alcohol. Patients taking monoamine oxidase inhibitors (MAOIs), for example *phenelzine*, should not take antihistamines because the MAOIs can exacerbate the sedative and anticholinergic effects of antihistamines. In addition, the first-generation antihistamines (*diphenhydramine* and others) with anticholinergic (antimuscarinic) actions may decrease the effectiveness of cholinesterase inhibitors (*donepezil*, *rivastigmine*, and *galantamine*) in the treatment of Alzheimer disease.

4. **Overdoses:** Although the margin of safety of H₁-receptor blockers is relatively high and chronic toxicity is rare, acute poisoning is

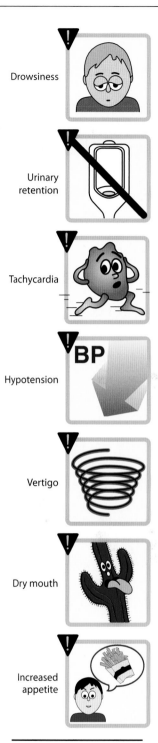

Drowsiness

Urinary retention

Tachycardia

BP
Hypotension

Vertigo

Dry mouth

Increased appetite

Figure 37.7
Some adverse effects observed with antihistamines. BP = blood pressure.

relatively common, especially in young children. The most common and dangerous effects of acute poisoning are those on the CNS, including hallucinations, excitement, ataxia, and convulsions. If untreated, the patient may experience a deepening coma and collapse of the cardiorespiratory system.

IV. HISTAMINE H$_2$-RECEPTOR BLOCKERS

Histamine H$_2$-receptor blockers have little, if any, affinity for H$_1$ receptors. Although antagonists of the histamine H$_2$ receptor (H$_2$ antagonists or H$_2$-receptor blockers) block the actions of histamine at all H$_2$ receptors, their chief clinical use is as inhibitors of gastric acid secretion in the treatment of ulcers and heartburn. The H$_2$-receptor blockers *cimetidine*, *ranitidine*, *famotidine*, and *nizatidine* are discussed in Chapter 40.

V. SEROTONIN

Serotonin is a neurotransmitter within the enteric nervous system and the CNS. It plays a role in vasoconstriction, inhibition of gastric secretion, and stimulation of smooth muscle contraction. Within the GI tract, it may serve as a local hormone to influence GI motility and secretion. Within the brain, the serotonergic neurons affect mood, appetite, body temperature regulation, and sleep. While serotonin has no therapeutic uses, selective serotonin agonists find clinical utility in the management of several disorders, such as depression and migraine headache.

A. Location, synthesis, and release of serotonin

1. **Location:** Serotonin is largely present within the enterochromaffin cells of the gastrointestinal tract. It is also found in storage granules in platelets and the raphe nuclei of the brainstem.

2. **Synthesis:** Serotonin (also known as 5-hydroxytryptamine, 5-HT) is synthesized from the amino acid L-tryptophan. L-Tryptophan undergoes hydroxylation of the indole ring to form L-5-hydroxytryptophan, followed by decarboxylation to form 5-hydroxytryptamine.

3. **Release of serotonin:** Following synthesis, serotonin is stored in vesicles and is released by exocytosis of the vesicle in response to an action potential. The activity of serotonin is terminated by uptake into the neuron and platelets. Metabolism occurs mainly via monoamine oxidase.

B. Mechanism of action

There are seven families of 5-HT receptors, designated by numeric subscripts 1 through 7. Most of these are G protein–coupled receptors, while the 5-HT$_3$ receptor is a ligand-gated cation channel. The 5-HT$_1$ and 5-HT$_2$ receptors have several subtypes denoted by letters (for example, 5-HT$_{2C}$). Serotonin has a wide range of effects that are mediated by the different types of serotonin receptors. For example, serotonin activity at 5-HT$_{2C}$ receptors in the CNS may cause a reduction in appetite, and stimulation of 5-HT$_3$ receptors in the GI tract and vomiting center may trigger emesis. [Note: 5-HT$_3$ receptor antagonists are highly effective for the management of chemotherapy-induced or postsurgical nausea and vomiting; see Chapter 40.]

C. Therapeutic Uses

Selective serotonin agonists have a variety of clinical indications, depending on the receptor specificity. Serotonin has a role in the pathophysiology of clinical depression, and agents such as selective serotonin reuptake inhibitors (SSRIs) and serotonin and norepinephrine reuptake inhibitors (SNRIs) are effective therapies for this condition (see Chapter 10). The clinical use of serotonin agonists in the management of migraine and obesity is further described below.

VI. DRUGS USED TO TREAT HEADACHE DISORDERS

The most common types of headaches are migraine, tension-type, and cluster headaches. Migraines can usually be distinguished from cluster headaches and tension-type headaches by the characteristics as shown in Figure 37.8. Patients with severe migraine headaches report one to five attacks per month of moderate to severe pain, which is usually unilateral. Headache disorders significantly affect quality of life and result in considerable health care costs. Management of headaches involves avoidance of headache triggers (for example, alcohol, chocolate, and stress) and use of abortive treatments for acute headaches, as well as prophylactic therapy in patients with frequent or severe migraines (Figure 37.9). Serotonin agonists (triptans and ergot alkaloids) are effective as abortive agents in the treatment of migraines.

A. Types of migraine

There are two main types of migraine headaches. The first, migraine without aura, is a severe, unilateral, pulsating headache that typically lasts from 2 to 72 hours. These headaches are often aggravated by physical activity and are accompanied by nausea, vomiting, photophobia (hypersensitivity to light), and phonophobia (hypersensitivity to sound). The majority of patients with migraine do not have aura.

	MIGRAINE	CLUSTER	TENSION TYPE
Family history	Yes	No	Yes
Sex	Females more often than males	Males more often than females	Females more often than males
Onset	Variable	During sleep	Under stress
Location	Usually unilateral	Behind or around one eye	Bilateral in band around head
Character and severity	Pulsating, throbbing	Excruciating, sharp, steady	Dull, persistent, tightening
Duration	2–72 hours per episode	15–90 minutes per episode	30 minutes to 7 days per episode
Associated symptoms	Visual auras, sensitivity to light and sound, pale facial appearance, nausea and vomiting	Unilateral or bilateral sweating, facial flushing, nasal congestion, lacrimation, pupillary changes	Mild intolerance to light and noise, anorexia

Figure 37.8
Characteristics of migraine, cluster, and tension-type headaches.

TRIPTANS
Almotriptan AXERT
Eletriptan RELPAX
Frovatriptan FROVA
Naratriptan AMERGE
Rizatriptan MAXALT, MAXALT-MLT
Sumatriptan IMITREX, ONZETRA, ZEMBRACE
Zolmitriptan ZOMIG

ERGOTS
Dihydroergotamine DHE 45, MIGRANAL
Ergotamine tartrate ERGOMAR

NSAIDs
Aspirin BAYER, BUFFERIN, ECOTRIN
Ibuprofen ADVIL, MOTRIN
Indomethacin INDOCIN
Ketorolac GENERIC ONLY
Naproxen ALEVE, ANAPROX, NAPROSYN

PROPHYLACTIC AGENTS
Anticonvulsants
β-Blockers
Calcium channel blockers
Tricyclic antidepressants

Figure 37.9
Summary of drugs used to treat migraine headache.

In the second type, migraine with aura, the headache is preceded by neurologic symptoms called auras, which can be visual, sensory, and/or cause speech or motor disturbances. Most commonly, these prodromal symptoms are visual (flashes, zigzag lines, and glare) and occur approximately 20 to 40 minutes before headache pain begins. In the 15% of migraine patients whose headache is preceded by an aura, the aura itself allows diagnosis. The headache in migraines with or without auras is similar. Women are threefold more likely than are men to experience either type of migraine.

B. Biologic basis of migraine headaches

The first manifestation of migraine with aura is a spreading depression of neuronal activity accompanied by reduced blood flow in the most posterior part of the cerebral hemisphere. This hypoperfusion gradually spreads forward over the surface of the cortex to other contiguous areas of the brain. The vascular alteration is accompanied by functional changes. The hypoperfusion persists throughout the aura and well into the headache phase. Patients who have migraine without aura do not show hypoperfusion. However, the pain of both types of migraine may be due to extracranial and intracranial arterial vasodilation, which leads to release of neuroactive molecules, such as substance P, neurokinin A, and calcitonin gene–related peptide.

C. Symptomatic treatment of acute migraine

Acute treatments can be classified as nonspecific (symptomatic) or migraine specific. Nonspecific treatment includes analgesics such as nonsteroidal anti-inflammatory drugs (NSAIDs) and antiemetics (for example, *prochlorperazine*) to control vomiting. Opioids are reserved as rescue medication when other treatments for a severe migraine are not successful. Migraine-specific therapy includes triptans and ergot alkaloids, which are $5\text{-}HT_{1B/1D}$ receptor and $5\text{-}HT_{1D}$ receptor agonists, respectively. It has been proposed that activation of $5\text{-}HT_1$ receptors by these agents leads either to vasoconstriction or to inhibition of the release of proinflammatory neuropeptides on the trigeminal nerve innervating cranial blood vessels.

1. **Triptans:** This class of drugs includes *almotriptan* [al-moe-TRIP-tan], *eletriptan* [el-e-TRIP-tan], *frovatriptan* [froe-va-TRIP-tan], *naratriptan* [nar-a-TRIP-tan], *rizatriptan* [rye-za-TRIP-tan], *sumatriptan* [soo-ma-TRIP-tan], and *zolmitriptan* [zole-ma-TRIP-tan]. *Sumatriptan* was the first available triptan, and is the prototype of this class. These agents rapidly and effectively abort or markedly reduce the severity of migraine headaches in about 70% of patients. The triptans are serotonin agonists, acting at a subgroup of serotonin receptors found on small peripheral nerves that innervate the intracranial vasculature. The nausea that occurs with *dihydroergotamine* and the vasoconstriction caused by *ergotamine* (see below) are much less pronounced with the triptans. *Sumatriptan* is given subcutaneously, intranasally, or orally (*sumatriptan* is also available in a combination product with *naproxen*). *Zolmitriptan* is available orally and by nasal spray. All other agents are taken orally. The onset of the parenteral drug *sumatriptan* is about 20 minutes, compared with 1 to 2 hours when the drug is administered orally.

The drug has a short duration of action, with an elimination half-life of 2 hours. Headache commonly recurs within 24 to 48 hours after a single dose of drug, but in most patients, a second dose is effective in aborting the headache. *Frovatriptan* is the longest-acting triptan, with a half-life of more than 24 hours. Individual response to triptans varies, and a trial of more than one triptan may be necessary before treatment is successful. Elevation of blood pressure and other cardiac events have been reported with triptan use. Therefore, triptans should not be administered to patients with risk factors for coronary artery disease without performing a cardiac evaluation prior to administration. Other adverse events with the use of triptans include pain and pressure sensations in the chest, neck, throat, and jaw. Dizziness and malaise have also been seen with the use of triptans.

2. **Ergot alkaloids:** *Ergotamine* [er-GOT-a-meen] and *dihydroergotamine* [dye-hye-droe-er-GOT-a-meen], a semisynthetic derivative of *ergotamine*, are ergot alkaloids approved for the treatment of migraine headaches. The action of the ergot alkaloids is complex, with ability to bind to 5-HT$_1$ receptors, α receptors, and dopamine receptors. 5-HT$_1$ receptors located on intracranial blood vessels are targets that cause vasoconstriction with the use of these agents. *Ergotamine* is currently available sublingually and is mostly effective when used in the early stages of the migraine. It is also available as an oral tablet or suppository containing both *ergotamine* and *caffeine*. *Ergotamine* is used with strict daily and weekly dosage limits due to its ability to cause dependence and rebound headaches. *Dihydroergotamine* is administered intravenously or intranasally and has an efficacy similar to that of *sumatriptan*. The use of *dihydroergotamine* is limited to severe cases of migraines. Nausea is a common adverse effect. *Ergotamine* and *dihydroergotamine* are contraindicated in patients with angina and peripheral vascular disease because they are significant vasoconstrictors.

3. **Nonspecific therapies:** Other therapies for acute migraine attacks include analgesics, antiemetics, nonsteroidal anti-inflammatory drugs, and corticosteroids.

D. Prophylaxis for migraine headache

Therapy to prevent migraine is indicated if the attacks occur two or more times a month and if the headaches are severe or complicated by serious neurologic signs. β-Blockers are the drugs of choice for migraine prophylaxis; however, calcium channel blockers, anticonvulsants (*topiramate* and *divalproex*), and tricyclic antidepressants have also shown effectiveness in migraine prevention (Figure 37.10).

E. Drugs for tension and cluster headache

Analgesics (NSAIDS, *acetaminophen*, *aspirin*) are used for symptom relief of tension headaches, and *caffeine* and *butalbital* are often combined with *acetaminophen* or *aspirin*. Triptans, along with inhalation of 100% oxygen, are used as first-line abortive strategies for cluster headache.

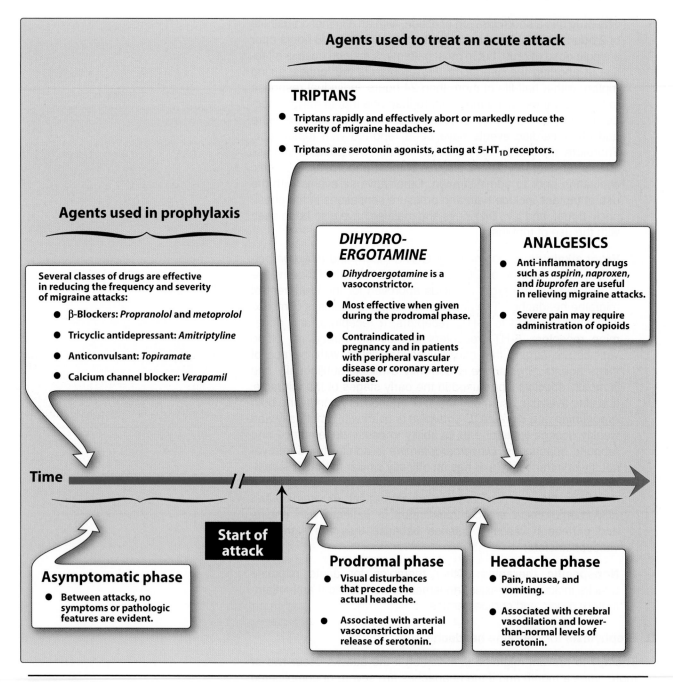

Figure 37.10
Drugs useful in the treatment and prophylaxis of migraine headaches.

VII. DRUGS FOR OBESITY

The term "obesity" is given to individuals with a body mass index (BMI) of 30 kg/m² or greater. Obesity is due in part to an energy imbalance; however, it is now well understood that genetics, metabolism, behavior, environment, culture, and socioeconomic status play a role in obesity, as well. Serotonin agonists have been used in the treatment of obesity for the appetite suppression that they produce. Drugs for obesity are considered effective if they demonstrate at least a 5% greater reduction in body weight as compared to placebo (no treatment). The majority of drugs approved to treat obesity have short-term indications for usage. A summary of medications for obesity is provided in Figure 37.11.

A. Serotonin agonists

The first serotonin agonists used for weight loss, *fenfluramine* and *dexflenfluramine*, were withdrawn from the market following an increase in potentially fatal adverse effects, including valvulopathy. Valvulopathy, which may lead to pulmonary hypertension, is linked to 5-HT$_{2B}$ receptors. *Lorcaserin* [lor-KAS-er-in] is a serotonin agonist with selectivity for the 5-HT$_{2C}$ serotonin receptor. In contrast to many other weight loss drugs, it is used for chronic weight management.

1. **Mechanism of action:** *Lorcaserin* selectively activates 5-HT$_{2C}$ receptors, which are almost exclusively found in the central nervous system. This activation, in turn, stimulates proopiomelanocortin (POMC) neurons, which activate melanocortin receptors, thereby causing a decrease in appetite (Figure 37.12). If a patient does not lose at least 5% of his or her body weight after 12 weeks of use, the drug should be discontinued.

2. **Pharmacokinetics:** *Lorcaserin* is extensively metabolized in the liver to two inactive metabolites that are then eliminated in the urine. *Lorcaserin* has not been studied for use in severe hepatic impairment and is not recommended in severe renal impairment.

3. **Adverse effects:** The most common adverse effects observed with *lorcaserin* are nausea, headache, dry mouth, dizziness, constipation, and lethargy. Although rare, mood changes and suicidal ideation can occur. The development of life-threatening serotonin syndrome or neuroleptic malignant syndrome has been reported with the use of serotonin agonists. Therefore, patients should be monitored for the emergence of these conditions while on *lorcaserin*. Because of the increased risk of serotonin syndrome, concomitant use of *lorcaserin* with selective serotonin reuptake inhibitors, serotonin–norepinephrine reuptake inhibitors, MAOIs, or other serotonergic drugs should be avoided. As mentioned above, valvulopathy has been associated with the use of 5-HT$_{2B}$ receptor agonists. Although the incidence of valvulopathy was not significantly increased in studies of *lorcaserin*, a 5-HT$_{2C}$ receptor agonist, patients should still be monitored for the development of this condition. For that reason, individuals with a history of heart failure should use this agent with caution.

B. Other agents for obesity

In addition to *lorcaserin*, several agents with varying mechanisms of action are available for weight loss and the management of obesity.

1. **Appetite suppressants:** *Phentermine* [FEN-ter-meen] and *diethylpropion* [dye-eth-ill-PROE-pee-on] are appetite suppressants. They exert pharmacologic action by increasing the release of norepinephrine and dopamine from the nerve terminals and by inhibiting reuptake of these neurotransmitters, thereby increasing

ANOREXIANTS	
Diethylpropion	TENUATE
Phentermine	ADIPEX-P
GLP-1 RECEPTOR AGONIST	
Liraglutide	SAXENDA
LIPASE INHIBITORS	
Orlistat	ALLI, XENICAL
SEROTONIN AGONISTS	
Lorcaserin	BELVIQ
COMBINATION DRUGS	
Bupropion/naltrexone	CONTRAVE
Phentermine/Topiramate	QSYMIA

Figure 37.11
Summary of drugs used in the treatment of obesity.

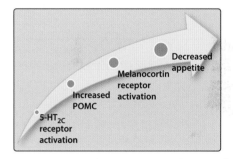

Figure 37.12
Lorcaserin mechanism of action. POMC = proopiomelanocortin.

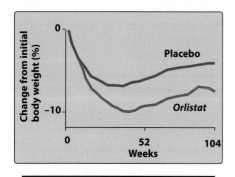

Figure 37.13
Effect of *orlistat* treatment on body
weight.

levels of neurotransmitters in the brain. The increase in norepinephrine signals a "fight-or-flight" response by the body, which,
in turn, decreases appetite. Tolerance to the weight loss effect
of these agents develops within weeks, and weight loss typically
plateaus. An increase in the dosage generally does not result
in further weight loss, and discontinuation of the drug is usually recommended once the plateau is reached. The anorexiants are classified as controlled substances due to the potential
for dependence or abuse. Dry mouth, headache, insomnia, and
constipation are common adverse effects. Heart rate and blood
pressure may be increased with these agents. Therefore, these
drugs should be avoided in patients with a history of uncontrolled
hypertension, cardiovascular disease, arrhythmias, heart failure,
or stroke. Concomitant use of anorexiants with monoamine oxidase inhibitors (MAOIs) or other sympathomimetics should be
avoided.

2. **Lipase inhibitor:** *Orlistat* [OR-lih-stat] is the only agent in a class
   of antiobesity drugs known as lipase inhibitors. It is indicated for
   weight loss or weight maintenance. *Orlistat* is a pentanoic acid
   ester that inhibits gastric and pancreatic lipases, thus decreasing
   the breakdown of dietary fat into smaller molecules that can be
   absorbed. Administration of *orlistat* decreases fat absorption by
   about 30%. The loss of calories from decreased absorption of fat
   is the main cause of weight loss. Figure 37.13 shows the effects
   of *orlistat* treatment. The clinical utility of *orlistat* is limited by gastrointestinal adverse effects, including oily spotting, flatulence with
   discharge, fecal urgency, and increased defecation. These effects
   may be minimized through a low-fat diet and the use of concomitant *cholestyramine*. *Orlistat* is contraindicated in pregnancy and
   in patients with chronic malabsorption syndrome or cholestasis.
   The drug also interferes with the absorption of fat-soluble vitamins
   and β-carotene. Patients should be advised to take a multivitamin
   supplement that contains vitamins A, D, E, and K and β-carotene.
   Orlistat can also interfere with the absorption of other medications,
   such as *amiodarone*, *cyclosporine*, and *levothyroxine*, and clinical
   response to these medications should be monitored if *orlistat* is
   initiated. The dose of *levothyroxine* should be separated from *orlistat* by at least 4 hours.

3. **Glucagon-like peptide-1 (GLP-1) receptor agonist:** *Liraglutide*
   is an injectable GLP-1 receptor agonist that is indicated for obesity.
   See Chapter 24 for a full discussion of GLP-1 receptor agonists.

4. **Combination therapy:** The combination of *phentermine* and *topiramate* has been approved for long-term use in the treatment of
   obesity. Initial studies of the anticonvulsant *topiramate* observed
   weight loss in patients taking the medication. Because of the
   sedating effects of *topiramate*, the stimulant *phentermine* was
   added to counteract sedation and promote additional weight loss.
   If a patient does not achieve a 5% weight loss after 12 weeks on
   the highest dose of this medication, then it should be discontinued. It is also important to note that this medication should not be
   stopped abruptly as seizures may be precipitated. *Topiramate* has
   been associated with birth defects including cleft palate, and, thus,

DRUG	TARGET	MECHANISM OF ACTION	PHARMACOKINETICS	ADVERSE EFFECTS
Bupropion + naltrexone	*Bupropion:* CNS–POMC neuron stimulation *Naltrexone:* CNS—blocks autoinhibitory feedback of the hypothalamic melanocortin system	Combination regulates the mesolimbic reward system and results in appetite suppression	Extensive metabolism through CYP2D6	Nausea, headache, dry mouth, dizziness, constipation, suicidal ideation
Liraglutide	GLP-1 receptor agonist	Slows gastric emptying and increases satiety	Excretion through the kidneys and metabolism in the liver	Nausea and vomiting, pancreatitis, hypoglycemia, acute gall bladder disease, elevated heart rate, suicidal ideation
Lorcaserin	CNS—5-HT$_{2C}$ receptor agonist	Appetite suppression	Extensive metabolism in the liver	Nausea, headache, dry mouth, dizziness, constipation, suicidal ideation, lethargy
Orlistat	GI system—inhibits gastric and pancreatic lipase	Fat absorption decreased by ~30%, which decreases overall caloric intake	Minimal systemic absorption	GI symptoms such as oily spotting, flatulence, fecal urgency, and increased defecation
Phentermine	CNS—increase in NE and dopamine release and reuptake inhibition	Appetite suppression	Excretion through the kidneys	Dry mouth, headache, insomnia, constipation Possible heart rate and blood pressure increases
Diethylpropion	CNS—increase in NE and dopamine release and reuptake inhibition	Appetite suppression	Excretion mainly through the kidneys	Dry mouth, headache, insomnia, constipation Possible heart rate and blood pressure increases
Phentermine + topiramate	*Phentermine:* CNS—increase in NE and dopamine release and reuptake inhibition *Topiramate:* CNS—increase in GABA	Appetite suppression and increased satiety	Excretion primarily through the kidneys with limited hepatic metabolism	Paresthesia, altered taste, dizziness, insomnia, dry mouth, constipation Contraindicated in pregnancy

Figure 37.14
Characteristics of the medications for obesity. CNS = central nervous system; GABA = γ-aminobutyric acid; GI = gastrointestinal; GLP = glucagon-like peptide; NE = norepinephrine; POMC = proopiomelanocortin.

the combination of *phentermine/topiramate* is contraindicated in pregnancy. *Bupropion* and *naltrexone* is another combination therapy approved for chronic weight management. Important characteristics of the medications for obesity are summarized in Figure 37.14.

Study Questions

Choose the ONE best answer.

37.1 A 43-year-old heavy machine operator complains of seasonal allergies. Which medication is most appropriate for management of his allergy symptoms?

A. Diphenhydramine
B. Doxylamine
C. Hydroxyzine
D. Fexofenadine

Correct answer = D. The use of first-generation H$_1$ antihistamines is contraindicated in the treatment of pilots and others who must remain alert. Because of its lower potential to induce drowsiness, fexofenadine may be recommended for individuals working in jobs in which wakefulness is critical.

37.2 Which statement concerning H_1 antihistamines is correct?

   A. Second-generation H_1 antihistamines are relatively free of adverse effects.

   B. Because of the established long-term safety of first-generation H_1 antihistamines, they are the first choice for allergic rhinitis.

   C. The motor coordination involved in driving an automobile is not affected by the use of first-generation H_1 antihistamines.

   D. H_1 antihistamines can be used in the treatment of acute anaphylaxis.

> Correct answer = A. Second-generation H_1 antihistamines are preferred over first-generation agents because they are relatively free of adverse effects. Driving performance is adversely affected by first-generation H_1 antihistamines. Epinephrine, not antihistamine, is an acceptable treatment for acute anaphylaxis. Second-generation H_1 antihistamines penetrate the blood–brain barrier to a lesser degree than do the first-generation drugs.

37.3 Which histamine receptor antagonist is known to enter the central nervous system readily and cause sedation?

   A. Hydroxyzine

   B. Cetirizine

   C. Desloratadine

   D. Loratadine

> Correct answer = A. Choices B, C, and D are all second-generation antihistamines that cross the blood–brain barrier to a much lesser extent than does hydroxyzine. Hydroxyzine is the only drug that crosses the blood–brain barrier easily.

37.4 Which drug is an H_1-receptor antagonist that also has serotonin receptor antagonism on the appetite center, with the ability to stimulate appetite?

   A. Hydroxyzine

   B. Loratadine

   C. Diphenhydramine

   D. Cyproheptadine

> Correct answer = D. Cyproheptadine has significant serotonin antagonism and is known to increase appetite.

37.5 Which drug for headache is contraindicated in patients with peripheral vascular disease?

   A. Ergotamine

   B. Aspirin

   C. Acetaminophen

   D. Naproxen

> Correct answer = A. Ergotamine is contraindicated in peripheral vascular disease because it is a significant vasoconstrictor.

37.6 A 29-year-old woman complains of migraine headaches associated with early onset vomiting. Currently, she uses ibuprofen as needed for her migraines, but it is not very effective. Which triptan would be ideal for this patient?

   A. Naratriptan

   B. Zolmitriptan

   C. Frovatriptan

   D. Almotriptan

> Correct answer = B. Although all of the triptans listed are available as an oral tablet, this patient suffers from vomiting associated with her migraines. Zolmitriptan and sumatriptan are available as an intranasal dosage form, which would be ideal for this patient.

37.7 A 35-year-old woman is having several severe migraines per month. The migraines are usually relieved with one or two doses of triptan drugs. Which is most appropriate for prophylaxis to reduce the frequency of her migraines?

   A. Dihydroergotamine

   B. Ibuprofen

   C. Propranolol

   D. Sumatriptan

> Correct answer = C. β-Blockers such as propranolol are used for prophylaxis to reduce the frequency of migraines. The other medications are all used to treat an acute migraine headache.

37.8 A 27-year-old married woman is asking about treatment options for obesity. She recently stopped taking her birth control medications, as she felt they were contributing to her weight gain. Which medication should be avoided in this patient?

A. Phentermine/topiramate

B. Orlistat

C. Diethylpropion

D. Lorcaserin

Correct answer = A. Although patients should not take any medications to lose weight during pregnancy, the topiramate component of this medication is especially dangerous, since it can be teratogenic. Because this patient stopped her birth control medicine, she is at risk of becoming pregnant and developing birth defects while also on this medication.

37.9 A fellow health care provider is concerned about prescribing orlistat to adolescent patients. Many of his adolescent patients are stopping the medication during the first month of treatment. Which side effect is the most likely reason the adolescents are stopping orlistat?

A. Valvulopathy

B. Suicidal ideation

C. Drowsiness

D. Flatulence

Correct answer = D. Flatulence is a very common side effect with orlistat, along with several other GI disturbances. For adolescents, these side effects may be embarrassing and difficult to manage. It is important to counsel patients about these gastrointestinal side effects with orlistat and recommend a low-fat diet as well as cholestyramine to counteract the effects should they become bothersome. The other side effects listed have been seen with other obesity medications, but not with orlistat.

37.10 A 38-year-old obese man with depression is considering a weight loss medication following several failed attempts with diet and exercise. Which medication could be considered in this individual?

A. Liraglutide

B. Bupropion + naltrexone

C. Orlistat

D. Lorcaserin

Correct answer = C. Only orlistat has not been associated with suicidal ideation. All of the other drugs listed may cause suicidal ideation and would not be advisable for an individual with depression. Also, with a history of depression, the patient may be taking a medication that could increase serotonin levels. The addition of lorcaserin, a serotonin receptor agonist, could lead to serotonin syndrome further excluding it from the list of possible options.

Anti-inflammatory, Antipyretic, and Analgesic Agents

Eric Dietrich and Amy Talana

38

I. OVERVIEW

Inflammation is a normal, protective response to tissue injury caused by physical trauma, noxious chemicals, or microbiologic agents. Inflammation is the body's effort to inactivate or destroy invading organisms, remove irritants, and set the stage for tissue repair. When healing is complete, the inflammatory process usually subsides. However, inappropriate activation of the immune system can result in inflammation and immune-mediated diseases such as rheumatoid arthritis (RA). Normally, the immune system can differentiate between self and nonself. In RA, white blood cells (WBCs) view the synovium as nonself and initiate an inflammatory attack. WBC activation leads to stimulation of T lymphocytes, which recruit and activate monocytes and macrophages. These cells secrete proinflammatory cytokines, including tumor necrosis factor (TNF)-α and interleukin (IL)-1, into the synovial cavity, ultimately leading to joint destruction and other systemic abnormalities characteristic of RA. In addition to T lymphocyte activation, B lymphocytes are also involved and produce rheumatoid factor and other autoantibodies to maintain inflammation. These defensive reactions cause progressive tissue injury, resulting in joint damage and erosions, functional disability, pain, and reduced quality of life. Pharmacotherapy for RA includes anti-inflammatory and/or immunosuppressive agents that modulate/reduce the inflammatory process, with the goals of reducing inflammation and pain, and halting or slowing disease progression. The agents discussed in this chapter (Figure 38.1) include nonsteroidal anti-inflammatory drugs (NSAIDs), *celecoxib, acetaminophen*, and disease-modifying antirheumatic drugs (DMARDs). Additionally, agents used for the treatment of gout are reviewed.

NSAIDs
Aspirin BAYER, BUFFERIN, ECOTRIN
Celecoxib CELEBREX
Diclofenac FLECTOR, PENNSAID, VOLTAREN
Diflunisal GENERIC ONLY
Etodolac GENERIC ONLY
Fenoprofen NALFON
Flurbiprofen GENERIC ONLY
Ibuprofen ADVIL, MOTRIN
Indomethacin INDOCIN
Ketorolac ACULAR, ACUVAIL
Ketoprofen GENERIC ONLY
Meclofenamate GENERIC ONLY
Mefenamic acid PONSTEL
Meloxicam MOBIC
Methyl salicylate WINTERGREEN OIL
Nabumetone GENERIC ONLY
Naproxen ALEVE, ANAPROX, NAPROSYN
Oxaprozin DAYPRO
Piroxicam FELDENE
Salsalate GENERIC ONLY
Sulindac GENERIC ONLY
Tolmetin GENERIC ONLY
OTHER ANALGESICS
Acetaminophen (Paracetamol) OFIRMEV, TYLENOL

Figure 38.1
Summary of anti-inflammatory drugs. NSAIDs = nonsteroidal anti-inflammatory drugs.

II. PROSTAGLANDINS

NSAIDs act through inhibition of the synthesis of prostaglandins. Thus, an understanding of NSAIDs requires comprehension of the actions and biosynthesis of prostaglandins—unsaturated fatty acid derivatives containing 20 carbons that include a cyclic ring structure. [Note: These compounds are sometimes referred to as eicosanoids; "eicosa" refers to the 20 carbon atoms.]

A. Role of prostaglandins as local mediators

Prostaglandins and related compounds are produced in minute quantities by virtually all tissues. They generally act locally on the tissues in which they are synthesized and are rapidly metabolized to inactive products at their sites of action. Therefore, prostaglandins do not circulate in the blood in significant concentrations. Thromboxanes and leukotrienes are related compounds that are synthesized from the same precursors as the prostaglandins.

B. Synthesis of prostaglandins

Arachidonic acid is the primary precursor of the prostaglandins and related compounds, and it is present as a component of the phospholipids of cell membranes. Free arachidonic acid is released from tissue phospholipids by the action of phospholipase A_2 via a process controlled by hormones and other stimuli. There are two major pathways in the synthesis of eicosanoids from arachidonic acid, the cyclooxygenase and the lipoxygenase pathways.

1. **Cyclooxygenase pathway:** Eicosanoids with ring structures (that is, prostaglandins, thromboxanes, and prostacyclins) are synthesized via the cyclooxygenase pathway. Two related isoforms of the cyclooxygenase enzymes exist. Cyclooxygenase-1 (COX-1) is responsible for the physiologic production of prostanoids, whereas cyclooxygenase-2 (COX-2) causes the elevated production of prostanoids that occurs in sites of chronic disease and inflammation. COX-1 is a constitutive enzyme that regulates normal cellular processes, such as gastric cytoprotection, vascular homeostasis, platelet aggregation, and reproductive and kidney functions. COX-2 is constitutively expressed in tissues such as the brain, kidney, and bone. Its expression at other sites is increased during states of chronic inflammation. Differences in binding site shape have permitted the development of selective COX-2 inhibitors (Figure 38.2). Additionally, expression of COX-2 is induced by inflammatory mediators like TNF-α and IL-1 but can also be pharmacologically inhibited by glucocorticoids (Figure 38.3), which may contribute to the significant anti-inflammatory effects of these drugs.

2. **Lipoxygenase pathway:** Alternatively, several lipoxygenases can act on arachidonic acid to form leukotrienes (Figure 38.3). Antileukotriene drugs, such as *zileuton*, *zafirlukast*, and *montelukast*, are treatment options for asthma (see Chapter 39).

DRUGS FOR RHEUMATOID ARTHRITIS
Abatacept ORENCIA
Adalimumab HUMIRA
Certolizumab CIMZIA
Etanercept ENBREL
Golimumab SIMPONI
Hydroxychloroquine PLAQUENIL
Infliximab INFLECTRA, REMICADE, RENFLEXIS
Leflunomide ARAVA
Methotrexate OTREXUP, TREXALL
Rituximab RITUXAN
Sarilumab KEVZARA
Sulfasalazine AZULFIDINE
Tocilizumab ACTEMRA
Tofacitinib XELJANZ

DRUGS FOR GOUT
Allopurinol ZYLOPRIM
Colchicine COLCRYS
Febuxostat ULORIC
Pegloticase KRYSTEXXA
Probenecid GENERIC ONLY

Figure 38.1 (continued)
Summary of anti-inflammatory drugs.

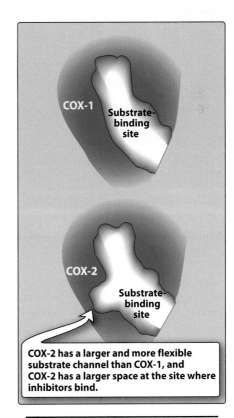

COX-2 has a larger and more flexible substrate channel than COX-1, and COX-2 has a larger space at the site where inhibitors bind.

Figure 38.2
Structural differences in active sites of cyclooxygenase (COX)-1 and COX-2.

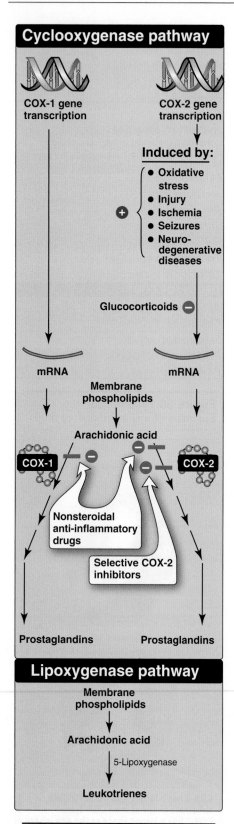

Figure 38.3
Synthesis of prostaglandins and
leukotrienes. COX = cyclooxygenase.

C. Actions of prostaglandins

Actions of prostaglandins are mediated by their binding to a variety of distinct G-coupled protein receptors in cell membranes. Prostaglandins and their metabolites act as local signals that fine-tune the response of a specific cell type. Their functions vary depending on the tissue and the specific enzymes within the pathway that are available at that particular site. For example, the release of thromboxane A_2 (TXA_2) from platelets during tissue injury triggers the recruitment of new platelets for aggregation and local vasoconstriction. However, prostacyclin (PGI_2), produced by endothelial cells, has opposite effects, inhibiting platelet aggregation and producing vasodilation. The net effect on platelets and blood vessels depends on the balance of these two prostanoids.

D. Therapeutic uses of prostaglandins

Prostaglandins have a major role in modulating pain, inflammation, and fever. They control many physiological functions, such as acid secretion and mucus production in the gastrointestinal (GI) tract, uterine contractions, and renal blood flow. Prostaglandins are among the chemical mediators released in allergic and inflammatory processes. Therefore, they find use for the disorders discussed below (Figure 38.4).

E. Alprostadil

Alprostadil [al-PROS-ta-dil] is a PGE_1 analog that is naturally produced in tissues such as seminal vesicles and cavernous tissues, in the placenta, and in the ductus arteriosus of the fetus. PGE_1 maintains the patency of the ductus arteriosus during pregnancy. The ductus closes soon after delivery to allow normal blood circulation between the lungs and the heart. In neonates with congenital heart conditions, infusion of *alprostadil* keeps the ductus open, allowing time until surgical correction is possible. *Alprostadil* is also used for erectile dysfunction (see Chapter 41).

F. Lubiprostone

Lubiprostone [loo-bee-PROS-tone] is a PGE_1 derivative indicated for the treatment of chronic idiopathic constipation, opioid-induced constipation, and irritable bowel syndrome with constipation. It stimulates chloride channels in the luminal cells of the intestinal epithelium, thereby increasing intestinal fluid secretion (see Chapter 40). Nausea and diarrhea are the most common adverse effects of *lubiprostone* (Figure 38.5). Nausea can be decreased if taken with food.

G. Misoprostol

Misoprostol [mye-soe-PROST-ole], a PGE_1 analog, is used to protect the mucosal lining of the stomach during chronic NSAID treatment. *Misoprostol* interacts with prostaglandin receptors on parietal cells within the stomach, reducing gastric acid secretion. Furthermore, *misoprostol* has a GI cytoprotective effect by stimulating mucus and bicarbonate production. This combination of effects decreases the incidence of NSAID-induced gastric ulcers. [Note: There is a combination product containing the NSAID *diclofenac* and *misoprostol*.] *Misoprostol* is also used off-label in obstetric settings for labor induction, since it increases uterine contractions by interacting with prostaglandin receptors in the uterus. *Misoprostol* has the potential to induce abortion. Therefore, the drug is contraindicated during pregnancy. Its use is limited by common adverse effects including diarrhea and abdominal pain.

H. Prostaglandin F$_{2\alpha}$ analogs

Bimatoprost [bih-MAT-oh-prost], *latanoprost* [la-TAN-oh-prost], *tafluprost* [TAF-loo-prost], and *travoprost* [TRAV-oh-prost] are PGF$_{2\alpha}$ analogs that are indicated for the treatment of open-angle glaucoma. By binding to prostaglandin receptors, they increase uveoscleral outflow, reducing intraocular pressure. They are administered as ophthalmic solutions once a day and are as effective as *timolol* or better in reducing intraocular pressure. *Bimatoprost* increases eyelash prominence, length, and darkness and is approved for the treatment of eyelash hypotrichosis. Ocular reactions include blurred vision, iris color change (increased brown pigmentation), increased number and pigment of eyelashes, ocular irritation, and foreign body sensation.

I. Prostacyclin (PGI$_2$) analogs

Epoprostenol [ee-poe-PROST-en-ol], the pharmaceutical form of naturally occurring prostacyclin, and the synthetic analogs of prostacyclin (*iloprost* [EYE-loe-prost] and *treprostinil* [tre-PROS-ti-nil]) are potent pulmonary vasodilators that are used for the treatment of pulmonary arterial hypertension. These drugs mimic the effects of prostacyclin in endothelial cells, producing a significant reduction in pulmonary arterial resistance with a subsequent increase in cardiac index and oxygen delivery. These agents have short half-lives. *Epoprostenol* and *treprostinil* are administered as a continuous intravenous infusion, and *treprostinil* is administered orally or via inhalation or subcutaneous infusion. Inhaled *iloprost* requires frequent dosing due to the short half-life (Figure 38.6). Dizziness, headache, flushing, and fainting are the most common adverse effects (Figure 38.7). Bronchospasm and cough can also occur after inhalation of *iloprost*.

III. NONSTEROIDAL ANTI-INFLAMMATORY DRUGS

NSAIDs are a group of chemically dissimilar agents that differ in their antipyretic, analgesic, and anti-inflammatory activities. The class includes derivatives of salicylic acid (*aspirin* [AS-pir-in], *diflunisal* [dye-FLOO-ni-sal], *salsalate* [SAL-sa-late]), propionic acid (*ibuprofen* [eye-bue-PROE-fen], *fenoprofen* [fen-oh-PROE-fen], *flurbiprofen* [flure-BI-proe-fen], *ketoprofen* [kee-toe-PROE-fen], *naproxen* [na-PROX-en], *oxaprozin* [ox-a-PROE-zin]), acetic acid (*diclofenac* [dye-KLOE-fen-ak], *etodolac* [ee-toe-DOE-lak], *indomethacin* [in-doe-METH-a-sin], *ketorolac* [kee-toe-ROLE-ak], *nabumetone* [na-BUE-me-tone], *sulindac* [sul-IN-dak], *tolmetin* [TOLE-met-in]), enolic acid (*meloxicam* [mel-OKS-i-kam], *piroxicam* [peer-OX-i-kam]), fenamates (*mefenamic* [me-fe-NAM-ik] *acid*,

PROSTAGLANDIN E1 ANALOGS
Alprostadil CAVERJECT, EDEX, MUSE, PROSTIN VR
Lubiprostone AMITIZA
Misoprostol CYTOTEC

PROSTAGLANDIN F2α ANALOGS
Bimatoprost LATISSE, LUMIGAN
Latanoprost XALATAN
Tafluprost ZIOPTAN
Travoprost TRAVATAN Z

PROSTACYCLIN ANALOGS
Epoprostenol FLOLAN, VELETRI
Iloprost VENTAVIS
Treprostinil ORENITRAM, REMODULIN, TYVASO

Figure 38.4
Summary of prostaglandin and *prostacyclin* analogs.

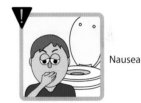
Nausea

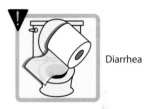
Diarrhea

Figure 38.5
Some adverse reactions to *lubiprostone*.

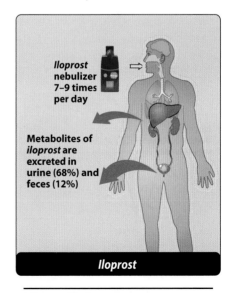

Iloprost nebulizer 7–9 times per day

Metabolites of *iloprost* are excreted in urine (68%) and feces (12%)

Iloprost

Figure 38.6
Administration and fate of *iloprost*.

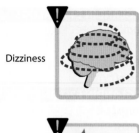

Dizziness

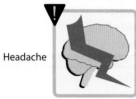

Headache

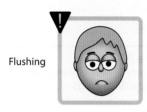

Flushing

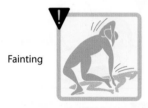

Fainting

Figure 38.7
Some adverse
reactions to *iloprost*.

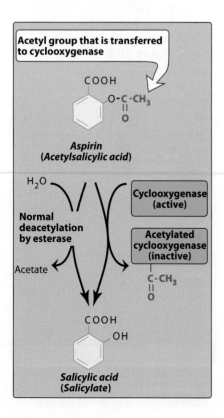

Acetyl group that is transferred
to cyclooxygenase

COOH

O-C-CH₃
‖
O

Aspirin
(Acetylsalicylic acid)

H₂O

Normal
deacetylation
by esterase

Acetate

Cyclooxygenase
(active)

Acetylated
cyclooxygenase
(inactive)

C-CH₃
‖
O

COOH
OH

Salicylic acid
(Salicylate)

meclofenamate [me-kloe-fen-AM-ate]), and the selective COX-2 inhibitor (*celecoxib* [sel-e-KOX-ib]). They act primarily by inhibiting the cyclooxygenase enzymes that catalyze the first step in prostanoid biosynthesis. This leads to decreased prostaglandin synthesis with both beneficial and unwanted effects. [Note: Differences in safety and efficacy of the NSAIDs may be explained by relative selectivity for the COX-1 or COX-2 enzyme. Inhibition of COX-2 is thought to lead to the anti-inflammatory and analgesic actions of NSAIDs, whereas inhibition of COX-1 is responsible for prevention of cardiovascular events and most adverse events.]

A. Aspirin and other NSAIDs

Aspirin can be thought of as a traditional NSAID, but it exhibits anti-inflammatory activity only at relatively high doses that are rarely used. It is used more frequently at lower doses to prevent cardiovascular events such as stroke and myocardial infarction (MI). *Aspirin* is often differentiated from other NSAIDs since it is an irreversible inhibitor of cyclooxygenase activity.

1. **Mechanism of action:** *Aspirin* is a weak organic acid that irreversibly acetylates and, thus, inactivates cyclooxygenase (Figure 38.8). The other NSAIDs are reversible inhibitors of cyclooxygenase. The NSAIDs, including *aspirin*, have three major therapeutic actions: they reduce inflammation (anti-inflammatory), pain (analgesic effect), and fever (antipyretic effect; Figure 38.9). However, not all NSAIDs are equally effective in each of these actions.

   a. **Anti-inflammatory actions:** Inhibition of cyclooxygenase diminishes the formation of prostaglandins and, thus, modulates aspects of inflammation mediated by prostaglandins. NSAIDs inhibit inflammation in arthritis, but they neither arrest the progression of the disease nor induce remission.

   b. **Analgesic action:** PGE₂ is thought to sensitize nerve endings to the action of bradykinin, histamine, and other chemical mediators released locally by the inflammatory process. Thus, by decreasing PGE₂ synthesis, the sensation of pain can be decreased. As COX-2 is expressed during times of inflammation and injury, it is thought that inhibition of this enzyme is responsible for the analgesic activity of NSAIDs. No single NSAID has demonstrated superior efficacy over another, and they are generally considered to have equivalent analgesic efficacy. The NSAIDs are used mainly for the management of mild to moderate pain arising from musculoskeletal disorders. One exception is *ketorolac*, which can be used for more severe pain, but for only a short duration.

   c. **Antipyretic action:** Fever occurs when the set-point of the anterior hypothalamic thermoregulatory center is elevated. This can be caused by PGE₂ synthesis, which is stimulated when endogenous fever-producing agents (pyrogens), such as cytokines, are released from WBCs that are activated by infection, hypersensitivity, malignancy, or inflammation. The

Figure 38.8
Metabolism of *aspirin* and acetylation of cyclooxygenase by *aspirin*.

NSAIDs lower body temperature in patients with fever by impeding PGE_2 synthesis and release, resetting the "thermostat" back toward normal. This rapidly lowers the body temperature of febrile patients by increasing heat dissipation through peripheral vasodilation and sweating. NSAIDs have no effect on normal body temperature.

2. Therapeutic uses

a. Anti-inflammatory and analgesic uses: NSAIDs are used in the treatment of osteoarthritis, gout, RA, and common conditions requiring analgesia (for example, headache, arthralgia, myalgia, and dysmenorrhea). Combinations of opioids and NSAIDs may be effective in treating pain caused by malignancy. Furthermore, the addition of NSAIDs may lead to an opioid-sparing effect, allowing for lower doses of opioids to be utilized. The salicylates exhibit analgesic activity at lower doses. Only at higher doses do these drugs show anti-inflammatory activity (Figure 38.10). For example, two 325-mg *aspirin* tablets administered four times daily produce analgesia, whereas 12 to 20 tablets per day produce both analgesic and anti-inflammatory activity.

b. Antipyretic uses: *Aspirin*, *ibuprofen*, and *naproxen* may be used to treat fever. [Note: *Aspirin* should be avoided in patients less than 19 years old with viral infections, such as varicella (chickenpox) or influenza, to prevent Reye syndrome—a syndrome that can cause fulminating hepatitis with cerebral edema, often leading to death.]

c. Cardiovascular applications: *Aspirin* irreversibly inhibits COX-1–mediated production of TXA_2, thereby reducing TXA_2-mediated vasoconstriction and platelet aggregation and the subsequent risk of cardiovascular events (Figure 38.11). The antiplatelet effects persist for the life of the platelet. Low doses of *aspirin* (75 to 162 mg—commonly 81 mg) are used prophylactically to reduce the risk of recurrent cardiovascular events, transient ischemic attacks (TIAs), stroke, and death in patients with a history of previous MI, TIA, or stroke. Chronic use of *aspirin* allows for continued inhibition as new platelets are generated. *Aspirin* is also used acutely to reduce the risk of death in acute MI and in patients undergoing certain revascularization procedures.

d. External applications: *Salicylic acid* is used topically to treat acne, corns, calluses, and warts. *Methyl salicylate* ("oil of wintergreen") is used externally as a cutaneous counterirritant in liniments, such as arthritis creams and sports rubs. *Diclofenac* is available in topical formulations (gel or solution) for treatment of osteoarthritis in the knees or hands. In addition, ocular formulations of *ketorolac* are approved for management of seasonal allergic conjunctivitis and inflammation and pain related to ocular surgery.

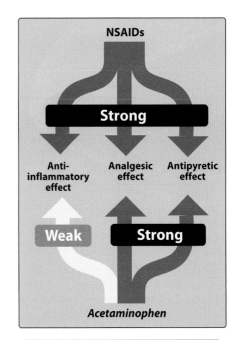

Figure 38.9
Actions of nonsteroidal anti-inflammatory drugs (NSAIDs) and *acetaminophen*.

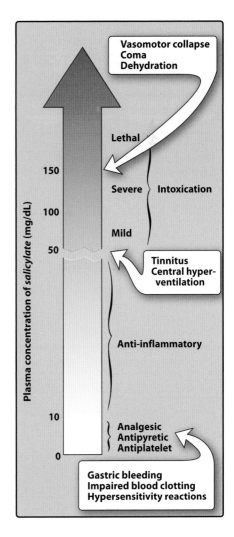

Figure 38.10
Dose-dependent effects of salicylate.

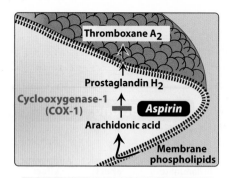

Figure 38.11
Aspirin irreversibly inhibits platelet cyclooxygenase-1.

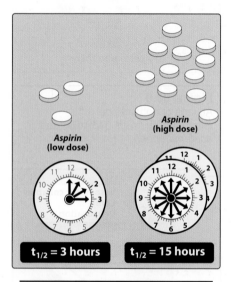

Figure 38.12
Effect of dose on the half-life of *aspirin*.

3. Pharmacokinetics

a. **Aspirin:** After oral administration, *aspirin* is rapidly deacetylated by esterases in the body to produce salicylate. Unionized salicylates are passively absorbed mainly from the upper small intestine. Salicylates (except for *diflunisal*) cross both the blood–brain barrier and the placenta and are absorbed through intact skin (especially *methyl salicylate*). Salicylate is converted by the liver to water-soluble conjugates that are rapidly cleared by the kidney, resulting in first-order elimination and a serum half-life of 3.5 hours. At anti-inflammatory dosages of *aspirin* (more than 4 g/day), the hepatic metabolic pathway becomes saturated, and zero-order kinetics are observed, leading to a half-life of 15 hours or more (Figure 38.12). Salicylate is secreted into the urine and can affect uric acid excretion. Therefore, *aspirin* should be avoided in gout, if possible, or in patients taking *probenecid*.

b. **Other NSAIDs:** Most NSAIDs are well absorbed after oral administration and circulate highly bound to plasma proteins. The majority are metabolized by the liver, mostly to inactivate metabolites. Few (for example, *nabumetone* and *sulindac*) have active metabolites. Excretion of active drug and metabolites is primarily via the urine.

4. **Adverse events:** Because of the adverse event profile, it is preferable to use NSAIDs at the lowest effective dose for the shortest duration possible.

a. **Gastrointestinal:** These are the most common adverse effects of NSAIDs, ranging from dyspepsia to bleeding. Normally, production of prostacyclin (PGI$_2$) inhibits gastric acid secretion, and PGE$_2$ and PGF$_{2\alpha}$ stimulate synthesis of protective mucus in both the stomach and small intestine. Agents that inhibit COX-1 reduce beneficial levels of these prostaglandins, resulting in increased gastric acid secretion, diminished mucus protection, and increased risk for GI bleeding and ulceration. Agents with a higher relative selectivity for COX-1 may have a higher risk for GI events compared to those with a lower relative selectivity for COX-1 (that is, higher COX-2 selectivity). NSAIDs should be taken with food or fluids to diminish GI upset. If NSAIDs are used in patients at high risk for GI events, proton pump inhibitors or *misoprostol* should be used concomitantly to prevent NSAID-induced ulcers (see Chapter 40).

b. **Increased risk of bleeding (antiplatelet effect):** As described above, *aspirin* inhibits COX-1–mediated formation of TXA$_2$ and reduces platelet aggregation for the lifetime of the platelet (3 to 7 days). Platelet aggregation is the first step in thrombus formation, and the antiplatelet effect of *aspirin* results in a prolonged bleeding time. For this reason, *aspirin* is often withheld for at least 1 week prior to surgery. NSAIDs other than *aspirin* are not utilized for their antiplatelet effect but can still prolong bleeding time, especially when combined with anticoagulants. Concomitant use of NSAIDs and *aspirin* can

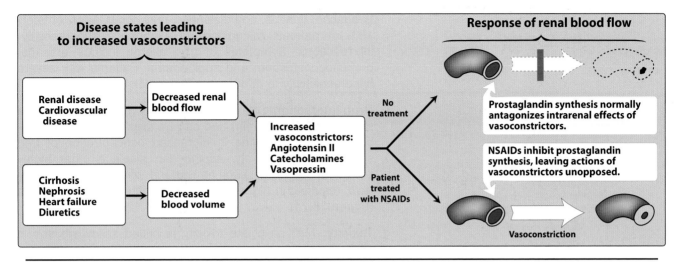

Figure 38.13
Renal effect of NSAID inhibition of prostaglandin synthesis. NSAIDs = nonsteroidal anti-inflammatory drugs.

prevent *aspirin* from binding to cyclooxygenase. Patients who take *aspirin* for cardioprotection should avoid concomitant NSAID use if possible or take *aspirin* at least 30 minutes prior to the NSAID.

c. **Renal effects:** NSAIDs prevent the synthesis of PGE$_2$ and PGI$_2$, prostaglandins that are responsible for maintaining renal blood flow (Figure 38.13). Decreased synthesis of prostaglandins can result in retention of sodium and water and may cause edema. Patients with a history of heart failure or kidney disease are at particularly high risk. These effects can also mitigate the beneficial effects of antihypertensive medications. In susceptible patients, NSAIDs have led to acute kidney injury.

d. **Cardiac effects:** Agents such as *aspirin*, with a very high degree of COX-1 selectivity at low doses, have a cardiovascular protective effect thought to be due to a reduction in the production of TXA$_2$. Agents with higher relative COX-2 selectivity have been associated with an increased risk for cardiovascular events, possibly by decreasing PGI$_2$ production mediated by COX-2. An increased risk for cardiovascular events, including MI and stroke, has been associated with all NSAIDs except *aspirin*. All NSAIDs carry a boxed warning regarding the increased risk for cardiovascular events. Use of NSAIDs, other than *aspirin*, is discouraged in patients with established cardiovascular disease. For patients with cardiovascular disease in whom NSAID treatment cannot be avoided, *naproxen* may be the least likely to be harmful.

e. **Other adverse effects:** NSAIDs are inhibitors of cyclooxygenases and, therefore, inhibit the synthesis of prostaglandins but not of leukotrienes. For this reason, NSAIDs should be used with caution in patients with asthma, as inhibition of prostaglandin synthesis can cause a shift toward leukotriene production and increase the risk of asthma exacerbations. Central nervous system (CNS) adverse events, such as

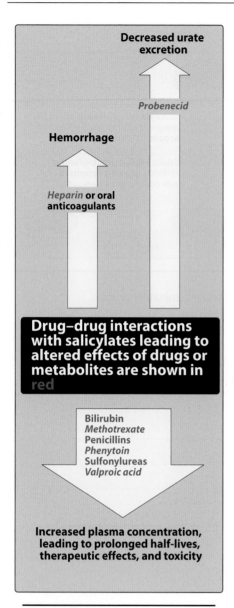

Decreased urate excretion

Probenecid

Hemorrhage

Heparin **or oral anticoagulants**

Drug–drug interactions with salicylates leading to altered effects of drugs or metabolites are shown in red

Bilirubin
Methotrexate
Penicillins
Phenytoin
Sulfonylureas
Valproic acid

Increased plasma concentration, leading to prolonged half-lives, therapeutic effects, and toxicity

Figure 38.14
Drugs interacting with salicylates.

headache, tinnitus, and dizziness, may occur. Approximately 15% of patients taking *aspirin* experience hypersensitivity reactions. Symptoms of true allergy include urticaria, bronchoconstriction, and angioedema. Patients with severe hypersensitivity to *aspirin* should avoid using NSAIDs.

f. **Drug interactions:** Salicylate is roughly 80% to 90% plasma protein bound (albumin) and can be displaced from protein-binding sites, resulting in increased concentration of free salicylate. Alternatively, *aspirin* can displace other highly protein-bound drugs, such as *warfarin*, *phenytoin*, or *valproic acid*, resulting in higher free concentrations of these agents (Figure 38.14).

g. **Toxicity:** Mild salicylate toxicity is called salicylism and is characterized by nausea, vomiting, marked hyperventilation, headache, mental confusion, dizziness, and tinnitus (ringing or roaring in the ears). When large doses of salicylate are administered, severe salicylate intoxication may result (see Figure 38.10). Restlessness, delirium, hallucinations, convulsions, coma, respiratory and metabolic acidosis, and death from respiratory failure may occur. Children are particularly prone to salicylate intoxication; ingestion of as little as 10 g of *aspirin* can be fatal.

h. **Pregnancy:** NSAIDs should be used in pregnancy only if benefits outweigh risks to the developing fetus. [Note: *Acetaminophen* is preferred if analgesic or antipyretic effects are needed during pregnancy.] In the third trimester, NSAIDs should generally be avoided due to the risk of premature closure of the ductus arteriosus.

B. **Celecoxib**

Celecoxib [SEL-e-KOX-ib], a selective COX-2 inhibitor, is significantly more selective for inhibition of COX-2 than COX-1 (Figure 38.15). Unlike the inhibition of COX-1 by *aspirin* (which is irreversible), the inhibition of COX-2 is reversible.

1. **Therapeutic uses:** *Celecoxib* is approved for the treatment of RA, osteoarthritis, and acute pain. *Celecoxib* has similar efficacy to NSAIDs in the treatment of pain.

2. **Pharmacokinetics:** *Celecoxib* is readily absorbed after oral administration. It is extensively metabolized in the liver by cytochrome P450 (CYP2C9), and the metabolites are excreted in feces and urine. The half-life is about 11 hours, and the drug may be dosed once or twice daily. The dosage should be reduced in those with moderate hepatic impairment, and *celecoxib* should be avoided in patients with severe hepatic or renal disease.

3. **Adverse effects:** Headache, dyspepsia, diarrhea, and abdominal pain are the most common adverse effects. *Celecoxib* is associated with less GI bleeding and dyspepsia than other NSAIDs. However, this benefit is lost when *aspirin* is added to *celecoxib* therapy. Patients who are at high risk of ulcers and require *aspirin* for cardiovascular prevention should avoid the use of *celecoxib*.

Like other NSAIDs, *celecoxib* has a similar risk for cardiovascular events. Patients who have had anaphylactoid reactions to *aspirin* or nonselective NSAIDs may be at risk for similar effects with *celecoxib*. Inhibitors of CYP2C9, such as *fluconazole*, may increase serum levels of *celecoxib*.

Figure 38.16 summarizes some of the therapeutic advantages and disadvantages of members of the NSAID family.

IV. ACETAMINOPHEN

Acetaminophen [a-SEET-a-MIN-oh-fen] (*N*-acetyl-*p*-aminophenol or APAP) inhibits prostaglandin synthesis in the CNS, leading to antipyretic and analgesic effects. *Acetaminophen* has less effect on cyclooxygenase in peripheral tissues (due to peripheral inactivation), which accounts for its weak anti-inflammatory activity. *Acetaminophen* does not affect platelet function or increase bleeding time. It is not considered an NSAID.

A. Therapeutic uses

Acetaminophen is used for the treatment of fever and the relief of pain. It is useful in patients with gastric complaints/risks with NSAIDs and those who do not require the anti-inflammatory action of NSAIDs. *Acetaminophen* is the analgesic/antipyretic of choice for children with viral infections or chickenpox (due to the risk of Reye syndrome with *aspirin*).

B. Pharmacokinetics

Acetaminophen is rapidly absorbed from the GI tract and undergoes significant first-pass metabolism. It is conjugated in the liver to form inactive glucuronidated or sulfated metabolites. A portion of *acetaminophen* is hydroxylated to form *N*-acetyl-*p*-benzoquinoneimine, or NAPQI, a highly reactive metabolite that can react with sulfhydryl groups and cause liver damage. At normal doses of *acetaminophen*, NAPQI reacts with the sulfhydryl group of glutathione produced by the liver, forming a nontoxic substance (Figure 38.17). *Acetaminophen* and its metabolites are excreted in urine. The drug is also available in intravenous and rectal formulations.

C. Adverse effects

At normal therapeutic doses, *acetaminophen* has few significant adverse effects. With large doses of *acetaminophen*, the available glutathione in the liver becomes depleted, and NAPQI reacts with the sulfhydryl groups of hepatic proteins (see Figure 38.17). Hepatic necrosis, a serious and potentially life-threatening condition, can result. Patients with hepatic disease, viral hepatitis, or a history of alcoholism are at higher risk of *acetaminophen*-induced hepatotoxicity. [Note: *N*-acetylcysteine is an antidote in cases of overdose (see Chapter 44).] *Acetaminophen* should be avoided in patients with severe hepatic impairment.

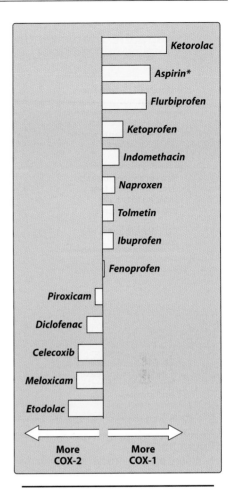

Figure 38.15
Relative selectivity of some commonly used NSAIDs. Data shown as the logarithm of their ratio of IC_{80} (drug concentration to achieve 80% inhibition of cyclooxygenase). *Aspirin* graphed for IC_{50} value due to it showing significantly more COX-1 selectivity at lower doses and graph using higher concentrations does not accurately reflect the usage or selectivity of *aspirin*.

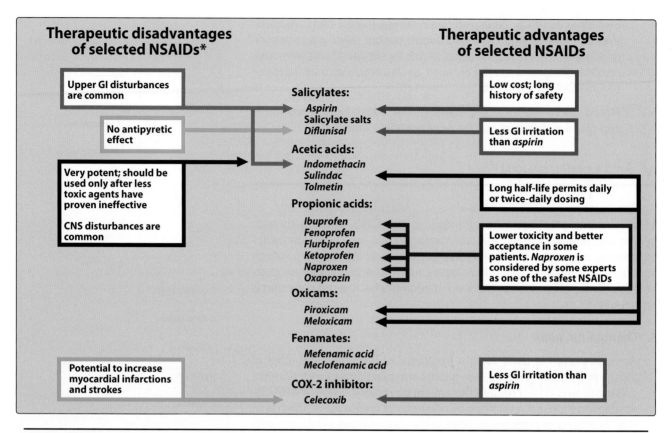

Figure 38.16
Summary of nonsteroidal anti-inflammatory agents (NSAIDs). *As a group, with the exception of *aspirin*, these drugs may
have the potential to increase risk of myocardial infarction and stroke. GI = gastrointestinal; CNS = central nervous system;
COX-2 = cyclooxygenase-2.

V. TRADITIONAL DISEASE-MODIFYING ANTIRHEUMATIC DRUGS

Traditional DMARDs (*methotrexate, hydroxychloroquine, leflunomide*, or
sulfasalazine) are used in the treatment of RA and have been shown to
slow the course of the disease, induce remission, and prevent further
destruction of the joints and involved tissues. Following diagnosis of RA,
these agents should be started as soon as possible to delay progression
of the disease. Monotherapy may be initiated with any of the traditional
DMARDs, although *methotrexate* is generally preferred. For patients
with inadequate response to monotherapy, a combination of traditional
DMARDs, or use of a TNF inhibitor or non-TNF biologic agent may be
needed. NSAIDs or glucocorticoids can also be used for their anti-inflammatory actions.

A. Methotrexate

Methotrexate [meth-oh-TREX-ate] is a folic acid antagonist that inhibits cytokine production and purine nucleotide biosynthesis, leading to
immunosuppressive and anti-inflammatory effects. It has become a
mainstay of treatment in patients with RA. Response to *methotrexate*

usually occurs within 3 to 6 weeks of starting treatment. Other traditional DMARDs, TNF inhibitors, or non-TNF biologic agents can be added to *methotrexate* if there is inadequate response to monotherapy with this agent. Doses of *methotrexate* required for RA treatment are much lower than those needed in cancer chemotherapy and are generally administered once weekly, thereby minimizing adverse effects. Common adverse effects of *methotrexate* when used for RA are mucosal ulceration and nausea. Cytopenias (particularly leukopenia), cirrhosis of the liver, and an acute pneumonia-like syndrome may occur with chronic administration. [Note: Supplementation with *folic acid* may improve tolerability of *methotrexate* and reduce GI and hepatic adverse effects.] Periodic liver function tests, complete blood counts, and monitoring for signs of infection are recommended. *Methotrexate* is contraindicated in pregnancy.

B. Hydroxychloroquine

Hydroxychloroquine [hye-drox-ee-KLOR-oh-kwin] is used for early, mild RA, and may be combined with *methotrexate*. Its mechanism of action in autoimmune disorders is unknown, and onset of effects takes 6 weeks to 6 months. *Hydroxychloroquine* has less adverse effects on the liver and immune system than other DMARDs. However, it may cause ocular toxicity, including irreversible retinal damage and corneal deposits, CNS disturbances, GI upset, and skin discoloration and eruptions.

C. Leflunomide

Leflunomide [le-FLOO-no-mide] is an immunomodulatory agent that preferentially causes cell arrest of the autoimmune lymphocytes through its action on dihydroorotate dehydrogenase (DHODH). After biotransformation, *leflunomide* becomes a reversible inhibitor of DHODH, an enzyme necessary for pyrimidine synthesis (Figure 38.18). *Leflunomide* may be used as monotherapy in patients who have intolerance or contraindications to use of *methotrexate* in RA, or it may be used in combination with *methotrexate* for patients with suboptimal response to *methotrexate* alone. Common adverse effects include headache, diarrhea, and nausea. Other effects are weight loss, allergic reactions, including a flu-like syndrome, skin rash, alopecia, and hypokalemia. The drug is not recommended in patients with liver disease as it can be hepatotoxic. *Leflunomide* is contraindicated in pregnancy. Monitoring parameters include signs of infection, complete blood count, electrolytes, and liver enzymes.

D. Sulfasalazine

Sulfasalazine [sul-fa-SAH-la-zeen] has recommendations for use similar to *leflunomide* in the treatment of RA. Its mechanism of action in treating RA is unclear. The onset of activity is 1 to 3 months, and it is associated with GI adverse effects (nausea, vomiting, anorexia) and leukopenia.

E. Glucocorticoids

Glucocorticoids (see Chapter 26) are potent anti-inflammatory drugs that are commonly used in patients with RA to provide symptom-

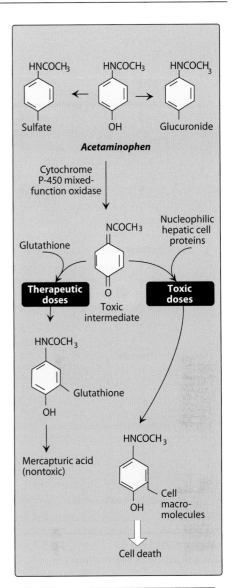

Figure 38.17
Metabolism of *acetaminophen*.

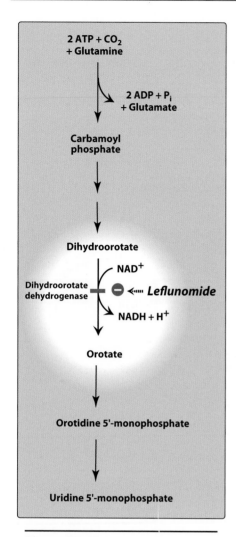

2 ATP + CO$_2$
+ Glutamine

2 ADP + P$_i$
+ Glutamate

Carbamoyl
phosphate

Dihydroorotate

NAD$^+$

Dihydroorotate
dehydrogenase ——⊖ ←···· **Leflunomide**

NADH + H$^+$

Orotate

Orotidine 5'-monophosphate

Uridine 5'-monophosphate

Figure 38.18
Site of action of *leflunomide*.

atic relief and bridge the time until other DMARDs become effective. Glucocorticoids should always be used at the lowest dose and for the shortest duration possible to avoid adverse effects associated with long-term use.

VI. BIOLOGIC DISEASE-MODIFYING ANTIRHEUMATIC DRUGS

IL-1 and TNF-α are proinflammatory cytokines involved in the pathogenesis of RA. When secreted by synovial macrophages, IL-1 and TNF-α stimulate synovial cells to proliferate and synthesize collagenase, thereby degrading cartilage, stimulating bone resorption, and inhibiting proteoglycan synthesis. The TNF-α inhibitors (*adalimumab, certolizumab, etanercept, golimumab,* and *infliximab*) are biologic DMARDs which have been shown to decrease signs and symptoms of RA, reduce progression of structural damage, and improve physical function. Clinical response can be seen within 2 weeks of therapy. TNF-α inhibitors are usually employed in RA after a patient has an inadequate response to traditional DMARDs. These agents may be used alone or in combination with traditional DMARDs. If a patient has failed monotherapy with one TNF-α inhibitor, a traditional DMARD may be added, or therapy with a non-TNF biologic agent or a different TNF-α inhibitor may be tried. TNF-α inhibitors should be used cautiously in those with heart failure, as they can cause and/or worsen preexisting heart failure. An increased risk of lymphoma and other cancers has been observed with the use of TNF-α inhibitors.

Biologic DMARDs include the TNF-α inhibitors, as well as the non-TNF biologic agents (*abatacept, rituximab, tocilizumab*). Like TNF-α inhibitors, non-TNF biologics are generally used in RA after a patient has an inadequate response to traditional DMARDs, and they may be used alone or in combination with traditional DMARDs. If a patient has failed monotherapy with one non-TNF biologic, a trial of another non-TNF biologic with or without *methotrexate* is warranted. Patients receiving biologic DMARDs are at increased risk for infections, such as tuberculosis, fungal opportunistic infections, and sepsis. [Note: TNF-α inhibitors and non-TNF biologic agents should not be used together due to the risk of severe infections.] Reactivation of hepatitis B may occur with the use of these agents. Live vaccinations should not be administered to patients taking any of the biologic DMARDs. Characteristics of the TNF-α inhibitors and non-TNF biologic therapies for the treatment of RA are outlined below. [Note: TNF-α inhibitors find use in a number of disorders, such as ulcerative colitis and Crohn disease (see Chapter 40), psoriasis, and ankylosing spondylitis.]

A. Adalimumab

Adalimumab [AY-da-LIM-ue-mab] is a recombinant monoclonal antibody that binds to TNF-α and interferes with its activity by blocking interaction of TNF-α with cell surface receptors. *Adalimumab* is administered subcutaneously weekly or every other week. It may cause headache, nausea, agranulocytosis, rash, reaction at the injection site, and increased risk of infections.

B. Certolizumab

Certolizumab [ser-toe-LIZ-oo-mab] is a humanized antibody that neutralizes biological actions of TNF-α. It is combined with polyethylene glycol (pegylated) and is administered every 2 weeks via subcutaneous injection. Adverse effects are similar to other TNF-α inhibitors.

C. Etanercept

Etanercept [ee-TAN-er-cept] is a genetically engineered fusion protein that binds to TNF-α, thereby blocking its interaction with cell surface TNF-α receptors. The combination of *etanercept* and *methotrexate* is more effective than *methotrexate* or *etanercept* alone in hindering the RA disease process, improving function, and achieving remission (Figure 38.19). *Etanercept* is given subcutaneously once weekly and is generally well tolerated.

D. Golimumab

Golimumab [goe-LIM-ue-mab] neutralizes the biological activity of TNF-α by binding to it and blocking its interaction with cell surface receptors. It is administered subcutaneously once a month in combination with *methotrexate*. *Golimumab* may increase hepatic enzymes.

E. Infliximab

Infliximab [in-FLIX-i-mab] is a chimeric monoclonal antibody composed of human and murine regions. The antibody binds specifically to human TNF-α and inhibits binding with its receptors. This agent is not indicated for monotherapy, as this leads to the development of anti-*infliximab* antibodies and reduced efficacy. *Infliximab* should be administered with *methotrexate*. *Infliximab* is administered as an IV infusion every 8 weeks. Infusion-related reactions, such as fever, chills, pruritus, and urticaria, may occur.

F. Abatacept

T lymphocytes need two interactions to become activated: 1) the antigen-presenting cell (macrophages or B cells) must interact with the receptor on the T cell and 2) the CD80/CD86 protein on the antigen-presenting cell must interact with the CD28 protein on the T cell. *Abatacept* [a-BAT-ah-cept] is a recombinant fusion protein and costimulation modulator that competes with CD28 for binding on CD80/CD86 protein, thereby preventing full T-cell activation and reducing the inflammatory response. *Abatacept* is administered as an IV infusion every 4 weeks. Common adverse effects include infusion-related reactions, headache, upper respiratory infections, and nausea.

G. Rituximab

In RA, B lymphocytes can perpetuate the inflammatory process in the synovium by 1) activating T lymphocytes, 2) producing autoantibodies and rheumatoid factor, and 3) producing proinflammatory cytokines, such as TNF-α and IL-1. *Rituximab* [ri-TUK-si-mab] is a chimeric murine/human monoclonal antibody directed against the CD20 antigen found on the surface of normal and malignant B lymphocytes. Administration of *rituximab* results in B-cell depletion.

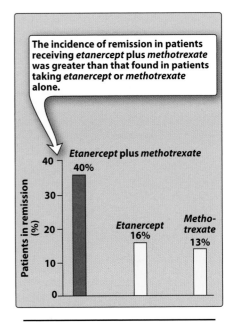

The incidence of remission in patients receiving *etanercept* plus *methotrexate* was greater than that found in patients taking *etanercept* or *methotrexate* alone.

Figure 38.19
Incidence of remission from the symptoms of RA after 1 year of therapy.

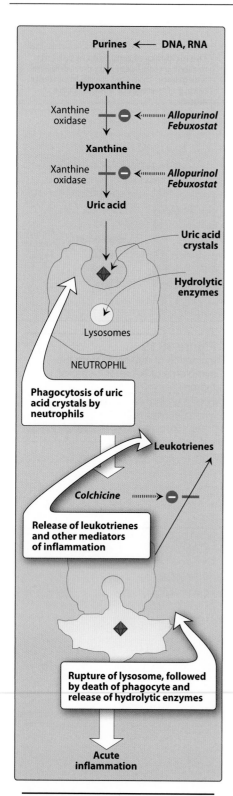

Figure 38.20
Role of uric acid in the inflammation of gout.

Rituximab is administered as an intravenous infusion every 16 to 24 weeks. To reduce infusion reactions, *methylprednisolone*, *acetaminophen*, and an antihistamine are administered prior to each infusion. Infusion reactions (urticaria, hypotension, and angioedema) are the most common complaints and typically occur during the first infusion.

H. Tocilizumab and sarilumab

Tocilizumab [toe-si-LIZ-ue-mab] and *sarilumab* [sar-IL-ue-mab] are recombinant monoclonal antibodies that bind to IL-6 receptors and inhibit activity of the proinflammatory cytokine IL-6. Both *tocilizumab* and *sarilumab* are administered as a subcutaneous injection every 2 weeks. *Tocilizumab* may also be administered as an intravenous infusion every 4 weeks. Adverse reactions to *tocilizumab* include elevated liver function tests, hyperlipidemia, neutropenia, hypertension, and infusion-related and injection site reactions. Adverse reactions for *sarilumab* are similar.

VII. OTHER DRUGS FOR RHEUMATOID ARTHRITIS

Janus kinases are intracellular enzymes that modulate immune cell activity in response to the binding of inflammatory mediators to the cellular membrane. *Tofacitinib* [toe-fa-SYE-ti-nib] is a synthetic small molecule that is an oral inhibitor of Janus kinases. It is indicated for the treatment of moderate to severe established RA in patients who have had an inadequate response or intolerance to *methotrexate*. Metabolism of *tofacitinib* is mediated primarily by CYP3A4, and dosage adjustments may be required if the drug is taken with potent inhibitors or inducers of this isoenzyme. Hemoglobin concentrations must be greater than 9 g/dL to start *tofacitinib* and must be monitored during therapy due to the risk for anemia. Likewise, lymphocyte and neutrophil counts should be checked prior to initiation of therapy and monitored during treatment. *Tofacitinib* treatment may also increase the risk for new primary malignancy and opportunistic infections. Due to long-term safety concerns, *tofacitinib* is usually reserved for patients who have inadequate response or intolerance to other agents. [Note: *Anakinra*, *azathioprine*, *cyclosporine*, *gold*, and *minocycline* are other agents used infrequently in the treatment of RA due to their adverse effect profile or the availability of other agents with more proven efficacy.]

VIII. DRUGS USED FOR THE TREATMENT OF GOUT

Gout is a metabolic disorder characterized by high levels of uric acid in the blood (hyperuricemia). Hyperuricemia can lead to deposition of sodium urate crystals in tissues, especially the joints and kidney. The deposition of urate crystals initiates an inflammatory process involving the infiltration of granulocytes that phagocytize the urate crystals (Figure 38.20). Acute flares of gout usually present as pain, swelling, tenderness, and redness in the affected joints (for example, big toe, knees, ankles, wrists, or elbows). The cause of hyperuricemia in gout is an imbalance between overproduction of uric acid and/or the inability to excrete uric acid renally. Most therapeutic strategies for gout involve lowering the uric acid level below the saturation point (6 mg/dL), thus preventing the deposition of urate crystals. This can be accomplished by interfering with uric acid synthesis or increasing uric acid excretion.

A. Treatment of acute gout

Acute gout attacks can result from a number of conditions, including excessive alcohol consumption, a diet rich in purines, and kidney disease. NSAIDs, corticosteroids, and *colchicine* are effective agents for the management of acute gouty arthritis. *Indomethacin* is considered the classic NSAID of choice, although all NSAIDs are likely to be effective in decreasing pain and inflammation. Intra-articular administration of corticosteroids (when only one or two joints are affected) is also appropriate in the acute setting, or systemic corticosteroids for more widespread joint involvement. Patients are candidates for prophylactic urate-lowering therapy if they have more than two attacks per year or they have chronic kidney disease, kidney stones, or tophi (deposit of urate crystals in the joints, bones, cartilage, or other body structures).

B. Treatment of chronic gout

Urate-lowering therapy for chronic gout aims to reduce the frequency of attacks and complications of gout. Treatment strategies include the use of xanthine oxidase inhibitors to reduce the synthesis of uric acid or use of uricosuric drugs to increase its excretion. Xanthine oxidase inhibitors (*allopurinol*, *febuxostat*) are first-line urate-lowering agents. Uricosuric agents (*probenecid*) may be used in patients who are intolerant to xanthine oxidase inhibitors or fail to achieve adequate response with those agents. [Note: Initiation of urate-lowering therapy can precipitate an acute gout attack due to rapid changes in serum urate concentrations. Medications for the prevention of an acute gout attack (low-dose *colchicine*, NSAIDs, or corticosteroids) should be initiated with urate-lowering therapy and continued for at least 6 months.]

C. Colchicine

Colchicine [KOL-chi-seen], a plant alkaloid, is used for the treatment of acute gouty attacks. It is neither a uricosuric nor an analgesic agent, although it relieves pain in acute attacks of gout.

1. **Mechanism of action:** *Colchicine* binds to tubulin, a microtubular protein, causing its depolymerization. This disrupts cellular functions, such as the mobility of neutrophils, thus decreasing their migration into the inflamed joint. Furthermore, *colchicine* blocks cell division by binding to mitotic spindles.

2. **Therapeutic uses:** The anti-inflammatory activity of *colchicine* is specific for gout, usually alleviating the pain of acute gout within 12 hours. [Note: *Colchicine* must be administered within 36 hours of onset of attack to be effective.] NSAIDs have largely replaced *colchicine* in the treatment of acute gouty attacks for safety reasons. *Colchicine* is also used as a prophylactic agent to prevent acute attacks of gout in patients initiating urate-lowering therapy.

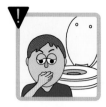

Nausea

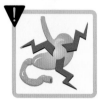

GI disturbance

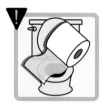

Diarrhea

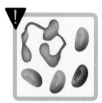

Agranulocytosis
Aplastic anemia

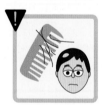

Alopecia

Figure 38.21
Some adverse
effects of *colchicine*.
GI = gastrointestinal.

3. **Pharmacokinetics:** *Colchicine* is administered orally and is rapidly absorbed from the GI tract. *Colchicine* is metabolized by hepatic CYP450 3A4 and other tissues. It undergoes enterohepatic recirculation and exhibits high interpatient variability in the elimination half-life. A portion of the drug is excreted unchanged in the urine.

4. **Adverse effects:** *Colchicine* may cause nausea, vomiting, abdominal pain, and diarrhea (Figure 38.21). Chronic administration may lead to myopathy, neutropenia, aplastic anemia, and alopecia. The drug should not be used in pregnancy and should be used with caution in patients with hepatic, renal, or cardiovascular disease. Dosage adjustments are required in patients taking CYP3A4 inhibitors (for example, *clarithromycin* and *itraconazole*) or P-gp inhibitors (for example, *amiodarone* and *verapamil*) and those with severe renal impairment.

D. Allopurinol

Allopurinol [al-oh-PURE-i-nole], a xanthine oxidase inhibitor, is a purine analog. It reduces the production of uric acid by competitively inhibiting the last two steps in uric acid biosynthesis that are catalyzed by xanthine oxidase (see Figure 38.20).

1. **Therapeutic uses:** *Allopurinol* is an effective urate-lowering therapy in the treatment of gout and hyperuricemia secondary to other conditions, such as that associated with certain malignancies (those in which large amounts of purines are produced, particularly after chemotherapy) or in renal disease.

2. **Pharmacokinetics:** *Allopurinol* is completely absorbed after oral administration. The primary metabolite alloxanthine (oxypurinol) is also a xanthine oxidase inhibitor with a half-life of 15 to 18 hours. Thus, effective inhibition of xanthine oxidase can be maintained with once-daily dosing. The drug and its active metabolite are excreted in the urine. Dose adjustment is needed if estimated glomerular filtration rate is less than 30 mL/min/1.73 m^2.

3. **Adverse effects:** *Allopurinol* is well tolerated by most patients. Hypersensitivity reactions, especially skin rashes, are the most common adverse reactions. The risk is increased in those with reduced renal function. Because acute attacks of gout may occur more frequently during the first several months of therapy, *colchicine*, NSAIDs, or corticosteroids can be administered concurrently.

E. Febuxostat

Febuxostat [feb-UX-oh-stat] is an oral xanthine oxidase inhibitor structurally unrelated to *allopurinol*. Its adverse effect profile is similar to that of *allopurinol*, although the risk for rash and hypersensitivity reactions may be reduced. *Febuxostat* does not have the same degree of renal elimination as *allopurinol* and thus requires less adjustment in those with reduced renal function. *Febuxostat* should be used with caution in patients with a history of heart disease or stroke, as this agent may be associated with a greater risk of these events as compared to *allopurinol*.

F. Probenecid

Probenecid [proe-BEN-a-sid] is an oral uricosuric drug. It is a weak organic acid that promotes renal clearance of uric acid by inhibiting the urate-anion exchanger in the proximal tubule. At therapeutic doses, it blocks proximal tubular reabsorption of uric acid. *Probenecid* should be avoided if the creatinine clearance is less than 50 mL/min. Adverse effects include nausea, vomiting, and dermatologic reactions, and, rarely, anemia or anaphylactic reactions.

G. Pegloticase

Pegloticase [peg-LOE-ti-kase] is a recombinant form of the enzyme urate oxidase or uricase. It acts by converting uric acid to allantoin, a water-soluble nontoxic metabolite that is excreted primarily by the kidneys. *Pegloticase* is indicated for patients with gout who fail treatment with standard therapies such as xanthine oxidase inhibitors. It is administered as an IV infusion every 2 weeks. Infusion-related reactions and anaphylaxis may occur with *pegloticase*, and patients should be premedicated with antihistamines and corticosteroids.

Study Questions

Choose the ONE best answer.

38.1 A 64-year-old man presents with mild to moderate musculoskeletal back pain. He states that he has tried acetaminophen without relief. His medical history includes diabetes, hypertension, hyperlipidemia, gastric ulcer (resolved), and coronary artery disease. Which is the most appropriate NSAID regimen to treat this patient's pain?

A. Celecoxib

B. Indomethacin and omeprazole

C. Naproxen and omeprazole

D. Naproxen

> Correct answer = C. This patient is at high risk of future ulcers, due to the history of gastric ulcer. Therefore, using a regimen that includes an agent that is more COX-2 selective or a proton pump inhibitor is warranted. Therefore, D is incorrect. Choices A and B are incorrect because this patient has significant cardiovascular risk and a history of coronary artery disease. Naproxen is thought of as the safest NSAID regarding cardiovascular disease, though it still can present risks. Therefore, C is correct as it uses the first-choice NSAID with the GI protection of a proton pump inhibitor.

38.2 Which statement is correct regarding the difference between acetaminophen and naproxen?

A. Acetaminophen has more anti-inflammatory effects compared with naproxen.

B. Acetaminophen has more GI side effects but less effects on bleeding compared with naproxen.

C. Acetaminophen has less risk for CV events compared with naproxen.

D. Acetaminophen has fewer antipyretic effects than naproxen.

> Correct answer = C. While acetaminophen inhibits prostaglandin synthesis via COX inhibition, it is inactivated peripherally so it is devoid of systemic GI, CV, and bleeding adverse effects which are hallmarks of NSAIDs like naproxen. However, as acetaminophen is active centrally, it is still able to maintain antipyretic effects similar to other NSAIDs.

38.3 Which statement correctly describes the proposed mechanism of cardioprotection from low-dose aspirin?

A. Aspirin preferentially inhibits COX-2 to lead to a relative reduction in thromboxane A_2 levels.

B. Aspirin preferentially inhibits COX-1 to lead to a relative reduction in thromboxane A_2 levels.

C. Aspirin preferentially inhibits COX-2 to lead to a relative reduction in prostacyclin levels.

D. Aspirin preferentially inhibits COX-1 to lead a relative reduction in prostacyclin levels.

> Correct answer = B. At low doses aspirin selectively inhibits COX-1, which reduces the production of thromboxane A_2, a substance that promotes vasoconstriction and platelet aggregation. COX-2 activity is thought to lead to relatively higher levels of prostacyclin which causes vasodilation and inhibits platelet aggregation. Selective COX-2 inhibitors, as well as all NSAIDs, may increase the risk for CV events by inhibiting the beneficial production of prostacyclin by COX-2, thereby leading to a relative imbalance of thromboxane A_2, and promoting platelet aggregation and vasoconstriction.

38.4 Which statement correctly describes the pathophysiologic actions of prostaglandins at a target tissue?

A. Promote vasoconstriction in the kidneys.
B. Promote sodium and water retention in the kidneys.
C. Decrease secretion of mucus at the lining of the stomach.
D. Decrease secretion of gastric acid in the stomach.

Correct answer = D. Prostaglandins, specifically PGE_2 and PGI_2, cause vasodilation in the renal arteries; a decrease in prostaglandins from NSAIDs can lead to vasoconstriction of renal arteries as well as sodium and water retention. In the stomach, PGI_2 inhibits gastric acid secretion, while PGE_2 and $PGF_{2\alpha}$ promote secretion of protective mucus at the stomach lining.

38.5 Which prostaglandin agent can be used to maintain the patency of the ductus arteriosus in neonates with congenital heart problems while awaiting surgery?

A. Misoprostol
B. Epoprostenol
C. Bimatoprost
D. Alprostadil

Correct answer = D. Misoprostol, a PGE_1 analog, is used for GI protection or labor induction. Epoprostenol, a PGI_2 analog, is used for the treatment of pulmonary arterial hypertension. Bimatoprost, a $PGF_{2\alpha}$ analog, is used topically in the eye for the treatment of open angle glaucoma or on the lashes for hypotrichosis. Alprostadil, a PGE_1 analog, is used to maintain patency of the ductus arteriosus in neonates with congenital heart problems. The drug can also be used for erectile dysfunction.

38.6 A 34-year-old woman with RA is planning for pregnancy. Which RA agents are absolutely contraindicated in pregnancy?

A. Abatacept and rituximab
B. Adalimumab and certolizumab
C. Infliximab and etanercept
D. Methotrexate and leflunomide

Correct answer = D. Both methotrexate and leflunomide are contraindicated in pregnancy. Data are limited in other RA agents to confirm or rule out teratogenicity in pregnancy. The risk of RA treatment on the developing fetus should be weighed against the benefits of improved RA symptoms with these therapies. Any adverse outcomes should be reported to the pregnancy registry.

38.7 Which agent for RA competes with CD28 to prevent full T-cell activation?

A. Sarilumab
B. Abatacept
C. Golimumab
D. Adalimumab

Correct answer = B. Abatacept is a costimulation modulator that competes with CD28 to prevent its binding on CD80/CD86 protein, resulting in reduced T-cell activation. Golimumab and adalimumab are both TNF-α inhibitors, and sarilumab is an IL-6 inhibitor.

38.8 Which statement correctly represents the mechanism of action of tofacitinib in the treatment of RA?

A. TNF-α inhibitor
B. Janus kinase inhibitor
C. IL-6 receptor blocker
D. Dihydrofolate reductase inhibitor

Correct answer = B. Tofacitinib is an inhibitor of Janus kinases 1, 3, and, to a lesser extent, 2. Methotrexate inhibits dihydrofolate reductase. Etanercept is an example of TNF-α inhibitor, and tocilizumab is an example of an IL-6 inhibitor.

38.9 A 54-year-old man with gout is found to have an issue with renal excretion of uric acid. Which drug is an oral agent that would target the cause of his acute gout attacks?

A. Allopurinol
B. Febuxostat
C. Probenecid
D. Pegloticase

Correct answer = C. Probenecid is a uricosuric agent that increases renal excretion by inhibiting the urate–anion exchanger in the proximal tubule, thereby blocking reabsorption of uric acid and facilitating its excretion. Allopurinol and febuxostat are xanthine oxidase inhibitors, which primarily act by decreasing uric acid production. Pegloticase works by increasing renal excretion of uric acid; however, it is an IV infusion.

38.10 A 64-year-old man presents with signs and symptoms of an acute gouty flare. Which strategy is the *least* likely to acutely improve his gout symptoms and pain?

A. Naproxen
B. Colchicine
C. Probenecid
D. Prednisone

Correct answer = C. Probenecid is a uricosuric agent indicated to lower serum urate levels to prevent gout attacks. It is not indicated during acute gout flares and should not be started until after the resolution of an acute attack. Naproxen, colchicine, and prednisone all represent viable treatment options that acutely reduce pain and inflammation associated with acute gout attacks.

Drugs for Disorders of the Respiratory System

Kyle Melin

39

I. OVERVIEW

Asthma, chronic obstructive pulmonary disease (COPD), and allergic rhinitis are commonly encountered respiratory disorders. Each of these conditions may be associated with a troublesome cough, which may be the only presenting complaint. Asthma is a chronic disease characterized by hyperresponsive airways that affects over 235 million patients worldwide. This disorder is underdiagnosed and undertreated, creating a substantial burden to individuals and families, and resulting in millions of emergency room visits. COPD is currently the fourth leading cause of death in the world, and is predicted to become the third leading cause of death by 2030. Allergic rhinitis is a common chronic disease and is characterized by itchy, watery eyes, runny nose, and a nonproductive cough that can significantly decrease quality of life. Each of these respiratory conditions may be managed with a combination of lifestyle changes and medications. Drugs used to treat respiratory conditions can be delivered topically to the nasal mucosa, inhaled into the lungs, or given orally or parenterally for systemic absorption. Local delivery methods, such as nasal sprays or inhalers, are preferred to target affected tissues while minimizing systemic adverse effects. Medications used to treat common respiratory disorders are summarized in Figure 39.1.

II. PREFERRED DRUGS USED TO TREAT ASTHMA

Asthma is a chronic inflammatory disease of the airways characterized by episodes of acute bronchoconstriction that cause shortness of breath, cough, chest tightness, wheezing, and rapid respiration.

A. Pathophysiology of asthma

Airflow obstruction in asthma is due to bronchoconstriction that results from contraction of bronchial smooth muscle, inflammation of the bronchial wall, and increased secretion of mucus (Figure 39.2). The underlying inflammation of the airways contributes to airway hyperresponsiveness, airflow limitation, respiratory symptoms, and disease

527

MEDICATION	INDICATION
SHORT-ACTING β₂ ADRENERGIC AGONISTS (SABAs)	
Albuterol PROAIR, PROVENTIL, VENTOLIN	Asthma, COPD
Levalbuterol XOPENEX	Asthma, COPD
LONG-ACTING β₂ ADRENERGIC AGONISTS (LABAs)	
Arformoterol BROVANA	COPD
Formoterol FORADIL, PERFOROMIST	Asthma, COPD
Indacaterol ARCAPTA	COPD
Olodaterol STRIVERDI RESPIMAT	COPD
Salmeterol SEREVENT	Asthma, COPD
INHALED CORTICOSTEROIDS	
Beclomethasone BECONASE AQ*, QVAR	Allergic rhinitis, Asthma, COPD
Budesonide PULMICORT, RHINOCORT*	Allergic rhinitis, Asthma, COPD
Ciclesonide ALVESCO, OMNARIS*, ZETONNA*	Allergic rhinitis, Asthma
Fluticasone FLONASE*, FLOVENT	Allergic rhinitis, Asthma, COPD
Mometasone ASMANEX, NASONEX*	Allergic rhinitis, Asthma
Triamcinolone NASACORT*	Allergic rhinitis, Asthma
LONG-ACTING β₂ ADRENERGIC AGONIST/CORTICOSTEROID COMBINATION	
Formoterol/budesonide SYMBICORT	Asthma, COPD
Formoterol/mometasone DULERA	Asthma, COPD
Salmeterol/fluticasone ADVAIR	Asthma, COPD
Vilanterol/fluticasone BREO ELLIPTA	COPD
SHORT-ACTING ANTICHOLINERGIC	
Ipratropium ATROVENT	Allergic rhinitis, Asthma, COPD
SHORT-ACTING β2 AGONIST/SHORT-ACTING ANTICHOLINERGIC COMBINATION	
Albuterol/ipratropium COMBIVENT RESPIMAT, DUONEB	COPD
LONG-ACTING ANTICHOLINERGIC (LAMA)	
Aclidinium TUDORZA PRESSAIR	COPD
Glycopyrrolate SEEBRI NEOHALER	COPD
Tiotropium SPIRIVA	Asthma, COPD
Umeclidinium INCRUSE ELLIPTA	COPD
LABA/LAMA COMBINATION	
Formoterol/glycopyrrolate BEVESPI AEROSPHERE	COPD
Indacaterol/glycopyrrolate UTIBRON NEOHALER	COPD
Vilanterol/umeclidinium ANORO ELLIPTA	COPD
Olodaterol/tiotropium STIOLTO RESPIMAT	COPD
LEUKOTRIENE MODIFIERS	
Montelukast SINGULAIR	Asthma, Allergic rhinitis
Zafirlukast ACCOLATE	Asthma
Zileuton ZYFLO CR	Asthma
ANTIHISTAMINES (H₁-RECEPTOR ANTAGONISTS)	
Azelastine ASTELIN*, ASTEPRO*	Allergic rhinitis
Cetirizine ZYRTEC	Allergic rhinitis
Desloratadine CLARINEX	Allergic rhinitis
Fexofenadine ALLEGRA	Allergic rhinitis
Loratadine CLARITIN	Allergic rhinitis
α-ADRENERGIC AGONISTS	
Oxymetazoline AFRIN, DRISTAN	Allergic rhinitis
Phenylephrine NEOSYNEPHRINE, SUDAFED PE	Allergic rhinitis
Pseudoephedrine SUDAFED	Allergic rhinitis
AGENTS FOR COUGH	
Benzonatate TESSALON PERLES	Cough suppressant
Codeine (with guaifenesin) VARIOUS	Cough suppressant/expectorant
Dextromethorphan VARIOUS	Cough suppressant
Dextromethorphan (with guaifenesin) VARIOUS	Cough suppressant/expectorant
Guaifenesin VARIOUS	Expectorant
OTHER AGENTS	
Benralizumab FASENRA	Asthma
Cromolyn NASALCROM*	Asthma, Allergic rhinitis
Mepolizumab NUCALA	Asthma
Omalizumab XOLAIR	Asthma
Reslizumab CINQAIR	Asthma
Roflumilast DALIRESP	COPD
Theophylline ELIXOPHYLLIN, THEO-24	Asthma, COPD

Figure 39.1
Summary of drugs affecting the respiratory system. *Indicates intranasal formulation. SABA = short-acting β₂ agonist; LABA = long-acting β₂ agonist; LAMA = long-acting muscarinic antagonist.

chronicity. Asthma attacks may be triggered by exposure to allergens, exercise, stress, and respiratory infections. Unlike COPD, cystic fibrosis, and bronchiectasis, asthma is usually not a progressive disease. However, if untreated, asthma may cause airway remodeling, resulting in increased severity and incidence of asthma exacerbations and/or death.

B. Goals of therapy

Drug therapy for long-term control of asthma is designed to reverse and prevent airway inflammation. The goals of asthma therapy are to decrease the intensity and frequency of asthma symptoms, prevent future exacerbations, and minimize limitations in activity related to asthma symptoms. First-line drug therapy based on classification of asthma is presented in Figure 39.3.

C. β_2-Adrenergic agonists

Inhaled β_2-adrenergic agonists directly relax airway smooth muscle. They are used for the quick relief of asthma symptoms, as well as adjunctive therapy for long-term control of the disease.

1. **Quick relief:** Short-acting β_2 agonists (SABAs) have a rapid onset of action (5 to 30 minutes) and provide relief for 4 to 6 hours. They are used for symptomatic treatment of bronchospasm, providing quick relief of acute bronchoconstriction. All patients with asthma should receive a SABA inhaler for use as needed. β_2 agonists have no anti-inflammatory effects, and they should not be used as monotherapy for patients with persistent asthma. However, monotherapy with SABAs may be appropriate for patients with mild, intermittent asthma or exercise-induced bronchospasm. Direct-acting β_2-selective agonists include *albuterol* [al-BYOO-ter-all] and *levalbuterol* [leh-val-BYOO-ter-all]. These agents provide significant bronchodilation with little of the undesired effect of α or β_1 stimulation (see Chapter 6). Adverse effects, such as tachycardia, hyperglycemia, hypokalemia, hypomagnesemia, and β_2-mediated skeletal muscle tremors are minimized with inhaled delivery versus systemic administration.

2. **Long-term control:** *Salmeterol* [sal-MEE-ter-all] and *formoterol* [for-MOE-ter-all] are long-acting β_2 agonists (LABAs) and chemical analogs of *albuterol*. *Salmeterol* and *formoterol* have a long duration of action, providing bronchodilation for at least 12 hours. Use of LABA monotherapy is contraindicated, and LABAs should be used only in combination with an asthma controller medication, such as an inhaled corticosteroid (ICS). ICS remain the long-term controllers of choice in asthma, and LABAs are considered to be useful adjunctive therapy for attaining control in moderate to severe asthma. Some LABAs are available as a combination product with an ICS (see Figure 39.1). Although both LABAs are usually used on a scheduled basis to control asthma, adults and adolescents with moderate persistent asthma can use the ICS/*formoterol* combination for relief of acute symptoms. Adverse effects of LABAs are similar to quick-acting β_2 agonists.

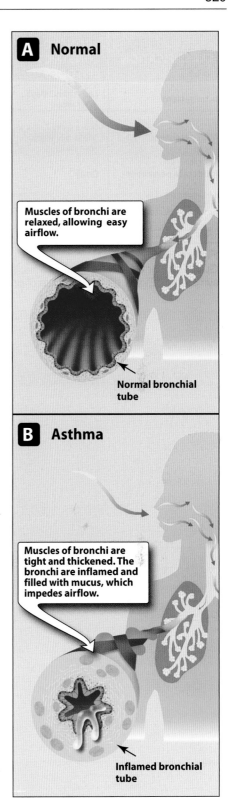

A Normal

Muscles of bronchi are relaxed, allowing easy airflow.

Normal bronchial tube

B Asthma

Muscles of bronchi are tight and thickened. The bronchi are inflamed and filled with mucus, which impedes airflow.

Inflamed bronchial tube

Figure 39.2
Comparison of bronchi of normal and asthmatic individuals.

CLASSIFICATION	BRONCHO-CONSTRICTIVE EPISODES	RESULTS OF PEAK FLOW OR SPIROMETRY	LONG-TERM CONTROL	QUICK RELIEF OF SYMPTOMS
Intermittent	Less than 2 days per week	Near normal*	No daily medication	Short-acting β₂ agonist
Mild persistent	More than 2 days per week, not daily	Near normal*	Low-dose ICS	Short-acting β₂ agonist
Moderate persistent	Daily	60%–80% of normal	Low-dose ICS + LABA OR Medium-dose ICS	Short-acting β₂ agonist ICS/*formoterol* is an alternative
Severe persistent	Continual	Less than 60% of normal	Medium-dose ICS + LABA OR High-dose ICS + LABA	Short-acting β₂ agonist ICS/*formoterol* is an alternative

Figure 39.3
Guidelines for the treatment of asthma. In all asthmatic patients, quick relief is provided by a SABA as needed for symptoms. *Eighty percent or more of predicted function. ICS = inhaled corticosteroid; LABA = long-acting β₂ agonist.

D. Corticosteroids

ICS are the drugs of choice for long-term control in patients with persistent asthma (Figure 39.3). Corticosteroids (see Chapter 26) inhibit the release of arachidonic acid through inhibition of phospholipase A_2, thereby producing direct anti-inflammatory properties in the airways (Figure 39.4). To be effective in controlling inflammation, these agents must be used regularly. Treatment of exacerbations or severe persistent asthma may require the addition of a short course of oral or intravenous corticosteroids.

1. **Actions on lung:** ICS therapy directly targets underlying airway inflammation by decreasing the inflammatory cascade (eosinophils, macrophages, and T lymphocytes), reversing mucosal edema, decreasing the permeability of capillaries, and inhibiting the release of leukotrienes. After several months of regular use, ICS reduce the hyperresponsiveness of the airway smooth muscle to a variety of bronchoconstrictor stimuli, such as allergens, irritants, cold air, and exercise.

2. **Routes of administration**

   a. **Inhalation:** The development of ICS has markedly reduced the need for systemic corticosteroid treatment to achieve control of asthma symptoms. However, as with all inhaled medications, appropriate inhalation technique is critical to the success of therapy (see section on Inhaler Technique).

   b. **Oral/systemic:** Patients with a severe exacerbation of asthma (status asthmaticus) may require intravenous *methylprednisolone* or oral *prednisone* to reduce airway inflammation. In most cases, suppression of the hypothalamic–pituitary–adrenal cortex axis does not occur during the oral *prednisone* "burst" (short course) typically prescribed for an asthma exacerbation. Thus, a dose taper is unnecessary prior to discontinuation.

3. **Adverse effects:** Oral or parenteral corticosteroids have a variety of potentially serious adverse effects (see Chapter 26), whereas ICS,

particularly if used with a spacer, have few systemic effects. ICS deposition on the oral and laryngeal mucosa can cause oropharyngeal candidiasis (due to local immune suppression) and hoarseness. Patients should be instructed to rinse the mouth in a "swish-and-spit" method with water following use of the inhaler to decrease the chance of these adverse events. Due to the potential for serious adverse effects, chronic maintenance with oral corticosteroids should be reserved for patients who are not controlled on an ICS.

III. ALTERNATIVE DRUGS USED TO TREAT ASTHMA

These drugs are useful for treatment of asthma in patients who are poorly controlled by conventional therapy or experience adverse effects secondary to corticosteroid treatment. These drugs should be used in conjunction with ICS therapy for most patients.

A. Leukotriene modifiers

Leukotrienes (LT) B_4 and the cysteinyl leukotrienes, LTC_4, LTD_4, and LTE_4, are products of the 5-lipoxygenase pathway of arachidonic acid metabolism and part of the inflammatory cascade. 5-Lipoxygenase is found in cells of myeloid origin, such as mast cells, basophils, eosinophils, and neutrophils. LTB_4 is a potent chemoattractant for neutrophils and eosinophils, whereas the cysteinyl leukotrienes constrict bronchiolar smooth muscle, increase endothelial permeability, and promote mucus secretion. *Zileuton* [zye-LOO-ton] is a selective and specific inhibitor of 5-lipoxygenase, preventing the formation of both LTB_4 and the cysteinyl leukotrienes. *Zafirlukast* [za-FIR-loo-kast] and *montelukast* [mon-te-LOO-kast] are selective antagonists of the cysteinyl leukotriene-1 receptor, and they block the effects of cysteinyl leukotrienes (Figure 39.4). These agents are approved for the prevention of asthma symptoms. They should not be used in situations where immediate bronchodilation is required. Leukotriene receptor antagonists have also shown efficacy for the prevention of exercise-induced bronchospasm.

1. **Pharmacokinetics:** These agents are orally active and highly protein bound. Food impairs the absorption of *zafirlukast*. The drugs undergo extensive hepatic metabolism. *Zileuton* and its metabolites are excreted in urine, whereas *zafirlukast*, *montelukast*, and their metabolites undergo biliary excretion.

2. **Adverse effects:** Elevations in serum hepatic enzymes may occur with these drugs, requiring periodic monitoring and discontinuation when enzymes exceed three to five times the upper limit of normal. Other effects include headache and dyspepsia. *Zafirlukast* is an inhibitor of cytochrome P450 (CYP) isoenzymes 2C8, 2C9, and 3A4, and *zileuton* inhibits CYP1A2. Coadministration with drugs that are substrates of these isoenzymes may result in increased effects and/or toxicity.

B. Cromolyn

Cromolyn [KRO-moe-lin] is a prophylactic anti-inflammatory agent that inhibits mast cell degranulation and release of histamine. It is an

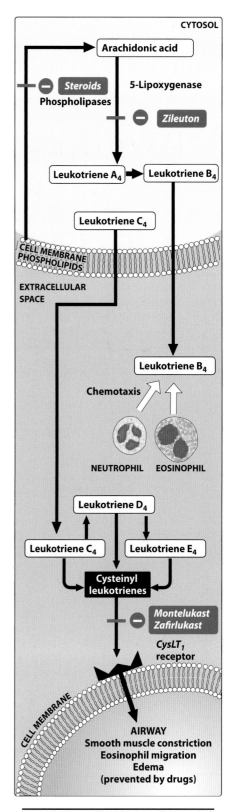

Figure 39.4
Sites of action for various respiratory medications. $CysLT_1$ = cysteinyl leukotriene-1.

alternative therapy for mild persistent asthma and is available as a nebulized solution. Because *cromolyn* is not a bronchodilator, it is not useful in managing an acute asthma attack. Due to its short duration of action, this agent requires dosing three or four times daily, which affects adherence and limits its use. Adverse effects are minor and include cough, irritation, and unpleasant taste.

C. Cholinergic antagonists

The anticholinergic agents block vagally mediated contraction of airway smooth muscle and mucus secretion (see Chapter 5). Inhaled *ipratropium* [IP-ra-TROE-pee-um], a short-acting quaternary derivative of *atropine*, is not recommended for the routine treatment of acute bronchospasm in asthma, as its onset is much slower than that of inhaled SABAs. However, it may be useful in patients who are unable to tolerate a SABA or patients with asthma–COPD overlap syndrome. *Ipratropium* also offers additional benefit when used with a SABA for the treatment of acute asthma exacerbations in the emergency department. *Tiotropium* [tye-oh-TROE-pee-um], a long-acting anticholinergic agent, can be used as an add-on treatment in adult patients with severe asthma and a history of exacerbations. Adverse effects such as xerostomia and bitter taste are related to local anticholinergic effects.

D. Theophylline

Theophylline [thee-OFF-i-lin] is a bronchodilator that relieves airflow obstruction in chronic asthma and decreases asthma symptoms. It may also possess anti-inflammatory activity, although the mechanism of action is unclear. Previously, the mainstay of asthma therapy, *theophylline* has been largely replaced with β_2 agonists and corticosteroids due to its narrow therapeutic window, adverse effect profile, and potential for drug interactions. Overdose may cause seizures or potentially fatal arrhythmias. *Theophylline* is metabolized in the liver and is a CYP1A2 and 3A4 substrate. It is subject to numerous drug interactions. Serum concentration monitoring should be performed when *theophylline* is used chronically.

E. Monoclonal antibodies

Omalizumab [OH-ma-LIZ-oo-mab] is a monoclonal antibody that selectively binds to human immunoglobulin E (IgE). This leads to decreased binding of IgE to its receptor on the surface of mast cells and basophils. Reduction in surface-bound IgE limits the release of mediators of the allergic response. The monoclonal antibodies *mepolizumab* [MEP-oh-LIZ-ue-mab], *benralizumab* [ben-ra-LIZ-ue-mab], and *reslizumab* [res-LIZ-ue-mab] are interleukin-5 (IL-5) antagonists. IL-5 is the major cytokine involved in recruitment, activation, and survival of eosinophils in eosinophilic asthma. These agents are indicated for the treatment of severe persistent asthma in patients who are poorly controlled with conventional therapy. Their use is limited by the high cost, route of administration (IV for *reslizumab* and subcutaneous for others), and adverse effect profile. Adverse effects include serious anaphylactic reactions (rare), arthralgias, fever, rash, and increased risk of infections. New malignancies have been reported.

IV. DRUGS USED TO TREAT CHRONIC OBSTRUCTIVE PULMONARY DISEASE

COPD is a chronic, irreversible obstruction of airflow that is usually progressive and characterized by persistent symptoms. These may include cough, excess mucus production, chest tightness, breathlessness, difficulty sleeping, and fatigue. Although symptoms are similar to asthma, the characteristic *irreversible* airflow obstruction of COPD is one of the most significant differences between the diseases. Smoking is the greatest risk factor for COPD and is directly linked to the progressive decline of lung function, as demonstrated by forced expiratory volume in one second (FEV_1). Smoking cessation should be recommended regardless of stage and severity of COPD, or the age of patient. Drug therapy for COPD is aimed at relief of symptoms and prevention of disease progression. Unfortunately, with currently available care, many patients still experience a decline in lung function over time.

A. Bronchodilators

Inhaled bronchodilators, including the β_2-adrenergic agonists and anticholinergic agents (muscarinic antagonists), are the foundation of therapy for COPD (Figure 39.5). These drugs increase airflow, alleviate symptoms, and decrease exacerbations. The long-acting bronchodilators, LABAs and long-acting muscarinic antagonists (LAMAs), are preferred as first-line treatment of COPD for all patients except those who are at low risk with less symptoms. LABAs include once-daily *indacaterol* [in-da-KA-ter-ol], *olodaterol* [OH-loe-DAT-er-ol], and *vilanterol* [vye-LAN-ter-ol], as well as the twice-daily inhaled formulations of *arformoterol*, *formoterol*, and *salmeterol*. *Aclidinium* [A-kli-DIN-ee-um], *tiotropium*, *glycopyrrolate* [GLYE-koe-PIR-oh-late], and *umeclidinium* [ue-ME-kli-DIN-ee-um]) are LAMAs. The combination

PATIENT GROUP	RECOMMENDED FIRST CHOICE	RECOMMENDED ESCALATION
A Low risk Fewer symptoms	**Bronchodilator:** **SABA** or **LABA** or **Short-acting anticholinergic** or **LAMA**	**Try alternative class**
B Low risk More symptoms	**Long acting bronchodilator:** **LABA** or **LAMA**	**LAMA + LABA**
C High risk Fewer symptoms	**LAMA**	**LAMA + LABA** or **LABA + ICS**
D High risk More symptoms	**LAMA + LABA**	**LAMA + LABA + ICS** (**May consider** *roflumilast* **if FEV$_1$ < 50% predicted and chronic bronchitis**)

Figure 39.5
Guidelines for the pharmacologic therapy of stable chronic obstructive pulmonary disease. FEV_1 = forced expiratory volume in 1 second; ICS = inhaled corticosteroid; LABA = long-acting β_2 agonist; LAMA = long-acting muscarinic antagonist; SABA = short-acting β_2 agonist.

of an anticholinergic and a β_2 agonist may be helpful in patients who have inadequate response to a single inhaled bronchodilator and are at risk of exacerbations.

B. Corticosteroids

The addition of an ICS to a long-acting bronchodilator may improve symptoms, lung function, and quality of life in COPD patients with FEV_1 of less than 60% predicted or patients with symptoms of both asthma and COPD. However, ICS treatment in COPD should be restricted to these patients, since use is associated with an increased risk of pneumonia. Although often used for acute exacerbations, oral corticosteroids are not recommended for long-term treatment of COPD.

C. Other agents

Roflumilast [roe-FLUE-mi-last] is an oral phosphodiesterase-4 inhibitor used to reduce exacerbations in patients with severe chronic bronchitis. Although its activity is not well defined in COPD, it is theorized to reduce inflammation by increasing levels of intracellular cAMP in lung cells. *Roflumilast* is not a bronchodilator and is not indicated for the relief of acute bronchospasm. Its use is limited by common adverse effects including weight loss, nausea, diarrhea, and headache. In COPD, the use of *theophylline* has largely been replaced by the more effective and tolerable long-acting bronchodilators.

V. INHALER TECHNIQUE

Appropriate inhaler technique differs between metered-dose inhalers (MDIs) and dry powder inhalers (DPIs). Proper technique is critical to the success of therapy, and inhaler technique should be assessed regularly.

A. Metered-dose inhalers and dry powder inhalers

MDIs have propellants that eject the active medication from the canister. Patients should be instructed to exhale before they actuate the inhaler, and then begin to inhale *slowly* as they press the canister and continue inhaling *slowly* and *deeply* throughout actuation. This technique avoids impaction of the medication onto the laryngeal mucosa and facilitates the drug reaching the site of action in the bronchial smooth muscle. A large fraction (typically 80% to 90%) of inhaled medication (for example, corticosteroids) is either deposited in the mouth and pharynx or swallowed (Figure 39.6). The remaining 10% to 20% of a dose of inhaled glucocorticoids that is not swallowed reaches the site of action in the airway. Use of appropriate technique with ICS reduces the risk of systemic absorption and adverse effects. DPIs require a different inhaler technique. Patients should be instructed to inhale *quickly* and *deeply* to optimize drug delivery to the lungs. Patients using any type of inhaled corticosteroid device should be instructed to rinse the mouth after use to prevent the development of oral candidiasis.

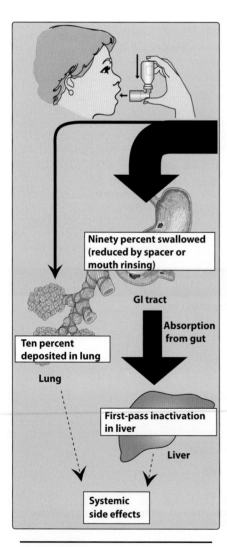

Ninety percent swallowed (reduced by spacer or mouth rinsing)

GI tract

Absorption from gut

Ten percent deposited in lung

Lung

First-pass inactivation in liver

Liver

Systemic side effects

Figure 39.6
Pharmacokinetics of inhaled glucocorticoids. GI = gastrointestinal.

B. Spacers

A spacer is a large-volume chamber attached to an MDI. The chamber reduces the velocity of the aerosol before entering the mouth, allowing large drug particles to be deposited in the device. The smaller, higher-velocity drug particles are less likely to be deposited in the mouth and more likely to reach the target airway tissue (Figure 39.7). Patients should be advised to wash and/or rinse spacers to reduce the risk of bacterial or fungal growth that may induce an asthma attack.

VI. DRUGS USED TO TREAT ALLERGIC RHINITIS

Rhinitis is an inflammation of the mucous membranes of the nose and is characterized by sneezing, itchy nose/eyes, watery rhinorrhea, nasal congestion, and sometimes a nonproductive cough. An attack may be precipitated by inhalation of an allergen (such as dust, pollen, or animal dander). The foreign material interacts with mast cells coated with IgE generated in response to a previous allergen exposure. The mast cells release mediators, such as histamine, leukotrienes, and chemotactic factors that promote bronchiolar spasm and mucosal thickening from edema and cellular infiltration. Antihistamines and/or intranasal corticosteroids are preferred therapies for allergic rhinitis.

A. Antihistamines

Oral antihistamines (H_1 receptor antagonists; see Chapter 37) have a fast onset of action and are useful for the management of symptoms of allergic rhinitis caused by histamine release, such as sneezing, watery rhinorrhea, and itchy eyes/nose. However, they are more effective for prevention of symptoms in mild or intermittent disease, rather than treatment once symptoms have begun. First-generation antihistamines, such as *diphenhydramine* and *chlorpheniramine*, are usually not preferred due to adverse effects, such as sedation, performance impairment, and other anticholinergic effects. The second-generation antihistamines (for example, *fexofenadine*, *loratadine*, *desloratadine*, *cetirizine*) are generally better tolerated. Ophthalmic and nasal antihistamine delivery devices are available for targeted, topical tissue delivery. Examples of topical intranasal antihistamines include *olopatadine* [OH-loe-PA-ta-deen] and *azelastine* [a-ZEL-uh-steen]. Intranasal antihistamines provide increased delivery of the drug with fewer adverse effects. Combinations of antihistamines with decongestants (see below) are effective when congestion is a feature of rhinitis, or when patients have no response or incomplete control of symptoms with intranasal corticosteroids.

B. Corticosteroids

Intranasal corticosteroids, such as *beclomethasone*, *budesonide*, *fluticasone*, *ciclesonide*, *mometasone*, and *triamcinolone*, are the most effective medications for treatment of allergic rhinitis. With an onset of action that ranges from 3 to 36 hours after first dose, intranasal corticosteroids improve sneezing, itching, rhinorrhea, and nasal congestion. Systemic absorption is minimal, and adverse effects of treatment are localized. These include nasal irritation, nosebleed,

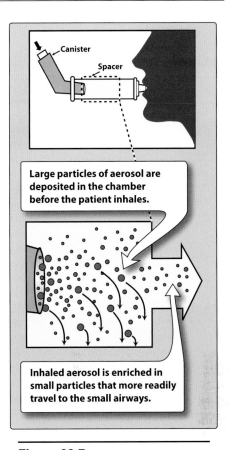

Figure 39.7
Effect of a spacer on the delivery of an inhaled aerosol.

sore throat, and, rarely, candidiasis. To minimize systemic absorption, patients should be instructed to avoid deep inhalation during administration into the nose, because the target tissue is the nose, not the lungs or the throat. For patients with chronic rhinitis, improvement may not be seen until 1 to 2 weeks after starting therapy.

C. α-Adrenergic agonists

Short-acting α-adrenergic agonists ("nasal decongestants"), such as *phenylephrine*, constrict dilated arterioles in the nasal mucosa and reduce airway resistance. Longer-acting *oxymetazoline* [OX-i-me-TAZ-oh-leen] is also available. When administered intranasally, these drugs have a rapid onset of action and show few systemic effects. However, intranasal formulations of α-adrenergic agonists should be used for no longer than 3 days due to the risk of rebound nasal congestion (rhinitis medicamentosa). For this reason, the α-adrenergic agents are not used in the long-term treatment of allergic rhinitis. Administration of oral α-adrenergic agonists results in a longer duration of action but also increased systemic effects, such as increased blood pressure and heart rate (see Chapter 6). As with intranasal formulations, regular use of oral α-adrenergic agonists (*phenylephrine* and *pseudoephedrine*) alone or in combination with antihistamines is not recommended.

D. Other agents

Intranasal *cromolyn* may be useful in allergic rhinitis, particularly when administered before contact with an allergen. To optimize the therapeutic effect, dosing should begin at least 1 to 2 weeks prior to allergen exposure. Although potentially inferior to other treatments, some leukotriene receptor antagonists are effective for allergic rhinitis as monotherapy or in combination with other agents. They may be a reasonable option in patients who also have asthma. An intranasal formulation of *ipratropium* is available to treat rhinorrhea associated with allergic rhinitis or the common cold. It does not relieve sneezing or nasal congestion.

VII. DRUGS USED TO TREAT COUGH

Coughing is an important defense mechanism of the respiratory system in response to irritants and is a common reason for patients to seek medical care. A troublesome cough may represent several etiologies, such as the common cold, sinusitis, or an underlying chronic respiratory disease. In some cases, cough may be an effective defense reflex against an underlying bacterial infection and should not be suppressed. Before treating cough, identification of its cause is important to ensure that antitussive treatment is appropriate. The priority should always be to treat the underlying cause of cough when possible.

A. Opioids

Codeine [KOE-deen], an opioid, decreases the sensitivity of cough centers in the central nervous system to peripheral stimuli and decreases mucosal secretion. These therapeutic effects occur at doses lower than those required for analgesia. However, common adverse effects, such as constipation, dysphoria, and fatigue, still occur. In addition, *codeine* has addictive potential, which limits its use, given increasing concerns with opioid addiction in the United States (see Chapter 14). *Dextromethorphan* [dex-troe-meth-OR-fan] is a synthetic derivative of *morphine* that has no analgesic effects in antitussive doses. It has a better adverse effect profile than does *codeine* and is equally effective for cough suppression. In low doses, *dextromethorphan* has a low addictive profile. However, it is also a potential drug of abuse, since it may cause dysphoria at high doses. *Guaifenesin* [gwye-FEN-e-sin], an expectorant, is available as a single-ingredient formulation and is commonly found in combination cough products with *codeine* or *dextromethorphan*.

B. Benzonatate

Unlike the opioids, *benzonatate* [ben-ZOE-na-tate] suppresses the cough reflex through peripheral action. It anesthetizes the stretch receptors located in the respiratory passages, lungs, and pleura. Adverse effects include dizziness, numbness of the tongue, mouth, and throat. These localized effects may be particularly problematic if the capsules are broken or chewed and the drug comes in direct contact with the oral mucosa.

Study Questions

Choose the ONE best answer.

39.1 A 12-year-old girl with asthma presents to the emergency room with complaints of cough, dyspnea, and wheezing after visiting a riding stable. Which is the most appropriate drug to rapidly reverse her bronchoconstriction?

A. Inhaled fluticasone
B. Inhaled beclomethasone
C. Inhaled albuterol
D. Intravenous propranolol

Correct answer = C. Inhalation of a rapid-acting β_2 agonist, such as albuterol, usually provides immediate bronchodilation. An acute asthmatic crisis often requires intravenous corticosteroids, such as methylprednisolone. Inhaled corticosteroids such as beclomethasone and fluticasone treat chronic airway inflammation but do not provide any immediate effect. Propranolol is a nonselective β-blocker and would aggravate the bronchoconstriction.

39.2 A 9-year-old girl has severe asthma that required three hospitalizations in the past year. She is now receiving therapy that has greatly reduced the frequency of severe attacks. Which drug is most likely responsible for this benefit?

A. Inhaled albuterol
B. Inhaled ipratropium
C. Inhaled fluticasone
D. Oral zafirlukast

Correct answer = C. Administration of an inhaled corticosteroid such as fluticasone significantly reduces the frequency of severe asthma attacks. This benefit is accomplished with minimal risk of the severe systemic adverse effects of oral corticosteroid therapy. The β_2 agonist albuterol is used to treat acute asthma symptoms. Ipratropium has more common use in COPD and sometimes in the acute management of acute asthma exacerbations. Zafirlukast may reduce the severity of attacks, but not to the same degree or consistency as fluticasone (or other corticosteroids).

39.3 A 68-year-old man has COPD with moderate airway obstruction. Despite using salmeterol twice daily, he reports continued symptoms of shortness of breath with mild exertion. Which agent is an appropriate addition to his current therapy?

A. Systemic corticosteroids
B. Albuterol
C. Tiotropium
D. Roflumilast

Correct answer = C. The addition of an anticholinergic bronchodilator to the LABA salmeterol would be appropriate and provide additional therapeutic benefit. Systemic corticosteroids are used to treat exacerbations in patients with COPD, but not recommended for chronic use. The addition of a SABA (albuterol) is less likely to provide additional benefit since the patient is already using medication with the same mechanism of action. Roflumilast is not indicated, since the patient only has moderate airway obstruction.

39.4 A 58-year-old woman with COPD has been hospitalized three times in the past year for COPD exacerbations. She reports only mild symptoms between exacerbations. Her regimen for the past year has included inhaled salmeterol twice daily and inhaled tiotropium once daily. Her current FEV$_1$ is below 60%. Which is an appropriate change in her drug therapy?

A. Discontinue the tiotropium.

B. Discontinue the salmeterol.

C. Change the salmeterol to a combination product that includes both a LABA and an inhaled corticosteroid (for example, salmeterol/fluticasone DPI).

D. Add theophylline.

Correct answer = C. The addition of an inhaled corticosteroid may provide additional benefit since the patient has significant airway obstruction and frequent exacerbations requiring hospitalization. It is not routinely recommended to discontinue a long-acting bronchodilator unless the patient experiences an adverse effect or experiences no therapeutic benefit. In this case, the patient reports mild symptoms in between exacerbations, suggesting she may benefit from both bronchodilators. Theophylline is an oral bronchodilator that is beneficial to some patients with stable COPD. However, because of its toxic potential, its use is not routinely recommended.

39.5 A 32-year-old man with a history of opioid addiction presents with cough due to a viral upper respiratory system infection. Which is appropriate symptomatic treatment for cough in this patient?

A. Guaifenesin/dextromethorphan

B. Guaifenesin/codeine

C. Benzonatate

D. Montelukast

Correct answer = C. Benzonatate suppresses the cough reflex through peripheral action and has no abuse potential. Dextromethorphan, an opioid derivative, and codeine, an opioid, both have abuse potential. Montelukast is not indicated for cough suppression.

39.6 Because of its anti-inflammatory mechanism of action, which drug requires regular administration for the treatment of asthma?

A. Tiotropium

B. Salmeterol

C. Mometasone

D. Albuterol

Correct answer = C. Inhaled corticosteroids have direct anti-inflammatory properties on the airways and require regular dosing to be effective. Tiotropium is used more frequently for the treatment of COPD. It does not have anti-inflammatory effects like the corticosteroids. Salmeterol and albuterol are both bronchodilators, but do not have anti-inflammatory properties.

39.7 Which agent is a preferred antihistamine for the management of allergic rhinitis?

A. Chlorpheniramine

B. Diphenhydramine

C. Phenylephrine

D. Cetirizine

Correct answer = D. Chlorpheniramine and diphenhydramine are first-generation antihistamines and are usually not a preferred treatment due to their increased risk of adverse effects, such as sedation, performance impairment, and other anticholinergic effects. Phenylephrine is short-acting α-adrenergic agonist ("nasal decongestant"). Cetirizine is a second-generation antihistamine and is generally better tolerated, making it a preferred agent for allergic rhinitis.

39.8 Which medication inhibits the action of 5-lipoxygenase and consequently the action of leukotriene B$_4$ and the cysteinyl leukotrienes?

A. Cromolyn

B. Zafirlukast

C. Zileuton

D. Montelukast

Correct answer = C. Zileuton is the only 5-lipoxygenase inhibitor available. While zafirlukast and montelukast both inhibit the effects of leukotrienes, they do so by blocking the receptor. Cromolyn inhibits mast cell degranulation and the release of histamine.

39.9 Which statement describes appropriate inhaler technique for a dry powder inhaler?

    A. Inhale slowly and deeply just before and throughout actuation of the inhaler.

    B. Use a large-volume chamber (spacer) to decrease deposition of drug in the mouth caused by improper inhaler technique.

    C. Inhale quickly and deeply to optimize drug delivery to the lungs.

    D. Rinse mouth in a "swish-and-spit" method with water prior to inhaler use to decrease the chance of adverse events.

> Correct answer = C. "Quick and deep" inhalation is required for effective use of a DPI. Inhaling "slowly and deeply" and the use of a spacer describe techniques associated with an MDI, not DPI. Rinsing the mouth may be appropriate for either type of inhaler if the medication being administered is an inhaled corticosteroid; however, this should always be done following inhaler use, not prior to use.

39.10 Which category of allergic rhinitis medications is most likely to be associated with rhinitis medicamentosa (rebound nasal congestion) with prolonged use?

    A. Intranasal corticosteroid

    B. Intranasal decongestant

    C. Leukotriene antagonist

    D. Oral antihistamine

> Correct answer = B. Intranasal decongestants should be used no longer than 3 days due to the risk of rebound nasal congestion (rhinitis medicamentosa). For this reason, the α-adrenergic agents should not be used in the long-term treatment of allergic rhinitis. The other agents may be used as chronic therapies.

Gastrointestinal and Antiemetic Drugs

40

Carol Motycka and Adonice Khoury

I. OVERVIEW

This chapter describes drugs used to treat six common medical conditions involving the gastrointestinal (GI) tract: 1) peptic ulcers and gastroesophageal reflux disease (GERD), 2) chemotherapy-induced emesis, 3) diarrhea, 4) constipation, 5) irritable bowel syndrome (IBS), and 6) and inflammatory bowel disease (IBD). Many drugs described in other chapters also find application in the treatment of GI disorders. For example, the *meperidine* derivative *diphenoxylate*, which decreases peristaltic activity of the gut, is useful in the treatment of severe diarrhea. Other drugs are used almost exclusively to treat GI tract disorders. For example, H_2 receptor antagonists and proton pump inhibitors (PPIs) are used to heal peptic ulcers.

II. DRUGS USED TO TREAT PEPTIC ULCER DISEASE AND GASTROESOPHAGEAL REFLUX DISEASE

The two main causes of peptic ulcer disease are infection with gram-negative <u>Helicobacter pylori</u> and the use of nonsteroidal anti-inflammatory drugs (NSAIDs). Increased hydrochloric acid (HCl) secretion and inadequate mucosal defense against gastric acid also play a role. Treatment approaches include 1) eradicating the <u>H. pylori</u> infection, 2) reducing secretion of gastric acid with the use of PPIs or H_2 receptor antagonists, and/or 3) providing agents that protect the gastric mucosa from damage, such as *misoprostol* and *sucralfate*. Figure 40.1 summarizes agents that are effective in treating peptic ulcer disease.

A. Antimicrobial agents

Patients with peptic ulcer disease (duodenal or gastric ulcers) who are infected with <u>H</u>. pylori require antimicrobial treatment. Infection with <u>H</u>. pylori is diagnosed via endoscopic biopsy of the gastric mucosa or various noninvasive methods, including serology, fecal antigen tests, and urea breath tests (Figure 40.2). Figure 40.3 shows a biopsy sample in which <u>H</u>. pylori is discovered on the gastric mucosa. Eradication of <u>H</u>. pylori with various combinations of antimicrobial drugs results in rapid healing of active ulcers and low recurrence rates (less than 15%, compared with 60% to 100% per year for ulcers healed with

ANTIMICROBIAL AGENTS
Amoxicillin GENERIC ONLY
Bismuth compounds PEPTO-BISMOL, KAOPECTATE
Clarithromycin BIAXIN
Metronidazole FLAGYL
Tetracycline GENERIC ONLY

H_2 – HISTAMINE RECEPTOR BLOCKERS
Cimetidine TAGAMET
Famotidine PEPCID
Nizatidine AXID
Ranitidine ZANTAC

PROTON PUMP INHIBITORS
Dexlansoprazole DEXILANT
Esomeprazole NEXIUM
Lansoprazole PREVACID
Omeprazole PRILOSEC
Pantoprazole PROTONIX
Rabeprazole ACIPHEX

PROSTAGLANDINS
Misoprostol CYTOTEC

ANTIMUSCARINIC AGENTS
Dicyclomine BENTYL

ANTACIDS
Aluminum hydroxide GENERIC ONLY
Calcium carbonate TUMS
Magnesium hydroxide MILK OF MAGNESIA
Sodium bicarbonate ALKA-SELTZER

MUCOSAL PROTECTIVE AGENTS
Bismuth subsalicylate PEPTO-BISMOL
Sucralfate CARAFATE

Figure 40.1
Summary of drugs used to treat peptic ulcer disease.

acid-reducing therapy alone). Currently, quadruple therapy of *bismuth subsalicylate*, *metronidazole*, and *tetracycline* plus a PPI is a recommended first-line option. This usually results in a 90% or greater eradication rate. Triple therapy consisting of a PPI combined with *amoxicillin* (*metronidazole* may be used in *penicillin*-allergic patients) plus *clarithromycin* is a preferred treatment when rates of *clarithromycin* resistance are low and the patient has no prior exposure to macrolide antibiotics.

B. H₂ receptor antagonists

Gastric acid secretion is stimulated by acetylcholine, histamine, and gastrin (Figure 40.4). The receptor-mediated binding of acetylcholine, histamine, or gastrin results in the activation of protein kinases, which in turn stimulates the H^+/K^+-adenosine triphosphatase (ATPase) proton pump to secrete hydrogen ions in exchange for K^+ into the lumen of the stomach. By competitively blocking the binding of histamine to H_2 receptors, these agents reduce the secretion of gastric acid. The four drugs used in the United States—*cimetidine* [si-MET-ih-deen], *famotidine* [fa-MOE-ti-deen], *nizatidine* [nye-ZA-ti-deen], and *ranitidine* [ra-NI-ti-deen]—inhibit basal, food-stimulated, and nocturnal secretion of gastric acid, reducing acid secretion by approximately 70%. *Cimetidine* was the first H_2 receptor antagonist. However, its utility is limited by its adverse effect profile and drug–drug interactions.

1. **Actions:** The histamine H_2 receptor antagonists act selectively on H_2 receptors in the stomach, without effects on H_1 receptors. They are competitive antagonists of histamine and are fully reversible.

2. **Therapeutic uses:** The use of these agents has decreased with the advent of PPIs.

    a. **Peptic ulcers:** All four agents are equally effective in promoting the healing of duodenal and gastric ulcers. However, recurrence is common if <u>H</u>. <u>pylori</u> is present and the patient is treated with these agents alone. Patients with NSAID-induced ulcers should be treated with PPIs, because these agents heal and prevent future ulcers more effectively than do H_2 receptor antagonists.

    b. **Acute stress ulcers:** These drugs are given as an intravenous infusion to prevent and manage acute stress ulcers associated with high-risk patients in the intensive care setting. However, because tolerance may occur with these agents, PPIs are also used for this indication.

    c. **Gastroesophageal reflux disease:** H_2 receptor antagonists are effective for the treatment of heartburn or GERD. H_2 receptor antagonists act by decreasing acid secretion; therefore, they may not relieve symptoms of heartburn for up to 45 minutes. Antacids more quickly and efficiently neutralize stomach acid, but their action is short lived. For these reasons, PPIs are now used preferentially in the treatment of GERD, especially for patients with severe and frequent heartburn.

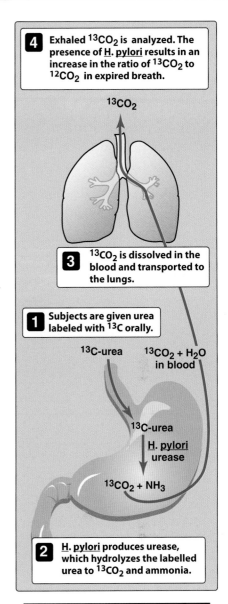

Figure 40.2
Urea breath test, one of several noninvasive methods for detecting presence of <u>Helicobacter</u> <u>pylori</u>.

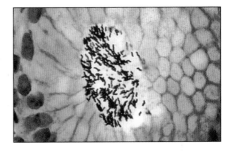

Figure 40.3
<u>Helicobacter</u> <u>pylori</u> in association with gastric mucosa.

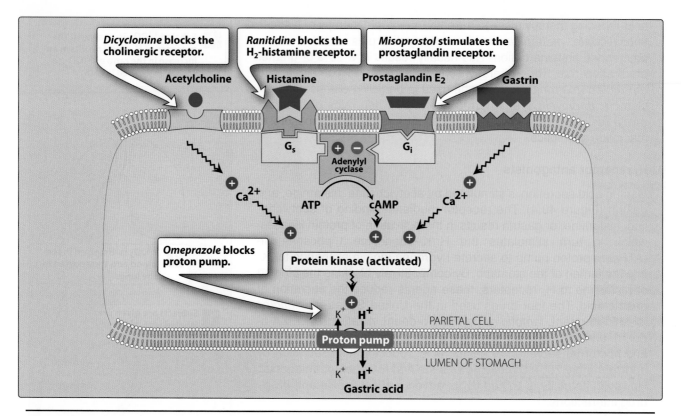

Figure 40.4
Effects of acetylcholine, histamine, prostaglandin E_2, and gastrin on gastric acid secretion by the parietal cells of stomach. G_s and G_i are membrane proteins that mediate the stimulatory or inhibitory effect of receptor coupling to adenylyl cyclase.

3. **Pharmacokinetics:** After oral administration, the H_2 receptor antagonists distribute widely throughout the body (including into breast milk and across the placenta) and are excreted mainly in the urine. *Cimetidine, ranitidine,* and *famotidine* are also available in intravenous formulations. The half-life of these agents may be increased in patients with renal dysfunction, and dosage adjustments are needed.

4. **Adverse effects:** In general, the H_2 receptor antagonists are well tolerated. However, *cimetidine* can have endocrine effects, such as gynecomastia and galactorrhea (continuous release/discharge of milk), because it acts as a nonsteroidal antiandrogen. Other central nervous system effects such as confusion and altered mentation occur primarily in elderly patients and after intravenous administration. H_2 receptor antagonists may reduce the efficacy of drugs that require an acidic environment for absorption, such as *ketoconazole. Cimetidine* inhibits several cytochrome P450 isoenzymes and can interfere with the metabolism of many drugs, such as *warfarin, phenytoin,* and *clopidogrel* (Figure 40.5).

C. Inhibitors of the H+/K+-ATPase proton pump

The PPIs bind to the H+/K+-ATPase enzyme system (proton pump) and suppress the secretion of hydrogen ions into the gastric lumen. The membrane-bound proton pump is the final step in the secretion of gastric acid (Figure 40.4). The available PPIs include *dexlansoprazole*

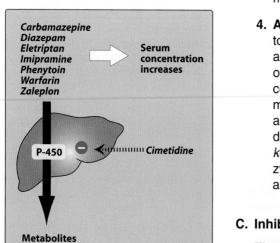

Figure 40.5
Drug interactions with *cimetidine.*

[DEX-lan-SO-pra-zole], *esomeprazole* [es-oh-MEH-pra-zole], *lansoprazole* [lan-SO-pra-zole], *omeprazole* [oh-MEH-pra-zole], *pantoprazole* [pan-TOE-pra-zole], and *rabeprazole* [rah-BEH-pra-zole].

1. **Actions:** These agents are prodrugs with an acid-resistant enteric coating to protect them from premature degradation by gastric acid. The coating is removed in the alkaline duodenum, and the prodrug, a weak base, is absorbed and transported to the parietal cell. There, it is converted to the active drug and forms a stable covalent bond with the H⁺/K⁺-ATPase enzyme. It takes about 18 hours for the enzyme to be resynthesized, and acid secretion is inhibited during this time. At standard doses, PPIs inhibit both basal and stimulated gastric acid secretion by more than 90%. An oral product containing *omeprazole* combined with *sodium bicarbonate* for faster absorption is also available.

2. **Therapeutic uses:** The PPIs are superior to the H₂ antagonists in suppressing acid production and healing ulcers. Thus, they are the preferred drugs for the treatment of GERD, erosive esophagitis, active duodenal ulcer, and pathologic hypersecretory conditions such as Zollinger-Ellison syndrome. PPIs reduce the risk of bleeding from ulcers caused by *aspirin* and other NSAIDs and may be used for prevention or treatment of NSAID-induced ulcers. PPIs are also used for stress ulcer prophylaxis and management. Finally, PPIs are combined with antimicrobial regimens used to eradicate H. pylori.

3. **Pharmacokinetics:** These agents are effective orally. For maximum effect, PPIs should be taken 30 to 60 minutes before breakfast or the largest meal of the day. [Note: *Dexlansoprazole* has a dual delayed-release formulation and can be taken without regard to food.] *Esomeprazole*, *lansoprazole*, and *pantoprazole* are available in intravenous formulations. Although the plasma half-life of these agents is only a few hours, they have a long duration of action due to covalent bonding with the H⁺/K⁺-ATPase enzyme. Metabolites of these agents are excreted in urine and feces.

4. **Adverse effects:** The PPIs are generally well tolerated. *Omeprazole* and *esomeprazole* may decrease the effectiveness of *clopidogrel* because they inhibit CYP2C19 and prevent the conversion of *clopidogrel* to its active metabolite. Concomitant use of these PPIs with *clopidogrel* is not recommended. PPIs may increase the risk of fractures, particularly if the duration of use is 1 year or greater (Figure 40.6). Prolonged acid suppression with PPIs (and H₂ receptor antagonists) may result in low vitamin B₁₂ because acid is required for its absorption in a complex with intrinsic factor. Elevated gastric pH may also impair the absorption of *calcium carbonate*. *Calcium citrate* is an effective option for calcium supplementation in patients on acid suppressive therapy, since absorption of the citrate salt is not affected by gastric pH. Diarrhea and Clostridium difficile colitis may occur in patients receiving PPIs. Patients must be counseled to discontinue PPI therapy and contact their physician if they have diarrhea for several days. Additional adverse effects may include hypomagnesemia and an increased incidence of pneumonia.

Nausea

Diarrhea

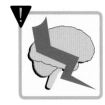
Headache

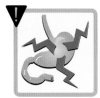
GI disturbance

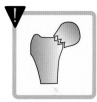
Bone Fractures (increased risk with long-term use: hip, wrist, and spine)

Figure 40.6
Some adverse effects of proton pump therapy. GI = gastrointestinal.

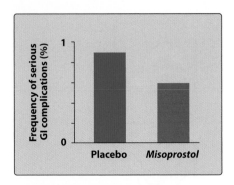

Figure 40.7
Misoprostol reduces serious gastrointestinal (GI) complications in patients with rheumatoid arthritis receiving NSAIDs.

D. Prostaglandins

Prostaglandin E, produced by the gastric mucosa, inhibits secretion of acid and stimulates secretion of mucus and bicarbonate (cytoprotective effect). A deficiency of prostaglandins is thought to be involved in the pathogenesis of peptic ulcers. *Misoprostol* [mye-soe-PROST-ole], an analog of prostaglandin E_1, is approved for the prevention of NSAID-induced gastric ulcers (Figure 40.7). Prophylactic use of *misoprostol* should be considered in patients who take NSAIDs and are at moderate to high risk of NSAID-induced ulcers, such as elderly patients and those with previous ulcers. *Misoprostol* is contraindicated in pregnancy, since it can stimulate uterine contractions and cause miscarriage. Dose-related diarrhea is the most common adverse effect and limits the use of this agent. Thus, PPIs are preferred agents for the prevention of NSAID-induced ulcers.

E. Antacids

Antacids are weak bases that react with gastric acid to form water and a salt to diminish gastric acidity. Because pepsin (a proteolytic enzyme) is inactive at a pH greater than 4, antacids also reduce pepsin activity.

1. **Chemistry:** Antacid products vary widely in their chemical composition, acid-neutralizing capacity, sodium content, and palatability. The efficacy of an antacid depends on its capacity to neutralize gastric HCl and on whether the stomach is full or empty. Food delays stomach emptying, allowing more time for the antacid to react and prolonging the duration of action. Commonly used antacids are combinations of salts of aluminum and magnesium, such as *aluminum hydroxide* and *magnesium hydroxide* [$Mg(OH)_2$]. *Calcium carbonate* [$CaCO_3$] reacts with HCl to form CO_2 and $CaCl_2$ and is also a commonly used preparation. Systemic absorption of *sodium bicarbonate* [$NaHCO_3$] can produce transient metabolic alkalosis and produce a significant sodium load. Therefore, this antacid is not recommended.

2. **Therapeutic uses:** Antacids are used for symptomatic relief of peptic ulcer disease, heartburn, and GERD. They should be administered after meals for maximum effectiveness. [Note: *Calcium carbonate* preparations are also used as calcium supplements for the prevention of osteoporosis.]

3. **Adverse effects:** *Aluminum hydroxide* tends to cause constipation, whereas *magnesium hydroxide* tends to produce diarrhea. Preparations that combine these agents aid in normalizing bowel function. Absorption of the cations from antacids (Mg^{2+}, Al^{3+}, Ca^{2+}) is usually not a problem in patients with normal renal function; however, accumulation and adverse effects may occur in patients with renal impairment.

F. Mucosal protective agents

Also known as cytoprotective compounds, these agents have several actions that enhance mucosal protection mechanisms, thereby preventing mucosal injury, reducing inflammation, and healing existing ulcers.

1. **Sucralfate:** This complex of *aluminum hydroxide* and sulfated sucrose binds to positively charged groups in proteins of both normal and necrotic mucosa. By forming complex gels with epithelial cells, *sucralfate* [soo-KRAL-fate] creates a physical barrier that protects the ulcer from pepsin and acid, allowing the ulcer to heal. Although *sucralfate* is effective for the treatment of duodenal ulcers and prevention of stress ulcers, its use is limited due to the need for multiple daily dosing, drug–drug interactions, and availability of more effective agents. Because it requires an acidic pH for activation, *sucralfate* should not be administered with PPIs, H_2 antagonists, or antacids. *Sucralfate* is well tolerated, but it can bind to other drugs and interfere with their absorption.

2. **Bismuth subsalicylate:** This agent is used as a component of quadruple therapy to heal H. pylori-related peptic ulcers. In addition to its antimicrobial actions, it inhibits the activity of pepsin, increases secretion of mucus, and interacts with glycoproteins in necrotic mucosal tissue to coat and protect the ulcer.

III. DRUGS USED TO CONTROL CHEMOTHERAPY-INDUCED NAUSEA AND VOMITING

Although nausea and vomiting occur in a variety of conditions (for example, motion sickness, pregnancy, and GI illnesses) and are always unpleasant for the patient, the nausea and vomiting produced by chemotherapeutic agents demands especially effective management. Nearly 70% to 80% of patients who undergo chemotherapy experience nausea and/or vomiting. Several factors influence the incidence and severity of chemotherapy-induced nausea and vomiting (CINV), including the specific chemotherapeutic drug (Figure 40.8); the dose, route, and schedule of administration; and patient variables. For example, young patients and women are more susceptible than older patients and men, and 10% to 40% of patients experience nausea and/or vomiting in anticipation of chemotherapy (anticipatory vomiting). CINV not only affects quality of life but can also lead to rejection of potentially curative chemotherapy. In addition, uncontrolled vomiting can produce dehydration, profound metabolic imbalances, and nutrient depletion.

A. Mechanisms that trigger vomiting

Two brainstem sites have key roles in the vomiting reflex pathway. The chemoreceptor trigger zone (CTZ) is located in the area postrema (a circumventricular structure at the caudal end of the fourth ventricle). It is outside the blood–brain barrier. Thus, it can respond directly to chemical stimuli in the blood or cerebrospinal fluid. The second important site, the vomiting center, which is located in the lateral reticular formation of the medulla, coordinates the motor mechanisms of vomiting. The vomiting center also responds to afferent input from the vestibular system, the periphery (pharynx and GI tract), and higher brainstem and cortical structures. The vestibular system functions mainly in motion sickness.

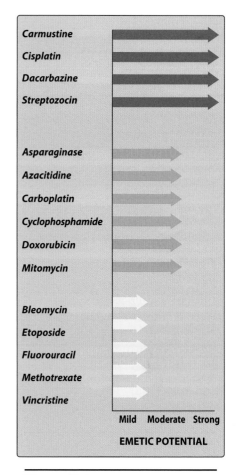

Figure 40.8
Comparison of emetic potential of anticancer drugs.

PHENOTHIAZINES

Prochlorperazine GENERIC ONLY

5-HT₃ SEROTONIN RECEPTOR ANTAGONISTS

Dolasetron ANZEMET

Granisetron SANCUSO, SUSTOL

Ondansetron ZOFRAN

Palonosetron ALOXI

SUBSTITUTED BENZAMIDES

Metoclopramide REGLAN

BUTYROPHENONES

Droperidol GENERIC ONLY

Haloperidol HALDOL

BENZODIAZEPINES

Alprazolam XANAX

Lorazepam ATIVAN

CORTICOSTEROIDS

Dexamethasone DECADRON

Methylprednisolone MEDROL

SUBSTANCE P/NEUROKININ-1 RECEPTOR ANTAGONIST

Aprepitant, Fosaprepitant EMEND

Netupitant* AKYNZEO

Rolapitant VARUBI

Figure 40.9
Summary of drugs used to treat CINV. *In combination with *palonosetron*.

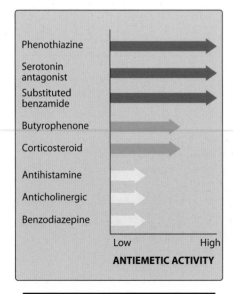

Figure 40.10
Efficacy of antiemetic drugs.

B. Emetic actions of chemotherapeutic agents

Chemotherapeutic agents can directly activate the medullary CTZ or vomiting center. Several neuroreceptors, including dopamine receptor type 2 and serotonin type 3 (5-HT₃), play critical roles. Often, the color or smell of chemotherapeutic drugs (and even stimuli associated with chemotherapy) can activate higher brain centers and trigger emesis. Chemotherapeutic drugs can also act peripherally by causing cell damage in the GI tract and by releasing serotonin from the enterochromaffin cells of the small intestine. Serotonin activates 5-HT₃ receptors on vagal and splanchnic afferent fibers, which then carry sensory signals to the medulla, leading to the emetic response.

C. Antiemetic drugs

Considering the complexity of the mechanisms involved in emesis, it is not surprising that antiemetics represent a variety of classes (Figure 40.9) and offer a range of efficacies (Figure 40.10). Anticholinergic drugs, especially the muscarinic receptor antagonist *scopolamine* and H₁-receptor antagonists, such as *dimenhydrinate*, *meclizine*, and *cyclizine*, are very useful in motion sickness but are ineffective against substances that act directly on the CTZ. The major categories of drugs used to control CINV include the following:

1. **Phenothiazines:** Phenothiazines, such as *prochlorperazine* [proe-klor-PER-ah-zeen], act by blocking dopamine receptors in the CTZ. *Prochlorperazine* is effective against low or moderately emetogenic chemotherapeutic agents (for example, *fluorouracil* and *doxorubicin*). Although increasing the dose improves antiemetic activity, adverse effects are dose limiting.

2. **5-HT₃ receptor blockers:** The 5-HT₃ receptor antagonists include *dolasetron* [dol-A-seh-tron], *granisetron* [gra-NI-seh-tron], *ondansetron* [on-DAN-seh-tron], and *palonosetron* [pa-low-NO-seh-tron]. These agents selectively block 5-HT₃ receptors in the periphery (visceral vagal afferent fibers) and in the CTZ. This class of agents is important in treating CINV, because of their superior efficacy and longer duration of action. These drugs can be administered as a single dose prior to chemotherapy (intravenously or orally) and are efficacious against all grades of emetogenic therapy. *Ondansetron* and *granisetron* prevent emesis in 50% to 60% of *cisplatin*-treated patients. These agents are also useful in the management of postoperative nausea and vomiting. 5-HT₃ antagonists are extensively metabolized by the liver; however, only *ondansetron* requires dosage adjustments in hepatic insufficiency. Excretion is via the urine. QT prolongation can occur with high doses of *ondansetron* and *dolasetron*. For this reason, the indication for CINV prophylaxis was withdrawn for intravenous *dolasetron*.

3. **Substituted benzamides:** One of several substituted benzamides with antiemetic activity, *metoclopramide* [met-oh-kloe-PRAH-mide], is effective at high doses against the emetogenic *cisplatin*, preventing emesis in 30% to 40% of patients and reducing emesis in the majority of patients. *Metoclopramide* accomplishes this through inhibition of dopamine in the CTZ. Antidopaminergic adverse effects, including extrapyramidal symptoms, limit long-

term high-dose use. *Metoclopramide* enhances gastric motility and is useful for patients with gastroparesis.

4. **Butyrophenones:** *Droperidol* [droe-PER-i-doll] and *haloperidol* [hal-oh-PER-i-doll] act by blocking dopamine receptors. The butyrophenones are moderately effective antiemetics. *Droperidol* had been used most often for sedation in endoscopy and surgery, usually in combination with opioids or benzodiazepines. However, it may prolong the QT_c interval and should be reserved for patients with inadequate response to other agents.

5. **Benzodiazepines:** The antiemetic potency of *lorazepam* [lor-A-ze-pam] and *alprazolam* [al-PRAH-zoe-lam] is low. Their beneficial effects may be due to their sedative, anxiolytic, and amnestic properties (see Chapter 9). These properties make benzodiazepines useful in treating anticipatory vomiting. Concomitant use of alcohol should be avoided due to additive CNS depressant effects.

6. **Corticosteroids:** *Dexamethasone* [dex-a-MEH-tha-sone] and *methylprednisolone* [meth-ill-pred-NIH-so-lone], used alone, are effective against mildly to moderately emetogenic chemotherapy. Most frequently, they are used in combination with other agents. Their antiemetic mechanism is not known, but it may involve blockade of prostaglandins.

7. **Substance P/neurokinin-1 receptor antagonists:** *Aprepitant* [ah-PRE-pih-tant], *netupitant* [net-UE-pi-tant], and *rolapitant* [roe-LA-pi-tant] target the neurokinin receptor in the vomiting center and block the actions of substance P. [Note: *Fosaprepitant* is a prodrug of *aprepitant* that is administered intravenously.] These oral agents are indicated for highly or moderately emetogenic chemotherapy regimens, and they are usually administered with *dexamethasone* and a 5-HT$_3$ antagonist. Unlike most 5-HT$_3$ antagonists, these agents are effective for the delayed phase of CINV, which occurs 24 hours or more after chemotherapy. *Aprepitant* and *rolapitant* undergo hepatic metabolism, primarily by CYP3A4. Coadministration with strong inhibitors or inducers of CYP3A4 (for example, *clarithromycin* or *St. John's wort*, respectively) should be avoided. *Aprepitant* is an inducer of CYP3A4 and CYP2C9, and it also exhibits dose-dependent inhibition of CYP3A4. Therefore, it may affect the metabolism of other drugs that are substrates of these isoenzymes and is subject to numerous drug interactions. *Rolapitant* is a moderate inhibitor of CYP2D6. Fatigue, diarrhea, abdominal pain, and hiccups are adverse effects of this class.

8. **Combination regimens:** Antiemetic drugs are often combined to increase efficacy or decrease toxicity (Figure 40.11). Corticosteroids, most commonly *dexamethasone*, increase antiemetic activity when given with high-dose *metoclopramide*, a 5-HT$_3$ antagonist, phenothiazine, butyrophenone, or a benzodiazepine. Antihistamines, such as *diphenhydramine*, are often administered in combination with high-dose *metoclopramide* to reduce extrapyramidal reactions or with corticosteroids to counter *metoclopramide*-induced diarrhea. Addition of a substance P/neurokinin-1 receptor antagonist to a 5-HT$_3$ antagonist and *dexamethasone* is beneficial in highly emetogenic regimens, especially those with delayed CINV.

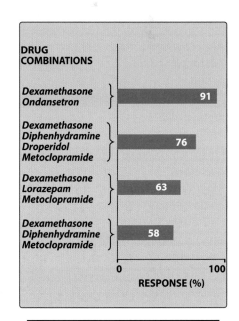

Figure 40.11
Effectiveness of antiemetic activity of some drug combinations against emetic episodes in the first 24 hours after *cisplatin* chemotherapy.

ANTIMOTILITY AGENTS

Diphenoxylate + atropine LOMOTIL

Loperamide IMODIUM A-D

ADSORBENTS

Aluminum hydroxide GENERIC ONLY

Methylcellulose CITRUCEL

AGENTS THAT MODIFY FLUID AND ELECTROLYTE TRANSPORT

Bismuth subsalicylate PEPTO-BISMOL

Figure 40.12
Summary of drugs used to treat diarrhea.

IV. ANTIDIARRHEALS

Increased motility of the GI tract and decreased absorption of fluid are major factors in diarrhea. Antidiarrheal drugs include antimotility agents, adsorbents, and drugs that modify fluid and electrolyte transport (Figure 40.12).

A. Antimotility agents

Two drugs that are widely used to control diarrhea are *diphenoxylate* [dye-fen-OKS-i-late] and *loperamide* [loe-PER-ah-mide]. Both are analogs of *meperidine* and have opioid-like actions on the gut. They activate presynaptic opioid receptors in the enteric nervous system to inhibit acetylcholine release and decrease peristalsis. At the usual doses, they lack analgesic effects. *Loperamide* is used for the general treatment of acute diarrhea, including traveler's diarrhea. Because these drugs can contribute to toxic megacolon, they should not be used in young children or in patients with severe colitis.

B. Adsorbents

Adsorbent agents, such as *aluminum hydroxide* and *methylcellulose* [METH-il-SEL-yoo-los], are used to control diarrhea. Presumably, these agents act by adsorbing intestinal toxins or microorganisms and/or by coating or protecting the intestinal mucosa. They are much less effective than antimotility agents, and they can interfere with the absorption of other drugs.

C. Agents that modify fluid and electrolyte transport

Bismuth subsalicylate, used for prevention and treatment of traveler's diarrhea, decreases fluid secretion in the bowel. Its action may be due to its salicylate component as well as its coating action. Adverse effects may include black tongue and black stools.

IRRITANTS and STIMULANTS

Bisacodyl CORRECTOL, DULCOLAX

Castor oil GENERIC ONLY

Senna EX-LAX, SENOKOT

BULK LAXATIVES

Methylcellulose CITRUCEL

Psyllium METAMUCIL

SALINE and OSMOTIC LAXATIVES

Lactulose CONSTULOSE, ENULOSE

Magnesium citrate CITROMA

Magnesium hydroxide MILK OF MAGNESIA

Polyethylene glycol GOLYTELY, MIRALAX

STOOL SOFTENERS

Docusate COLACE

LUBRICANT LAXATIVES

Glycerin suppositories GENERIC ONLY

Mineral oil GENERIC ONLY

Figure 40.13
Summary of drugs used to treat constipation.

V. LAXATIVES

Laxatives are commonly used in the treatment of constipation to accelerate the motility of the bowel, soften the stool, and increase the frequency of bowel movements. These drugs are classified on the basis of their mechanism of action (Figure 40.13). Laxatives increase the potential for loss of pharmacologic effect of poorly absorbed, delayed-acting, and extended-release oral preparations by accelerating their transit through the intestines. They may also cause electrolyte imbalances when used chronically. Many of these drugs have a risk of dependency for the user.

A. Irritants and stimulants

1. **Senna:** This agent is a widely used stimulant laxative. Its active ingredient is a group of sennosides, a natural complex of anthraquinone glycosides. Taken orally, *senna* causes evacuation of the bowels within 6 to 12 hours. It also causes water and electrolyte secretion into the bowel. In combination products with a *docusate*-containing stool softener, it is useful in treating opioid-induced constipation.

2. **Bisacodyl:** Available as suppositories and enteric-coated tablets, *bisacodyl* [bis-ak-oh-dil] is a potent stimulant of the colon. It acts directly on nerve fibers in the mucosa of the colon.

3. **Castor oil:** This agent is broken down in the small intestine to ricinoleic acid, which is very irritating to the stomach and promptly increases peristalsis. Pregnant patients should avoid *castor oil* because it may stimulate uterine contractions. Use of *castor oil* is generally not recommended due to poor palatability and potential for GI adverse effects.

B. Bulk laxatives

The bulk laxatives include hydrophilic colloids (from indigestible parts of fruits and vegetables). They form gels in the large intestine, causing water retention and intestinal distension, thereby increasing peristaltic activity. Similar actions are produced by *methylcellulose*, psyllium seeds, and bran. They should be used cautiously in patients who are immobile because of their potential for causing intestinal obstruction. *Psyllium* can reduce the absorption of other oral drugs, and administration of other agents should be separated from *psyllium* by at least two hours.

C. Saline and osmotic laxatives

Saline cathartics, such as *magnesium citrate* and *magnesium hydroxide*, are nonabsorbable salts (anions and cations) that hold water in the intestine by osmosis. This distends the bowel, increasing intestinal activity and producing defecation in a few hours. Electrolyte solutions containing *polyethylene glycol* (*PEG*) are used as colonic lavage solutions to prepare the gut for radiologic or endoscopic procedures. *PEG* powder for solution without electrolytes is also used as a laxative and has been shown to cause less cramping and gas than other laxatives. *Lactulose* is a semisynthetic disaccharide sugar that acts as an osmotic laxative. It cannot be hydrolyzed by GI enzymes. Oral doses reach the colon and are degraded by colonic bacteria into lactic, formic, and acetic acids. This increases osmotic pressure, causing fluid accumulation, colon distension, soft stools, and defecation. *Lactulose* is also used for the treatment of hepatic encephalopathy, due to its ability to reduce ammonia levels.

D. Stool softeners (emollient laxatives or surfactants)

Surface active agents that become emulsified with the stool produce softer feces and ease passage of stool. These include *docusate sodium* and *docusate calcium*. They may take days to become effective and are often used for prophylaxis rather than acute treatment. Stool softeners should not be taken concomitantly with *mineral oil* because of the potential for absorption of the *mineral oil*.

E. Lubricant laxatives

Mineral oil and *glycerin suppositories* are lubricants and act by facilitating the passage of hard stools. *Mineral oil* should be taken orally in an upright position to avoid its aspiration and potential for lipid or lipoid pneumonia.

IBS-C AGENTS
Linaclotide LINZESS
Lubiprostone AMITIZA
IBS-D AGENTS
Alosetron LOTRONEX
Eluxadoline VIBERZI
Rifaximin XIFAXAN
AGENTS FOR IBS-C AND IBS-D
Dicyclomine BENTYL
Hyoscyamine ANASPAZ, LEVBID, LEVSIN

Figure 40.14
Summary of drugs used to treat irritable bowel syndrome. IBS-C = irritable bowel syndrome with constipation; IBS-D = irritable bowel syndrome with diarrhea.

F. Chloride channel activators

Lubiprostone [loo-bee-PROS-tone] works by activating chloride channels to increase fluid secretion in the intestinal lumen. This eases the passage of stools and causes little change in electrolyte balance. *Lubiprostone* is used in the treatment of chronic constipation and irritable bowel syndrome with constipation (IBS-C), particularly because tolerance or dependency has not been associated with this drug. Also, drug–drug interactions are minimal because metabolism occurs quickly in the stomach and jejunum.

VI. IRRITABLE BOWEL SYNDROME

Irritable bowel syndrome (IBS) is characterized by chronic abdominal pain and altered bowel habits in the absence of an organic cause. IBS may be classified as constipation predominant (IBS-C), diarrhea predominant (IBS-D), or a combination of both. Diet and psychosocial modifications play an important role in management of the disease, as well as drug therapy (Figure 40.14). Key characteristics of medications used for the treatment of IBS-C and IBS-D are provided in Figure 40.15.

VII. DRUGS USED TO TREAT INFLAMMATORY BOWEL DISEASE

Inflammatory bowel disease (IBD) is a group of idiopathic chronic intestinal conditions characterized by immune-mediated GI tract inflammation in response to bacterial antigens in the intestinal lumen. The most common

DRUG	INDICATION	MECHANISM OF ACTION	ADVERSE EFFECTS
Linaclotide	IBS-C*	Increases intestinal fluid secretion via increased cGMP	Diarrhea, abdominal pain, flatulence, and abdominal distention Do not use in children < 17 years old
Lubiprostone	Women with IBS-C*	Chloride channel activator	Nausea and vomiting, dyspepsia, headache, dizziness, and hypotension
Alosetron	Women with severe IBS-D	5-HT$_3$ antagonist	Constipation, nausea and vomiting, heartburn, ischemic colitis (rare)
Eluxadoline	IBS-D	μ-Opioid receptor agonist	Constipation, abdominal pain, nausea, pancreatitis (rare) Possible risk of dependence and overdose
Rifaximin	Short-term use in IBS-D	Decreases bacterial load (structural analog of *rifampin*)	Nausea, fatigue, headache, dizziness, peripheral edema, and risk of <u>Clostridium difficile</u> infection
Dicyclomine	IBS-C and IBS-D	Antimuscarinic; decreases GI spasms and motility	Anticholinergic effects such as drowsiness and dry mouth
Hyoscyamine	IBS-C and IBS-D	Antimuscarinic; decreases GI spasms and motility	Anticholinergic effects such as drowsiness and dry mouth Overdose may produce hallucinations, arrhythmias, and nausea and vomiting

Figure 40.15
Characteristics of drugs used to treat irritable bowel syndrome. cGMP = cyclic guanosine monophosphate; IBS-C = irritable bowel syndrome with constipation; IBS-D = irritable bowel syndrome with diarrhea; GI = gastrointestinal.
*Also indicated for the treatment of chronic constipation.

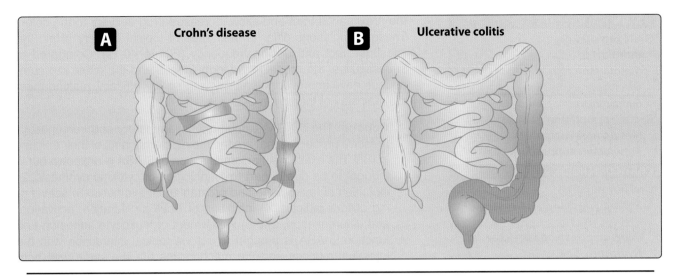

Figure 40.16
Distribution patterns of disease with **(A)** skip lesions in Crohn's disease and **(B)** continuous involvement of the colon, beginning with the rectum, in ulcerative colitis.

subtypes of IBD are Crohn's disease (CD) and ulcerative colitis (UC). CD can affect any portion of the GI tract from the mouth to the anus in a noncontinuous fashion and is characterized by transmural inflammation. UC usually affects the rectum. It may extend continuously to affect other parts of the colon, and is characterized by inflammation limited to the mucosal layer (Figure 40.16). Severity, extent of disease, and risk of complications guide treatment of IBD. Remission of IBD can be induced with the use of rectal and oral 5-aminosalicylates (5-ASAs), corticosteroids (rectal, oral locally delivered and systemic), and biologic agents (TNF-α inhibitors, α-4 integrin inhibitors, and the IL-12/23 inhibitor *ustekinumab*). Drugs used to maintain remission are the same as those used for induction. The immunomodulators (*azathioprine*, *6-mercaptopurine*, and *methotrexate*) are additional agents used in the maintenance of remission in IBD. Figure 40.17 summarizes agents used in the treatment of IBD.

A. 5-Aminosalicylates

Two types of 5-ASA compounds exist, the azo compounds and the *mesalamine* compounds. The azo compounds are prodrugs that consist of a 5-ASA molecule bound via an azo (N=N) bond to another molecule. These include *balsalazide* [bal-SAL-a-zide], *olsalazine* [ole-SAL-a-zeen], and *sulfasalazine* [SUL-fa-SAL-a-zeen]. The oral *mesalamine* [me-SAL-a-meen] compounds consist of single 5-ASA molecules enclosed within an enteric coat or a semipermeable membrane. The first 5-ASA agent used in the treatment of IBD, *sulfasalazine*, is a prodrug consisting of 5-ASA linked to sulfapyridine. Colonic bacteria cleave *sulfasalazine* to produce 5-ASA (*mesalamine*) and sulfapyridine (Figure 40.18). When it became known that 5-ASA was responsible for the efficacy of *sulfasalazine* while sulfapyridine was mainly responsible for its adverse effects, unlinked 5-ASA formulations were produced. However, unlinked 5-ASA is rapidly absorbed, with only 20% reaching the site of action in the terminal ileum and colon. Therefore, other azo bonded compounds and various formulations of *mesalamine* were developed to limit absorption of 5-ASA in

5-AMINOSALICYLATES

Oral Formulation
Balsalazide COLAZAL, GIAZO
Mesalamine ASACOL, PENTASA
Olsalazine DIPENTUM
Sulfasalazine AZULFIDINE
Rectal Formulation
Mesalamine enema ROWASA
Mesalamine suppository CANASA

CORTICOSTEROIDS

Oral Formulation
Budesonide delayed-release
ENTOCORT EC
Budesonide extended-release UCERIS
Hydrocortisone CORTEF
Prednisone DELTASONE
Methylprednisolone MEDROL
Intravenous Formulation
Hydrocortisone SOLU-CORTEF
Methylprednisolone SOLU-MEDROL
Rectal Formulation
Budesonide foam UCERIS RECTAL
Hydrocortisone suppository
ANUCORT-HC
Hydrocortisone enema CORTENEMA
Hydrocortisone foam CORTIFOAM

BIOLOGIC AGENTS

TNF-α Inhibitors
Adalimumab HUMIRA
Certolizumab CIMZIA
Golimumab SIMPONI
Infliximab REMICADE
α4-Integrin Inhibitors
Vedolizumab ENTYVIO
IL-12/23 Inhibitor
Ustekinumab STELARA

IMMUNOMODULATORS

Azathioprine IMURAN
6-Mercaptopurine GENERIC ONLY
Methotrexate VARIOUS

Figure 40.17
Agents used in the treatment of IBD.

the proximal GI tract and allow increased drug delivery to the colon. These formulations differ in their sites of topical delivery within the intestinal tract and dosing frequency (Figure 40.19). Compared to *sulfasalazine*, the *mesalamine* formulations and the other azo compounds have improved tolerability with similar efficacy, making them the mainstay of therapy in UC.

1. **Actions:** The 5-ASAs exhibit anti-inflammatory and immunosuppressive properties that are the main determinants of their efficacy in IBD. The exact mechanism of action of 5-ASA is unknown but is thought to be due in part to 1) inhibition of cytokine synthesis, 2) inhibition of leukotriene and prostaglandin synthesis, 3) scavenging of free radicals, 4) inhibition of T-cell proliferation, activation, and differentiation, and 5) impairment of leukocyte adhesion and function. 5-ASA is thought to act via topical interaction with the intestinal mucosa and the mechanisms are the same with both oral and rectal administration.

2. **Therapeutic uses:** The 5-ASA drugs are the mainstay of treatment in UC. All 5-ASA formulations and *sulfasalazine* are indicated in UC for induction and maintenance of remission. Current guidelines recommend these agents as first line for mild–moderate disease. Use of 5-ASA drugs in CD is limited due to a general lack of efficacy.

3. **Pharmacokinetics:** 5-ASA (*mesalamine*) pharmacokinetics are variable and dependent on route of administration (for example, rectal vs. oral), type of oral formulation (see Figure 40.19), and disease activity. Absorption of 5-ASA increases with more severe disease and decreases with decreasing pH. In UC, 5-ASAs work by local effect. Therefore, the 5-ASA preparations deliver drug to the colon for maximal intestinal exposure. Absorption of rectally administered *mesalamine* and systemic exposure depends on rectal retention time. Due to the topical mechanism of action, differences in systemic exposure are not related to efficacy but may be important for adverse effects. *Sulfasalazine* is administered orally, with the sulfapyridine component having significant absorption (60% to 80%).

4. **Adverse effects:** Adverse effects of *sulfasalazine* occur in up to 45% of patients, with the majority due to the sulfapyridine component. Headache, nausea, and fatigue are most common and are dose related. Serious reactions include hemolytic anemia, myelosuppression, hepatitis, pneumonitis, nephrotoxicity, fever, rash, and Stevens-Johnson syndrome. Treatment should be discontinued at the first sign of skin rash or hypersensitivity. *Sulfasalazine* reversibly impairs male fertility. *Sulfasalazine* also inhibits intestinal folate absorption, and folate supplementation is recommended with chronic use. The newer *mesalamine* formulations are well tolerated; headache and dyspepsia are the most common adverse effects. Rarely, acute interstitial nephritis may occur and renal function should be monitored in patients receiving *mesalamine*. Watery diarrhea occurs in up to 20% of patients treated with *olsalazine*. Some formulations of *mesalamine* depend on pH for their release (see Figure 40.19) and coadministration of drugs that increase pH

(for example, PPIs, H$_2$ receptor antagonists, and antacids) may result in increased systemic absorption and premature release of 5-ASA before reaching the site of action. Concomitant use should be avoided or another formulation of 5-ASA that is non-pH dependent should be used (for example, *olsalazine, balsalazide*).

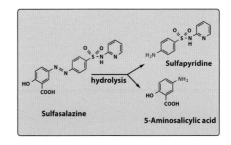

Figure 40.18
Sulfasalazine metabolism.

B. Corticosteroids

Corticosteroids are used in IBD for their anti-inflammatory effects as they are in other inflammatory conditions (see Chapter 26). Although very effective at inducing remission in IBD, long-term maintenance with corticosteroids should be avoided due to the deleterious effects of chronic use. Rectal formulations (for example, *hydrocortisone* enema and *budesonide* foam) have fewer adverse effects than systemic steroids but use is limited to left-sided disease in UC. Enteric-release preparations of oral *budesonide* deliver corticosteroid to a portion of inflamed intestine. This agent has minimal systemic adverse effects due to low bioavailability resulting from extensive first-pass hepatic metabolism. Delayed-release *budesonide* delivers drug to the terminal ileum and proximal large bowel and is used in ileocecal CD. Extended-release *budesonide* delivers drug throughout the colon and is used in UC patients with pancolitis. Although systemic exposure is less than other corticosteroids, the use of *budesonide* in extended maintenance of remission is limited due to concerns with long-term use.

C. Biologic agents

The TNF-α inhibitors, α-4 integrin inhibitors, and the IL-12/23 inhibitor *ustekinumab* are biologic agents used in the management of IBD. Use of these agents is associated with an increased risk for infection. Patients should be evaluated for tuberculosis and treatment for latent TB should be considered prior to use of these drugs. Many of

DRUG	BRAND(S)	ROUTE	DOSING FREQUENCY	FORMULATION	SITE OF DELIVERY
Balsalazide	Colazal	PO	Three times daily	5-ASA azo bonded to inert carrier molecule; release dependent on cleavage by colonic bacteria	Colon
Mesalamine	Apriso	PO	Once daily	pH-dependent (≥ 6) delayed release with extended-release matrix core	Colon
	Asacol, Asacol HD	PO	Three times daily	pH-dependent (≥ 7) delayed release	Distal ileum, colon
	Canasa	Rectal	Once daily	Suppository	Rectum
	Lialda	PO	Once daily	pH-dependent (≥ 7) delayed-release multimatrix system	Distal ileum, colon
	Pentasa	PO	Four times daily	Ethyl cellulose membrane controlled-release micropellets	Entire small intestine, colon
	Rowasa	Rectal	Once daily	Liquid enema	Rectum, sigmoid colon
Olsalazine	Dipentum	PO	Twice daily	5-ASA azo bonded to another 5-ASA molecule; release dependent on cleavage by colonic bacteria	Colon

Figure 40.19
5-Aminosalicylate formulations.

these agents have other therapeutic indications such as rheumatoid arthritis (see Chapter 38) or psoriasis (see Chapter 43). The actions, pharmacokinetics, and adverse effects of these drugs in other conditions are similar in IBD.

1. **TNF-α inhibitors:** TNF-α inhibitors are parenteral agents that are effective for both induction and maintenance of remission in IBD. *Infliximab* [in-FLIX-ih-mab] and *adalimumab* [AY-da-LIM-ue-mab] are indicated in both moderate–severe CD and UC. *Certolizumab* [SER-toe-LIZ-oo-mab] is indicated for moderate–severe CD, and *golimumab* [goe-LIM-ue-mab] is indicated for moderate–severe UC. The TNF-α inhibitors are generally reserved as second-line agents in patients with UC who have failed 5-ASAs, are unresponsive to or dependent on corticosteroids, or who present with more severe disease. In CD, the TNF-α inhibitors have a first-line role in patients with moderate–severe disease and those at higher risk of progression and worse outcomes. These agents are associated with the development of immunogenicity and antidrug antibodies that can result in loss of response in a significant proportion of patients.

2. **α-4 integrin inhibitors:** α-4 Integrins are adhesion molecules that promote leukocyte migration to sites of inflammation. Use of α-4 integrin inhibitors reduces lymphocyte migration into the intestinal mucosa and inflammation. The use of α-4 integrin inhibitors in IBD is reserved for disease refractory to TNF-α inhibitors. *Vedolizumab* [VE-doe-LIZ-ue-mab] exhibits specific binding to α-4/β-7 integrin and is indicated for refractory UC and CD. The most common adverse reactions include headache, arthralgia, nausea, fatigue, and musculoskeletal pain.

3. **IL-12/23 inhibitor:** *Ustekinumab* [YOO-sti-KIN-ue-mab] inhibits the cytokines IL-12 and IL-23 involved in lymphocyte activation. It is indicated for psoriasis, psoriatic arthritis, and induction and maintenance of remission in CD in patients refractory to or intolerant of TNF-α inhibitors, immunomodulators, or corticosteroids. Common adverse effects include headache, arthralgia, infection, nausea, and nasopharyngitis.

D. Immunomodulators

The immunomodulator drugs most often used in IBD are *methotrexate* and the thiopurines *azathioprine* and *6-mercaptopurine* (*6-MP*). *Methotrexate* (*MTX*) also has therapeutic applications in cancer, rheumatoid arthritis, and psoriasis (see Chapters 35, 38, and 43) and *azathioprine* is sometimes used in kidney transplant (see Chapter 36). The actions, pharmacokinetics, and adverse effects of the immunomodulators in other conditions are similar in IBD.

1. **Methotrexate:** *MTX* is a structural analogue of folic acid that inhibits the production of folinic acid. The exact mechanism of action in CD is unknown. Only intramuscular or subcutaneous administration of *MTX* has efficacy in CD. *MTX* is a recommended monotherapy option for maintenance of remission in CD, but is not recommended in maintenance for UC. Common adverse effects of *MTX* are headache, nausea, vomiting, abdominal discomfort,

serum aminotransferase elevations, and rash. Daily administration of folic acid is effective at reducing the incidence of GI adverse effects and is recommended in patients receiving *MTX*.

2. **Thiopurines:** The thiopurines *azathioprine* and *6-mercaptopurine* (*6-MP*) are oral medications that have corticosteroid-sparing effects in patients with UC and CD. They are considered first line as monotherapy for maintenance of remission. Use of thiopurines in IBD is limited by concerns of toxicity, including bone marrow suppression and hepatotoxicity. Monitoring of complete blood counts and liver function tests is recommended in all patients treated with a thiopurine.

Study Questions

Choose the ONE best answer.

40.1 A 68-year-old patient with cardiac failure is diagnosed with ovarian cancer. She begins using cisplatin but becomes nauseous and suffers from severe vomiting. Which drug would be most effective to counteract the emesis in this patient without exacerbating her cardiac problem?

A. Droperidol
B. Dolasetron
C. Prochlorperazine
D. Palonosetron

Correct answer = D. Palonosetron is a 5-HT$_3$ antagonist that is effective against drugs with high emetogenic activity, such as cisplatin. Although dolasetron is also in this category, its propensity to affect the heart makes it a poor choice for this patient. Droperidol is only a moderately effective antiemetic and has the potential to prolong the QTc interval, so it is not preferred in this patient. The antiemetic effect of prochlorperazine, a phenothiazine, is most beneficial against anticancer drugs with moderate to low emetogenic properties.

40.2 A 45-year-old woman complains of severe persistent heartburn and an unpleasant, acid-like taste in her mouth. The clinician suspects that she has gastroesophageal reflux disease. Which drug is most appropriate?

A. An antacid such as aluminum hydroxide
B. Dicyclomine
C. Granisetron
D. Esomeprazole

Correct answer = D. It is appropriate to treat this patient with a proton-pump inhibitor (PPI) to reduce acid production and promote healing. An H$_2$ receptor antagonist might also be effective, but the PPIs are preferred. An antacid would decrease gastric acid, but its effects are short lived compared to those of the PPIs and H$_2$ receptor antagonists. Dicyclomine is an antimuscarinic drug that is mainly used as an antispasmodic for IBS. The 5-HT$_3$ receptor antagonist granisetron is an antiemetic, and not appropriate for the treatment of GERD.

40.3 A couple celebrating their 30th wedding anniversary are given a trip to Peru to visit Machu Picchu. Because of past experiences while traveling, they ask their doctor to prescribe an agent in case they experience diarrhea. Which drug would be effective?

A. Omeprazole
B. Loperamide
C. Famotidine
D. Lubiprostone

Correct answer = B. Loperamide is the only drug that has antidiarrheal activity. Omeprazole is a proton-pump inhibitor, famotidine antagonizes the H$_2$ receptor to reduce acid production, and lubiprostone is indicated for chronic constipation or IBS-C.

40.4 A 27-year-old woman who is 34 weeks' pregnant is on bed rest and is experiencing mild constipation. Which drug is most appropriate for her?

A. Castor oil
B. Docusate
C. Mineral oil
D. Loperamide

Correct answer = B. Although its effects are not immediate, docusate may be used for mild constipation and is generally considered safe in pregnancy. Castor oil should not be used in pregnancy because of its ability to cause uterine contractions. Mineral oil should not be used in bedridden patients due to the possibility of aspiration. Loperamide is used for diarrhea, not constipation.

40.5 Which drug has been known to cause discoloration of the tongue?

    A. Amoxicillin

    B. Omeprazole

    C. Bismuth subsalicylate

    D. Lubiprostone

Correct answer = C. Bismuth subsalicylate compounds may cause a harmless black discoloration of the tongue. The other agents have not been associated with this effect.

40.6 An elderly woman with a recent history of myocardial infarction is seeking a medication to help treat her occasional heartburn. She is currently taking several medications, including aspirin, clopidogrel, simvastatin, metoprolol, and lisinopril. Which drug should be avoided in this patient?

    A. Calcium citrate

    B. Famotidine

    C. Omeprazole

    D. Ranitidine

Correct answer = C. Omeprazole may possibly decrease the efficacy of clopidogrel because it inhibits the conversion of clopidogrel to its active form.

40.7 Extrapyramidal symptoms (EPS) have been associated with which drug?

    A. Metoclopramide

    B. Sucralfate

    C. Aprepitant

    D. Bisacodyl

Correct answer = A. Only metoclopramide has been associated with EPS. This is due to its ability to inhibit dopamine activity.

40.8 Which agent for gastrointestinal problems is contraindicated in pregnancy?

    A. Calcium carbonate

    B. Famotidine

    C. Lansoprazole

    D. Misoprostol

Correct answer = D. Misoprostol, a synthetic prostaglandin analog, is contraindicated in pregnancy because it may stimulate uterine contractions. The other medications may be used during pregnancy for the treatment of heartburn (common in pregnancy) or peptic ulcer disease.

40.9 A patient presents with a 2-month history of crampy right lower quadrant abdominal pain. Results of endoscopy are consistent with moderate Crohn's disease involving the terminal ileum and proximal large intestine. Which drug is best to initiate in this patient at this time?

    A. Extended-release budesonide

    B. Delayed-release budesonide

    C. Mesalamine enema

    D. Ustekinumab

Correct answer = B. Delayed-release budesonide is indicated in Crohn's disease because it releases in the terminal ileum and proximal large bowel and is effective in inducing remission. Extended-release budesonide, although effective at inducing remission, is only indicated in ulcerative colitis because it does not release in the small bowel and would not be expected to be effective in this patient's ileal disease. Mesalamine enema is only effective on the distal large intestine. Ustekinumab is only indicated in patients who are refractory or intolerant to TNF-α inhibitors.

40.10 A patient with a history of ulcerative colitis well controlled on mesalamine (Apriso) presents with epigastric pain and dark tarry stools. He is found to have a duodenal ulcer and is prescribed esomeprazole for 8 weeks. At follow-up 2 weeks later, his epigastric pain and dark tarry stools are resolved. However, he reports having increased lower abdominal pain and increased stool frequency. Which change in drug therapy is appropriate at this time?

    A. Change esomeprazole to omeprazole due to interaction with mesalamine (Apriso).

    B. Discontinue esomeprazole.

    C. Change mesalamine (Apriso) to mesalamine (Asacol).

    D. Change mesalamine (Apriso) to olsalazine (Dipentum).

Correct Answer = D. The patient seems to be having increased symptoms of ulcerative colitis after starting the PPI, esomeprazole. The pH-dependent release formulations of mesalamine have a significant interaction with the PPIs, which may lead to early release and loss of efficacy. A is incorrect because omeprazole is expected to have the same interaction. B is incorrect because this patient still requires therapy with a PPI. C is incorrect because Asacol is also pH-dependent release and is likely to be affected. D is correct because olsalazine is not pH dependent and release relies on cleavage by colonic bacteria.

Drugs for Urologic Disorders

Katherine Vogel Anderson and Kaylie Smith

41

I. OVERVIEW

Erectile dysfunction (ED) and benign prostatic hyperplasia (BPH) are common urologic disorders in males. ED is the inability to maintain penile erection for the successful performance of sexual activity. ED has many physical and psychological causes, including vascular disease, diabetes, medications, depression, and sequelae to prostatic surgery. It is estimated to affect more than 30 million men in the United States. BPH is nonmalignant enlargement of the prostate, which occurs naturally as men age. As the prostate grows in size, lower urinary tract symptoms develop, which can significantly impact a patient's quality of life. A summary of drugs for ED and BPH is provided in Figure 41.1.

II. DRUGS USED TO TREAT ERECTILE DYSFUNCTION

Therapy for ED includes penile implants, intrapenile injections of *alprostadil*, intraurethral suppositories of *alprostadil*, and oral phosphodiesterase-5 (PDE-5) inhibitors. Because of the efficacy, ease of use, and safety of PDE-5 inhibitors, these drugs are first-line therapy for ED.

A. Phosphodiesterase-5 inhibitors

Four PDE-5 inhibitors *sildenafil* [sil-DEN-a-fil], *vardenafil* [var-DEN-na-fil], *tadalafil* [ta-DAL-a-fil], and *avanafil* [a-VAN-a-fil] are approved for the treatment of ED. [Note: *Sildenafil* and *tadalafil* are also indicated to treat pulmonary hypertension, although the dosage regimen differs for this indication.] All four PDE-5 inhibitors are equally effective in treating ED, and the adverse effect profiles of the drugs are similar. However, these agents differ in the duration of action and the effects of food on drug absorption.

1. **Mechanism of action:** Sexual stimulation results in smooth muscle relaxation of the corpus cavernosum, increasing the inflow of blood (Figure 41.2). The mediator of this response is nitric oxide (NO). NO activates guanylyl cyclase, which forms cyclic guanosine monophosphate (cGMP) from guanosine triphosphate. cGMP produces smooth muscle relaxation through a reduction in the intracellular Ca^{2+} concentration. The duration of action of

DRUGS FOR ERECTILE DYSFUNCTION
Alprostadil MUSE, CAVERJECT, EDEX
Avanafil STENDRA
Sildenafil VIAGRA
Tadalafil CIALIS
Vardenafil LEVITRA, STAXYN

α BLOCKERS
Alfuzosin UROXATRAL
Doxazosin CARDURA
Prazosin MINIPRESS
Silodosin RAPAFLO
Tamsulosin FLOMAX
Terazosin HYTRIN

5 α-REDUCTASE INHIBITORS
Dutasteride AVODART
Finasteride PROPECIA, PROSCAR

COMBINATION PRODUCT
Dutasteride/tamsulosin JALYN

Figure 41.1
Summary of drugs used for the treatment of urologic disorders.

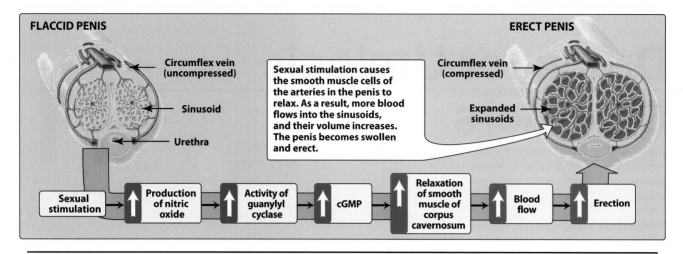

Figure 41.2
Mechanism of penile erection. cGMP = cyclic guanosine monophosphate.

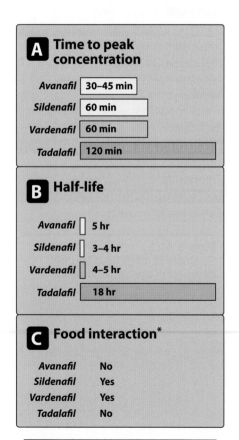

Figure 41.3
Some properties of
phosphodiesterase inhibitors.
*Delay in time to reach peak drug
concentration when taken with high-
fat foods.

cyclic nucleotides is controlled by the action of PDE. At least 11 isozymes of PDE have been characterized. *Sildenafil, vardenafil, tadalafil,* and *avanafil* inhibit PDE-5, the isozyme responsible for degradation of cGMP in the corpus cavernosum. The action of PDE-5 inhibitors is to increase the flow of blood into the corpus cavernosum at any given level of sexual stimulation. At recommended doses, PDE-5 inhibitors have no effect in the absence of sexual stimulation.

2. **Pharmacokinetics:** *Sildenafil* and *vardenafil* have similar pharmacokinetic properties. Both drugs should be taken approximately 1 hour prior to anticipated sexual activity, with erectile enhancement observed for up to 4 hours after administration. Thus, administration of *sildenafil* and *vardenafil* must be timed appropriately with regard to anticipated sexual activity. The absorption of both drugs is delayed by consumption of a high-fat meal. *Vardenafil* is also available in an orally disintegrating tablet (ODT) formulation, which is not affected by a high-fat meal. However, the bioavailability of the ODT formulation may be decreased by water, and therefore, the ODT should be placed under the tongue and not administered with liquids. The *vardenafil* ODT provides a higher systemic bioavailability than the *vardenafil* film-coated oral tablet, and these products are not interchangeable. *Tadalafil* has a slower onset of action (Figure 41.3) than *sildenafil* and *vardenafil*, but a significantly longer half-life of approximately 18 hours. As such, it is approved for once-daily dosing (in addition to as-needed dosing). This results in enhanced erectile function for up to 36 hours. Furthermore, the absorption of *tadalafil* is not clinically influenced by food. The timing of sexual activity is less critical for *tadalafil* because of its prolonged duration of effect. Of all the PDE-5 inhibitors, *avanafil* has the quickest onset of action. It should be taken 30 minutes prior to sexual activity. All PDE-5 inhibitors are metabolized by the cytochrome P450 3A4 (CYP3A4) isoenzyme. Dosage adjustments for *sildenafil, tadalafil,* and *vardenafil* are recommended in patients with mild to moderate hepatic dysfunction. PDE-5 inhibitors should be avoided in patients with severe hepatic

impairment. For patients with severe renal dysfunction, the dose of *sildenafil* and *tadalafil* should be reduced, and daily-dose *tadalafil* and as needed *avanafil* are contraindicated in these patients.

3. **Adverse effects:** The most frequent adverse effects of the PDE-5 inhibitors are headache, flushing, dyspepsia, and nasal congestion. These effects are generally mild, and men with ED rarely discontinue treatment because of side effects. Disturbances in color vision (loss of blue/green discrimination) may occur with PDE-5 inhibitors, likely due to inhibition of PDE-6 (a PDE found in the retina that is important in color vision). *Tadalafil*, however, does not appear to disrupt PDE-6, and reports of changes in color vision have been rare with this medication. The incidence of these reactions appears to be dose dependent. Sudden hearing loss has also been reported with the use of PDE-5 inhibitors, perhaps due to changes in sinus pressure because of vasodilation. *Tadalafil* has been associated with back pain and myalgias, likely because of inhibition of PDE-11, an enzyme found in skeletal muscle. There is an inherent cardiac risk associated with sexual activity. Therefore, PDE-5 inhibitors should be used with caution in patients with a history of cardiovascular disease or those with strong risk factors for cardiovascular disease. PDE-5 inhibitors should not be used more than once per day for the treatment of ED. All of the PDE-5 inhibitors have the potential to cause priapism (a painful, prolonged erection). Although this is a rare side effect, it is a medical emergency.

4. **Drug interactions:** Because of the ability of PDE-5 inhibitors to potentiate the hypotensive activity of NO, administration of these medications in combination with organic nitrates (for example, *nitroglycerin* products, *isosorbide dinitrate*, or *isosorbide mononitrate*) is contraindicated. PDE-5 inhibitors may produce additive blood pressure–lowering effects when used in patients taking α-adrenergic antagonists for treatment of hypertension and/or alleviation of symptoms associated with BPH. The combination of PDE-5 inhibitors and α-adrenergic antagonists should be used with caution. Patients should be on a stable dose of the α-adrenergic antagonist prior to the initiation of the PDE-5 inhibitor, and the PDE-5 inhibitor should be started at a low dose if this combination is used. Doses of PDE-5 inhibitors may need to be reduced in the presence of potent inhibitors of CYP3A4, such as *clarithromycin*, *ritonavir*, and other protease inhibitors. Because of QT prolongation, the combination of *vardenafil* and *dronedarone* should be avoided.

B. Alprostadil

Alprostadil [al-PRAHST-uh-dill] is synthetic prostaglandin E1 (PGE1). In the penile tissue, PGE1 allows for relaxation of the smooth muscle in the corpus cavernosum. *Alprostadil* is available as an intraurethral suppository and an injectable formulation. Although PDE-5 inhibitors are considered first-line therapy for the treatment of ED, *alprostadil* may be used for patients who are not candidates for oral therapies. In contrast to oral agents, *alprostadil* acts locally, which may reduce the occurrence of adverse effects.

1. **Mechanism of action:** *Alprostadil* causes smooth muscle relaxation by an unknown mechanism. It is believed that *alprostadil* increases concentrations of cyclic adenosine monophosphate (cAMP) within cavernosal tissue. As a result, protein kinase is activated, allowing trabecular smooth muscle relaxation and dilation of cavernosal arteries. Increased blood flow to the erection chamber compresses venous outflow, so that blood is entrapped and erection may occur.

2. **Pharmacokinetics:** Systemic absorption of *alprostadil* is minimal. If any *alprostadil* is systemically absorbed, it is quickly metabolized. The onset of action of *alprostadil* is 5 to 10 minutes when given as a urethral suppository and 2 to 25 minutes when administered by injection. The resulting erection may last for 30 to 60 minutes, or longer, depending upon the particular patient.

3. **Adverse effects:** Since *alprostadil* is not systemically absorbed, adverse systemic effects are rare. However, hypotension or headache is a possibility due to PGE1-induced vasodilation. Locally, adverse effects of *alprostadil* include penile pain, urethral pain, and testicular pain. Bleeding from the insertion or injection of *alprostadil* is rare. Hematoma, ecchymosis, and rash are possible from *alprostadil* injection, although these adverse effects are also rare. *Alprostadil* administration may lead to priapism.

III. BENIGN PROSTATIC HYPERPLASIA

Three classes of medications are used to treat BPH: α_1-adrenergic antagonists, 5-α reductase inhibitors, and PDE-5 inhibitors.

A. α1-Adrenergic antagonists

Terazosin [ter-AY-zoe-sin], *doxazosin* [dox-AY-zoe-sin], *tamsulosin* [tam-SUE-loh-sin], *alfuzosin* [al-FUE-zoe-sin], and *silodosin* [sil-oh-DOE-sin] are selective competitive blockers of the α_1 receptor. All five agents are indicated for the treatment of BPH (Figure 41.1). *Prazosin* is an α-blocker that is used off-label in the treatment of BPH. However, current guidelines do not endorse the use of *prazosin* for BPH. Please refer to Chapter 7 for a discussion of α-blockers in the setting of hypertension.

1. **Mechanism of action:** α_{1A} receptors are found in the prostate, α_{1B} receptors are found in the prostate and vasculature, and α_{1D} receptors are found in the vasculature. By blocking the α_{1A} and α_{1B} receptors in the prostate, the α-blockers cause prostatic smooth muscle relaxation, which leads to improved urine flow. *Doxazosin*, *terazosin*, and *alfuzosin* block α_{1A} and α_{1B} receptors, whereas *tamsulosin* and *silodosin* are more selective for the α_{1A} receptor. Because *doxazosin*, *terazosin*, and *alfuzosin* block α_{1B} receptors, these agents decrease peripheral vascular resistance and lower arterial blood pressure by causing relaxation of both arterial and venous smooth muscle. In contrast, *tamsulosin* and *silodosin* have

less of an effect on blood pressure because they are more selective for the prostate-specific α_{1A} receptor.

2. **Pharmacokinetics:** The α-blockers are well absorbed following oral administration. When taken with food, the absorption of *tamsulosin*, *alfuzosin*, and *silodosin* is increased. Therefore, for best efficacy, these agents should be taken with food or after a meal, typically supper. *Doxazosin*, *alfuzosin*, *tamsulosin*, and *silodosin* are metabolized through the cytochrome P450 system. *Silodosin* is also a substrate for P-glycoprotein (P-gp). *Terazosin* is metabolized in the liver, but not through the CYP system. In general, the α-blockers have a half-life of 8 to 22 hours, with peak effects 1 to 4 hours after administration. *Silodosin* requires dosage adjustment in renal impairment and is contraindicated in patients with severe renal dysfunction.

3. **Adverse effects:** α-Blockers may cause dizziness, a lack of energy, nasal congestion, headache, drowsiness, and orthostatic hypotension. Because *tamsulosin* and *silodosin* are more selective for the α_{1A} receptors found on the smooth muscle of the prostate, they have relatively minimal effects on blood pressure, although dizziness and orthostasis may occur. By blocking α receptors in the ejaculatory ducts and impairing smooth muscle contraction, inhibition of ejaculation and retrograde ejaculation have been reported. Several of these agents have a caution about "floppy iris syndrome," a condition in which the iris billows in response to intraoperative eye surgery (Figure 41.4).

4. **Drug interactions:** Drugs that inhibit CYP3A4 and CYP2D6 (for example, *verapamil*, *diltiazem*) may increase the plasma concentrations of *doxazosin*, *alfuzosin*, *tamsulosin*, and *silodosin*, whereas drugs that induce the CYP450 system (for example, *carbamazepine*, *phenytoin*, and *St. John's wort*) may decrease plasma concentrations. *Alfuzosin* may prolong the QT interval, so it should be used with caution with other drugs that cause QT prolongation (for example, class III antiarrhythmics). Because *silodosin* is a substrate for P-gp, drugs that inhibit P-gp, such as *cyclosporine*, may increase *silodosin* concentrations.

B. 5-α Reductase inhibitors

Finasteride [fin-AS-ter-ide] and *dutasteride* [doo-TAS-ter-ride] inhibit 5-α reductase. Compared to the α-blockers, which provide patients with relief from BPH symptoms within 7 to 10 days, these agents may take up to 12 months to relieve symptoms.

1. **Mechanism of action:** Both *finasteride* and *dutasteride* inhibit the enzyme 5-α reductase, which is responsible for converting *testosterone* to the more active *dihydrotestosterone* (DHT). DHT is an androgen that stimulates prostate growth. By reducing DHT, the prostate shrinks and urine flow improves. Compared with *finasteride*, *dutasteride* is more potent and causes a greater decrease in DHT. In order for the 5-α reductase inhibitors to be effective, the prostate must be enlarged. Since it takes several months for 5-α reductase inhibitors to reduce the prostate size, it is appropriate to use these agents in combination with an α-blocker to provide

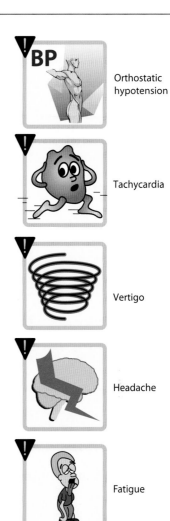

Figure 41.4
Some adverse effects commonly observed with nonselective α-blockers.

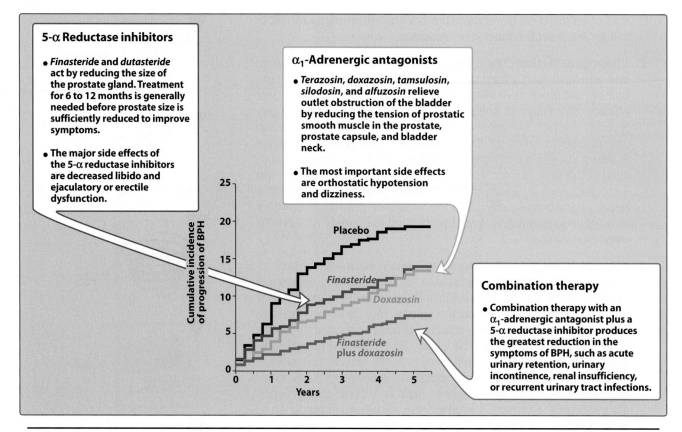

5-α Reductase inhibitors

- *Finasteride* and *dutasteride* act by reducing the size of the prostate gland. Treatment for 6 to 12 months is generally needed before prostate size is sufficiently reduced to improve symptoms.

- The major side effects of the 5-α reductase inhibitors are decreased libido and ejaculatory or erectile dysfunction.

α₁-Adrenergic antagonists

- *Terazosin, doxazosin, tamsulosin, silodosin,* and *alfuzosin* relieve outlet obstruction of the bladder by reducing the tension of prostatic smooth muscle in the prostate, prostate capsule, and bladder neck.

- The most important side effects are orthostatic hypotension and dizziness.

Combination therapy

- Combination therapy with an α₁-adrenergic antagonist plus a 5-α reductase inhibitor produces the greatest reduction in the symptoms of BPH, such as acute urinary retention, urinary incontinence, renal insufficiency, or recurrent urinary tract infections.

Figure 41.5
Therapy for benign prostatic hyperplasia (BPH).

relief of symptoms. *Dutasteride* and *tamsulosin* are available as a combination product for this indication. Figures 41.5 and 41.6 summarize important differences between these two classes of agents. *Finasteride* and *dutasteride* are also used for alopecia, since a reduction in scalp and serum DHT prevents hair loss.

2. **Pharmacokinetics:** Food does not affect the absorption of *finasteride* or *dutasteride*. Both agents are highly protein bound and metabolized by the CYP450 system. The mean plasma elimination half-life of *finasteride* is 6 to 16 hours, while the terminal elimination half-life of *dutasteride* is 5 weeks once steady-state concentrations are achieved (which is typically after 6 months of therapy).

	α₁-ADRENERGIC ANTAGONISTS	5 α-REDUCTASE INHIBITORS
Decrease in prostate size	No	Yes
Peak onset	2–4 weeks	6–12 months
Decrease in PSA	No	Yes
Sexual dysfunction	+	++
Hypotensive effects	++	–
Commonly used drugs	*Tamsulosin* and *alfuzosin*	*Finasteride* and *dutasteride*

Figure 41.6
Comparisons of treatment for BPH. PSA = prostate-specific antigen.

3. **Adverse effects:** The 5-α reductase inhibitors cause sexual side effects, such as decreased ejaculate, decreased libido, ED, gynecomastia, and oligospermia. *Finasteride* and *dutasteride* are teratogenic. Women who are pregnant or of childbearing age should not handle or ingest either agent, as this may lead to serious birth defects involving the genitalia in a male fetus. Although both agents are metabolized by the CYP450 system, drug interactions are rare. It is not ideal to use a 5-α reductase inhibitor with *testosterone*, since both *finasteride* and *dutasteride* inhibit the conversion of *testosterone* to its active form, DHT.

C. Phosphodiesterase-5 inhibitor

Tadalafil is the only PDE-5 inhibitor approved for the treatment of BPH. PDE-5 is present in the prostate and bladder. As such, inhibition of PDE-5 by *tadalafil* allows for vasodilation and relaxation of the smooth muscle of the prostate and bladder, which thereby improves symptoms of BPH.

Study Questions

Choose the ONE best answer.

41.1 Which is CORRECT regarding the mechanism of action of phosphodiesterase-5 (PDE-5) inhibitors?

    A. PDE-5 inhibitors increase prostaglandin production.

    B. PDE-5 inhibitors enhance the effect of nitric oxide.

    C. PDE-5 inhibitors cause vasoconstriction of the erection chamber.

    D. PDE-5 inhibitors antagonize cyclic GMP.

> Correct answer = B. PDE-5 inhibitors enhance the effect of nitric oxide by preventing the breakdown of cGMP. PDE-5 inhibitors do not affect prostaglandin production. Although blood is drawn to the erection chamber, PDE-5 inhibitors allow for this via vasodilation, not vasoconstriction. PDE-5 inhibitors prevent the breakdown of cGMP but do not antagonize its action.

41.2 When selecting between the available PDE-5 inhibitors for treatment of ED, which is an important consideration?

    A. Tadalafil has the shortest half-life of the PDE-5 inhibitors.

    B. Sildenafil should be given with food to increase absorption.

    C. Vardenafil ODT doses are not equal to film-coated vardenafil doses.

    D. Avanafil should be taken at least 1 hour before intercourse.

> Correct answer = C. The ODT dosage form of vardenafil provides a high systemic concentration of vardenafil, which is higher than that provided by the film-coated tablets. As such, the doses are not interchangeable. Tadalafil has the longest half-life of all PDE-5 inhibitors. Food may delay sildenafil absorption. Avanafil has the quickest onset of action and may be taken 30 minutes before intercourse.

41.3 A patient who is taking a PDE-5 inhibitor for ED is diagnosed with angina. Which antianginal medication would be of particular concern in this patient?

    A. Metoprolol

    B. Diltiazem

    C. Amlodipine

    D. Nitroglycerin

> Correct answer = D. Nitrates, such as nitroglycerin, can cause life-threatening hypotension when taken with PDE-5 inhibitors. While metoprolol, diltiazem, and amlodipine may all lower blood pressure, the interaction with PDE-5 inhibitors is not relevant.

41.4 Which BEST describes the mechanism of action of alprostadil?

    A. Alprostadil blocks cGMP.

    B. Alprostadil blocks nitric oxide.

    C. Alprostadil increases PDE-5.

    D. Alprostadil increases cAMP.

> Correct answer = D. Through an unknown mechanism, alprostadil (a synthetic prostaglandin) increases levels of cAMP, causing smooth muscle relaxation. Alprostadil does not affect cGMP, nitric oxide, or PDE-5.

41.5 Which is CORRECT regarding local administration of alprostadil?

A. Local administration of alprostadil allows for low systemic absorption.

B. Local administration of alprostadil increases the chance of drug interactions.

C. Local administration of alprostadil is accomplished by application of a cream.

D. Local administration of alprostadil causes changes in color vision.

Correct answer = A. Local administration of alprostadil allows for minimal systemic absorption. This makes alprostadil associated with few drug interactions. Alprostadil is administered by injection or urethral suppository, not a cream. Because there is little systemic absorption, and alprostadil does not affect PDE-6, changes in color vision are not likely.

41.6 Which is the BEST description of the mechanism of action of dutasteride?

A. Dutasteride blocks 5-α reductase.

B. Dutasteride blocks α_{1A} receptors.

C. Dutasteride blocks PDE-5.

D. Dutasteride blocks α_{1A} and α_{1B} receptors.

Correct answer = A. Dutasteride blocks 5-α reductase. Dutasteride does not affect α_{1A} receptors, α_{1B} receptors, or PDE-5.

41.7 A patient is worried about starting terazosin because he is very sensitive to side effects of medications. Which adverse effect would be most expected in this patient?

A. Erectile dysfunction

B. Gynecomastia

C. Dizziness

D. Vomiting

Correct answer = C. Because of the α-blocking properties, terazosin commonly causes dizziness (this may be related to orthostatic hypotension). ED and gynecomastia would be unexpected with α-blockers. While most any drug may cause nausea and vomiting, terazosin is much more likely to cause dizziness.

41.8 Which describes an important difference between terazosin and tamsulosin?

A. Terazosin blocks α_{1A} receptors, whereas tamsulosin blocks α_{1A} and α_{1B} receptors.

B. Terazosin blocks α_{1A} and α_{1B} receptors, whereas tamsulosin blocks α_{1A} receptors.

C. Terazosin blocks 5-α reductase, whereas tamsulosin blocks PDE-5.

D. Terazosin must be taken with food, whereas tamsulosin can be taken on an empty stomach.

Correct answer = B. Tamsulosin is more selective for the α_{1A} receptor, found in the prostate. Terazosin blocks α_{1A}; however, terazosin also blocks α_{1B}. Neither one blocks 5-α reductase nor PDE-5. Tamsulosin should be taken with food, while terazosin does not need to be taken with food.

41.9 Which is CORRECT regarding finasteride?

A. Finasteride is associated with significant hypotension.

B. Finasteride is associated with birth defects.

C. Finasteride is effective within 2 weeks of initiation.

D. Finasteride is renally eliminated.

Correct answer = B. Because finasteride inhibits the conversion of testosterone to its active form, it may cause significant developmental defects in the male genitalia of a developing fetus. As such, it is contraindicated in pregnancy. Unlike the α-blockers, the 5-α reductase inhibitors are not associated with hypotension. Finasteride may take up to 12 months before it is effective. Finasteride is metabolized via CYP450 and is not renally eliminated.

41.10 A 70-year-old man with BPH and an enlarged prostate continues to have urinary symptoms after an adequate trial of tamsulosin. Dutasteride is added to his therapy. In addition to tamsulosin, he is also taking hydrochlorothiazide, testosterone, and vardenafil as needed before intercourse. Which of his medications could have an interaction with dutasteride?

A. Hydrochlorothiazide

B. Tamsulosin

C. Testosterone

D. Vardenafil

Correct answer = C. Because dutasteride prevents the conversion of testosterone to the more active form, DHT, these medications have an interaction. Essentially, dutasteride prevents testosterone from "working." Hydrochlorothiazide does not interfere with the metabolism of dutasteride, and dutasteride does not have any effect on the blood pressure–lowering effects of hydrochlorothiazide. Tamsulosin is appropriate in combination with a 5-α reductase inhibitor when the prostate is enlarged. Vardenafil is only prescribed as needed, and the two drugs do not have a pharmacokinetic interaction.

Drugs for Anemia

Lori Dupree

42

I. OVERVIEW

Anemia is defined as a below-normal plasma hemoglobin concentration resulting from a decreased number of circulating red blood cells or an abnormally low total hemoglobin content per unit of blood volume. General signs and symptoms of anemia include fatigue, palpitations, shortness of breath, pallor, dizziness, and insomnia. Anemia can be caused by chronic blood loss, bone marrow abnormalities, hemolysis, infections, malignancy, endocrine deficiencies, renal failure, and a number of other disease states. A large number of drugs cause toxic effects on blood cells, hemoglobin production, or erythropoietic organs, which, in turn, may cause anemia. Nutritional anemias are caused by dietary deficiencies of substances such as iron, *folic acid*, and vitamin B_{12} (*cyanocobalamin*) that are necessary for normal erythropoiesis. Individuals with a genetic predisposition to anemia, such as sickle cell disease, can benefit from pharmacologic treatment with actions beyond nutritional supplementation, such as *hydroxyurea*. Anemia can be temporarily corrected by transfusion of whole blood. A summary of agents used for the treatment of anemias is provided in Figure 42.1.

TREATMENT OF ANEMIA
Cyanocobalamin (B₁₂)
Darbepoetin ARANESP
Epoetin alfa EPOGEN, PROCRIT
Folic acid GENERIC ONLY
Iron INFED, VENOFER, OTHERS
TREATMENT OF NEUTROPENIA
Filgrastim NEUPOGEN, ZARXIO
Pegfilgrastim NEULASTA
Sargramostim LEUKINE
Tbo-filgrastim GRANIX
TREATMENT OF SICKLE CELL ANEMIA
Hydroxyurea DROXIA, HYDREA

Figure 42.1
Summary of drugs for the treatment of anemia.

II. AGENTS USED TO TREAT ANEMIAS

A. Iron

Iron is stored in the intestinal mucosal cells, liver, spleen, and bone marrow as ferritin (an iron–protein complex) and delivered to the marrow for hemoglobin production by transferrin, a transport protein. Iron deficiency, the most common nutritional deficiency, results from a negative iron balance due to depletion of iron stores and/or inadequate intake, such as acute or chronic blood loss, menstruating or pregnant women, or periods of accelerated growth in children. In addition to general signs and symptoms of anemia, iron deficiency anemia may cause pica (hunger for ice, dirt, paper, etc.), koilonychias (upward curvature of the finger and toe nails), and soreness and cracking at the corners of the mouth.

1. **Mechanism of action:** Supplementation with elemental iron corrects the iron deficiency. The CDC recommends 150 to 180 mg/day of oral elemental iron administered in divided doses two to three times daily for patients with iron deficiency anemia.

2. **Pharmacokinetics:** Iron is absorbed after oral administration. Acidic conditions in the stomach keep iron in the reduced ferrous form, which is the more soluble form. Iron is then absorbed in the duodenum. [Note: The amount absorbed depends on the current body stores of iron. If iron stores are adequate, less iron is absorbed. If stores are low, more iron is absorbed.] The relative percentage of iron absorbed decreases with increasing doses. Oral preparations include *ferrous sulfate*, *ferrous fumarate*, *ferrous gluconate*, *polysaccharide–iron complex*, and *carbonyl iron* formulations. The percentage of elemental iron varies in each oral iron preparation (Figure 42.2). Parenteral formulations of iron, such as *iron dextran*, *sodium ferric gluconate*, *ferumoxytol*, *ferric carboxymaltose*, and *iron sucrose*, are also available. While parenteral administration treats iron deficiency rapidly, oral administration may take several weeks.

3. **Adverse effects:** Gastrointestinal (GI) disturbances caused by local irritation (abdominal pain, constipation, nausea, diarrhea) and dark stools are the most common adverse effects of oral iron supplements. Parenteral iron formulations may be used in those who cannot tolerate or inadequately absorb oral iron, as well as those receiving *erythropoietin* with hemodialysis or chemotherapy. Fatal hypersensitivity and anaphylactoid reactions can occur in patients receiving parenteral iron (mainly *iron dextran* formulations). A test dose should be administered prior to *iron dextran*. In addition, intravenous iron should be used cautiously in the

IRON FORMULATION	BRAND NAME(S)	ELEMENTAL IRON (%)	NOTES
Ferrous gluconate	Fergon, Ferro-Tab	12	• Less elemental iron, but similar tolerability to *ferrous sulfate*
Ferric ammonium citrate	Iron citrate	18	• Less bioavailable than ferrous salts • Must be reduced to ferrous form in the intestine
Ferrous sulfate	Fer-in-Sol, Feratab	20	• Most common oral iron supplement • Low cost with good effectiveness and tolerability
Ferrous sulfate, anhydrous	Slow-Fe	30	• Extended-release formulation of *ferrous sulfate* (once-daily dosing) • Higher cost than *ferrous sulfate*
Ferrous fumarate	Ferretts, Ferrimin, Hemocyte	33	• Similar effectiveness and tolerability to *ferrous sulfate* • Almost no taste compared to other iron salts
Carbonyl iron	Icar, Feosol	100	• Microparticles of purified iron • Dissolves in the stomach to form HCl salt to be absorbed • Less toxic than iron salts due to slower absorption rate (continued iron release for 1 to 2 days)
Polysaccharide-iron complex	Bifera, NovaFerrum, Nu-Iron 150	100	• Tasteless and odorless • Once-daily elemental iron dose similar to twice-daily *ferrous sulfate*

Figure 42.2
Characteristics of various iron formulations.

presence of active infections. [Note: Iron is essential for bacterial growth.]

B. Folic acid (folate)

The primary use of *folic acid* is in treating deficiency states that arise from inadequate levels of the vitamin. Folate deficiency may be caused by 1) increased demand (for example, pregnancy and lactation), 2) poor absorption caused by pathology of the small intestine, 3) alcoholism, or 4) treatment with drugs that are dihydrofolate reductase inhibitors (for example, *methotrexate* and *trimethoprim*), drugs that directly inhibit DNA synthesis (for example, *azathioprine* and *zidovudine*), or drugs that reduce folate absorption (for example, *phenytoin* and *phenobarbital*). A primary result of *folic acid* deficiency is megaloblastic anemia (large-sized red blood cells), which is caused by diminished synthesis of purines and pyrimidines. This leads to an inability of erythropoietic tissue to make DNA and, thereby, proliferate (Figure 42.3). [Note: To avoid neurological complications of vitamin B_{12} deficiency, it is important to evaluate the basis of the megaloblastic anemia prior to instituting therapy. Both vitamin B_{12} and folate deficiency can cause similar symptoms.]

Folic acid is rapidly absorbed in the jejunum unless abnormal pathology is present. Oral *folic acid* administration is nontoxic and at high doses, excess vitamin is excreted in the urine. Rare hypersensitivity reactions to parenteral injections have been reported.

C. Cyanocobalamin and hydroxocobalamin (vitamin B_{12})

Deficiencies of vitamin B_{12} can result from either low dietary levels or, more commonly, poor absorption of the vitamin due to the failure of gastric parietal cells to produce intrinsic factor (as in pernicious anemia), or a loss of activity of the receptor needed for intestinal uptake of the vitamin. Nonspecific malabsorption syndromes or gastric resection can also cause vitamin B_{12} deficiency. In addition to general signs and symptoms of anemia, vitamin B_{12} deficiency anemia may cause tingling (pins and needles) in the hands and feet, difficulty walking, dementia, and, in extreme cases, hallucinations, paranoia, or schizophrenia. [Note: *Folic acid* administration alone reverses the hematologic abnormality and, thus, masks the vitamin B_{12} deficiency, which can then proceed to severe neurologic dysfunction and disease. The cause of megaloblastic anemia needs to be determined in order to be specific in terms of treatment. Therefore, megaloblastic anemia should not be treated with *folic acid* alone but, rather, with a combination of *folic acid* and *vitamin B_{12}*.]

The vitamin may be administered orally (for dietary deficiencies), intramuscularly, or deep subcutaneously (for pernicious anemia). Intramuscular *hydroxocobalamin* [hye-drox-oh-koe-BAL-a-min] is preferred since it has a rapid response, is highly protein bound, and maintains longer plasma levels. In patients with malabsorption, such as in bariatric surgery (surgical treatment for obesity), vitamin B_{12} supplementation as *cyanocobalamin* [sye-an-oh-koe-BAL-a-min] is required daily in high oral doses or monthly by the parenteral route. This vitamin is nontoxic even in large doses. In pernicious anemia, therapy must be continued for life.

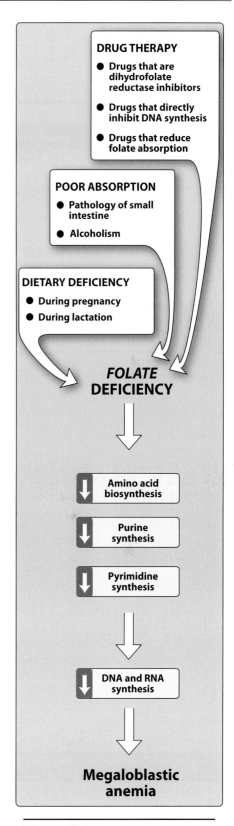

Figure 42.3
Causes and consequences of *folic acid* depletion.

D. Erythropoietin and darbepoetin

Peritubular cells in the kidneys respond to hypoxia and synthesize and release *erythropoietin* [ee-rith-ro-POI-eh-tin; EPO], a glycoprotein. EPO stimulates stem cells to differentiate into proerythroblasts and promotes the release of reticulocytes from the marrow and initiation of hemoglobin formation. Thus, EPO regulates red blood cell proliferation and differentiation in bone marrow. Human *erythropoietin* (*epoetin alfa*), produced by recombinant DNA technology, is effective in the treatment of anemia caused by end-stage renal disease, human immunodeficiency virus infection, bone marrow disorders, prematurity, and malignancy. A long-acting form of *erythropoietin*, *darbepoetin* [dar-be-POE-e-tin], has a half-life about three times that of *epoetin alfa* due to the addition of two carbohydrate chains. These agents are well tolerated and are administered intravenously in renal dialysis patients or subcutaneously for other indications. Side effects such as blood pressure elevation and arthralgia may occur in some cases. [Note: The former may be due to increases in peripheral vascular resistance and/or blood viscosity.] In addition, iron supplementation may be required to ensure an adequate response.

When *epoetin alfa* is used to target hemoglobin concentrations over 11 g/dL, serious cardiovascular events (such as thrombosis and severe hypertension), increased risk of death, shortened time to tumor progression, and decreased survival have been observed. The recommendations for all patients receiving *epoetin alfa* or *darbepoetin* include a minimum effective dose that does not exceed a hemoglobin level of 12 g/dL, and a hemoglobin level that does not rise by more than 1 g/dL over a 2-week period. Additionally, if the hemoglobin level exceeds 10 g/dL, doses of *epoetin alfa* or *darbepoetin* should be reduced or treatment should be discontinued. Neither agent has any value in the acute treatment of anemia due to their delayed onset of action.

III. AGENTS USED TO TREAT NEUTROPENIA

Myeloid growth factors or granulocyte colony-stimulating factors (G-CSF), such as *filgrastim* [fil-GRAS-tim], *tbo-filgrastim*, and *pegfilgrastim* [peg-fil-GRAS-tim], and granulocyte-macrophage colony-stimulating factors (GM-CSF), such as *sargramostim* [sar-GRA-moe-stim], stimulate granulocyte production in the marrow to increase neutrophil counts and reduce the duration of severe neutropenia. These agents are typically used prophylactically to reduce the risk of neutropenia following chemotherapy and bone marrow transplantation. *Filgrastim* and *sargramostim* can be dosed either subcutaneously or intravenously, whereas *tbo-filgrastim* and *pegfilgrastim* are dosed subcutaneously only. The main difference between the available agents is in the frequency of dosing. *Filgrastim*, *tbo-filgrastim*, and *sargramostim* are dosed once a day beginning 24 to 72 hours after chemotherapy, until the absolute neutrophil count (ANC) reaches 5000 to 10,000/µL. *Pegfilgrastim* is a pegylated form of G-CSF, resulting in a longer half-life when compared to the other agents, and is administered 24 hours after chemotherapy, as a single dose, rather than once daily. Monitoring of ANC is typically not necessary with *pegfilgrastim*. There is no evidence to show superiority of one agent over another in terms of efficacy, safety, or tolerability. Bone pain is a common adverse effect with these agents.

IV. AGENTS USED TO TREAT SICKLE CELL DISEASE

A. Hydroxyurea

Hydroxyurea [hye-DROX-ee-yoo-ree-ah] is an oral ribonucleotide reductase inhibitor that can reduce the frequency of painful sickle cell crises (Figure 42.4). In sickle cell disease, *hydroxyurea* increases fetal hemoglobin (HbF) levels, thus diluting the abnormal hemoglobin S (HbS). Polymerization of HbS is delayed and reduced in treated patients, so that painful crises are not caused by sickled cells blocking capillaries and causing tissue anoxia. A clinical response may take three to six months. Important side effects of *hydroxyurea* include bone marrow suppression and cutaneous vasculitis. It is important that *hydroxyurea* is administered under the supervision of a provider experienced in the treatment of sickle cell disease. *Hydroxyurea* is also used off-label to treat acute myelogenous leukemia, psoriasis, and polycythemia vera.

Figure 42.5 provides a summary of medications used in the management of anemia.

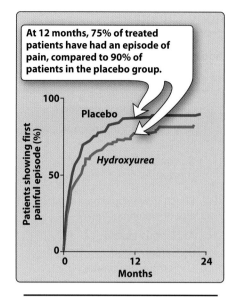

Figure 42.4
Effect of treatment with *hydroxyurea* on the percentage of sickle cell patients experiencing first painful episode.

MEDICATION	ADVERSE EFFECTS	DRUG INTERACTIONS	MONITORING PARAMETERS
TREATMENT OF ANEMIA			
Cyanocobalamin/B_{12}	Injection site pain Arthralgia Dizziness Headache Nasopharyngitis Anaphylaxis	Proton pump inhibitors—may decrease oral absorption of vitamin B_{12}	Vitamin B_{12} Folate Iron
Erythropoietin/epoetin alfa	Edema Pruritus Nausea/vomiting Hypertension CVA Thrombosis	*Darbepoetin alfa*—duplication of therapy can lead to increased adverse events	H/H Serum ferritin Blood pressure
Darbepoetin alfa	Edema Dyspnea Hypertension CVA Thrombosis	*Epoetin alfa*—duplication of therapy can lead to increased adverse events	H/H Serum ferritin Blood pressure
Folic acid	Bad taste in mouth Nausea Confusion Irritability	*Cholestyramine*—may interfere with absorption	CBC Serum folate
Iron	Pruritus N/V/D Headache Anaphylaxis	*Deferoxamine*—chelates iron *Dimercaprol*—chelates iron	H/H Serum iron TIBC Transferrin Reticulocyte count
TREATMENT OF SICKLE CELL ANEMIA			
Hydroxyurea	Myelosuppression Skin ulcer Secondary leukemia Elevated liver enzymes	HIV medications—*hydroxyurea* can decrease CD4 counts Salicylates—increase bleeding risk *Probenecid*—↑ uric acid	CBC

Figure 42.5
Medications for the management of anemia. CBC = complete blood count; CVA = cerebrovascular accident; H/H = hemoglobin and hematocrit; N/V/D = nausea/vomiting/diarrhea; TIBC = total iron binding capacity.

Study Questions

Choose the ONE best answer.

42.1 Which is an appropriate treatment for a nutritional anemia that presents as a hunger for ice and/or upward curvature of the fingernails?

  A. Vitamin B_{12} (cyanocobalamin)
  B. Folic acid
  C. Vitamin D
  D. Iron

Correct answer = D. Vitamin B_{12}, folic acid, and iron deficiencies all contribute to anemia, but iron deficiency is associated with pica (hunger for ice or dirt) and koilonychias (upward curvature of toenails/fingernails). Vitamin D deficiency does exist but does not cause anemia.

42.2 Which iron supplement contains the highest percentage of elemental iron?

  A. Ferrous sulfate
  B. Carbonyl iron
  C. Ferrous gluconate
  D. Ferric ammonium citrate

Correct answer = B. Ferrous sulfate contains 20% (or 30% in the anhydrous formulation), ferrous gluconate contains 12%, and ferric ammonium citrate contains 18% of elemental iron. These are all well below the percent of elemental iron in carbonyl iron, which contains 100% elemental iron.

42.3 A 56-year-old woman is discovered to have megaloblastic anemia. Her past medical history is significant for alcoholism. Which would be the best treatment option for this patient?

  A. Oral vitamin B_{12}
  B. Parenteral vitamin B_{12}
  C. Oral folic acid
  D. Oral vitamin B_{12} with oral folic acid

Correct answer = D. The patient has a history of alcoholism, which would suggest folic acid deficiency anemia. However, folic acid administration alone reverses the hematologic abnormality and masks possible vitamin B_{12} deficiency, which can then proceed to severe neurologic dysfunction and disease. The cause of megaloblastic anemia needs to be determined in order to be specific in terms of treatment. Therefore, megaloblastic anemia should not be treated with folic acid alone but, rather, with a combination of folic acid and vitamin B_{12}.

42.4 A 60-year-old woman presents to her primary care physician complaining of dizziness and fatigue. Following laboratory testing, the patient is diagnosed with iron deficiency anemia, and oral iron supplementation is needed. Which would be the most appropriate dosing regimen for the patient?

  A. Ferrous fumarate 325 mg once daily
  B. Ferrous gluconate 256 mg once daily
  C. Polysaccharide–iron complex 150 mg two to three times daily
  D. Ferrous sulfate 325 mg two to three times daily

Correct answer = D. The recommended dose of iron supplementation in iron deficiency anemia is typically about 150 mg of elemental iron in two to three divided doses. Extended-release formulations (such as polysaccharide–iron complex) may be dosed once daily. Ferrous sulfate 325 mg contains approximately 65 mg of elemental iron, ferrous fumarate 325 mg contains about 107 mg elemental iron, ferrous gluconate 256 mg contains approximately 30 mg elemental iron, and polysaccharide–iron complex 150 mg contains 150 mg elemental iron.

42.5 A 63-year-old female patient with anemia secondary to chronic kidney disease and a hemoglobin level of 8.6 g/dL is treated with epoetin alfa. Eight days after the initial dose of epoetin alfa, the patient's hemoglobin is 10.5 g/dL. Which would be the next step in the management of this patient's anemia?

  A. Discontinue epoetin alfa
  B. Discontinue epoetin alfa and initiate darbepoetin
  C. Continue epoetin alfa
  D. Increase the dose of epoetin alfa

Correct answer = A. Hemoglobin has increased to more than 10 g/dL and more than 1 g/dL in 2 weeks, so epoetin alfa should be discontinued or the dose reduced. Switching to darbepoetin, continuing epoetin alfa, or increasing the dose of epoetin alfa would continue to increase hemoglobin and lead to increased risk of cardiovascular events.

42.6 Which drug would be beneficial to reduce the frequency of painful crises in a patient with sickle cell disease?

A. Epoetin alfa
B. Filgrastim
C. Hydroxyurea
D. Sargramostim

Correct answer = C. Clinical evidence supports the use of hydroxyurea for reducing the frequency and severity of painful sickle cell crises during the course of sickle cell disease. Epoetin alfa helps increase hemoglobin and red blood cell production in anemias secondary to chronic kidney disease, HIV, bone marrow disorders, and other disorders. Filgrastim and sargramostim stimulate granulocyte production in the marrow to increase the neutrophil counts and reduce the duration of severe neutropenia.

42.7 After completing his last cycle of chemotherapy, a 68-year-old man received a dose of pegfilgrastim prophylactically to reduce his risk of neutropenia. Twenty-four hours later, he returned to clinic to receive an additional dose of pegfilgrastim and was told he did not need another dose. Which would explain the rationale behind this recommendation?

A. Absolute neutrophil count is above 1000/μL
B. Pegfilgrastim is given as single dose
C. Next dose of pegfilgrastim is due 72 hours after the first dose
D. Next dose of pegfilgrastim is due 48 hours after the first dose

Correct answer = B. Pegfilgrastim is a pegylated form of G-CSF and has a longer half-life; therefore, it is administered as a single dose with no additional doses needed. Monitoring of the ANC is not necessary with pegfilgrastim due to the pharmacokinetics of the drug.

42.8 A patient has been taking ferrous sulfate 325 mg twice daily for two weeks and is complaining of a bad taste after each dose. Which once-daily, oral iron formulations would improve tolerability and provide a similar total daily dose of elemental iron as twice-daily ferrous sulfate?

A. Ferric ammonium citrate 25 mg
B. Ferrous gluconate 100 mg
C. Ferrous sulfate, anhydrous 142 mg
D. Polysaccharide–iron complex 150 mg

Correct answer = D. Once-daily polysaccharide–iron complex (150 mg = 150 mg elemental iron) is tasteless and odorless, with a similar total daily dose of elemental iron as ferrous sulfate 325 mg twice daily (130 mg elemental iron/day). Once-daily ferric ammonium citrate 25 mg (4.5 mg elemental iron) is less bioavailable than twice-daily ferrous sulfate. Ferrous sulfate and ferrous gluconate have similar tolerability, but once-daily ferrous gluconate has less elemental iron (12 mg elemental iron). Ferrous sulfate, anhydrous has better tolerability with the extended-release formulation, but has less elemental iron (43 mg elemental iron) administered once daily compared to twice daily ferrous sulfate.

42.9 Which patient with iron deficiency anemia would need the parenteral form of iron replacement?

A. 22-year-old woman with heavy menstrual periods
B. 58-year-old man with end stage renal disease on hemodialysis
C. 32-year-old woman in the first trimester of pregnancy
D. 40-year-old man with a diabetic foot infection

Correct answer = B. Clinical evidence supports the use of parenteral iron over oral iron in hemodialysis patients due to a significantly greater increase in hemoglobin levels and lower incidence of treatment-related adverse events. Parenteral iron is also preferred in patients who cannot tolerate oral iron or who have iron malabsorption. Patients with heavy menstrual periods, who are pregnant, or who have chronic disease states, such as diabetes, and infections, should be administered an initial trial of oral iron.

42.10 An 81-year-old woman presents to the emergency department with progressive weakness, fatigue, confusion, and reports of seeing people in her house who were trying to hurt her but who were not physically present. Her physical exam was positive for pallor but negative for koilonychias or cracking at the corners of the mouth. Which deficiency would be the highest priority in this patient's workup?

A. Vitamin B_{12}
B. Iron
C. Folate
D. Calcium

Correct answer = A. Based on the presentation of confusion and hallucinations, vitamin B_{12} deficiency should be considered the highest priority. Second priority would be to assess folate deficiency, since symptoms are similar to vitamin B_{12} deficiency. Iron would be the third priority due to the patient's age, even without the presence of koilonychias or cracking of the mouth. Last priority would be to assess age-related deficiencies in calcium, which could lead to fatigue as well as muscle cramps, poor appetite, and abnormal heart rhythms.

Drugs for Dermatologic Disorders

Stacey Curtis and Cary Mobley

43

I. OVERVIEW

The skin is a complex and dynamic organ comprised of cells, tissues, and biomolecules that coordinate to provide many interdependent functions, including protection from environmental insults from noxious chemicals, infectious pathogens, and ultraviolet radiation, as well as serving vital functions in wound repair, sensation, thermoregulation, and vitamin D synthesis. This chapter focuses on drugs that are used for some of the more common skin conditions including psoriasis, acne, rosacea, infections, pigmentation disorders, and alopecia. Drugs for acne, superficial bacterial infections, and rosacea are summarized in Figure 43.1. [Note: Agents for fungal infections of the skin are covered in the chapter on antifungals (see Chapter 33).]

II. TOPICAL PREPARATIONS

The skin is composed of two main layers, the epidermis and the dermis (Figure 43.2). The epidermis is composed of several layers of keratinocytes, with the outermost layer, the stratum corneum, serving as the primary barrier to external insults. The dermis, located between the epidermis and the subcutaneous tissue, is composed of connective tissue and contains many specialized structures, such as sweat glands, sebaceous glands, hair follicles, and blood vessels. Defects in skin structure and function induced by genetics and by environmental insults can lead to numerous dermatological conditions, many of which can be controlled or cured with the use of drug therapy.

Use of topical agents for treatment of dermatologic disorders is not only convenient but also can minimize systemic adverse effects. Common topical dosage forms include sprays, powders, lotions, creams, pastes, gels, ointments, and foams. The choice of which dosage form to use for a particular condition involves factors such as occlusiveness, ease of application, patient acceptance, and drug potency. The choice also includes consideration of stratum corneum thickness and integrity, as well as the type, location, and extent of the lesions being treated.

AGENTS FOR ACNE	
Adapalene	DIFFERIN
Azelaic acid	AZELEX
Benzoyl peroxide	VARIOUS
Clindamycin	CLEOCIN
Dapsone	ACZONE
Doxycycline	DORYX
Erythromycin	VARIOUS
Isotretinoin	VARIOUS
Minocycline	VARIOUS
Salicylic acid	VARIOUS
Tazarotene	TAZORAC
Tretinoin	RETIN-A

AGENTS FOR SUPERFICIAL BACTERIAL INFECTIONS	
Bacitracin	VARIOUS
Gentamicin	VARIOUS
Mupirocin	BACTROBAN
Neomycin	VARIOUS
Polymyxin	VARIOUS
Retapamulin	ALTABAX

AGENTS USED FOR ROSACEA	
Azelaic acid	FINACEA
Brimonidine	MIRVASO
Doxycycline	ORACEA
Metronidazole	METROGEL
Oxymetazoline	RHOFADE
Pimecrolimus	ELIDEL
Sulfacetamide sodium	VARIOUS

Figure 43.1
Summary of drugs for acne, superficial bacterial infections, and rosacea.

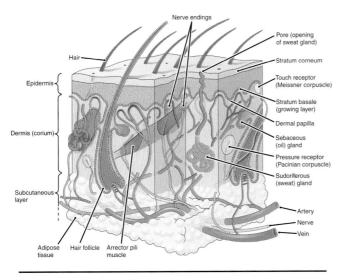

Figure 43.2
Cross section of the skin.

III. AGENTS FOR ACNE

Acne vulgaris (common acne) is a common skin disorder that occurs in about 85% of individuals 12 to 24 years of age, coinciding with an increase in androgen production. [Note: Use of oral contraceptives may help decrease circulating levels of free androgen and reduce symptoms of acne in females (see Chapter 25).] It begins with excessive proliferation and adhesion of skin cells that form a keratin plug (microcomedone), which closes the hair follicle (Figure 43.3). Within the closed hair follicle, skin cells are shed and sebum production continues. This causes the follicle to dilate to form a comedone.

The sebum serves as a nutrient for the proliferation of <u>Propionibacterium acnes</u>, which along with other factors, triggers an inflammatory response that causes the formation of a pustule or papule—the pimple. If this progresses, the follicular wall can rupture, leading to the formation of an inflamed nodule. Different medications can be used alone or in combination to affect one or more of these pathological components to clear the acne lesions.

A. Antibiotics

Topical and oral antibiotics are commonly used in acne, with oral antibiotics reserved for moderate-to-severe acne. The use of antibiotics in acne is based not only on their antibacterial effects but also on antiinflammatory properties, which can be significant for some antibiotics, such as the tetracyclines. The most common topical antibiotics used are *clindamycin* [klin-da-MYE-sin] (solution or gel) and *erythromycin* [er-ITH-roe-MYE-sin] (cream, gel, or lotion). The most common oral antibiotics used for acne are the tetracyclines, *doxycycline* [DOX-i-SYE-kleen] and *minocycline* [mi-no-SYE-kleen], and the macrolides, *erythromycin* and *azithromycin* [a-ZITH-roe-MYE-sin]. Topical forms tend to be well tolerated. For oral tetracyclines, common adverse effects are gastrointestinal disturbances and photosensitivity, and for the macrolides, gastrointestinal disturbances are common. The most

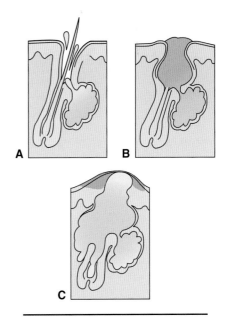

Figure 43.3
Acne vulgaris. **A.** Normal sebaceous gland and hair follicle. **B.** Comedone formation. **C.** Pustule formation.

significant concern in the use of both topical and oral antibiotics is the development of bacterial resistance. Some measures that can be taken to limit the development of resistance include using antibiotics only in combination with other acne agents, using oral antibiotics for the shortest time possible, and using low-dose oral antibiotics (subantimicrobial dosing) when possible. Also, once acne lesions are clear, patients should follow with topical maintenance therapy with effective nonantibiotic topical agents, such as *benzoyl peroxide* and the retinoids. Antibiotics are covered in more detail in the chapters on anti-infective therapy (see Chapter 30).

B. Azelaic acid

Azelaic [aze-eh-LAY-ik] *acid* is a naturally occurring dicarboxylic acid that has antibacterial activity against P. acnes through its ability to inhibit protein synthesis. It also exhibits anti-inflammatory activity, inhibits the division and differentiation of keratinocytes, and shows comedolytic activity. *Azelaic acid* exhibits a lightening effect on hyperpigmented skin, which makes it useful in patients who experience dyspigmentation as a consequence of inflammatory acne. It is available as a cream and a gel, and the major adverse effects are mild and transient pruritus, burning, stinging and tingling.

C. Benzoyl peroxide

Benzoyl peroxide [BEN-zoyl per-OX-ide] is a commonly used topical medication that improves acne primarily through its bactericidal action, where its oxidizing activity is lethal for P. acnes. It shows no bacterial resistance. The agent also reduces inflammation and has comedolytic activity. It is available in topical washes, foams, creams, and gels. The major adverse effects are dry skin, irritation, and bleaching of bedding and clothing. It may also cause contact dermatitis in some patients.

D. Dapsone

Dapsone [DAP-sone] is a sulfone that exhibits both anti-inflammatory and antibacterial activity and is effective at reducing inflammatory acne lesion counts, with some reduction in noninflammatory lesions as well. The anti-inflammatory activity derives partly from its ability to interfere with neutrophilic function and to reduce the production of tumor necrosis factor-α (TNF-α) by mononuclear cells. *Dapsone* is available as a topical gel with the most common adverse effects being transient oiliness, dryness, and erythema, which may be at least in part due to the nondrug part of the formulation.

E. Retinoids

Retinoids are vitamin A derivatives that interact with retinoid receptors to regulate gene expression in a manner that normalizes keratinocyte differentiation and reduces hyperproliferation (giving them comedolytic activity). They also reduce sebum production and inflammation. These diverse effects make retinoids useful for acne, as well as a variety of other conditions, including psoriasis and severe rosacea. For acne vulgaris, the topical retinoids *tretinoin* [TRET-i-no-in], *adapalene* [a-DAP-a-leen], and *tazarotene* [ta-ZAR-oh-teen] are used for mild and moderate forms, whereas the oral retinoid *isotretinoin* [eye-so-TRET-i-no-in] is reserved for severe nodular forms of acne.

Adverse effects of the topical retinoids include erythema, desquamation, burning, and stinging. These effects often decrease with time. Other potential adverse effects include dry mucous membranes and photosensitivity. Patients should be cautioned to wear sunscreen. Though their systemic absorption is generally limited, use should be avoided during pregnancy, particularly topical *tazarotene*, which is the most teratogenic of the three topical retinoids for acne. Oral *isotretinoin*, used in severe acne, has potentially serious adverse effects including psychiatric effects and birth defects. It is contraindicated in women who are pregnant or intend to become pregnant.

F. Salicylic acid

Topical *salicylic* [sal-i-SIL-ik] *acid*, a β-hydroxy acid, penetrates the pilosebaceous unit and works as an exfoliant to clear comedones. Its comedolytic effects are not as pronounced as those of the retinoids. The drug has mild anti-inflammatory activity and is keratolytic at higher concentrations. *Salicylic acid* is used as a treatment for mild acne and is available in many over-the-counter facial washes and medicated treatment pads. Mild skin peeling, dryness, and local irritation are adverse effects.

G. Sulfacetamide sodium

Sulfacetamide sodium [SUL-fa-SET-a-mide SOE-dee-um] interferes with bacterial growth and is often combined with sulfur, a keratolytic agent. The combination is used to treat inflammatory acne lesions when present. It is also used to treat rosacea (see below). The product is available as cleanser, cream, foam, gel, lotion, pads, suspension, and a wash. The most common adverse effects include contact dermatitis, erythema, pruritus, Stevens-Johnson syndrome, and xeroderma.

IV. AGENTS FOR SUPERFICIAL BACTERIAL INFECTIONS

Several gram-positive and gram-negative bacteria can cause various superficial skin infections, such as folliculitis and impetigo, as well as deeper infections, such as erysipelas and cellulitis. In more severe cases, these infections can lead to ulceration and systemic infections. This section covers topical antibacterial agents that can be used for the treatment and prevention of certain superficial skin infections.

A. Bacitracin

Bacitracin [bas-i-TRAY-sin] is a peptide antibiotic active against many gram-positive organisms. It is used mainly in topical formulations; if used systemically, it is toxic. *Bacitracin* is mostly used for the prevention of skin infections after burns or minor scrapes. It is frequently found in combination products with *neomycin* and/or *polymyxin* (see below). It is available as an ointment.

B. Gentamicin

Gentamicin [GEN-ta-MYE-sin] interferes with bacterial protein synthesis targeting gram-negative organisms. This agent is often used

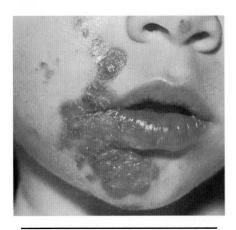

Figure 43.4
Impetigo on the face.

in combination with other agents to treat skin infections caused by gram-negative organisms. It is available as a cream and an ointment. Topical use of this agent rarely causes systemic side effects.

C. Mupirocin

Mupirocin [mue-PIR-oh-sin] is a protein synthesis inhibitor targeting gram-positive organisms. It is useful in treating impetigo (a contagious skin infection caused by streptococci or staphylococci; Figure 43.4) and other serious gram-positive skin infections, including infections caused by *methicillin*-resistant <u>Staphylococcus aureus</u>. It is available as a cream and an ointment. [Note: Intranasal *mupirocin* may be used to eradicate colonization with *methicillin*-resistant <u>S. aureus</u> and reduce the risk of infection in hospitalized patients.] The most common adverse effects are pruritus, skin rash, and burning.

D. Neomycin

Neomycin [nee-oh-MY-sin] interferes with bacterial protein synthesis and is active primarily against gram-negative organisms, with some activity against gram-positive organisms. This agent is often formulated with other topical anti-infectives, such as *bacitracin* and *polymyxin* to treat skin infections. The combination is available as an ointment. Common adverse effects associated with the combination agents include contact dermatitis, erythema, rash, and urticaria.

E. Polymyxin

Polymyxin [paw-lee-MIX-in] *B* is a cyclic hydrophobic peptide that disrupts the bacterial cell membrane of gram-negative organisms. As noted above, it is commonly combined with *bacitracin* ("double antibiotic") and *neomycin* with *bacitracin* ("triple antibiotic") in topical products used for the prevention of skin infections after minor skin trauma. These combinations are available as ointments.

F. Retapamulin

Retapamulin [RE-te-PAM-ue-lin] is a protein synthesis inhibitor active against gram-positive organisms. It is indicated for the treatment of impetigo. The only available dosage form is an ointment, and the most common adverse effects are pruritus and skin irritation.

V. AGENTS USED FOR ROSACEA

Rosacea is a common inflammatory disorder affecting the central portion of facial skin. Common clinical features include facial erythema (flushing) and inflammatory lesions that are similar to acne lesions. The signs, symptoms, and severity determine the treatment for this disorder. *Azelaic acid* is one potential treatment for rosacea. Other topical and oral products for rosacea are described below.

A. Brimonidine

Brimonidine [bri-MOE-ni-deen] is an alpha$_2$ adrenoceptor agonist that reduces erythema through vasoconstriction. It is available as a gel and its major adverse effects are burning, localized warm feeling, and flushing. [Note: *Brimonidine* ophthalmic solution is used for the treatment of glaucoma.]

B. Doxycycline

Doxycycline [DOX-i-SYE-kleen] is an antibacterial agent used orally at low doses, where it exerts its effects on rosacea, not by killing bacteria, but rather through its anti-inflammatory effects. It is available as a capsule and tablet, and its major adverse effects include diarrhea, nausea, dyspepsia, and nasopharyngitis.

C. Metronidazole

Metronidazole [me-troe-NI-da-zole] is an antibacterial agent used topically for rosacea. It is believed to work in rosacea through anti-inflammatory or immunosuppressive effects, rather than through its antibacterial effects. It is available as a cream, gel, and lotion, and its major adverse effects are burning, erythema, skin irritation, xeroderma, and acne vulgaris.

D. Oxymetazoline

Oxymetazoline [ox-e-meh-TAZ-oh-leen] is an α_1 adrenoceptor agonist that reduces erythema through vasoconstriction. It is available as a cream, and its major adverse effects are application site dermatitis, worsening inflammatory lesions, site pruritus, site erythema, and a burning sensation.

E. Pimecrolimus

Pimecrolimus [pim-e-KROE-li-mus] is a topical calcineurin inhibitor/immunosuppressant agent that decreases inflammation. It is available as a cream, and its major adverse effects are burning, irritation, pruritus, and erythema.

VI. AGENTS FOR PIGMENTATION DISORDERS

The color of skin is derived from melanin produced by melanocytes in the basal layer of the epidermis. When the melanocytes are damaged, the melanin levels are affected, which ultimately leads to pigmentation disorders. If the body does not make enough melanin, the skin gets lighter (hypopigmentation). If the body makes too much melanin, the skin gets darker (hyperpigmentation). Pigmentation disorders can be widespread and affect many areas of the skin or they can be localized. Agents used for pigmentation disorders are discussed below and summarized in Figure 43.5.

A. Hydroquinone

Hydroquinone [HYE-droe-KWIN-one] is a topical skin-whitening agent that reduces hyperpigmentation associated with freckles and melasma (brown to gray-brown patches on the skin; Figure 43.6). It is often used in combination with topical retinoids to treat the signs

AGENTS FOR PIGMENTATION DISORDERS
Hydroquinone GENERIC ONLY
Methoxsalen GENERIC ONLY
Tazarotene AVAGE

AGENTS FOR PSORIASIS
Acitretin SORIATANE
Adalimumab HUMIRA
Apremilast OTEZLA
Brodalumab SILIQ
Calcipotriene DOVONEX
Calcitriol VECTICAL
Certolizumab pegol CIMZIA
Coal tar VARIOUS
Etanercept ENBREL
Golimumab SIMPONI
Guselkumab TREMFYA
Infliximab REMICADE
Ixekizumab TALTZ
Methotrexate VARIOUS
Salicylic acid VARIOUS
Secukinumab COSENTYX
Tazarotene TAZORAC
Ustekinumab STELARA

AGENTS FOR ALOPECIA
Finasteride PROPECIA
Minoxidil ROGAINE

Figure 43.5
Summary of drugs for pigmentation disorders, psoriasis, and alopecia.

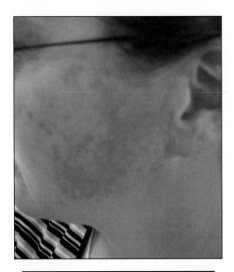

Figure 43.6
Melasma on the face.

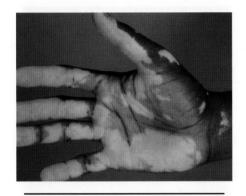

Figure 43.7
The palm is frequently affected by vitiligo.

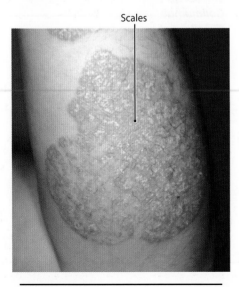

Scales

Figure 43.8
Psoriasis. A large, scaly, erythematous plaque.

of photoaging. The mechanism of action of *hydroquinone* is through inhibition of the tyrosinase, an enzyme required for melanin synthesis. *Hydroquinone* lightens the skin temporarily and is commonly used as a 4% preparation. It should not be used in higher concentrations, or in excessive quantities for an extended duration, as it is associated with possible carcinogenicity. The most common adverse effect is local skin irritation.

B. Methoxsalen

Methoxsalen [meth-OX-a-len] is a psoralen photoactive agent that stimulates melanocytes and is used as a repigmentation agent for patients with vitiligo (Figure 43.7). It must be photoactivated by UV radiation to form a DNA adduct inhibiting DNA replication by a method called PUVA (psoralen plus UVA radiation). *Methoxsalen* inhibits cell proliferation and promotes cell differentiation of epithelial cells. Topical *methoxsalen* may be used for small patches of vitiligo, and oral therapy is used for more widespread disease. Because of the possibilities for aging of the skin and carcinogenicity, it is used with caution.

C. Tazarotene

Tazarotene is a topical retinoid, which decreases hyperpigmentation, and is sometimes used to treat the signs of photoaging. It is available as a cream, foam, and gel. The most common adverse effects include itching, burning, erythema, rash, and dryness.

VII. AGENTS FOR PSORIASIS

Psoriasis is a chronic autoimmune skin disease that manifests as epidermal hyperplasia and dermal inflammation, which can range from mild to disabling. It is a condition that has significant genetic associations and it tends to wax and wane, with flare-ups that can be triggered by a number of environmental factors including stress and skin trauma. There are several forms of psoriasis, with the most common form being plaque psoriasis. Plaque psoriasis is characterized by the presence of sharply demarcated, thick, erythematous plaques that are usually covered by dry silvery-white scales (Figure 43.8). The plaques range in size from 1 square centimeter to several square centimeters. In mild-to-moderate cases, these plaques cover less than 5% of the body surface area, but in more severe cases, they can cover more than 20% of the body. Therapies may target inflammation and the abnormal immune response, as well as epidermal hyperproliferation.

A. Apremilast

Apremilast [a-PRE-mi-last] is an oral agent approved for moderate to severe plaque psoriasis. It works by inhibiting phosphodiesterase-4, which ultimately leads to reduced production of several inflammatory mediators in psoriasis. The most common adverse effects are diarrhea, nausea, and headache. Depression may also occur. Strong CYP450 inducers (for example, *carbamazepine*, *phenytoin*) may reduce the efficacy of *apremilast*, and coadministration is not recommended.

B. Biologic agents

Biologics are agents isolated from natural sources, including humans, animals, and microorganisms. They can be composed of sugars, proteins, or nucleic acids or complex combinations of these substances. The biologics approved for psoriasis are all injectable, antibody-based proteins produced by recombinant DNA technology. They are used for moderate-to-severe psoriasis and their mechanism of action results from their interaction with specific cytokines that induce or mediate T-cell effector function, which is important in autoimmune diseases such as psoriasis. For example, several biologics target TNF-α, which plays multiple roles in psoriasis pathogenesis, including the stimulation of keratinocyte proliferation, neutrophils, and the release of proinflammatory cytokines. The TNF-α blockers include *etanercept* [ee-TAN-er-sept], *infliximab* [in-FLIKS-e-mab], *adalimumab* [a-da-LIM-yoo-mab], *certolizumab pegol* [ser-toe-LIZ-oo-mab PEG-ol], and *golimumab* [goe-LIM-ue-mab]. Biologics that target other cytokines important in psoriasis pathogenesis include the anti-IL-12/IL-23 medication, *ustekinumab* [YOO-sti-KIN-ue-mab]; the anti-IL-23 medication, *guselkumab* [gue-sel-KOO-mab]; and the anti-IL-17A medications, *secukinumab* [SEK-ue-KIN-ue-mab], *ixekizumab* [IX-ee-KIZ-ue-mab], and *brodalumab* [broe-DAL-ue-mab]. Though each agent has specific potential risks and adverse effects, among the adverse effects that they share include injection or infusion reactions and increased risk of infections due to their suppression of the immune system. In addition, because they are foreign proteins, there is a risk for the development of antidrug antibodies, which may affect efficacy over the course of therapy.

C. Keratolytic agents

Keratolytic agents such as *coal tar* and *salicylic acid* are effective in localized psoriasis, especially on the scalp. They improve corticosteroid penetration. *Coal tar* inhibits excessive skin cell proliferation and may also have anti-inflammatory effects. Because it is cosmetically unappealing, *coal tar* may have a low acceptance rate among patients and, consequently, its use has been largely supplanted by the newer topical agents.

D. Methotrexate

Methotrexate [meth-oh-TREX-ate] is the most commonly used systemic therapy for psoriasis. The drug is used in more severe forms of psoriasis and the primary mechanism of action is due to immunosuppressive activity, resulting from its ability to reduce DNA synthesis in cells of the immune system, particularly T lymphocytes. *Methotrexate* is available in oral and injectable dosage forms. Among the common potential adverse effects are nausea, diarrhea, mouth ulcers, hair loss, and skin rashes. The primary long-term risk is the potential for liver damage, and therefore, periodic liver function tests are required for patients using *methotrexate*.

E. Retinoids

Retinoids normalize keratinocyte differentiation and reduce hyperproliferation and inflammation. *Tazarotene* is a topical retinoid used

LOW STRENGTH	INTERMEDIATE STRENGTH	HIGH STRENGTH	VERY HIGH STRENGTH
Alclometasone dipropionate 0.05% (c, o)	Betamethasone dipropionate 0.05% (c)	Amcinonide 0.1% (c, l, o)	Betamethasone dipropionate 0.05% (o, g)
Clocortolone pivalate 0.1% (c)	Desonide 0.05% (c, l, o)	Betamethasone dipropionate, augmented 0.05% (c, l)	Clobetasol propionate 0.05% (c, g, o)
Fluocinolone acetonide 0.01% solution (s)	Desoximetasone 0.05% (c)	Desoximetasone 0.05% (o)	Diflorasone diacetate 0.05% (o)
Hydrocortisone base or acetate 0.25% to 2.5% (o, c)	Fluocinolone acetonide 0.025% (c, o)	Diflorasone diacetate 0.05% (o, c)	Fluocinonide 0.1% (c)
Triamcinolone acetonide 0.025% (c, l, o)	Flurandrenolide 0.025 to 0.5% (c, o)	Fluocinonide 0.05% (c, g, o, s)	Flurandrenolide 0.05% (l)
	Fluticasone propionate 0.005% to 0.05% (o, c)	Halcinonide 0.1% (c, o)	Halobetasol 0.05% (c, o)
	Hydrocortisone butyrate 0.1% (c, o, s)	Triamcinolone acetonide 0.5% (c, o)	
	Hydrocortisone valerate 0.2% (c, o)		
	Mometasone furoate 0.1% (c, o, l)		
	Triamcinolone acetonide 0.1% to 0.2% (c, o)		

Figure 43.9
Potency of various topical corticosteroids. c = cream; g = gel; o = ointment; s = solution.

for the treatment of plaque psoriasis. Adverse effects are similar to other topical retinoids described for acne. *Acitretin* [a-si-TRE-tin] is a second-generation retinoid used orally in the treatment of pustular forms of psoriasis. Similar to oral *isotretinoin* used in acne, *acitretin* is teratogenic and women must avoid pregnancy for at least 3 years after the use of this drug (due to its long duration of teratogenic potential). Ethanol is contraindicated with this agent. Cheilitis, pruritus, peeling skin, and hyperlipidemia are common adverse effects.

F. Topical corticosteroids

Topical corticosteroids have been a mainstay of psoriasis therapy for over 50 years, and are used in many other skin conditions as well. The available agents differ in potencies and are formulated in a variety of dosage forms, including solutions, lotions, creams, ointments, gels, and shampoo (Figure 43.9). Upon binding to intracellular corticosteroid receptors, these agents produce numerous effects that can be beneficial for psoriasis, including anti-inflammatory, antiproliferative, immunosuppressive, and vasoconstrictive effects. Potential adverse effects, especially with the long-term use of potent corticosteroids, include skin atrophy, striae, acneiform eruptions, dermatitis, local infections, and hypopigmentation. In children, excessive use of potent agents applied to a large surface area can cause systemic toxicity, including possible depression of the hypothalamic–pituitary–adrenal axis and growth retardation.

G. Vitamin D analogues

Calcipotriene [kal-sih-poh-TRY-een] and *calcitriol* [kal-si-TRYE-ol] are synthetic vitamin D_3 derivatives used topically to treat plaque psoriasis. They inhibit keratinocyte proliferation, enhance keratinocyte differentiation, and inhibit inflammation. *Calcipotriene* is available in cream, ointment, solution, and foam formulations, and *calcitriol* is available as an ointment. Potential adverse effects include itching, dryness, burning, irritation, and erythema.

VIII. AGENTS FOR ALOPECIA

Alopecia (baldness) is the partial or complete loss of hair from areas where hair normally grows. The most common type of hair loss is androgenic alopecia (also known as male pattern baldness), which can occur in men or women. Trichogenic agents are used to stimulate hair growth and slow the progression of hair loss.

A. Finasteride

Finasteride [fih-NAH-steh-ride] is an oral 5-α reductase inhibitor that blocks conversion of testosterone to the potent androgen 5-α dihydrotestosterone (DHT). High levels of DHT can cause the hair follicle to miniaturize and atrophy. *Finasteride* decreases scalp and serum DHT concentrations, thus inhibiting a key factor in the etiology of androgenic alopecia. [Note: *Finasteride* is used in higher doses for the treatment of benign prostatic hyperplasia (see Chapter 41).] Adverse effects include decreased libido, decreased ejaculation, and erectile dysfunction. The drug should not be used or handled in pregnancy, as it can cause hypospadias in a male fetus. Like *minoxidil*, use must be continued to maintain therapeutic benefits.

B. Minoxidil

Minoxidil [min-OX-i-dil], originally used as a systemic antihypertensive, was noted to have the adverse effect of increased hair growth. This adverse effect was turned into a therapeutic application in the treatment of alopecia. For hair loss, the drug is available as a nonprescription topical foam or solution, without systemic hypotensive effects. *Minoxidil* is effective at halting hair loss in both men and women and may produce hair growth in some patients. Although the mechanism of action is not fully known, it is believed to act, at least in part, by shortening the rest phase of the hair cycle. The drug must be used continuously to maintain effects on hair growth. The main adverse effects include erythema and pruritus.

Study Questions

Choose the ONE best answer.

43.1 Which is correct regarding the use of isotretinoin in the treatment of acne?

A. It is used topically in the treatment of acne.
B. It acts primarily on the corticosteroid receptors.
C. It is used for milder forms of acne.
D. It is contraindicated in pregnancy.

Correct answer = D. Isotretinoin is an oral retinoid reserved for more severe forms of acne. Retinoic acids play an important role in mammalian embryogenesis. Excessive amounts of retinoids such as isotretinoin have been shown to cause teratogenicity, but the exact molecular mechanism is not known.

43.2 Which drug is a topically applied antibiotic that is thought to work through anti-inflammatory effects to treat rosacea?

A. Brimonidine
B. Doxycycline
C. Metronidazole
D. Benzoyl peroxide

Correct answer = C. Metronidazole is an antibacterial agent used topically for rosacea. It is believed to work in rosacea through anti-inflammatory or immunosuppressive effects. Doxycycline is also used for its anti-inflammatory effects, but is used orally rather than topically.

43.3 Which drug is taken orally for more severe forms of psoriasis?

A. Etanercept
B. Calcipotriene
C. Tazarotene
D. Methotrexate

Correct answer = D. Methotrexate is the most commonly used systemic therapy for psoriasis. It is used in more severe forms of psoriasis and is available as an oral tablet and injection.

43.4 Which is correct regarding trichogenic agents?

A. Topically applied minoxidil is known for its hypotensive effects.
B. Once hair regrowth has been established with topically applied minoxidil, hair growth will be maintained after discontinuing its use.
C. Finasteride inhibits the 5-α reductase enzyme that controls the production of DHT from testosterone.
D. Both oral and topical minoxidil are commonly used for alopecia.

Correct answer = C. Androgenic alopecia is associated with DHT concentrations, and finasteride is known to inhibit the 5-α reductase enzyme required for the formation of DHT from testosterone. Only topical minoxidil is used for the treatment of alopecia. Both minoxidil and finasteride must be continued to maintain effects on hair growth.

43.5 A 12-year-old child has extensive psoriatic lesions covering his back. Which topical therapy would, with continuous use, most likely prevent him from reaching his full adult height?

A. Clobetasol propionate
B. Salicylic acid
C. Calcipotriene
D. Calcitriol

Correct answer = A. Excessive use of potent corticosteroids applied to a large surface area can cause systemic toxicity, including growth retardation.

43.6 A 17-year-old female has darkened spots on her face following resolution of acne lesions. Which agent is the best choice to treat her acne, if one of the goals of therapy is to lighten these spots?

A. Benzoyl peroxide
B. Azelaic acid
C. Clindamycin
D. Dapsone

Correct answer = B. Azelaic acid exhibits a lightening effect on hyperpigmented skin, which makes it useful in patients who experience dyspigmentation as a consequence of inflammatory acne. The other agents do not lighten the skin.

43.7 A 26-year-old woman is diagnosed with pustular psoriasis. She is getting married in 1 year and she would like to become pregnant and start a family within a year of her marriage. Which agent should be avoided for treatment of her psoriasis because the duration of its teratogenic potential may affect her plans for pregnancy?

A. Methotrexate
B. Triamcinolone acetonide
C. Infliximab
D. Acitretin

Correct answer = D. Acitretin is teratogenic and women must avoid pregnancy for at least 3 years after the use of this drug (due to the long duration of teratogenic potential).

43.8 A patient has been using topical minoxidil to manage his baldness for several years, but now wants to stop using the medication. What is the likely consequence of discontinuing this medication?

A. Hair loss will resume.
B. Hair growth will be maintained.
C. Hair color will start to turn gray.
D. Blood pressure will increase.

Correct answer = A. Topical minoxidil must be used continuously to maintain effects on hair growth. Minoxidil does not affect hair color, and topical minoxidil does not affect blood pressure.

43.9 A 16-year-old female has mild acne on her face. Which agent is the least appropriate choice for treating her acne?

A. Benzoyl peroxide
B. Topical clindamycin
C. Oral doxycycline
D. Adapalene

Correct answer = C. Oral antibiotics, such as doxycycline, are reserved for moderate to severe acne.

43.10 Which topical antibacterial agent targets gram-negative bacteria?

A. Gentamicin
B. Bacitracin
C. Mupirocin
D. Retapamulin

Correct answer = A. Gentamicin interferes with bacterial protein synthesis targeting gram-negative organisms and is often used in combination with other agents to treat skin infections caused by gram-negative organisms.

Clinical Toxicology

44

Dawn Sollee and Emily Jaynes Winograd

I. OVERVIEW

For thousands of years, poisons and the study of them (toxicology) have been woven into the rich fabric of the human experience. Homer and Aristotle described the poison arrow; Socrates was executed with poison hemlock; lead poisoning may have helped bring down the Roman Empire; Marilyn Monroe, Elvis Presley, and Michael Jackson all fatally overdosed on prescription medications. Toxins can be inhaled, insufflated (snorted), orally ingested, injected, and absorbed dermally (Figure 44.1). An understanding of the varied mechanisms of toxicity helps to develop an approach to treatment. This chapter provides an overview of the emergent management of the poisoned patient, as well as a brief review of some of the more common and interesting toxins, their mechanisms, clinical presentations, and clinical management.

II. EMERGENCY TREATMENT OF THE POISONED PATIENT

The first principle in the management of the poisoned patient is to treat the patient, not the poison. Airway, breathing, and circulation are assessed and addressed initially, along with any other immediately life-threatening toxic effect (for example, profound increases or decreases in blood pressure, heart rate, respirations, or body temperature, or any dangerous dysrhythmias). Acid/base and electrolyte disturbances, *acetaminophen* and salicylate blood levels, and results of other appropriate drug screens can be further assessed as laboratory results are obtained. After administering oxygen, obtaining intravenous access, and placing the patient on a cardiac monitor, the poisoned patient with altered mental status should be considered for administration of the "coma cocktail." The coma cocktail consists of intravenous dextrose to treat hypoglycemia, a possible toxicological cause of altered mental status, *naloxone* to treat possible opioid or *clonidine* toxicity, and *thiamine* for ethanol-induced Wernicke encephalopathy.

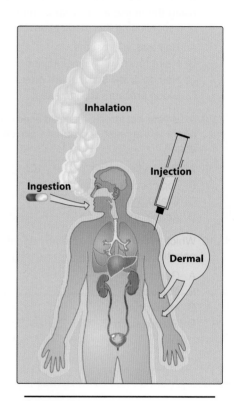

Figure 44.1
Routes of exposure for toxins.

A. Decontamination

Once the patient is stabilized, decontamination can occur. This may include flushing the eyes with saline or tepid water to a neutral pH for ocular exposures, rinsing the skin for dermal exposures, and/or gastrointestinal (GI) decontamination with gastric lavage, activated charcoal, or whole bowel irrigation (utilizing a polyethylene glycol electrolyte balanced solution) for ingestions. Therapy should be administered preferably within 1 hour of ingestion. Several substances do not adsorb to activated charcoal (for example, lead and other heavy metals, *iron, lithium, potassium*, and alcohols), limiting the use of activated charcoal unless there are coingested products.

B. Elimination enhancement

1. **Hemodialysis:** The elimination of some medications/toxins may be enhanced by hemodialysis if certain properties are met, such as low protein binding, small volume of distribution, small molecular weight, and water solubility of the toxin. Examples of medications or substances that can be removed with hemodialysis include methanol, ethylene glycol, salicylates, *theophylline, phenobarbital*, and *lithium*.

2. **Urinary alkalinization:** Alkalinization of the urine enhances the elimination of salicylates or *phenobarbital*. Increasing the urine pH with intravenous *sodium bicarbonate* transforms the drug into an ionized form that prevents reabsorption, thereby trapping it in the urine to be excreted by the kidney. The goal urine pH is 7.5 to 8, while ensuring the serum pH does not exceed 7.55.

3. **Multiple-dose activated charcoal:** Multiple-dose activated charcoal enhances the elimination of certain drugs (for example, *theophylline, phenobarbital, digoxin, carbamazepine*). Activated charcoal is extremely porous and has a high surface area, which creates a gradient across the lumen of the gut. Medications traverse from areas of high concentration to low concentration, promoting absorbed medication to cross back into the gut to be adsorbed by the activated charcoal. In addition, activated charcoal blocks the reabsorption of medications that undergo enterohepatic recirculation (such as *phenytoin*), by adsorbing the substance to the activated charcoal (Figure 44.2). Bowel sounds must be present prior to each activated charcoal dose to prevent obstruction.

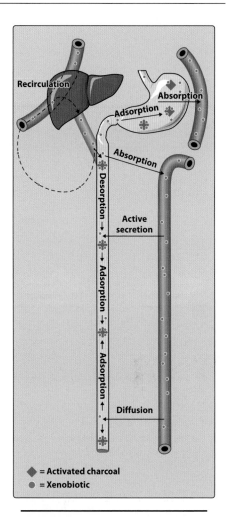

Figure 44.2
Mechanism of multiple-dose activated charcoal.

III. SELECT PHARMACEUTICAL AND OCCUPATIONAL TOXICITIES

A. Acetaminophen

Acetaminophen produces toxicity when normal metabolic pathways become saturated, leading to the production of a hepatotoxic metabolite (*N*-acetyl-*p*-benzoquinone imine, NAPQI) (Figure 44.3). After therapeutic doses of *acetaminophen*, the liver generates glutathione, which detoxifies NAPQI. However, in overdose, glutathione is depleted, leaving the metabolite to produce toxicity. There are four

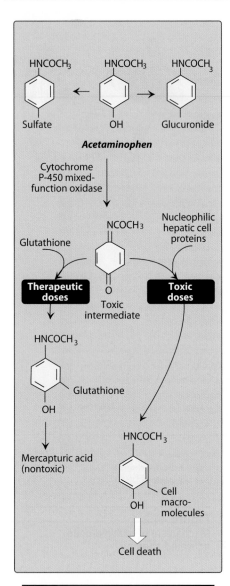

Figure 44.3
Metabolism of *acetaminophen*.

Phase 1 (0 to 24 hours): loss of appetite, nausea, vomiting, general malaise

Phase 2 (24 to 72 hours): abdominal pain, increased liver enzymes

Phase 3 (72 to 96 hours): liver necrosis, jaundice, encephalopathy, renal failure, death

Phase 4 (> 4 days to 2 weeks): complete resolution of symptoms and organ failure

Figure 44.4
Phases of *acetaminophen* toxicity.

phases typically describing *acetaminophen* toxicity (Figure 44.4). The antidote for *acetaminophen* toxicity, *N-acetylcysteine* (*NAC*), works as a glutathione precursor and glutathione substitute, and assists with sulfation. *NAC* may also function as an antioxidant to aid in recovery. *NAC* is most effective when initiated within 8 to 10 hours of ingestion. The Rumack-Matthew nomogram (Figure 44.5), which is based on the time of ingestion and the serum *acetaminophen* level, is utilized after an acute ingestion to determine if *NAC* therapy is needed. The nomogram is helpful to predict *acetaminophen* toxicity when levels can be obtained between 4 and 24 hours postingestion.

B. Alcohols

1. **Methanol (wood alcohol) and ethylene glycol:** Methanol is found in products like windshield washer fluid and model airplane fuel. Ethylene glycol is most commonly found in radiator antifreeze. These primary alcohols are relatively nontoxic and mainly cause central nervous system (CNS) depression. However, methanol and ethylene glycol are oxidized to toxic products: formic acid in the case of methanol, and glycolic, glyoxylic, and oxalic acids in the case of ethylene glycol. *Fomepizole* [foe-MEP-i-zole] inhibits this oxidative pathway by blocking alcohol dehydrogenase. [Note: Ethanol is an alternative if *fomepizole* is not available.] It prevents the formation of toxic metabolites and allows the parent alcohols to be excreted by the kidney (Figure 44.6). Hemodialysis is often utilized to remove the toxic acids that are already produced. In addition, cofactors are administered to encourage metabolism to nontoxic metabolites (*folate* for methanol, *thiamine* and *pyridoxine* for ethylene glycol). If untreated, methanol ingestion may produce blindness, metabolic acidosis, seizures, and coma. Ethylene glycol ingestion may lead to renal failure, hypocalcemia, metabolic acidosis, and heart failure.

2. **Isopropanol (rubbing alcohol, isopropyl alcohol):** This secondary alcohol is metabolized to acetone via alcohol dehydrogenase. Acetone cannot be further oxidized to carboxylic acids, and therefore, acidemia does not occur. Because isopropyl alcohol is not metabolized to a toxic metabolite, no antidote is necessary to treat an isopropyl alcohol ingestion. Isopropanol is a known CNS depressant (approximately twice as intoxicating as ethanol) and GI irritant. Treatment centers on supportive care.

C. Carbon monoxide

Carbon monoxide is a colorless, odorless, and tasteless gas. It is a natural by-product of the combustion of carbonaceous materials, and common sources of this gas include automobiles, poorly vented furnaces, fireplaces, wood-burning stoves, kerosene space heaters, house fires, charcoal grills, and generators. Following inhalation, carbon monoxide rapidly binds to hemoglobin to produce carboxyhemoglobin. The binding affinity of carbon monoxide to hemoglobin is 230 to 270 times greater than that of oxygen. Consequently, even low concentrations of carbon monoxide in the air can produce significant levels of carboxyhemoglobin. In addition, bound carbon monoxide increases hemoglobin affinity for oxygen at the other oxygen-binding sites. This

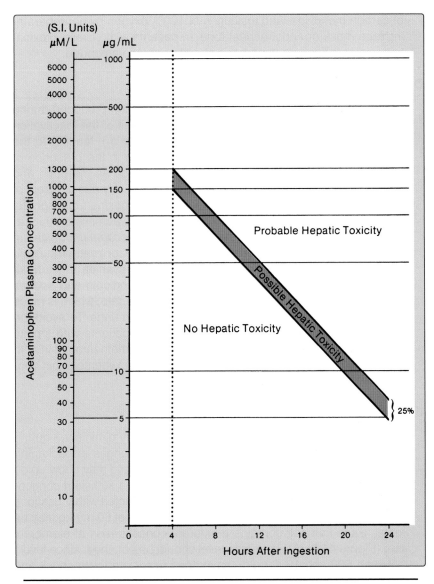

Figure 44.5
Rumack-Matthew nomogram for *acetaminophen* poisoning. *Acetaminophen* concentration plotted vs. time after exposure to predict potential toxicity and antidote use. Reprinted from B. H. Rumack. *Acetaminophen* overdose in children and adolescents. *Pediatr. Clin. North Am.* 33: 691 (1986), with permission.

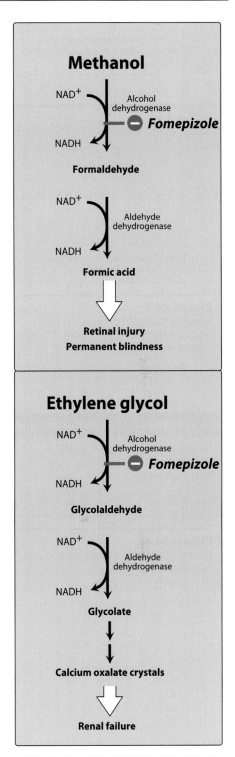

Figure 44.6
Metabolism of methanol and ethylene glycol.

high-affinity binding of oxygen prevents the unloading of oxygen at the tissues, further reducing oxygen delivery (Figure 44.7). The presence of this highly oxygenated blood may produce "cherry red" skin. Carbon monoxide toxicity can also occur following inhalation or ingestion of methylene chloride found in paint strippers. Once absorbed, methylene chloride is metabolized to carbon monoxide through the hepatic cytochrome P450 pathway. The symptoms of carbon monoxide intoxication are consistent with hypoxia, including headache, dyspnea, lethargy, confusion, and drowsiness. Higher exposure levels can lead to seizures, coma, and death. The management of a carbon monoxide–poisoned patient includes prompt removal from the source

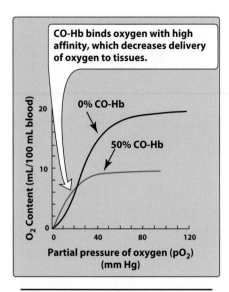

Figure 44.7
Effect of carbon monoxide on the oxygen affinity of hemoglobin. CO-Hb = carbon monoxyhemoglobin.

Content	Elemental iron (%)
Ferrous fumarate	33
Ferrous gluconate	12
Ferrous sulfate	20

Figure 44.8
Elemental iron contained in various iron preparations.

of carbon monoxide, and institution of 100% oxygen by nonrebreathing face mask or endotracheal tube. In patients with severe intoxication, oxygenation in a hyperbaric chamber is recommended.

D. Cyanide

Cyanide is one of the toxic products of combustion produced during house fires. Its principal toxicity occurs as a result of the inactivation of the enzyme cytochrome oxidase (cytochrome a_3), leading to the inhibition of cellular respiration. Therefore, even in the presence of oxygen, tissues with a high oxygen demand such as the brain and heart are adversely affected. Death can occur quickly due to arrest of oxidative phosphorylation and production of adenosine triphosphate. The antidote, *hydroxocobalamin* (vitamin B_{12a}), is administered intravenously to bind the cyanide and produce *cyanocobalamin* (vitamin B_{12}) without the adverse effects of hypotension or methemoglobin production seen with older antidotes. The older cyanide antidote kit consists of *sodium nitrite* to form cyanomethemoglobin and *sodium thiosulfate* to accelerate the production of thiocyanate, which is much less toxic than cyanide and is quickly excreted in urine. To avoid the oxygen carrying capacity becoming too low in patients with smoke inhalation and cyanide toxicity, the induction of methemoglobin with *sodium nitrite* should be avoided unless the carboxyhemoglobin concentration is less than 10%.

E. Iron

The incidence of pediatric iron toxicity has greatly diminished during the past two decades due to education and changes in packaging and labeling of iron products. Iron is radiopaque and may show up on an abdominal radiograph if the product contains a sufficient concentration of elemental iron. Toxic effects can be expected with ingestions as little as 20 mg/kg of elemental iron, and doses of 60 mg/kg may be lethal. Each iron salt contains a different concentration of elemental iron (Figure 44.8). A serum iron level should be obtained, since levels between 500 and 1000 µg/dL have been associated with shock and levels higher than 1000 µg/dL with death. Patients with iron toxicity usually present with nausea, vomiting, and abdominal pain. Depending on the amount of elemental iron ingested, the patient may experience a latent period or may progress quickly to hypovolemia, metabolic acidosis, hypotension, and coagulopathy. Ultimately, hepatic failure and multisystem failure, coma, and death may occur. *Deferoxamine* [defer-OKS-a-meen], an iron-specific chelator, binds free iron, creating ferrioxamine, which is excreted in the urine. Hypotension may occur if rapid intravenous boluses of *deferoxamine* are administered instead of a continuous infusion.

F. Lead

Lead is ubiquitous in the environment, with sources of exposure including old paint, drinking water, industrial pollution, food, and contaminated dust. Most chronic exposure to lead occurs with inorganic lead salts, such as those in paint used in housing constructed prior to 1978. Adults absorb about 10% of ingested lead, whereas children absorb about 40%. Inorganic forms of lead are initially distributed to the soft tissues and more slowly redistribute to bone, teeth, and hair. Lead impairs bone formation and causes increased calcium deposition in long bones visible on x-ray. Ingested lead is radiopaque and may appear on an abdominal radiograph if present in the GI tract. Lead has an apparent blood half-life of about 1 to 2 months, whereas its half-life in the bone is 20 to 30 years. Chronic exposure to lead can have serious effects on several tissues (Figure 44.9). Early symptoms of lead toxicity can include discomfort and constipation (and, occasionally, diarrhea), whereas higher exposures can produce painful intestinal spasms. CNS effects from lead include headaches, confusion, clumsiness, insomnia, fatigue, and impaired concentration. As the disease progresses, clonic convulsions and coma can occur. Death is rare, given the ability to treat lead intoxication with chelation therapy. Blood levels of 5 to 20 μg/dL in children have been shown to lower IQ in the absence of other symptoms. Finally, lead can cause hypochromic, microcytic anemia as a result of a shortened erythrocyte life span and disruption of heme synthesis.

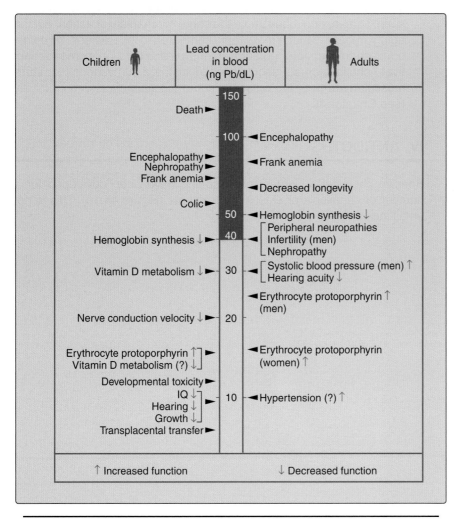

Figure 44.9
Comparison of effects of lead on children and adults. From the Centers for Disease Control and Prevention. http://wonder.cdc.gov/.

POISON	ANTIDOTE(S)
Acetaminophen	*N-Acetylcysteine*
Anticholinergic agents (antihistamines, etc.)	*Physostigmine*
Arsenic	*Dimercaprol, succimer (dimercaptosuccinic acid, DMSA), dimercaprol*
Benzodiazepine	*Flumazenil*
Carbon monoxide	**Oxygen (± hyperbaric chamber)**
Cyanide	*Hydroxocabalamin,* **sodium nitrite, and** *sodium thiosulfate*
Dabigatran	*Idarucizumab*
Digitalis	*Digoxin-immune Fab*
Heparin	*Protamine sulfate*
Hydrofluoric acid	*Calcium*
Iron	*Deferoxamine*
Isoniazid **and** *Gyromitra* **mushrooms**	*Pyridoxine*
Lead	*Calcium disodium edetate, dimercaprol, succimer (dimercaptosuccinic acid, DMSA)*
Methanol and ethylene glycol	*Fomepizole*
Methemoglobinemia	*Methylene blue*
Opiates, *clonidine*	*Naloxone*
Organophosphates, nerve gases	*Atropine, pralidoxime*
Warfarin	*Vitamin K1 (phytonadione)*

Figure 44.10
Common antidotes.

Multiple chelators can be utilized in the treatment of lead toxicity. When levels are greater than 45 µg/dL, but less than 70 µg/dL in children, *succimer* (*dimercaptosuccinic acid [DMSA]*), an oral chelator, is the treatment of choice. With lead levels greater than 70 µg/dL or if encephalopathy is present, dual parenteral therapy is required with *dimercaprol* given intramuscularly and *calcium disodium edetate* given intravenously. *Dimercaprol* is suspended in peanut oil and should not be given to those with a peanut allergy.

G. Organophosphate and carbamate insecticides

These insecticides exert their toxicity through inhibition of acetylcholinesterase, with subsequent accumulation of excess acetylcholine producing nicotinic (mydriasis, fasciculations, muscle weakness, tachycardia, hypertension) and muscarinic (diarrhea, urination, miosis, bradycardia, bronchorrhea, emesis, lacrimation, salivation) effects. Carbamates reversibly bind to acetylcholinesterase, whereas organophosphates undergo an aging process to ultimately irreversibly inactivate the enzyme. Organophosphate nerve agents, such as sarin, soman, and tabun, have the same mechanism of action, but the aging process is much more rapid compared to insecticides. *Atropine*, a muscarinic receptor antagonist, and *pralidoxime*, an oxime to reactivate cholinesterase, should be administered intravenously or intramuscularly to treat the muscarinic and nicotinic effects, respectively (see Chapter 4).

IV. ANTIDOTES

Specific chemical antidotes for poisoning have been developed for a number of chemicals or classes of toxicants (Figure 44.10). This is not an all-inclusive list.

Study Questions

Choose the ONE best answer.

44.1 A 3-year-old boy is brought to the emergency department by his mother, who reports that he has been crying continuously and "does not want to play or eat" for the past few days. She also states that he has not had regular bowel movements, with mostly constipation and occasional diarrhea, and frequently complains of abdominal pain. The child now has an altered level of consciousness, is difficult to arouse, and begins to seize. The clinician rules out infection and other medical causes. Upon questioning, the mother states that the house is in an older neighborhood, that her house has not been remodeled or repainted since the 1940s, and that the paint is chipping around the windows and doors. The child is otherwise breathing on his own and urinating normally. Which toxin would you expect to be producing such severe effects in this child?

A. Iron
B. Lead
C. Carbon monoxide
D. Cyanide

Correct answer = B. Lead poisoning is common among children in older homes painted before lead was removed from paint. Paint chips with lead are easily ingested by toddlers, and excessively high lead levels can lead to the signs and symptoms described plus clumsiness, confusion, headaches, coma, constipation, intestinal spasms, and anemia. Death is rare when chelation therapy is instituted. Iron can produce abdominal pain, but more often would cause diarrhea, vomiting, and volume loss. Carbon monoxide would affect the entire household, depending on the source. Clinical effects from carbon monoxide would include headache, nausea, and CNS depression. If he had cyanide poisoning, death would have occurred quickly following respiratory arrest of oxidative phosphorylation and production of adenosine triphosphate, but this child has been exhibiting symptoms over several days.

44.2 A 41-year-old male jeweler presents to the emergency department after he was found unconscious on the floor of the shop by a coworker. The coworker states that the patient complained of being cold this morning around 8 AM (the central heat was broken, and the outdoor temperature was 34°F) and that since noon, he had been complaining of headache, drowsiness, confusion, and nausea. The clinician notices that he has cherry red skin. What is the most likely toxin causing his signs and symptoms?

A. Ethylene glycol
B. Cyanide
C. Acetaminophen
D. Carbon monoxide

Correct answer = D. Although watch makers and other professionals who use electroplating may be at higher risk for cyanide exposure because many plating baths use cyanide-containing ingredients (for example, potassium cyanide), this patient shows signs of carbon monoxide poisoning, such as cherry red skin, headache, confusion, nausea, and drowsiness leading to unconsciousness. The history also leads us to believe that this person may have been using a space heater to stay warm, which would be consistent with the description. A carboxyhemoglobin level should be obtained to confirm the exposure. Cyanide in low doses from such an occupational exposure can present with loss of consciousness, flushing, headache, and confusion. Chronically, workers may develop a rash after handling cyanide solutions. Also, an odor of bitter almonds may be present. An arterial blood gas and a venous blood gas could be obtained and compared to determine if cyanide is present (a lack of oxygen extraction would be present on the venous side). Ethylene glycol toxicity may cause alterations in mental status, but the history did not include anything suggesting a toxic alcohol ingestion. Acetaminophen toxicity is not consistent with this presentation.

44.3 A 50-year-old migrant field worker comes to the emergency department and complains of diarrhea, tearing, nausea and vomiting, and sweating. The clinician notices that he looks generally anxious and has fine fasciculations in the muscles of the upper chest as well as pinpoint pupils. Which antidote should he receive first?

A. N-acetylcysteine
B. Sodium nitrite
C. Deferoxamine
D. Atropine

Correct answer = D. Atropine is appropriate for this patient, who has symptoms consistent with organophosphate (insecticide) poisoning. The mnemonic DUMBBELS (diarrhea, urination, miosis, bronchorrhea/bradycardia, emesis, lacrimation, salivation) can be used to remember the signs and symptoms of cholinergic toxicity. An anticholinergic antidote, atropine, controls these muscarinic symptoms, whereas the antidote pralidoxime treats the nicotinic symptoms like fasciculations (involuntary muscle quivering or twitching). N-acetylcysteine is the antidote for acetaminophen overdose and acts as a sulfhydryl donor. Sodium nitrite is one of the antidotes included in the old cyanide antidote kit (sodium nitrite and sodium thiosulfate). Deferoxamine is the chelating agent for iron.

44.4 A 45-year-old man presented to the emergency department 18 hours after ingesting an unknown product. On presentation, he is tachycardic, hypertensive, tachypneic, and complaining of flank pain. A metabolic panel is obtained, and the patient has a large anion gap acidosis, an increased creatinine, and hypocalcemia. Which substance was most likely ingested?

A. Methanol
B. Acetaminophen
C. Ethylene glycol
D. Iron

Correct answer = C. Ethylene glycol produces a metabolic acidosis from the toxic metabolites. The formation of calcium oxalate crystals, which can be found on urinalysis, leads to hypocalcemia and renal failure. The treatment regimen for this patient would include intravenous fomepizole, if some of the parent compound was still present, and hemodialysis. Methanol may produce a metabolic acidosis as well, but its target organ of toxicity is the eyes instead of the kidneys as with ethylene glycol. Acetaminophen toxicity may produce upper quadrant pain within the first 24 hours, but vital sign abnormalities are not usually found during this time frame. Iron toxicity may also produce a metabolic acidosis and tachycardia. However, hypocalcemia does not occur.

44.5 A 27-year-old woman presents to the emergency department 6 hours after reportedly ingesting 20 tablets of acetaminophen 500 mg. An acetaminophen level is drawn, but it has to be sent out to another lab and will not return for another 6 hours. What is the most appropriate next step in management of this patient?

A. Administer a dose of activated charcoal.
B. Start empirical N-acetylcysteine therapy.
C. Wait for the level to return and then decide what to do.
D. Draw a NAPQI level.

Correct answer = B. N-acetylcysteine should be started empirically on the basis of the history, and then, once the level returns and is plotted on the Rumack-Matthew nomogram, a final decision on whether to continue therapy can be made. Activated charcoal would not be of any benefit 6 hours post-acetaminophen ingestion. The optimal time frame to give N-acetylcysteine is within 8 to 10 hours postingestion. So, waiting on the level to return would put the patient more than 12 hours postingestion. Therefore, initiation of N-acetylcysteine therapy should happen, if possible during the optimal time frame. Clinicians are unable to draw a NAPQI level and therefore cannot utilize this to guide therapy.

44.6 A 15-year-old girl presents to the emergency department with CNS depression. She is slightly bradycardic and slightly hypotensive. Upon further questioning, the mother admits that the patient was found with an open bottle of clonidine. Which antidote might be beneficial for this patient?

A. Flumazenil
B. Atropine
C. Deferoxamine
D. Naloxone

Correct answer = D. Naloxone has a reversal rate of the CNS effects of approximately 50% in clonidine ingestions. Flumazenil reverses benzodiazepines and has no effect on clonidine. Atropine is an anticholinergic agent and would not improve the CNS depression. Deferoxamine is the chelator for iron.

44.7 A 45-year-old woman presents to the emergency department with a complaint of persistent vomiting. The patient appears intoxicated, but an ethanol level returns as negative and her basic metabolic panel is unremarkable. Which substance did she probably ingest?

A. Isopropyl alcohol
B. Methanol
C. Ethylene glycol
D. Ethanol

Correct answer = A. Isopropyl alcohol produces twice as much CNS depression as ethanol and is known to cause GI distress. Isopropyl alcohol is metabolized to acetone, so a metabolic acidosis does not result (which is in contrast to the acidosis generated by methanol and ethylene glycol). The ethanol level was negative, eliminating ethanol as an ingestion.

44.8 A 5-year-old boy is brought in to the healthcare facility for being irritable and failure to thrive. He is drowsy, and his vital signs are normal. The doctor diagnoses him with lead toxicity when the blood lead level returns as 75 µg/dL. Which chelator regimen should be started?

A. Dimercaprol
B. Calcium disodium edetate
C. Both dimercaprol and calcium disodium edetate
D. Succimer

Correct answer = C. Dual parenteral therapy with dimercaprol and calcium disodium edetate is indicated if encephalopathy is present, or if the lead level is greater than 70 µg/dL in a child. Dimercaprol intramuscular therapy is initiated 4 hours prior to the intravenous administration of calcium disodium edetate when both medications are required. Succimer (dimercaptosuccinic acid, DMSA) is utilized when the lead level is greater than 45 µg/dL but less than 70 µg/dL, without encephalopathy.

44.9 A healthy 2-year-old boy ingested one of his mother's 2 mg clonazepam tablets 1 hour ago. The child presented to the emergency department with CNS depression but a normal heart rate and blood pressure. His bedside glucose check is also normal. Which antidote might be helpful?

A. Flumazenil

B. Naloxone

C. Physostigmine

D. Fomepizole

Correct answer = A. Flumazenil is a competitive benzodiazepine antagonist that reverses the CNS depression from benzodiazepines such as clonazepam. After flumazenil administration, resedation usually occurs, since the duration of the benzodiazepine is longer than that of the flumazenil. Naloxone reverses the effects from opioids and clonidine, not benzodiazepines. Physostigmine is the antidote for anticholinergic toxicity. Fomepizole is the antidote for methanol or ethylene glycol toxicity.

44.10 A 47-year-old man with a history of a seizure disorder, maintained on phenytoin, presented to the emergency department with salicylate toxicity. The salicylate level was 50 mg/dL (15 to 35 mg/dL therapeutic range) and the phenytoin level was 15 mg/L (10 to 20 mg/L therapeutic range). What therapy can be considered to enhance the elimination of salicylate without impacting the phenytoin?

A. Multiple doses of activated charcoal

B. Urinary alkalinization

C. Whole bowel irrigation

D. Urinary acidification

Correct answer = B. Urinary alkalinization enhances the elimination of the salicylate but does not affect the therapeutic phenytoin level. Multiple doses of activated charcoal would lower the concentration of both medications, rendering the phenytoin subtherapeutic. Whole bowel irrigation is another GI decontamination modality involving administration of large quantities (up to 2 L/h in adults) of a polyethylene glycol–balanced electrolyte solution via a nasogastric tube until the patient generates clear rectal effluent.

Index

Note: Page numbers followed by '*f*' indicate figures. TRADE NAMES of drugs are shown in capital letters and *generic names* are shown in italics. Page numbers in bold indicate **main discussions**. Page numbers followed by '*e*' indicate electronic chapters

ALBENZA. *See Albendazole*
Albiglutide, 311*f*
Albumin, as drug-binding protein, 10
Albuterol, 73*f,* **84**, 85, 528*f,* 529
  mechanism of action of, 26–27
Alcaftadine, 493*f,* 496–497
Alcohol, **586**. *See also* Ethanol
ALDACTONE. *See Spironolactone*
Aldosterone, 341
  and blood pressure regulation, 204, 205*f*
  synthesis of, 340
Aldosterone antagonists, **226–227**, 231*f*
  for heart failure, 238
  site of action of, 219*f*
Alemtuzumab, 103*f,* 481*f,* 483*f,* **484–485**
Alendronate, 348*f,* 349, 349*f*
ALEVE. *See Naproxen*
ALFENTA. *See Alfentanil*
Alfentanil, 180*f,* **186**
Alfuzosin, 91*f,* **98–99**, 557*f,* 560–561
ALIMTA. *See Pemetrexed*
ALINIA. *See Nitazoxanide*
Alirocumab, 287*f*
Aliskiren, 203*f,* 211–212
Alkalinization, urine, 585
ALKERAN. *See Melphalan*
Alkylating agents, 454*f,* **465–467**, 466*f*
ALLEGRA. *See Fexofenadine*
Allergic and inflammatory conditions, H₁ antihistamines, 495–496
Allergic rhinitis
  antihistamines for, 535
  corticosteroids for, 535–536
  drugs used to treat, **535–536**, 527
Allergy, histamine role in, 494
ALLI. *See Orlistat*
Allograft, 483
Allopurinol, 508*f,* **524**
Almotriptan, 500–501, 500*f*
Alogliptin, 311*f,* 320–321
Alopecia, agents for, 577*f,* **581**
ALORA. *See Estradiol (transdermal)*
Alosetron, 550*f*
ALOXI. *See Palonosetron*
Alprazolam, 116*f,* **121**, 546*f,* 547
  adverse effects of, 121*f*
  anxiolytic effects of, 118
Alprostadil, **510**, 511*f,* 557, 557*f,* **559–560**
  adverse effects of, 560
  mechanism of action of, 560
  pharmacokinetics of, 560
ALSUMA. *See Sumatriptan*
ALTABAX. *See Retapamulin*
ALTACE. *See Ramipril*
Alteplase (tPA), 268*f,* 283
ALTOPREV. *See Lovastatin*
Aluminum hydroxide, 544–545, 548, 548*f*
  for peptic ulcer disease, 540*f*
ALVESCO. *See Ciclesonide*
Alzheimer disease, 56–57
  drug treatment for, 103*f*
Amantadine, 103*f,* 436*f,* 443
AMARYL. *See Glimepiride*
AMBIEN. *See Zolpidem*
Amebiasis, **604e–607e**
Amebicides, mixed, **605e–606e**
AMERGE. *See Naratriptan*
American sleeping sickness. *See* Trypanosomiasis
AMICAR. *See Aminocaproic acid*
AMIDATE. *See Etomidate*
Amikacin, 384*f*
Amiloride, 203*f,* 208, 218*f,* **227**
γ-Aminobutyric acid (GABA), 104–105, 105*f*
  benzodiazepines, 116–117, 117*f*
  as neurotransmitter, 45
  in Parkinson disease, 105–106, 106*f*
Aminocaproic acid, 268*f,* 283*f,* 284
Aminoglycosides, 384*f,* **388–390**, 413*f*
  absorption of, 389, 390*f*
  administration and fate of, 390*f*
  adverse effects of, 390, 390*f*

allergic reactions, 390
antibacterial spectrum of, 389
distribution of, 11, 389
drug interactions with, 69
elimination of, 390
mechanism of action of, 388–389
nephrotoxicity of, 390
neuromuscular paralysis caused by, 390
ototoxicity of, 390
pharmacokinetics of, 389–390
resistance to, 389
therapeutic applications of, 389*f*
Aminopenicillins, 369
5-Aminosalicylates (5-ASAs), **551–553**, 552*f,* 553*f*
  actions of, 552
  adverse effects of, 552–553
  pharmacokinetics of, 552
  therapeutic uses of, 552
Aminosalicylic acid, 413*f*
Amiodarone, 248*f,* **254–255**
AMITIZA. *See Lubiprostone*
Amitriptyline, 128*f,* 132, 136*f*
Amlodipine, 203*f,* 212, 259*f,* 262–263
Amnesia
  anterograde, benzodiazepine-induced, 118
  benzodiazepine-induced, 119
Amobarbital, 116*f. See also* Barbiturates
Amoxapine, 128*f,* 136*f*
Amoxicillin, 368*f*–369*f,* 369, 377, 377*f*
  for peptic ulcer disease, 540*f*
AMOXIL. *See Amoxicillin*
Amphetamine, 73*f,* **85**, 194*f,* **197–199**, 197*f,* **596e**
  actions of, 198
  adverse effects of, 199, 199*f*
  cardiovascular effects, 199
  CNS effects, 199
  contraindications, 199
  gastrointestinal system effects, 199
  mechanism of action of, 79, 79*f,* 197
  pharmacokinetics of, 199
  therapeutic uses, 198–199
Amphotericin B, **423–425**, 423*f*
  administration and fate, 425*f*
  adverse effects, 425, 426*f*
  antifungal spectrum, 424–425
  mechanism of action, 423–424
  model of pore formation, 425*f*
  pharmacokinetics, 425
  resistance, 425
Ampicillin, 361*f,* 361*f,* 368*f*–369*f,* 369
AMPYRA. *See Dalfampridine*
Amylin analog, synthetic, 316
Amyotrophic lateral sclerosis (ALS), drug treatment for, 103*f,* 114
AMYTAL. *See Amobarbital*
ANADROL. *See Oxymetholone*
ANAFRANIL. *See Clomipramine*
Anakinra, 522
Analgesia
  and *morphine,* 182
  therapeutic use of, 184*f*
Analgesics, 161*f. See also* Opioid(s)
  NSAIDs as (*see* Nonsteroidal anti-inflammatory drugs (NSAIDs))
Anaphylactic shock, *epinephrine* for, 80
Anaphylaxis, histamine role in, 494
ANAPROX. *See Naproxen*
ANASPAZ. *See Hyoscyamine*
Anastrozole, 454*f,* **471**
ANCEF. *See Cefazolin*
ANCOBON. *See Flucytosine*
Ancylostoma duodenale, 618*e*
ANDRODERM. *See Testosterone (patch)*
ANDROGEL. *See Testosterone (topical)*
Androgen(s), 326*f,* **335–337**
  adverse effects of, 336–337
  mechanism of action of, 335
  pharmacokinetics of, 336
  secretion of, 335
  therapeutic uses of, 335–336
  unapproved uses of, 335–336

ANDROID. *See Methyltestosterone*
ANECTINE. *See Succinylcholine*
Anemia. *See also* Sickle cell disease
  agents used to treat, 565*f,* **565–568**, 569, 569*f*
  causes of, 565
  chloramphenicol-induced, 394
  definition of, 565
  hemolytic, 406
  management of, 569*f*
  megaloblastic, 407, 567, 567*f*
  nutritional, 565
Anesthesia, 161, 161*f*
  adjuncts, 176–177
    actions of, 177*f*
    analgesia, 177
    anxiety, 177
    gastrointestinal medications, 176
    PONV medications, 176–177
  induction of, 163
  inhalation, 163–168
    alveolar wash-in, 165
    alveolar-to-venous partial pressure gradient, 166
    cardiac output, 165–166
    characteristics of, 169*f*
    common features of, 163–164
    desflurane, 167
    fat, 166
    isoflurane, 167
    malignant hyperthermia, 168
    mechanism of action, 167
    nitrous oxide, 168
    potency, 164
    sevoflurane, 167
    skeletal muscles, 166
    solubility in blood, 165
    uptake and distribution, 164–166
    vessel-poor group, 166
    vessel-rich group, 166
    washout, 166
  intravenous, 169–172
    barbiturates, 171
    benzodiazepines, 171
    dexmedetomidine, 172
    effect of reduced cardiac output, 170
    etomidate, 172
    induction, 170
    ketamine, 172
    opioids, 172
    propofol, 170–171
    recovery, 170
  levels of sedation, 161, 162*f*
  local, 174–176
    actions of, 174
    allergic reactions, 175
    duration of action, 175
    local anesthetic systemic toxicity, 175–176
    metabolism, 175
    onset of, 175
    pharmacologic properties of, 176*f*
    potency of, 175
  maintenance of, 163
  neuromuscular blockers, 173
  recovery of, 163
  stages of general, 162–163
  therapeutic disadvantages and advantages, 173*f*
  therapeutic use of, 184*f*
Anesthetic(s)
  general (*see* General anesthetic(s))
  inhaled, 161, 164–165
  intravenous, 169–172
  local (*see* Local anesthetic(s))
Angina pectoris
  β-blockers for, 95, 99*f*
  characteristics of, 259, 265*f*
  classic, 259
  and concomitant diseases, 260
  drugs used to treat, 260 (*see also* Antianginal drugs)
  effort-induced, 259–260

N

Figure Credits

Figure 1.21. Modified from H. P. Range and M. M. Dale. Pharmacology. Churchill Livingstone (1987).

Figure 1.23. Modified from Figure 6-3, Libby: Braunwald's Heart Disease: A Textbook of Cardiovascular Medicine, 8th ed. Philadelphia, PA, Saunders (2007).

Figure 3.3. Reprinted from B. J. Cohen and K. L. Hull. Memmler's Structure and Function of the Human Body, 11th ed. Philadelphia, PA, Wolters Kluwer (2016), with permission.

Figure 6.9. Modified from M. J. Allwood, A. F. Cobbold, and J. Ginsburg. Peripheral vascular effects of noradrenaline, isopropyl-noradrenaline and dopamine. Br. Med. Bull. 19: 132 (1963).

Figure 6.11. Modified from M. J. Allwood, A. F. Cobbold, and J. Ginsburg. Peripheral vascular effects of noradrenaline, isopropyl-noradrenaline and dopamine. Br. Med. Bull. 19: 132 (1963).

Figure 8.13. Modified from R. Young. Update on Parkinson's disease. Am. Fam. Physician 59: 2155 (1999).

Figure 9.5. Modified from A. Kales. Excertpa Medical Congress Series 899: 149 (1989).

Figure 9.6. From data of E. C. Dimitrion, A. J. Parashos, and J. S. Giouzepas. Drug Invest. 4: 316 (1992).

Figure 12.9. From Science Source, New York, NY.

Figure 12.10. Modified from K. J. Meador, G. A. Baker, N. Browning, et al. Cognitive function at 3 years of age after fetal exposure to antiepileptic drugs. N. Engl. J. Med. 360: 1597 (2009).

Figure 14.11. Modified from T. R. Kosten and P. G. O'Connor. Management of drug and alcohol withdrawal. N. Engl. J. Med. 348: 1786 (2003).

Figure 15.4. Modified from N. L. Benowitz. Pharmacologic aspects of cigarette smoking and nicotine addiction. N. Engl. J. Med. 319: 1318 (1988).

Figure 15.5. Modified from B. J. Materson. Drug Ther. 157 (1985).

Figure 18.6. Modified from J. B. King, A. P. Bress, A. D. Reese, M. A. Munger. Neprilysin inhibition in heart failure with reduced ejection fraction: a clinical review. Pharmacotherapy 35: 823 (2015).

Figure 18.7. Modified from P. Deedwania. Selective and specific inhibition of If with ivabradine for the treatment of coronary artery disease or heart failure. Drugs. 73: 1569 (2013).

Figure 18.10. Modified from M. Jessup and S. Brozena. N. Engl. J. Med. 348: 2007 (2003).

Figure 18.11. Modified from C. W. Yancy, et al. 2017 ACC/AHA/HFSA Focused Update of the 2013 ACCF/AHA Guideline for the Management of Heart Failure: a report of the American College of Cardiology/American Heart Association Task Force on Clinical Practice Guidelines and the Heart Failure Society of America. Circulation. 136: 1 (2017).

Figure 19.3. Modified from J. A. Beven and J. H. Thompson. Essentials of Pharmacology. Philadelphia, PA, Harper and Row (1983).

Figure 22.6. Data from M. K. S. Leow, C. L. Addy, and C. S. Mantzoros. Clinical review 159: human immunodeficiency virus/highly active antiretroviral therapy-associated metabolic syndrome: clinical presentation, pathophysiology, and therapeutic strategies. J. Clin. Endocrinol. Metab. 88: 1961 (2003).

Figure 22.7. Data from D. J. Schneider, P. B. Tracy, and B. E. Sobel. Hosp. Pract. 107 (1998).

Figure 23.2. Modified from B. G. Katzung. Basic and Clinical Pharmacology. Appleton and Lange (1987).

Figure 23.6. From R. R. Preston and T. E. Wilson. Lippincott Illustrated Reviews: Physiology. Philadelphia, PA, Lippincott Williams & Wilkins (2013).

Figure 23.11. Modified from K. Okamura, H. Ikenoue, and A. Shiroozu. Reevaluation of the effects of methylmercaptoimidazole and propylthiouracil in patients with Graves' hyperthyroidism. J. Clin. Endocrinol. Metab. 65: 719 (1987).

Figure 24.5. Modified from M. C. Riddle. Postgrad. Med. 92: 89 (1992).

Figure 24.7. Modified from I. R. Hirsch. Insulin analogues. N. Engl. J. Med. 352: 174 (2005).

Figure 24.9. Data from O. B. Crofford. Diabetes control and complications. Annu. Rev. Med. 46: 267 (1995).

Figure 25.9. Data from the Guttmacher Institute. Contraceptive use in the United States. Available at https://www.guttmacher.org/fact-sheet/contraceptive-use-united-states.

Figure 26.7. Data from K. G. Saag, R. Koehnke, and J. R. Caldwell, et al. Low dose long-term corticosteroid therapy in rheumatoid arthritis: an analysis of serious adverse events. Am. J. Med. 96: 115 (1994).

Figure 32.4. Data from D. A. Evans, K. A. Maley, and V. A. McRusick. Genetic control of isoniazid metabolism in man. Br. Med. J. 2: 485 (1960).

Figure 32.5. Data from P. J. Neuvonen, K. T. Kivisto, and P. Lehto. Clin. Pharm. Ther. 50: 499 (1991).

Figure 32.12. Modified from Y. Nivoix, D. Leveque, and R. Herbrecht, et al. The enzymatic basis of drug-drug interactions with systemic triazole antifungals. Clin. Pharmacokinet. 47: 779 (2008).

Figure 34.5. Data from Surveillance for Viral Hepatitis—United States 2015. Available at https://www.cdc.gov/hepatitis/statistics/2015surveillance/commentary.htm

Figure 34.14. Data from H. H. Balfour. Antiviral drugs. N. Engl. J. Med. 340: 1255 (1999).

Figure 35.4. Reprinted from Dr. Thomas George, MD, with permission.

Figure 35.6. Modified from N. Kartner and V. Ling. Multidrug resistance in cancer. Sci. Am. (1989).

Figure 37.9. Data from D. D. Dubose, A. C. Cutlip, and W. D. Cutlip. Migraines and other headaches: an approach to diagnosis and classification. Am. Fam. Physician 51: 1498 (1995).

Figure 38.15. Data from T. D. Warner, F. Giuliano, I. Vojnovic, et al. Nonsteroid drug selectivities for cyclo-oxygenase-1 rather than cyclo-oxygenase-2 are associated with human gastrointestinal toxicity: a full in vitro analysis. Proc. Natl. Acad. Sci. U. S. A. 96: 7563 (1999).

Figure 40.2. Modified from D. R. Cave. Therapeutic approaches to recurrent peptic ulcer disease. Hosp. Pract. 27(9A): 33–49, 199 (1992). With permission from Taylor & Francis Ltd, www.tandfonline.com.

Figure 40.5. Modified with permission from F. E. Silverstein, D. Y. Graham, and J. R. Senior. Misoprostol reduces serious gastrointestinal complications in patients with rheumatoid arthritis receiving nonsteroidal anti-inflammatory drugs. A randomized, double-blind, placebo-controlled trial. Ann. Intern. Med. 123: 241 (1995).

Figure 40.6. Data from S. M. Grunberg and P. J. Hesketh. Control of chemotherapy-induced emesis. N. Engl. J. Med. 329: 1790 (1993).

Figure 40.7. Modified from F. E. Silverstein, D. Y. Graham, J. R. Senior. Misoprostol reduces serious gastrointestinal complications in patients with rheumatoid arthritis receiving nonsteroidal antiinflammatory drugs. A randomized, double-blind, placebocontrolled trial. Ann. Intern. Med. 123: 241 (1995).

Figure 40.8. Data from S. Bilgrami and B. G. Fallon. Chemotherapy-induced nausea and vomiting. Easing patients' fear and discomfort with effective antiemetic regimens. Postgrad. Med. 94: 55 (1993).

Figure 43.6. Reprinted from S. Jensen. Pocket Guide for Nursing Health Assessment: A Best Practice Approach, 2nd ed. Philadelphia, PA, Wolters Kluwer (2015), with permission.

Figure 44.5. Reprinted from B. H. Rumack. Acetaminophen overdose in children and adolescents. Pediatr. Clin. North Am. 33: 691 (1986), with permission.

Figure 44.9. From the Centers for Disease Control and Prevention. Available at http://wonder.cdc.gov/, with permission.

Figure 45.13. From the Centers for Disease Control and Prevention; National Center for Health Statistics. National Vital Statistics System, mortality. CDC WONDER. Atlanta, GA, US Department of Health and Human Services, CDC (2016). Available at https://wonder.cdc.gov/.